Instructional Course Lectures

Volume XXXIX 1990

American Academy
of Orthopaedic Surgeons

Instructional Course Lectures

Volume XXXIX 1990

Edited by
Walter B. Greene, MD
Professor of Orthopaedic Surgery and Pediatrics
Division of Orthopaedics
The University of North Carolina School of Medicine
Chapel Hill, North Carolina

With 790 illustrations

American Academy
of Orthopaedic Surgeons

American Academy of Orthopaedic Surgeons

Instructional Course Lectures
Volume XXXIX

Director of Communications and Publications: Mark W. Wieting
Assistant Director, Publications: Marilyn L. Fox, PhD
Senior Editor: Wendy O. Schmidt
Medical Editor: Bruce A. Davis
Publications Secretary: Monica M. Trocker

Design: James Buddenbaum Design, Wilmette, Illinois
Typesetting: Impressions, Inc., Madison, Wisconsin
Printing: Mack Printing Company, Easton, Pennsylvania
Stock: Acid-free Warrenflo

Contributors

Robert S. Adelaar, MD, Professor of Surgery, Medical College of Virginia, Richmond, Virginia

Jorge E. Alonso, MD, Assistant Professor of Surgery/Orthopaedic Trauma, The University of Alabama, Birmingham, Alabama

Thomas P. Andriacchi, PhD, The Claude N. Lambert, MD–Helen S. Thomson Professor and Director, Section of Orthopedic Research, Department of Orthopedic Surgery, Rush-Presbyterian–St. Luke's Medical Center, Chicago, Illinois

James Aronson, MD, Associate Professor, Department of Orthopaedics, University of Arkansas for Medical Sciences, Little Rock, Arkansas

George S. Bassett, MD, Assistant Professor of Orthopaedics, University of Southern California School of Medicine, Children's Hospital of Los Angeles, Los Angeles, California

Fred Behrens, MD, Professor of Orthopaedic Surgery, Case Western Reserve University, Director, Department of Orthopaedics, MetroHealth Medical Center, Cleveland, Ohio

Norman E. Beisaw, MD, Professor of Orthopaedic Surgery, St. Vincent Hospital, University of Massachusetts Medical School, Worcester, Massachusetts

Daniel R. Benson, MD, Professor, Chief of Spine Service, Department of Orthopaedic Surgery, University of California–Davis, Sacramento, California

J. David Blaha, MD, Associate Professor, Department of Orthopedic Surgery, Chief, Section of Arthritis Surgery, West Virginia University Medical Center, Morgantown, West Virginia

Lawrence B. Bone, MD, Assistant Professor of Orthopaedics and General Surgery, State University of New York at Buffalo, Buffalo, New York

John H. Bowker, MD, Professor and Associate Chairman, Department of Orthopaedics and Rehabilitation, University of Miami School of Medicine, Medical Director, Jackson Memorial Rehabilitation Center, Miami, Florida

Michael J. Brennan, MD, Assistant Professor, Department of Orthopaedics, Milwaukee County Medical Complex, Milwaukee, Wisconsin

Andrew R. Burgess, MD, Director of Orthopaedic Traumatology, Maryland Institute for Emergency Medical Services Systems, Assistant Professor of Surgery, University of Maryland School of Medicine, Baltimore, Maryland

William E. Burkhalter, MD, Professor and Associate Chairman for Clinical Affairs, Chief, Division of Hand Surgery, University of Miami School of Medicine, Department of Orthopaedics and Rehabilitation, Miami, Florida

Jason Calhoun, MD, Assistant Professor, Division of Orthopaedic Surgery, Department of Surgery, University of Texas Medical Branch, Galveston, Texas

Michael W. Chapman, MD, Professor and Chairman, Department of Orthopaedics, University of California–Davis, Sacramento, California

George Cierny III, MD, Associate Professor of Surgery, Crawford Long Hospital, Department of Orthopaedics, Emory University School of Medicine, Atlanta, Georgia

Jose Cobos, MD, Research Associate, Division of Orthopaedic Surgery, Department of Surgery, University of Texas Medical Branch, Galveston, Texas

Robert H. Cofield, MD, Consultant in Orthopedics, Mayo Clinic, Professor, Mayo Medical School, Rochester, Minnesota

John Cone, MD, Associate Professor of Surgery, University of Arkansas for Medical Sciences, Little Rock, Arkansas

Fred G. Corley, MD, Associate Professor of Orthopaedics, University of Texas Medical School, San Antonio, Texas

Michael J. Coughlin, MD, Orthopaedic Surgeon, Boise, Idaho, Associate Clinical Professor of Surgery, Division of Orthopaedics and Rehabilitation, Oregon Health Sciences University, Portland, Oregon

Andrea Cracchiolo III, MD, Professor, Division of Orthopaedic Surgery, University of California, Los Angeles School of Medicine, Los Angeles, California

Laurence E. Dahners, MD, Associate Professor, Division of Orthopaedics, University of North Carolina School of Medicine, Chapel Hill, North Carolina

Lorraine J. Day, MD, Associate Professor of Orthopedic Surgery, University of California, San Francisco, California

Bradley C. Edgerton, MD, Orthopaedic Surgeon, Durango, Colorado

Eugene A. Elia, MD, Clinical Assistant Professor, Department of Orthopaedics, University of Pennsylvania, Philadelphia, Pennsylvania

John L. Esterhai, Jr, MD, Associate Professor of Orthopaedic Surgery, University of Pennsylvania School of Medicine, Philadelphia, Pennsylvania

Robert H. Fitzgerald, Jr, MD, Professor and Chairman, Department of Orthopaedic Surgery, Wayne State University, Detroit, Michigan

Larry F. Frevert, MD, Resident, Department of Orthopaedic Surgery, University of Arkansas for Medical Sciences, Little Rock, Arkansas

James R. Gage, MD, Director, Kinesiology Laboratory, Newington Children's Hospital, Associate Professor of Orthopaedics, University of Connecticut Medical School, Newington, Connecticut

Bertram Goldberg, MD, Associate Professor, University of Colorado Health Sciences Center, Denver, Colorado, Orthopaedic Surgeon, Englewood, Colorado

John S. Gould, MD, Professor and Chairman, Department of Orthopaedic Surgery, Medical College of Wisconsin, Milwaukee, Wisconsin

S. Ashby Grantham, MD, Professor of Clinical Orthopaedic Surgery, Columbia University College of Physicians and Surgeons, Columbia-Presbyterian Medical Center, New York, New York

Stuart A. Green, MD, Clinical Professor of Orthopaedic Surgery, University of California, Irvine, California, Program Director, Problem Fracture Service, Rancho Los Amigos Medical Center, Downey, California

Anthony G. Gristina, MD, Professor, Section of Orthopedic Surgery, Wake Forest University Medical Center, Winston-Salem, North Carolina

Stephen F. Gunther, MD, Chairman, Department of Orthopaedic Surgery, Washington Hospital Center, Professor, Department of Orthopaedic Surgery, George Washington University, Washington, DC, Professor, Department of Surgery, Uniformed Services University of Health Sciences, Bethesda, Maryland

Ramon B. Gustilo, MD, Professor, University of Minnesota, Chairman, Department of Orthopaedics, Hennepin County Medical Center, Minneapolis, Minnesota

John H. Harp, Jr, BSCE, Research Engineer, Department of Orthopaedics, Arkansas Children's Hospital, Little Rock, Arkansas

William H. Harris, MD, Clinical Professor of Orthopaedics, Harvard Medical School, Chief, Hip and Implant Unit, Massachusetts General Hospital, Boston, Massachusetts

Stephen L. Henry, MD, Instructor, Department of Orthopaedic Surgery, University of Louisville School of Medicine, Louisville, Kentucky

R. Bruce Heppenstall, MD, Professor and Chief of Orthopaedic Surgery, Hospital of the University of Pennsylvania, Chief of Orthopaedic Surgery, Veterans Administration, Philadelphia, Pennsylvania

James L. Hughes, MD, Chairman, Department of Orthopaedics, University of Mississippi Medical Center, Jackson, Mississippi

Gregory K. Johnson, MD, Chief Resident, Department of Orthopaedic Surgery, Stanford University Hospital, Palo Alto, California

Kenneth A. Johnson, MD, Professor of Orthopaedic Surgery, Mayo Clinic Scottsdale, Scottsdale, Arizona

Kenneth D. Johnson, MD, Associate Professor, Department of Orthopaedics and Rehabilitation, Vanderbilt University, Medical Center North, Nashville, Tennessee

Jesse B. Jupiter, MD, Associate Orthopaedic Surgeon, The Massachusetts General Hospital, Assistant Professor of Orthopaedic Surgery, Harvard Medical School, Boston, Massachusetts

Timothy L. Keenen, MD, Assistant Professor of Orthopedics, Oregon Health Sciences University, Portland, Oregon

Loren L. Latta, PhD, Professor and Director of Research, University of Miami School of Medicine, Department of Orthopaedics and Rehabilitation, Miami, Florida

Charles S. Levy, MD, Chairman, Infectious Diseases, Washington Hospital Center, Associate Professor of Medicine, George Washington University, Washington, DC

Paul A. Lotke, MD, Professor of Surgery, Department of Orthopaedics, Hospital of the University of Pennsylvania, Philadelphia, Pennsylvania

Jon Mader, MD, Professor of Internal Medicine, Division of Infectious Diseases, University of Texas Medical Branch, Galveston, Texas

Roger A. Mann, MD, Director Foot Fellowship, Associate Clinical Professor of Orthopaedic Surgery, University of California School of Medicine, San Francisco, California, Oakland, California

Thomas W. McNeill, MD, Associate Professor, Rush College of Medicine, Chicago, Illinois

John W. Michael, MEd, CPO, Assistant Clinical Professor, Duke University Medical Center, Director, Department of Prosthetics and Orthotics, Durham, North Carolina

Michael E. Miller, MD, Associate Professor, Chief of Orthopaedic Trauma, Department of Orthopaedic Surgery, Emory University School of Medicine, Chief of Orthopaedic Surgery, Grady Memorial Hospital, Atlanta, Georgia

David G. Murray, MD, Professor, Department of Orthopedic Surgery, State University of New York, Health Science Center, College of Medicine, Syracuse, New York

Paul T. Naylor, MD, Chief Resident, Department of Orthopedic Surgery, Wake Forest University Medical Center, Winston-Salem, North Carolina

Carl L. Nelson, MD, Professor and Chairman, Head, Section of Adult Reconstruction, Department of Orthopaedic Surgery, University of Arkansas for Medical Sciences, Little Rock, Arkansas

Ruth L. Nelson, MD, Instructor, Department of Orthopaedic Surgery, University of Arkansas for Medical Sciences, General Orthopaedics, Little Rock, Arkansas

Silvia Ōunpuu, MS, Kinesiologist, Kinesiology Laboratory Coordinator, Newington Children's Hospital, Newington, Connecticut

Guy D. Paiement, MD, Assistant Clinical Professor of Surgery, Universite de Montreal/Hopital du Sacre-Coeur, Montreal, PQ, Canada

Dror Paley, MD, Assistant Professor, Division of Orthopaedic Surgery, University of Maryland Hospital, Baltimore, Maryland

Michael J. Patzakis, MD, Professor of Orthopaedic Surgery, University of Southern California School of Medicine, Los Angeles, California

John C. Pearce, MD, Orthopaedic Surgeon, Austin, Texas

Jacquelin Perry, MD, Consultant, Centinela Hospital Biomechanics Laboratory, Chief, Pathokinesiology, Rancho Los Amigos Medical Center, Professor, Orthopedics, University of Southern California, Downey, California

Michael S. Pinzur, MD, Associate Professor of Orthopaedics and Rehabilitation, Loyola University Medical Center, Director, Special Teams for Amputations, Mobility, Prosthetics/Orthotics (STAMPS), Hines Veterans Administration Hospital, Maywood, Illinois

Charles A. Rockwood, Jr, MD, Professor and Chairman Emeritus, University of Texas Health Science Center, San Antonio, Texas

David Seligson, MD, Professor, Department of Orthopaedics, University of Louisville, Louisville, Kentucky

Michael J. Shereff, MD, Associate Professor, Department of Orthopaedic Surgery, New York University School of Medicine, Associate Director, Orthopaedic Foot and Ankle Service, Hospital for Joint Diseases Orthopaedic Institute, New York, New York

Peter J. Stern, MD, Clinical Professor of Orthopaedic Surgery, University of Cincinnati College of Medicine, Cincinnati, Ohio

James B. Stiehl, MD, Assistant Professor of Orthopaedic Surgery, Medical College of Wisconsin, Milwaukee County Medical Complex, Milwaukee, Wisconsin

David H. Sutherland, MD, Professor of Surgery/Orthopaedics and Rehabilitation, University of California, San Diego Medical School, Chief of Orthopaedic Surgery, Children's Hospital & Health Center, San Diego, California

Vernon T. Tolo, MD, Head, Division of Orthopaedics, Children's Hospital of Los Angeles, Professor of Orthopaedics, University of Southern California School of Medicine, Los Angeles, California

Dean T. Tsukayama, MD, Assistant Professor of Medicine, University of Minnesota, Medical Director, Musculoskeletal Sepsis Unit, Section of Infectious Disease, Hennepin County Medical Center, Minneapolis, Minnesota

Lawrence X. Webb, MD, Associate Professor, Department of Orthopedic Surgery, Wake Forest University Medical Center, Winston-Salem, North Carolina

Sara Jane Wessinger, RN, Research Nurse, Orthopaedic Biomechanics Laboratory, Massachusetts General Hospital, Boston, Massachusetts

Gerald R. Williams, MD, Assistant Instructor, Department of Orthopaedic Surgery, University of Texas Health Science Center, San Antonio, Texas

Frank C. Wilson, MD, Professor, Chief, Division of Orthopaedics, University of North Carolina School of Medicine, Chapel Hill, North Carolina

Edwin MacKenzie Wyman, MD, Orthopedic Resident, University of Massachusetts Medical Center, Worcester, Massachusetts

Joseph B. Zagorski, MD, Clinical Professor, Co-Director Special Fracture Clinic, Department of Orthopaedics and Rehabilitation, University of Miami School of Medicine, South Miami, Florida

Gregory A. Zych, DO, Associate Professor, Department of Orthopaedics and Rehabilitation, University of Miami School of Medicine, Miami, Florida

Preface

Instructional Course Lectures at the annual meeting of the American Academy of Orthopaedic Surgery have been presented since 1942. Although initially the lectures were viewed with some scepticism, the excellence of this educational format was quickly recognized. A natural extension of these presentations was to preserve and amplify their usefulness by publication. The first volume based on the courses, *Lectures on Peace and War Orthopaedic Surgery*, was published in 1943. With few exceptions, a volume of selected topics from the Instructional Course Lectures has been published annually.

Although format, content, and publisher have changed over the years, the central focus of the series remains unchanged. The purpose of the *Instructional Course Lectures* volume is to provide a high quality, written discussion of selected topics pertinent to patient care and the practice of orthopaedic surgery. Volume 39 seeks to continue that tradition with 72 chapters on 14 subjects selected from the instructional course lectures presented at the 1989 Annual Meeting. Inspecting the table of contents will quickly demonstrate the breadth and depth of subjects included. Some chapters are thorough reviews and updates in the surgical and medical management of problems that have always been part of orthopaedic surgery. Others provide information about new techniques of analysis and treatment.

The quality of this volume is a credit to the contributors and to the publications staff of the Academy. Each primary author has previously been recognized by the Instructional Course Lectures Committee and the course coordinators as having special experience and expertise in his or her subject. For their additional time, energy, and commitment, I would like to thank all the authors for sharing their research and experience.

It has been a great pleasure to work with the publications staff of the Academy. They can be accurately described as a very professional but patient group who wants to produce excellent work. In particular, I would like to note Marilyn L. Fox, PhD, who directed the development and publication of Volume 39; and Bruce A. Davis, who managed the editorial process. They were ably assisted by Wendy O. Schmidt, who reviewed manuscripts and layout for technical accuracy and stylistic consistency; Monica Trocker, who coordinated word processing and correspondence with the authors; and Mark W. Wieting, who is the Director of the Academy's Department of Communications and Publications.

Thanks are also due to committee members, Joseph S. Barr, Jr, MD; Frank H. Bassett III, MD; Robert E. Eilert, MD; Hugh S. Tullos, MD, who helped formulate the 1989 instructional courses; and to Kathie Niesen of the Academy staff, who does such a fine job in organizing the Instructional Courses and attending to the many details that ensure their continued success and improvement.

Finally, I would like to acknowledge my wife, Debby. Her support is instrumental in all of my work.

To paraphrase Francis Bacon, learning is a great pleasure, and I hope you enjoy reading and learning from this *Instructional Course Lectures* volume as much as I have.

Walter B. Greene, MD
Chapel Hill, North Carolina
Chairman, Committee on Instructional Courses

Joseph S. Barr, Jr, MD
Boston, Massachusetts

Frank H. Bassett III, MD
Durham, North Carolina

Robert E. Eilert, MD
Denver, Colorado

Hugh S. Tullos, MD
Houston, Texas

Contents

The Adult Foot

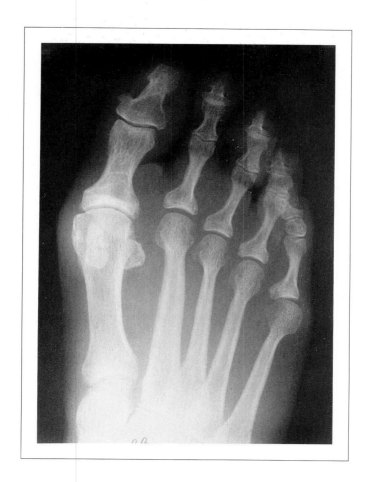

Decision-Making in Bunion Surgery

Roger A. Mann, MD

Introduction

The decision-making process starts with a careful history and a physical examination. The importance of the history is to determine the patient's main problem. At times, although a patient has a significant deformity, the main complaint is pain under the second metatarsal head or a painful second hammertoe. In about 75% of my cases, the chief complaint of a patient with a hallux valgus deformity is pain over the medial eminence. The history should also include a description of the shoes worn, noting any modifications that the patient has made. A work history is important, because surgery should be deferred if the patient stands all day, especially if the work involves physical labor, repeated squatting, or lifting from the floor. An athletic history is also important because bunion surgery may leave the patient with a straighter toe but a less functional foot.

The patient's expectations must be evaluated carefully to eliminate any misconceptions regarding foot surgery—notions gleaned from such sources as misleading advertisements and radio talk shows. The true nature of the problem must be explained to the patient. Patients often believe that after foot surgery they will be able to wear any type of shoe. In my experience, one third of patients have unrestricted shoe wear be-

fore surgery. After surgery, two thirds have unrestricted shoe wear, which leaves one third of patients still limited in their choice of shoes.

Other problems associated with bunion surgery, including possible joint pain or stiffness, recurrence of deformity, nerve entrapment, and development of a plantar callus under the second metatarsal head caused by shortening or dorsiflexion of the first metatarsal, should be discussed before surgery to allow the patient to make an informed decision.

The physical examination begins by observing the feet while the patient is standing. An assessment of the longitudinal arch is made, and the degree of deformity

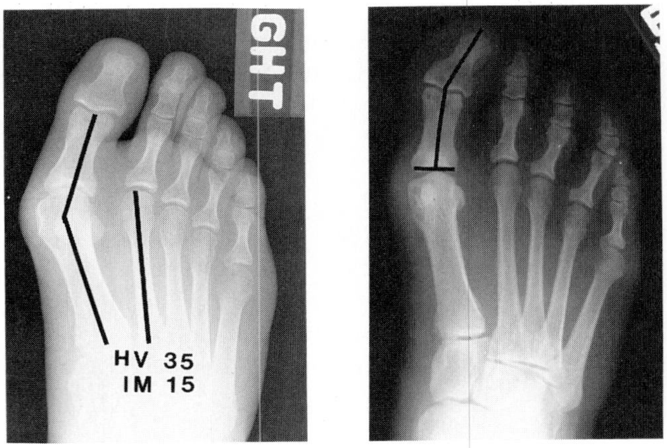

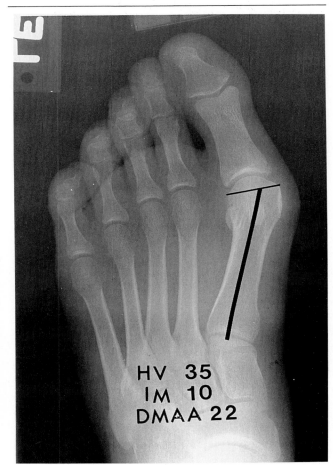

Fig. 1 **Left**, Hallux valgus angle is measured by angle subtended by the line bisecting the proximal phalanx and the first metatarsal and the intermetatarsal angle by a line bisecting the first and second metatarsals. **Right**, The interphalangeal angle is measured by a line bisecting the proximal and distal phalanges.

Fig. 2 The distal metatarsal articular angle (DMAA) is determined by drawing a line transversely connecting the proximal edge of the articular surface related to a line bisecting the long axis of the first metatarsal.

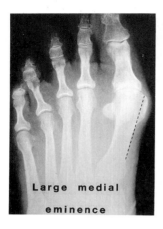
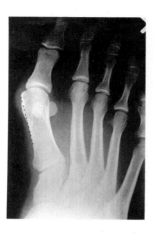

Fig. 3 **Left**, Large medial eminence. **Right**, Small medial eminence.

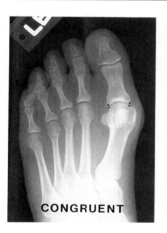
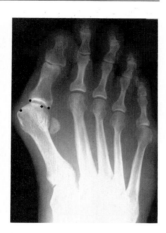

Fig. 4 **Left**, Congruent joint. **Right**, Incongruent joint—note lateral subluxation of the proximal phalanx on the metatarsal head.

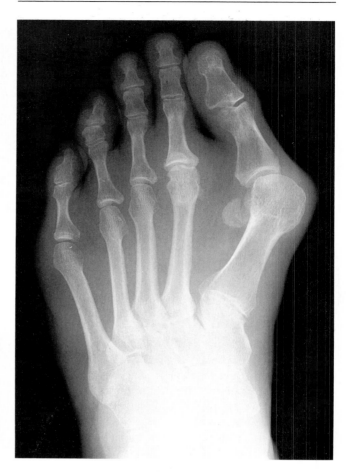

Fig. 5 Oblique metatarsocuneiform joint.

of the hallux and lesser toes is observed. The range of motion of the ankle, subtalar, transverse tarsal, and metatarsophalangeal joints is noted, comparing one limb with the other. The mobility of the first metatarsocuneiform joint is tested by dorsiflexion and plantar flexion of the metatarsal. This measurement is somewhat subjective in nature, and the two feet should be compared.

The presence and location of any plantar callosities should be noted. A callus beneath the second metatarsal head may be associated with loss of weightbearing by the first metatarsal secondary to an advanced hallux valgus, with dislocation of the second metatarsophalangeal joint, or with a hypermobile first metatarsocuneiform joint.

The first metatarsophalangeal joint should be carefully examined, noting the range of motion in the po-

sition of the deformity, and also observing what occurs as the toe is realigned. If the degree of dorsiflexion is abruptly diminished as the joint is realigned, this should alert the surgeon to the fact that if the proximal phalanx is fully corrected on the metatarsal head there may be a significant loss of dorsiflexion at the metatarsophalangeal joint.

The medial eminence is examined to determine whether a significant bursa is present and if the dorsomedial nerve is painful. The degree of pronation of the hallux should be noted, because advanced pronation precludes certain types of bunion repair.

The circulatory status of the foot is carefully determined, and Doppler pressures obtained if there is any question. Sensation is examined to screen for a peripheral neuropathy.

Radiographic Evaluation

Weightbearing radiographs are obtained and the following observations made: hallux valgus angle, presence of hallux valgus interphalangeus, intermetatarsal

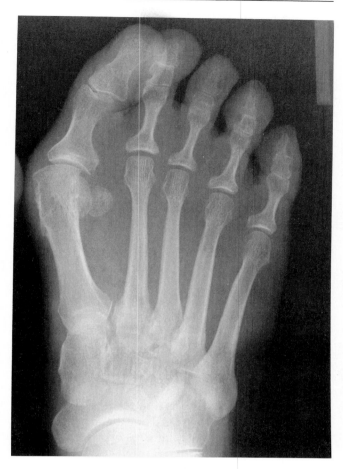

Fig. 6 The lateral facet at the lateral base of the metatarsal prevents closure of the intermetatarsal angle without osteotomy.

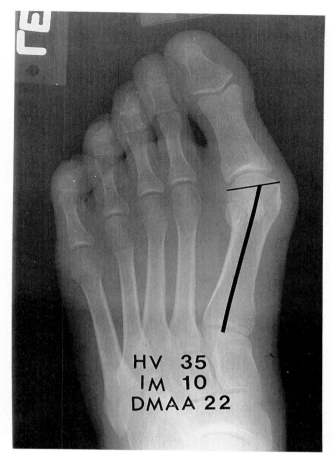

HV 35
IM 10
DMAA 22

Fig. 7 Hallus valgus deformity secondary primarily to lateral sloping of the distal metatarsal articular surface.

angle, alignment of the distal metatarsal articular angle (DMAA), degree of sesamoid displacement, size of the medial eminence, whether the metatarsophalangeal joint is congruent or incongruent, the shape of the metatarsocuneiform joint, and the presence of joint narrowing.

The hallux valgus angle is obtained by measuring the angle subtended by a line bisecting the proximal phalanx and the metatarsal, the interphalangeal angle by a line bisecting the proximal and distal phalanges, and the intermetatarsal angle by a line bisecting the first and second metatarsals (Fig. 1). The DMAA is the relationship between the articular surface of the metatarsal head and the longitudinal axis of the first metatarsal. The angle lies between a line transversely connecting the proximal edge of the articular surface and a line that bisects the long axis of the first metatarsal (Fig. 2). The degree of sesamoid displacement—the relationship of the fibular sesamoid to the lateral aspect of the metatarsal head—is in part related to the degree of pronation of the hallux and the degree of the valgus deformity. The size of the medial eminence is determined by drawing a line along the medial aspect of the metatarsal shaft (Fig. 3). The alignment of the metatarsophalangeal joint is expressed as congruent or incongruent depending on whether the joint is subluxated or not.[1] This is determined, using a radiograph, by placing dots at the medial and lateral edges of the articular surface on both the metatarsal head and the proximal phalanx. If the two pairs of dots are parallel to each other, the joint is congruent. If not, the joint is incongruent or subluxated (Fig. 4). The shape of the metatarsocuneiform joint varies, depending in part on the angle of the anteroposterior radiograph. In patients with a hypermobile metatarsocuneiform joint, the joint tends to be more oblique (Fig. 5). Occasionally a lateral facet is present that obstructs closure of the intermetatarsal angle (Fig. 6).

Clinical Significance of Radiographic Findings

The clinical relevance of the radiographic findings and their surgical implications must be fully understood when planning hallux valgus surgery in order for the orthopaedist to decide which surgical procedure is ap-

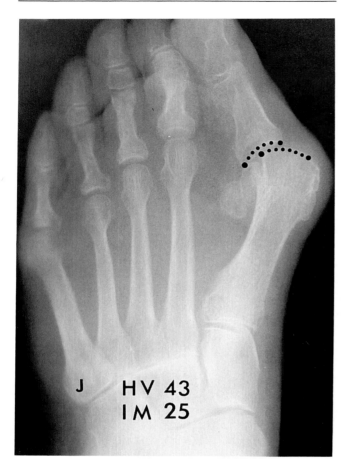

J   H V 43
    I M 25

Fig. 8 Incongruent metatarsophalangeal joint but with a small DMAA. The proximal phalanx can be rotated back onto the metatarsal head, producing satisfactory correction of the hallux valgus deformity.

propriate for each type of hallux valgus deformity. Note, however, that the radiographic findings must always be correlated with the physical findings.

Hallux valgus interphalangeus measures the lateral deviation intrinsic to the hallux itself. Normally this angle is 15 degrees or less but it is quite variable—6 to 24 degrees.[2] If it exists as an isolated entity, which is usually the case, a proximal phalangeal osteotomy will give adequate correction. If it coexists with a hallux valgus deformity, then correction of the metatarsophalangeal joint alone may not completely correct the deformity and the addition of a phalangeal osteotomy should be considered.

The hallux valgus angle measures the lateral deviation of the proximal phalanx on the metatarsal head. The hallux valgus angle is normally less than 20 degrees. Although this is an important measurement, it must be correlated with whether the metatarsophalangeal joint is congruent or incongruent as well as with the DMAA. If the joint is congruent, the proximal phalanx is cen-

tered on the articular surface of the metatarsal head. In an incongruent joint, the proximal phalanx is displaced or subluxated laterally in relation to the articular surface of the metatarsal head. The DMAA, which relates the angle of the distal articular surface to the long axis of the metatarsal, normally slopes laterally 0 to 10 degrees. Precise measurement of this angle may be difficult because the borders of the articular surface are somewhat indistinct.

The clinical significance of these measurements is that the entire hallux valgus deformity may result from a laterally sloping metatarsal head with a congruent joint (Fig. 7). If this is the case, any attempt to move the proximal phalanx around on the articular surface of the metatarsal head would only disrupt the normal relationship between these two articular surfaces. To attempt this would probably cause stiffness of the metatarsophalangeal joint or recurrence of the deformity after the articular surfaces have realigned themselves. This type of deformity calls either for some type of distal metatarsal osteotomy to realign the articular surface of the metatarsal shaft or for a phalangeal osteotomy and removal of the medial eminence.

If the metatarsophalangeal joint is incongruent, then the proximal phalanx can be rotated back over the distal articular surface and satisfactory alignment can be achieved, providing the distal articular surface is not sloped too far laterally (Fig. 8). If the DMAA is more than 20 degrees and the joint is incongruent, then the proximal phalanx can be repositioned over the metatarsal head, but the residual deformity should be corrected with a compensating phalangeal osteotomy (Fig. 9). If these anatomic deformities are recognized when planning the surgery, an incomplete correction can be avoided.

The intermetatarsal angle measures the relationship between the first and second metatarsals. The intermetatarsal angle is normally less than 10 degrees. Several factors affect the magnitude of the intermetatarsal angle, including pressure of the proximal phalanx against the metatarsal head and the inherent anatomic alignment. This alignment depends partly on the mobility of the metatarsocuneiform joint. As the proximal phalanx drifts into valgus, it puts pressure against the metatarsal head, pushing it medially and widening the intermetatarsal angle. In some cases, in which the intermetatarsal angle was wide to begin with, wearing of narrow shoes has pushed the phalanx into valgus. It has been demonstrated that the intermetatarsal angle corrects about 5 degrees after a distal soft-tissue bunion repair.[3] This apparently means that with relief of the medial pressure generated by the proximal phalanx against the metatarsal head, there is enough mobility at the metatarsocuneiform joint to permit this correction to occur. If the intermetatarsal angle does not correct when a distal soft-tissue procedure is carried out, it means the intermetatarsal angle is fixed, and the

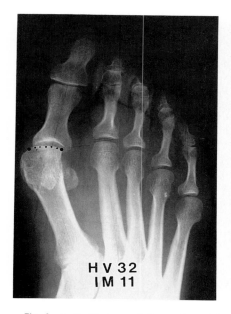
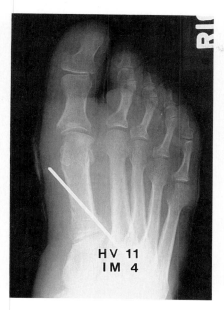
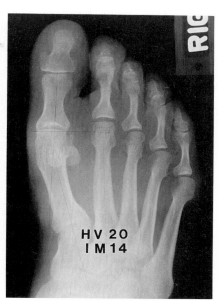

Fig. 9 **Left**, Moderate hallux valgus deformity but with a DMAA of 20 degrees. **Center**, Immediately postoperative radiograph with metatarsophalangeal joint held open. **Right**, Postoperative result with residual hallux valgus angle of 20 degrees because of the high DMAA.

distal soft-tissue procedure cannot succeed when a fixed bony deformity is present. The determination as to whether the intermetatarsal angle will correct can be made radiographically only when a lateral facet is present at the base of the metatarsal. If a facet is present, usually the intermetatarsal angle cannot be corrected without a metatarsal osteotomy.

The sesamoids are normally positioned beneath the metatarsal head. In the anteroposterior radiograph, about 20% to 30% of the lateral aspect of the fibular sesamoid is exposed. In patients with hallux valgus, there is increased exposure of the fibular sesamoid because pressure from the proximal phalanx has pushed the metatarsal head off the sesamoid sling. The degree of exposure of the sesamoids depends on the severity of the hallux valgus and the degree of pronation of the hallux.

The size of the medial eminence is judged by how far it protrudes medially beyond a line drawn along the medial aspect of the metatarsal shaft. A hallux valgus deformity may be associated with a small or large medial eminence. From a surgical standpoint, it is important to note the size of the medial eminence because in hallux valgus surgery correction is achieved not by removing a portion of the articular surface with the medial eminence but by realigning the metatarsophalangeal joint.

The obliquity of the metatarsocuneiform joint is variable. The mobility of this joint cannot be determined radiographically but rather is based on clinical examination. As pointed out previously, patients with a hy-

permobile first metatarsocuneiform joint tend to have a more obliquely configured joint.

Arthrosis of the metatarsophalangeal joint is not usually a significant factor in patients with hallux valgus, but, when present to a significant degree with joint narrowing and osteophyte formation, a primary hallux valgus repair may be precluded because it would only increase the joint's stiffness.

Overview of Hallux Valgus Surgery

The basic purpose of hallux valgus surgery is to correct the deformity and maintain a biomechanically functional foot. Unfortunately, despite our best efforts, this goal cannot always be achieved. Bunion procedures in general consist of soft-tissue procedures about the first metatarsophalangeal joint, distal metatarsal osteotomies, proximal metatarsal osteotomies, phalangeal osteotomies, arthrodeses, and implants. A combination of procedures is frequently required to produce a satisfactory result.

The distal soft-tissue procedure about the first metatarsophalangeal joint involves releasing the lateral joint capsule, plicating the medial joint capsule, and excising the medial eminence. Release of the lateral joint capsule consists of releasing the adductor hallucis from its insertion into the proximal phalanx and cutting the transverse metatarsal ligament and the lateral joint capsule, without removing the fibular sesamoid. This procedure gives the most predictable result when carried out for a mild to moderate deformity, that is, when

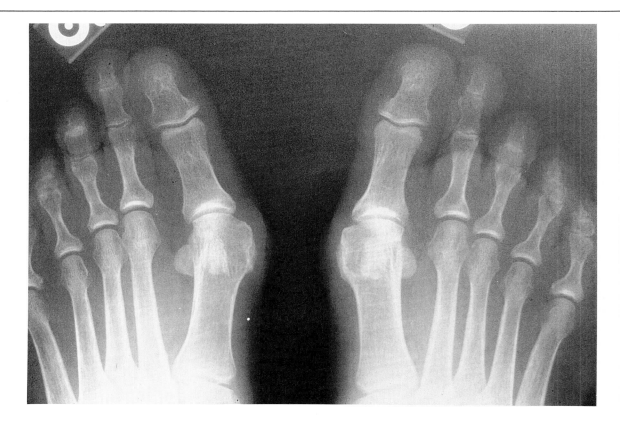

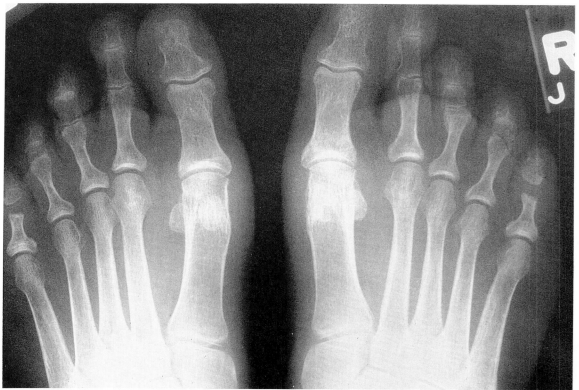

Fig. 10 **Top**, Preoperative radiograph of bilateral hallux valgus deformity. **Bottom**, Postoperative radiograph after distal soft-tissue procedure.

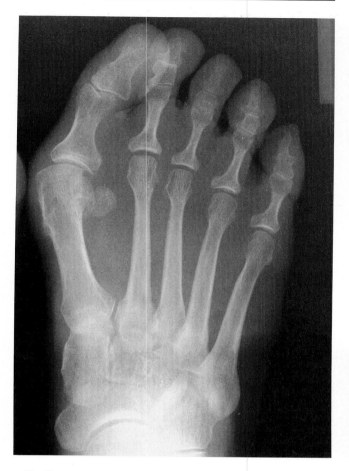

Fig. 11 Recurrent hallux valgus deformity after a distal soft-tissue procedure. Because of a fixed intermetatarsal angle, the procedure failed. A proximal metatarsal osteotomy is required to correct a fixed intermetatarsal angle.

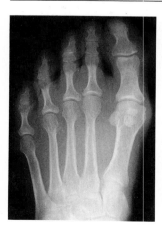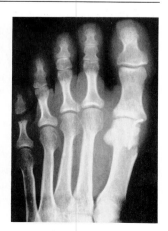

Fig. 12 **Left**, Radiograph of a hallux valgus deformity with a congruent joint. **Right**, Postoperative radiograph after a chevron procedure. Note pin fixation.

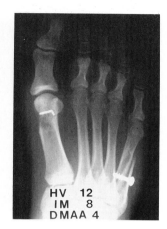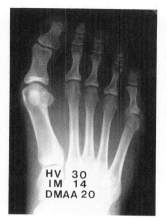

Fig. 13 **Left**, Hallux valgus deformity with a congruent joint and a DMAA of 20 degrees. **Right**, Postoperative result after chevron procedure with a medial closing wedge that corrected the DMAA to 4 degrees.

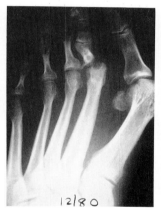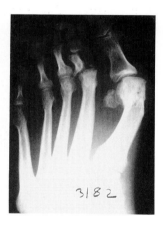

Fig. 14 **Left**, Severe hallux valgus deformity. **Right**, Incomplete correction of the deformity utilizing a chevron osteotomy.

the metatarsophalangeal joint is incongruent, the hallux valgus angle is less than 30 degrees, and the intermetatarsal angle is less than 14 degrees.[3,4] The correction depends on how well the proximal phalanx can be repositioned on the metatarsal head, and whether the first and second metatarsals are flexible enough to permit correction of the intermetatarsal angle after the pressure from the proximal phalanx against the metatarsal head has been relieved (Fig. 10). If the intermetatarsal angle is rigid and will not correct, a soft-tissue procedure will fail and the deformity will recur (Fig. 11).

The two principal distal metatarsal osteotomy procedures are the chevron[5,6] and Mitchell procedures.[7,8] These procedures correct the deformity in slightly different ways. The chevron translates the metatarsal head

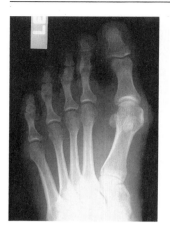
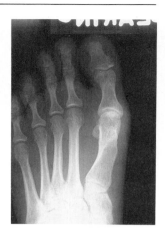

Fig. 15 **Left,** Hallux valgus deformity. **Right,** Satisfactory correction after a Mitchell procedure.

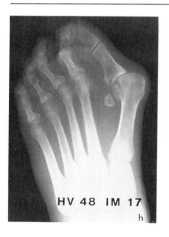
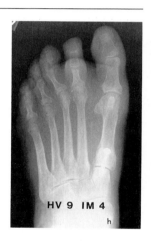

HV 48 IM 17
h

HV 9 IM 4
h

Fig. 16 **Left,** Severe hallux valgus deformity. **Right,** Postoperative correction after a distal soft-tissue procedure and proximal metatarsal osteotomy.

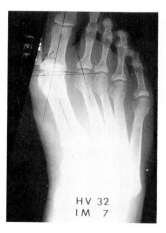
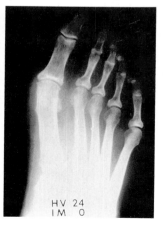

HV 32
IM 7

HV 24
IM 0

Fig. 17 **Left,** Hallux valgus deformity with a DMAA of 35 degrees. **Right,** Incomplete correction of the hallux valgus because of large DMAA. When this type deformity is present, an Akin procedure must be utilized to bring about full correction.

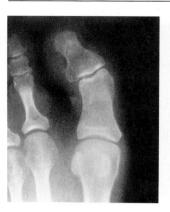
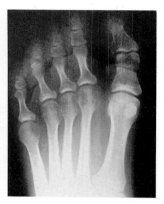

Fig. 18 **Left,** Hallux valgus interphalangeus. **Right,** Satisfactory correction after an Akin procedure.

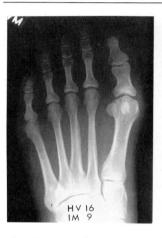
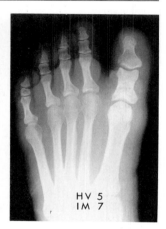

HV 16
IM 9

HV 5
IM 7

Fig. 19 **Left,** Hallux valgus deformity with a congruent joint and a large medial eminence. **Right,** Satisfactory correction utilizing an Akin procedure and excision of the medial eminence.

laterally 3 to 5 mm, which narrows the foot (Fig. 12). If a medial closing wedge osteotomy is added to the procedure by removing 1 to 2 mm of bone from the proximal chevron cut, the distal articular surface can be realigned and a hallux valgus with a congruent joint but abnormal DMAA can be corrected (Fig. 13). If the intermetatarsal angle is too large, approximately 15 degrees or more, the chevron osteotomy usually cannot correct it, nor can it correct a hallux valgus deformity of more than 35 degrees or a toe that is severely pronated (Fig. 14). The Mitchell osteotomy is similar to the chevron osteotomy but has the ability to correct a greater degree of intermetatarsal angle and hallux valgus deformity (Fig. 15).

The proximal metatarsal osteotomy can achieve the greatest degree of correction of the intermetatarsal angle, but it should be combined with a distal soft-tissue procedure to correct the hallux valgus deformity (Fig.

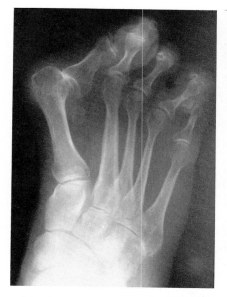
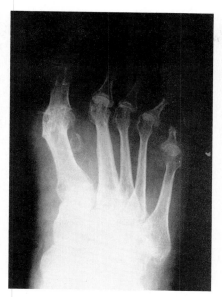
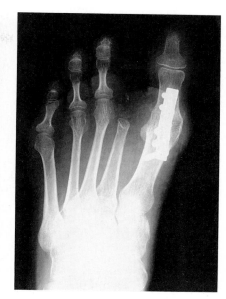

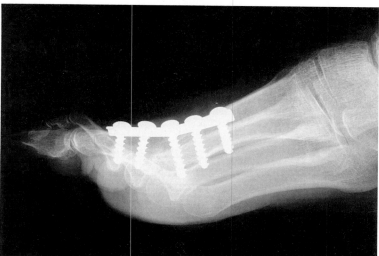

Fig. 20 **Top left,** Severe hallux valgus deformity with dislocation of the metatarsophalangeal joint. **Top center,** Satisfactory result after an arthrodesis of the metatarsophalangeal joint. **Top right,** Arthrodesis utilizing a quarter tubular plate. **Bottom,** Lateral radiograph demonstrating utilization of a quarter tubular plate.

16). This procedure is used to correct more severe deformities. If the distal metatarsal articular angle is more than 20 degrees, a phalangeal osteotomy may be required to gain full correction (Fig. 17). There are three basic proximal metatarsal osteotomies—a closing wedge, an opening wedge, and a crescent-shaped cut. I prefer the crescent-shaped osteotomy because it is the most stable and involves little or no shortening. The closing wedge results in some shortening, and sometimes causes dorsiflexion of the distal metatarsal when the osteotomy site is closed. The opening wedge osteotomy is somewhat unstable and has a further disadvantage in that, by lengthening the first metatarsal in a patient with a severe hallux valgus deformity, further tension is placed across the already tight metatarso-

phalangeal joint. This tension makes it difficult to maintain correction.

The osteotomy of the proximal phalanx[9] corrects a hallux valgus interphalangeus (Fig. 18). If the problem is a hallux valgus with a congruent joint and the DMAA is less than 15 degrees, a phalangeal osteotomy with removal of the medial eminence will produce a satisfactory result (Fig. 19). Although the phalangeal osteotomy cannot correct any deformity of the metatarsophalangeal joint, it is used in conjunction with other procedures, such as the chevron or proximal osteotomy combined with a distal soft-tissue procedure. It is used to achieve full correction when the distal metatarsal articular angle is more than 15 to 20 degrees.

An arthrodesis of the metatarsophalangeal joint is a

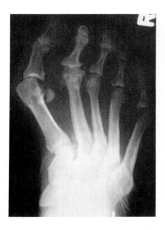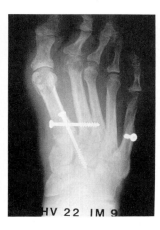

Fig. 21 **Left**, Hallux valgus deformity associated with a hypermobile first metatarsocuneiform joint, hallux valgus of 45 degrees and intermetatarsal angle of 15 degrees. **Right**, Satisfactory postoperative correction utilizing a distal soft-tissue procedure and metatarsocuneiform arthrodesis.

very reliable procedure that is useful in patients with severe deformity associated with joint stiffness and loss of motion. When a patient has degenerative joint disease that is too advanced for a reconstructive procedure, an arthrodesis produces a functional foot that will not deteriorate with time (Fig. 20).

I believe that use of Silastic implants in primary bunion surgery is rarely indicated. Patients with advanced arthritis, who do not desire an arthrodesis, may be considered for an implant. A basic principle, however, is that the implant cannot by itself maintain the correction. It is imperative that the intermetatarsal angle be corrected with an osteotomy and that the metatarsophalangeal joint be realigned when the implant is inserted. Any attempt to rely on the implant to correct the hallux valgus and the intermetatarsal angle will fail.

Fusion of the metatarsocuneiform joint in conjunction with hallux valgus surgery is indicated when hypermobility of the first metatarsocuneiform joint exists (Fig. 21). Although many patients demonstrate some hypermobility, I reserve this procedure for patients whose hypermobility is of such a degree that the patient has a significant callus beneath the second metatarsal head caused by a loss of weightbearing from the hypermobile first ray. The problem with a first metatarsocuneiform fusion is the degree of rigidity that it produces within the foot. Conversely, if a patient with marked hypermobility does not undergo a first metatarsocuneiform fusion, there is a significant possibility of recurrence of the deformity.

Decision-Making in Hallux Valgus Surgery

On the basis of the preceding material, the following algorithm is offered as a guide in selecting a procedure

to be used to correct a hallux valgus deformity (Fig. 22). Although it is based on the abnormal anatomy in patients with hallux valgus and on the results of various procedures as described in the literature, by its very nature it is somewhat arbitrary. The purpose of the algorithm is to provide the reader with a logical approach to bunion surgery, an approach that has stood the test of time. It is not exhaustive. Other procedures not included in this classification can also produce satisfactory results.

The first decision that must be made is whether the joint is congruent, incongruent, or has degenerative joint disease. Having made this decision, let us look at what procedures can be carried out for the congruent joint. The congruent joint can be corrected by using a chevron (Fig. 12) or an Akin procedure (Fig. 19), along with excision of the medial eminence. In these procedures we are dealing with a proximal phalanx that is centered over the metatarsal head, but needs to be realigned by an extra-articular procedure. If the distal metatarsal articular surface is sloped laterally more than 20 degrees, realignment is best achieved by the chevron procedure. To this a medial closing-wedge osteotomy is added to realign the distal articular surface to the long axis of the metatarsal and correct the abnormality (Fig. 13). If the DMAA is less than 15 degrees, the Akin procedure and medial eminence excision can also produce a satisfactory result. If a hallux valgus interphalangeus is present, the Akin procedure is the procedure of choice (Fig. 18).

For a patient with an incongruent joint and an intermetatarsal angle of less than 15 degrees and a hallux valgus angle of less than 30 degrees, the chevron procedure, the distal soft-tissue procedure with or without a proximal osteotomy, or a Mitchell procedure can produce satisfactory results. Generally speaking, for a patient beyond 50 years of age the chevron does not give as good a result as it does for a younger patient. The distal soft-tissue procedure can also give a satisfactory result, but in approximately 60% to 70% of the cases a crescent-shaped osteotomy must be added to adequately correct the intermetatarsal angle and prevent recurrence. The Mitchell procedure can also give a satisfactory result in this group of patients.

As noted in Figure 22, for patients with an intermetatarsal angle of more than 15 degrees and a hallux valgus angle of less than 40 degrees, the chevron procedure probably cannot reliably produce a satisfactory result. The distal soft-tissue procedure with a proximal crescent-shaped osteotomy and Mitchell will, and as such should be considered the procedures of choice.

If the intermetatarsal angle is more than 20 degrees and the hallux valgus angle is more than 40 degrees, a severe deformity exists and the Mitchell procedure will not produce a reliable result. With this degree of deformity, an arthrodesis or a distal soft-tissue procedure

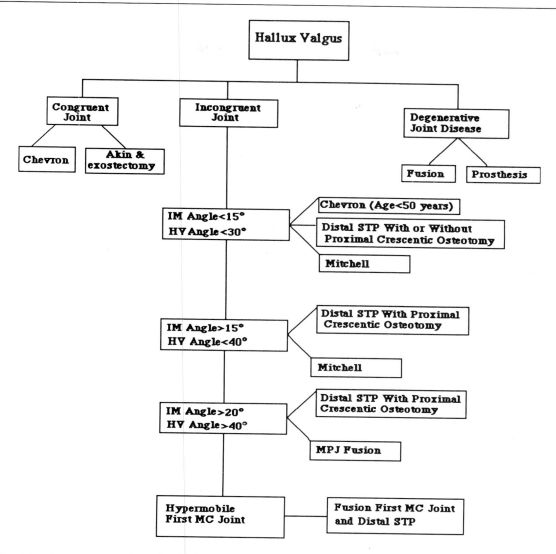

Fig. 22 Algorithm that presents a scheme for decision-making in hallux valgus surgery.

with a proximal crescent-shaped osteotomy will produce satisfactory alignment.

If there is hypermobility of the first metatarsocuneiform joint, then a fusion of the first metatarsocuneiform joint, along with a distal soft-tissue procedure, will produce a satisfactory result.

If degenerative joint disease is present, then fusion or an implant can be considered. As mentioned previously, I believe that an arthrodesis will give a better long-term result than will a prosthetic replacement.

Acknowledgment

The figures shown in this chapter are reproduced with permission from Roger A. Mann, MD.

References

1. Piggott H: The natural history of hallux valgus in adolescence and early adult life. *J Bone Joint Surg* 1960;42B:749–760.
2. Steel MW III, Johnson KA, DeWitz MA, et al: Radiographic measurements of the normal adult foot. *Foot Ankle* 1980;1:151–158.
3. Mann RA, Coughlin MJ: Hallux valgus: Etiology, anatomy, treatment and surgical considerations. *Clin Orthop* 1981;157:31–41.
4. Mann RA: *Surgery of the Foot.* St Louis, CV Mosby, 1988, pp 89–98.
5. Corless JR: A modification of the Mitchell procedure, abstract. *J Bone Joint Surg* 1976;58B:138.
6. Johnson KA, Cofield RH, Morrey BF: Chevron osteotomy for hallux valgus. *Clin Orthop* 1979;142:44–47.
7. Carr CR, Boyd BM: Correctional osteotomy for metatarsus primus varus and hallux valgus. *J Bone Joint Surg* 1968;50A:1353–1367.
8. Mitchell CL, Fleming JL, Allen R, et al: Osteotomy-bunionectomy for hallux valgus. *J Bone Joint Surg* 1958;40A:41–60.
9. Akin OF: The treatment of hallux valgus: A new operative procedure and its results. *Med Sentinel* 1925;33:678.

Hallux Rigidus

Roger A. Mann, MD

Hallux rigidus results from degenerative changes in the first metatarsophalangeal joint. As the degenerative process advances, the first metatarsophalangeal joint becomes enlarged and increasingly painful and rigid as motion, especially dorsiflexion, is lost. First described by Davies-Colley[1] in 1887 as hallux flexus, the condition was later termed hallux rigidus by Cotterill.[2]

The etiology of hallux rigidus is secondary to degenerative arthritis. The cause of the arthritis is trauma, such as an intra-articular fracture, compression of the joint surfaces (turf toe), previous osteochondritic lesion of the first metatarsal head, or, in by far the largest number of cases, is of unknown etiology. Published studies have not linked levels of physical activity to the development of hallux rigidus.

Initially, hallux rigidus is associated with pain and synovitis of the metatarsophalangeal joint. The articular cartilage on the metatarsal head undergoes variable but progressive degeneration during this period. As the condition continues, osteophytes develop, mainly about the dorsomedial, dorsal, and lateral aspects of the head. Rarely do osteophytes occur directly medially or on the plantar aspect. The articular surface between the sesamoids and the metatarsal head is infrequently involved. As the osteophytes increase in size, dorsiflexion of the metatarsophalangeal joint is no longer possible because of the mechanical barrier they create. Occasionally the dorsal osteophyte becomes so large that the hallux is held in plantar flexion; hence the term hallux flexus. In its more advanced state, if the plantar flexion of the hallux continues, the first metatarsal becomes elevated. This has led to the term metatarsus primus elevatus.

The articular cartilage of the proximal phalanx, although not primarily affected, undergoes some changes. Although these are never as severe as those in the metatarsal head, occasionally a dorsal osteophyte on the proximal phalanx occurs and, in some cases, it may fracture. The loss of dorsiflexion of the metatarsophalangeal joint increases stress on the interphalangeal joint, and can cause hyperextension of the joint. This hyperextension can cause a callus to develop beneath the condyles of the proximal phalanx and become symptomatic.

The patient is initially aware of pain and swelling of the metatarsophalangeal joint, associated with the synovitis and early degenerative changes. As the osteophytes develop, progressive enlargement of the metatarsal head makes shoe fitting a problem (Fig. 1). As the degree of dorsiflexion decreases, the mechanical obstruction of the proximal phalanx causes dorsal pain. This is a serious problem for athletes, especially if running is a main activity. Eventually even walking becomes uncomfortable. Often neuritic symptoms, such as tingling and numbness, develop, caused by pressure on the dorsomedial cutaneous nerve to the great toe. Physical examination reveals varying degrees of enlargement of the metatarsal head with synovial thickening. A small abrasion or ulceration may develop over the dorsal prominence, caused by pressure from footwear (Fig. 1). Although the ridge of bone is sensitive to palpation, maximum pain often occurs along the lateral aspect of the joint, where a prominent exostosis is frequently present. The range of motion is decreased, mainly in dorsiflexion, and forced dorsiflexion often reproduces the patient's symptoms. Plantar flexion is decreased because stretching of the extensor hallucis longus tendon and joint capsule over the dorsal osteophytes is painful. There may be some dysesthesias over the dorsomedial cutaneous nerve, and if there is a large osteophyte along the lateral aspect of the metatarsal head, the superficial branch of the deep peroneal nerve may also be sensitive. A significant degree of hallux valgus is rare.

Radiographic findings are consistent with degenerative arthritis of the metatarsophalangeal joint. The lateral view reveals the extent of the dorsal exostosis and of joint-space narrowing (Fig. 2). Careful evaluation of the lateral radiograph reveals how much joint space remains. The dorsal half of the joint space may be absent while the lower half is maintained. An exostosis may be present on the dorsal aspect of the proximal phalanx, which occasionally is fractured through its base. The anteroposterior radiograph reveals the squaring-off of the joint, the narrowing of the joint space, and the degree of lateral osteophyte formation (Fig. 3). Joint-space narrowing is difficult to evaluate on the anteroposterior view because the osteophytes overlap. The sesamoids are rarely involved in the degenerative process.

Conservative management of hallux rigidus begins with symptomatic treatment consisting of nonsteroidal anti-inflammatory medications for the synovitis phase, along with appropriate footwear. A stiff-soled shoe to decrease dorsiflexion of the metatarsophalangeal joint is often helpful. Orthoses are commercially available that make the forepart of the shoe more rigid. Because these orthoses occupy space, the toe box of the shoe

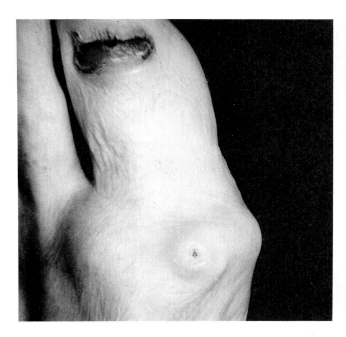
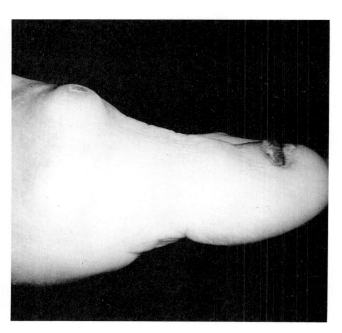

Fig. 1 Left, Note the marked enlargement of the first metatarsophalangeal joint in this patient with hallux rigidus. A small ulceration has formed secondary to pressure from the shoe. **Right,** The lateral view demonstrates the large dorsal osteophytes which have formed. These increase the bulk of the joint and also limit dorsiflexion.

must be large enough to accommodate the enlarged metatarsophalangeal joint and the orthotic device. An extra-depth shoe is often useful. As the disease process continues, occasionally an intra-articular injection of a steroid preparation may afford temporary relief.

If the pain becomes too disabling, surgical intervention may provide a satisfactory solution. Decision-making in the initial surgical treatment of hallux rigidus is based on the type and extent of abnormality. As a rule, the main problem at that time is the impingement of the proximal phalanx against the dorsal osteophytes. As the initial treatment for this problem, a cheilectomy should be strongly considered.

Cheilectomy

A cheilectomy, by removing the dorsal 20% to 30% of the metatarsal head, relieves the dorsal impingement, and provides increased dorsiflexion, significant pain reduction, and decreased bulk of the joint. It further offers the advantage that if the result is unsatisfactory, a salvage procedure, such as an arthrodesis, a Keller procedure, a bipolar implant, or a phalangeal osteotomy, can easily be performed.

The main indication for a cheilectomy is a symptomatic hallux rigidus secondary to osteophyte formation about the metatarsal head. If a lateral radiograph shows

that reasonable joint space exists in the plantar half of the metatarsophalangeal joint, I believe the procedure has a good chance of success. If no joint space is present, I would consider an arthrodesis, which produces a satisfactory long-term result and still leaves the patient with a functional foot. For the older patient, with limited ambulatory needs, a Keller procedure, along with debulking of the metatarsal head, can be done. Although the use of Silastic implants is tempting, they rarely withstand the stress placed on them by the active person interested in sports. The hemiarthroplasty has been losing favor because of breakdown of the material, erosion of the prosthesis into the bone, and synovitis. Bipolar implants may produce acceptable long-term results in the less active individual.

Surgical Technique

A cheilectomy is carried out through a dorsal incision centered over the metatarsophalangeal joint. The joint capsule is incised on either side of the extensor hallucis longus tendon. The plane between the capsule and synovium is developed and as complete a synovectomy as possible is carried out, dorsally, medially, and laterally.

The proximal phalanx is sharply plantar flexed to permit inspection of the joint. The large dorsal ridge of bone is readily identified, along with the lateral osteophytes. The articular cartilage often proves to be significantly more destroyed than the radiograph would

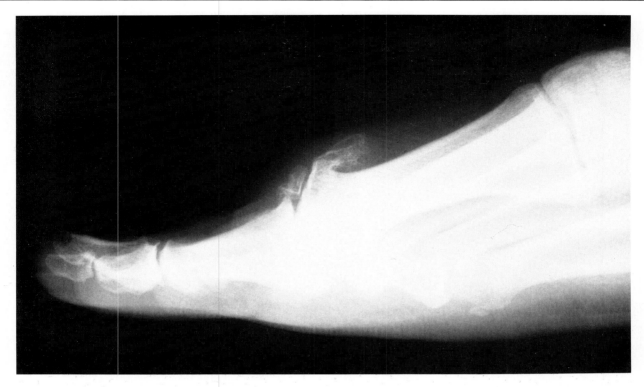

Fig. 2 Lateral radiograph demonstrating the large dorsal exostosis on the metatarsal head, along with a loose body in the dorsal joint space.

lead one to suspect. The dorsal one third to one half of the articular cartilage may be absent, exposing subchondral bone, or it may no longer be firmly attached to bone. The phalangeal cartilage often presents some fibrillation but is rarely damaged. The metatarsal sesamoid articulation should be inspected. Significant abnormality in this articulation is rare.

The amount of bone to be removed from the metatarsal head is dictated by the size of the dorsal exostosis and the degree of articular cartilage destruction. If degeneration of the articular cartilage is not significant and the main problem is the dorsal exostosis, then about 20% of the dorsal aspect of the metatarsal head is removed along with the exostosis. Using a small osteotome, excess bone is removed on a slope, starting distally at the metatarsal head, and ending just proximal to the origin of the osteophyte. If articular cartilage degeneration is significant, a greater amount of metatarsal head is removed.

As a general rule, I start the metatarsal head resection just dorsal to the edge of what appears to be viable articular cartilage. In severe cases, as much as one third of the dorsal aspect of the metatarsal head is removed (Fig. 4). I advise being somewhat aggressive in resecting bone. The lateral osteophytes are removed in line with the metatarsal shaft, and the dorsal, medial, and lateral corners of the metatarsal head are rounded (Fig. 5).

After the bone has been excised, it should be possible to dorsiflex the metatarsophalangeal joint about 70 degrees. If this degree of dorsiflexion cannot be achieved, it is probable that insufficient bone has been removed (Fig. 6). Loose fragments of bone, articular cartilage, and synovial tissue are then irrigated out of the joint, and bone wax is applied to the raw bone surfaces. The joint capsule and skin are closed in separate layers.

A tight compression dressing is applied for 12 to 18 hours, followed by a lighter-weight dressing for ten days. The patient wears a wooden shoe for walking. Sutures are removed at ten days, and the patient is then encouraged to wear a soft flexible shoe or sandal. Active and passive motion of the metatarsophalangeal joint for five minutes every hour while the patient is awake is encouraged. The patient will be hesitant at first, but, with encouragement, range of motion is increased over the ensuing weeks. If patients are not encouraged to pursue range of motion, it will not be obtained. For this reason, weekly visits are necessary. After two to three months, most of the motion that will be achieved is present; however, improvement of generalized reaction about the metatarsophalangeal joint in the form of soft-tissue thickening and swelling may continue for as long as six months.

The results following a cheilectomy as documented in a series by Mann and Clanton[3] revealed complete

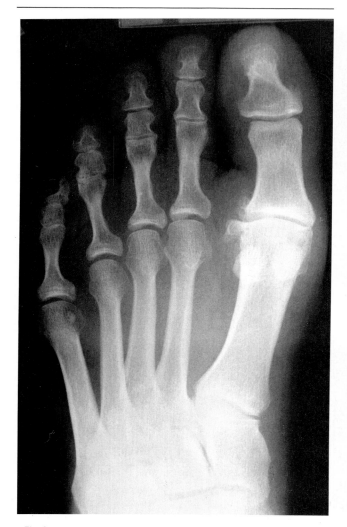

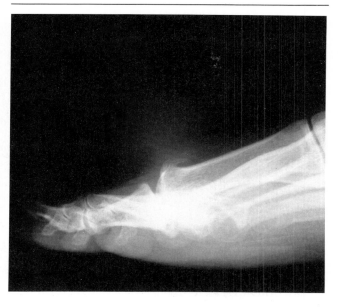

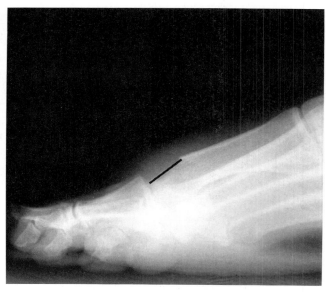

Fig. 3 Anteroposterior radiograph demonstrating the squaring off of the joint and the large osteophytes present along the lateral aspect of the joint.

Fig. 4 **Top,** Lateral radiograph demonstrating large dorsal osteophyte. **Bottom,** Postoperative radiograph demonstrating that the dorsal 25% to 30% of the metatarsal head has been excised when carrying out a cheilectomy.

relief of pain in 22 of 31 patients. Six others had significant relief, two had no relief, and one was made worse. The range of motion averaged 29 degrees before surgery and 48 degrees after. It should be noted that five metatarsophalangeal joints had no increased motion and three lost motion. In discussing the cheilectomy with patients before surgery, it is important to remind them that they have a joint with degenerative arthritis. The surgery relieves the dorsal impingement, which is the main cause of their pain, but obviously does not eliminate the degenerative changes. The surgery will relieve pain and improve range of motion, but because degenerative arthritis is present in the joint, vigorous activities may still cause some pain. As mentioned previously, the main advantage of the cheilectomy is that it is a simple and reliable procedure that, for the majority of patients, results in good pain relief and increased function.

Arthrodesis of the Metatarsophalangeal Joint

If the patient is not a candidate for a cheilectomy or if the cheilectomy fails to achieve a satisfactory result, I favor an arthrodesis of the metatarsophalangeal joint. Although there are many ways to achieve an arthrodesis, I prefer using a dorsal plate, which provides rigid fixation and permits immediate postoperative ambulation in a wooden shoe. Although the plate is applied to the dorsal surface, which is the compression side,

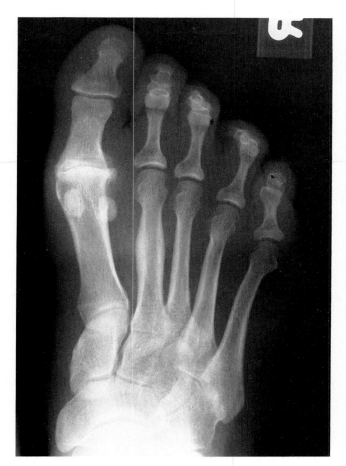 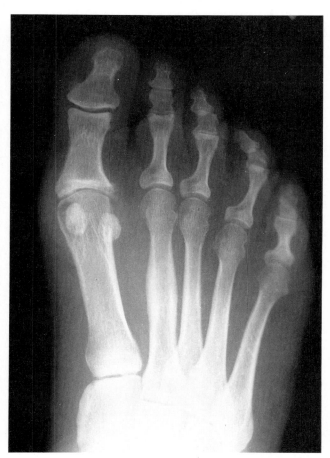

Fig. 5   Left, Preoperative radiograph demonstrating the large exostosis on the lateral side of the metatarsal head. **Right**, Postoperative radiograph demonstrating the appearance after removal of the osteophytes about the metatarsal head and particularly the lateral aspect.

the forces applied across the joint do not seem to be of sufficient magnitude to disrupt the fixation.

Surgical Technique

The metatarsophalangeal joint is approached dorsally, moving the extensor hallucis longus tendon medially or laterally. A synovectomy is carried out, and the collateral ligaments are cut to facilitate exposure to the metatarsal head. About 5 mm of the distal portion of the metatarsal head is removed with a small power saw. The base of the proximal phalanx is then freed of its soft-tissue attachments. The hallux is held in approximately 15 degrees of valgus and 15 degrees of dorsiflexion in relation to the plantar surface of the foot, or approximately 30 degrees of dorsiflexion in relation to the first metatarsal shaft. Holding the proximal phalanx in proper alignment and looking at the cut end of the metatarsal head permits the alignment of the phalangeal osteotomy to be appreciated. An osteotomy in the proximal phalanx made parallel to that in the metatarsal head can usually achieve proper align-

ment of the metatarsophalangeal joint. The cut surfaces are approximated and the alignment is carefully checked. If the alignment is not correct, another cut is made to reposition the toe. Any exostosis remaining is removed to debulk the joint. The cut surfaces are held together, and two crossed Kirschner wires are inserted to maintain the position. At this point the alignment of the hallux should be 15 degrees of valgus, 15 degrees of dorsiflexion in relation to the plantar surface of the foot, and neutral rotation. If not, the toe must be repositioned.

Fixation is achieved with a one quarter-tubular, five- or six-hole compression plate placed on the dorsal surface so that at least two screws are placed into the proximal phalanx. The plate usually must be bent slightly to allow dorsiflexion at the metatarsophalangeal joint. The plate is fixed to the bone with 3.5-mm cortical screws. The screws in the proximal phalanx are placed first and the others are then inserted into the metatarsal to produce compression (Fig. 7). The skin is closed and a compression dressing applied for 12 to

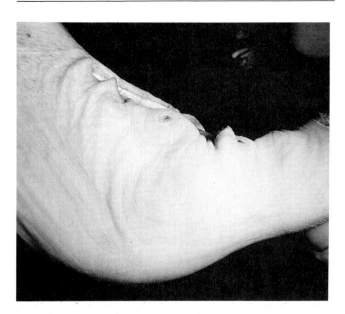

Fig. 6 Intraoperative picture demonstrating that 70 degrees of dorsiflexion should be obtained intraoperatively, and, if not, more bone should be excised from the dorsal aspect of the metatarsal head.

18 hours, after which a light dressing is applied. The patient is allowed to walk, wearing a wooden shoe. Union usually occurs in ten to 12 weeks.

After arthrodesis, patients are free of pain and can function at a rather high level. They can walk, play golf, and ride a bicycle without limitations. Racket sports and jogging may present a problem for some patients after a fusion. Women can wear shoes with a 1½- to 2-inch heel without problems. The only problem following an arthrodesis in proper position is that 30% to 40% of patients will develop degenerative change of the interphalangeal joint. This is rarely of clinical significance.

Keller Procedure

The use of the Keller procedure in older, less active patients with hallux rigidus can produce a satisfactory, although variable, result. The variability results because the base of the proximal phalanx is removed, significantly impairing the weightbearing function of the first metatarsal through loss of the windlass mechanism. Transfer of pressure to the second metatarsal may result, which can give rise to rather disabling second metatarsalgia. Another problem associated with the Keller procedure is that the great toe can drift into various positions, mainly dorsiflexion and valgus, because of inadequate stabilization of the proximal phalanx. The Keller procedure, however, can always be converted to a fusion, which will usually produce a satisfactory end

result. I have used the Keller procedures in older individuals who are not particularly active on their feet in order to debulk the joint and at the same time relieve the patient's pain.

Surgical Technique

The surgical technique of a Keller procedure is through a dorsal approach. The extensor tendon is moved medially or laterally and the joint capsule opened. A synovectomy is carried out. The metatarsal head is debulked, usually in line with the metatarsal shaft. This differs from the cheilectomy, in which the dorsal 20% to 30% of the metatarsal head is removed. The proximal 20% to 30% of the proximal phalanx is removed in order to decompress the metatarsophalangeal joint. If possible, the short flexors should be reattached to the base of the proximal phalanx, although poor tissue quality may make this impossible. In some cases a longitudinal small Steinmann pin is used to stabilize the metatarsophalangeal joint and to act as a spacer during the first three to four weeks after surgery. During this time, the patient can walk, wearing a wooden shoe. To restore joint motion, passive motion is encouraged following removal of the pin.

Proximal Phalangeal Osteotomy

The proximal phalangeal osteotomy[4] is used in younger patients to relieve plantar flexion at the metatarsophalangeal joint. The phalangeal osteotomy dorsiflexes the proximal phalanx, relieving plantar flexion of the hallux brought about by the dorsal osteophytes on the metatarsal head. This procedure, although sound in theory, does not alleviate the abnormal anatomy in the way that the cheilectomy does. For this reason, I prefer to carry out a cheilectomy. If insufficient dorsiflexion is achieved after a cheilectomy, then a proximal phalangeal osteotomy may be considered.

Surgical Technique

Through a dorsal approach, a wedge of bone whose base is directed dorsally is removed. This allows the toe to be brought into 25 to 30 degrees of dorsiflexion in relation to the metatarsal shaft. Because the toe is no longer held in a plantar-flexed position, some of the dorsal impingement is relieved. I believe that if the proximal phalangeal osteotomy is carried out, a significant cheilectomy should not be carried out concurrently. A cheilectomy performed at the same time would result in too much stiffness because the osteotomy site would have to heal before starting range-of-motion exercises, thereby stiffening the joint and defeating the procedure's purpose. After surgery, the patient wears a wooden shoe until the osteotomy site heals sufficiently to permit motion.

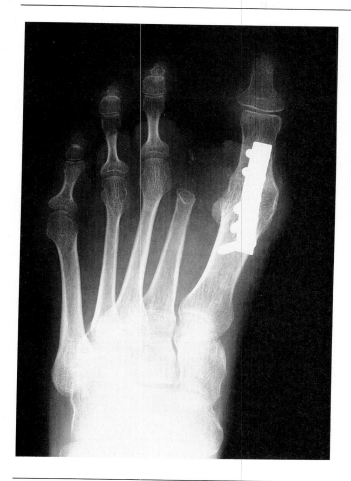

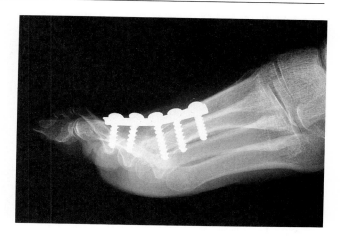

Fig. 7 Left, Postoperative radiograph demonstrating the appearance of the plate in the anteroposterior view. **Right**, Appearance of the plate in the lateral view.

Silastic Implant

Although use of a double-stemmed Silastic implant can be considered in the treatment of hallux rigidus, it should not be used in patients who will subject it to significant stress. This includes most individuals involved in any type of sporting activities.

Surgical Technique

The surgical technique involves a dorsal approach to the metatarsophalangeal joint, with the extensor tendon moved medially or laterally. Sufficient bone is removed from the metatarsal head and proximal phalanx to permit reaming of the medullary canals and insertion of the prosthesis. The metatarsal head is debulked of the proliferative bone. When inserting a prosthesis, it is important to avoid too much tension, because of inadequate bone resection, or too much medial or lateral stress. After surgery, the patient wears a wooden shoe for walking. Once the wound has healed, active and passive range of motion are encouraged. Immobilization is discontinued after approximately four weeks.

References

1. Davies-Cooley: Contraction of the metatarso-phalangeal joint of the great toe, abstract. *Br Med J* 1887;1:728.
2. Cotterill JM: Condition of stiff great toe in adolescents. *Edinb Med J* 1887;33:459–462.
3. Mann RA, Clanton T0: Hallux rigidus: Treatment by cheilectomy. *J Bone Joint Surg* 1988;7OA:400–406.
4. Moberg E: A simple operation for hallux rigidus. *Clin Orthop* 1979;142:55–56.

Sesamoid Pain: Causes and Surgical Treatment

Michael J. Coughlin, MD

Introduction

Located within the tendons of the flexor hallucis brevis, the sesamoids of the first metatarsophalangeal joint play a significant role in the function of the hallux by absorbing most of the weightbearing stresses on the medial forefoot, protecting the tendon of the flexor hallucis longus in its exposed position, and increasing the mechanical advantage of the flexor hallucis brevis.[1] Although isolated abnormalities of the sesamoid occur infrequently, disruption of normal mechanics because of arthritis,[1-6] trauma,[1,2,4,7-18] infection,[19-25] osteochondritis,[2,10,13,26-29] or sesamoiditis[3,10,26,27,29-31] can lead to significant disability.

Anatomy

Sesamoid abnormalities are rare, but isolated injury or degeneration may cause significant dysfunction of the first metatarsophalangeal joint. To fully appreciate the nature of the clinical problems as well as the indications for surgical treatment, an understanding of the pertinent anatomy and function of the sesamoid mechanism is necessary. The intrinsic musculature and sesamoid mechanism of the hallux differentiate the first ray from the lateral toes. The dorsal surfaces of the sesamoids articulate with plantar facets of the first metatarsal head. A crista, or intersesamoidal ridge, separates the medial and lateral metatarsal facets (Fig. 1). The intersesamoidal ridge stabilizes the sesamoid complex. In advanced cases of hallux valgus, when the sesamoid complex is dislocated from the metatarsal, the intersesamoidal ridge atrophies and may even be obliterated.

The sesamoids are connected to the base of the proximal phalanx through extensions of the flexor hallucis brevis tendon (the plantar plate) and are suspended by a sling-like mechanism composed of the metatarsophalangeal collateral ligaments and the sesamoid ligaments (Fig. 2). The plantar aponeurosis inserts into the sesamoids and joint capsule, affording a static plantar-flexion force at the metatarsophalangeal joint. The flexor hallucis brevis, through the sesamoid mechanism, provides the only effective plantar-flexion force at the metatarsophalangeal joint.

The adductor hallucis tendon, which inserts into the lateral aspect of the proximal phalanx and into the lateral sesamoid, stabilizes the sesamoid mechanism lat-

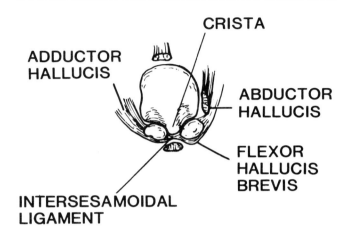

Fig. 1 Cross section of first metatarsal head demonstrating sesamoids and the intersesamoidal ridge. (Reproduced with permission from Mann RA, Coughlin MJ: Hallux valgus and complications of hallux valgus, in *Surgery of the Foot*, ed 5. St. Louis, CV Mosby, 1986.)

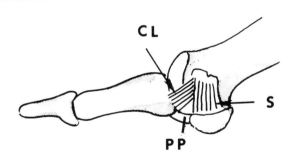

Fig. 2 The sesamoids and collateral ligaments (CL) provide medial and lateral stability to the metatarsophalangeal joint. PP, Plantar plate. (Reproduced with permission from Mann RA, Coughlin MJ: Hallux valgus and complications of hallux valgus, in *Surgery of the Foot*, ed 5. St. Louis, CV Mosby, 1986.)

erally. The abductor hallucis tendon, through its insertion into the plantar medial base of the proximal phalanx, as well as the medial sesamoid, stabilizes the sesamoid mechanism medially. Further stability is provided by the intersesamoidal ligament, which connects the sesamoids and forms the base of a canal enveloping the flexor hallucis longus tendon.

The sesamoids are entirely intratendinous except dorsally where they articulate with the head of the first metatarsal. When a person is standing, the sesamoids are located slightly proximal to the metatarsal head. With dorsiflexion of the hallux, the sesamoids are pulled distally, thereby protecting the otherwise exposed plantar surface of the first metatarsal head. During the act of rising onto the toes, the sesamoids (especially the medial sesamoid) absorb the main weightbearing stresses for the medial forefoot. The medial sesamoid is located slightly more distally[4,20] and is slightly larger than the lateral sesamoid. Orr[32] calculated that the average width of the tibial sesamoid is 9 to 11 mm. Its length averages 12 to 15 mm. The fibular sesamoid is smaller and averages 7 to 9 mm wide and 9 to 10 mm long.

The ossification of the hallucal sesamoids occurs between 7 and 10 years of age.[1,2,4] Often, the ossification of the sesamoids occurs from multiple ossification centers, and this may be the cause of bipartite or tripartite sesamoids.[1]

Radiographic Examination

Routine radiographs provide limited information concerning the sesamoids. On the dorsal plantar view, the metatarsal head typically overlaps both sesamoids, often obscuring detail. On a lateral projection, the sesamoids overlap each other. The fibular sesamoid is best demonstrated on a lateral oblique radiograph (Fig. 3, top) which profiles this sesamoid between the first and second metatarsal heads. Richardson[33] described a tibial sesamoid view (Fig. 3, bottom left). To isolate the medial sesamoid, the radiograph is taken with the foot in the lateral position and with the metatarsophalangeal joint extended 50 degrees. The roentgen beam is angled 15 degrees cephalad while centered over the first metatarsal head. The most useful radiograph, however, is the axial sesamoid view (Fig. 3, bottom right), which often clarifies the diagnosis.[2,13,29,34]

In the symptomatic patient with normal radiographic findings, a bone scan may be useful. Increased uptake on a bone scan[2,26,33] may indicate sesamoid abnormality. Often a bone scan will demonstrate increased uptake before changes, such as sclerosis, fragmentation, or disintegration, can be detected radiographically.

Physical Examination

The subjective symptoms in a patient with a symptomatic sesamoid include discomfort or pain in the toe-off phase of gait. Objective clinical findings include restricted range of motion, pain on movement or direct palpation, diminished strength in either dorsal or plantar flexion, localized metatarsophalangeal swelling, and/or development of plantar callosities. A mild metatarsophalangeal joint synovitis may accompany sesamoid abnormalities.

Assessment of hallux alignment is important, as the great toe may deviate medially or laterally with sesamoid abnormalities, or after sesamoid resection. An adjacent digital nerve may be compressed by either the tibial or fibular sesamoid, causing radicular symptoms or numbness. A positive Tinel's sign may be elicited by palpation in the area of the sesamoids.

Sesamoid Abnormalities

Hallux Valgus

Pronation of the great toe often occurs as the magnitude of the hallux valgus increases. As the toe migrates into valgus, the first metatarsal deviates into a varus position. With increased deformity, the head of the first metatarsal progressively subluxates off of the sesamoid mechanism. The sesamoid mechanism retains its anatomic relationship to the second metatarsal, because it is tethered by the transverse metatarsal ligament and the conjoined adductor hallucis tendon. Thus, in hallux valgus, the tibial sesamoid assumes a position under the metatarsal head and receives all weightbearing forces transmitted through the first metatarsal head. The fibular sesamoid, however, is often displaced into the first intermetatarsal space, where it no longer receives weightbearing forces.

For this displacement to occur, the intersesamoidal ridge must be eroded (Fig. 4). Radiographs often show a partial attrition of the intersesamoidal ridge in a moderate hallux valgus deformity. With severe deviation, complete erosion of the ridge occurs. The adductor hallucis tendon, because of its insertion onto the plantar lateral base of the proximal phalanx and the lateral sesamoid, adds a rotational force (pronation) to the hallux as the valgus deformity increases.

With hallux valgus surgery, the orientation of the sesamoids can be adequately corrected, undercorrected, or overcorrected. One should attempt to realign the articulation of the sesamoids with the two plantar facets of the first metatarsal. Often this is accomplished by releasing the contracted adductor hallucis tendon and lateral capsular structures. Occasionally, a lateral sesamoidectomy is performed. These procedures may allow the tibial sesamoid to be relocated to the medial facet of the first metatarsal. However, an unstable situation can occur because the intersesamoidal ridge has been eroded and the medial facet is no longer a stable articulating surface. Either recurrent lateral sesamoid migration with the development of hallux valgus or medial migration of the tibial sesamoid associated with a hallux varus deformity may occur (Fig. 5). Maintenance of surgical correction with semirigid dressings may be necessary until the correction stabilizes.

A fibular sesamoid should only be resected where a

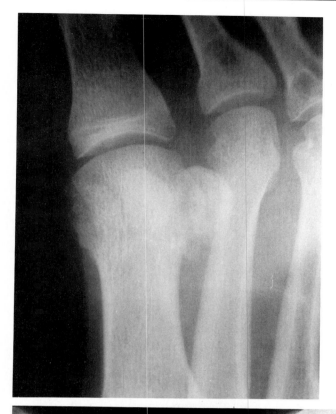

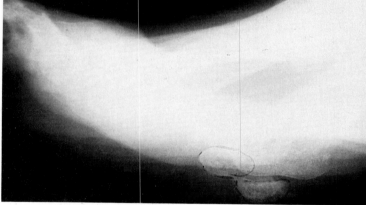

Fig. 3 **Top,** Lateral oblique radiograph of the sesamoids. **Bottom left,** Oblique radiograph demonstrating tibial sesamoids. **Bottom right,** Axial view of sesamoids demonstrating cystic degenerative changes in the first metatarsal head.

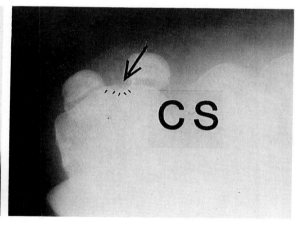

significant lateral contracture remains after a complete lateral soft-tissue release has been performed or if significant degenerative changes of the lateral sesamoid prevent adequate metatarsophalangeal joint motion with realignment of the toe. Postoperative medial dislocation of the tibial sesamoid and hallux varus deformity have been reported after a McBride-type bunionectomy that includes a fibular sesamoidectomy.[35] This problem is more common with hallux valgus deformities of more than 40 degrees. Complete erosion of the intersesamoidal ridge, coupled with an extremely tight intrinsic mechanism, may lead to a potentially unstable situation. An excessive exostectomy and overly aggressive reefing of the medial capsule may then lead to a postoperative hallux varus deformity.

Arthritis

Degenerative arthritis of the metatarsal sesamoid articulation has been reported.[1-6] Arthritis may be associated with hallux rigidus, rheumatoid arthritis, and other systemic arthritides, or local degenerative arthritis of one or both sesamoids may occur (Fig. 6). Scranton and Rutkowski[5] documented erosion of cartilage in cases of progressive sesamoid chondromalacia that eventually required surgical resection. Degenerative arthritis of the sesamoids may be a logical pro-

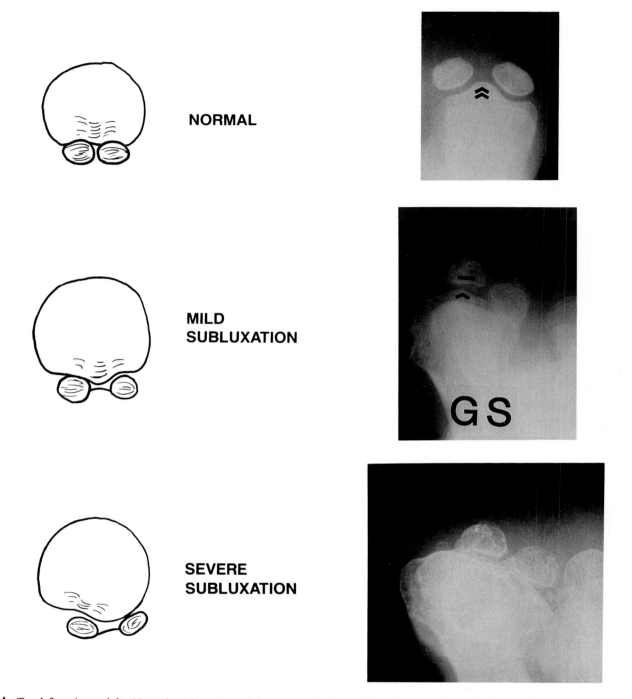

NORMAL

MILD SUBLUXATION

SEVERE SUBLUXATION

Fig. 4 Top left and **top right,** Normal axial position of the sesamoids. **Center left** and **center right,** Moderate hallux valgus associated with moderate sesamoid subluxation. **Bottom left** and **bottom right,** Severe hallux valgus associated with severe sesamoid subluxation.

gression of early sesamoiditis, chondromalacia, or localized trauma to the sesamoids. Swelling and erythema are often demonstrated on physical examination. Other characteristic findings are restricted metatarsophalangeal joint motion, pain on localized palpation, and pain with forced dorsiflexion of the joint.

Nonsurgical care may alleviate discomfort in walking. A stiff insole, a rocker outer sole, and metatarsal padding may reduce metatarsophalangeal joint motion and diminish pain, and a nonsteroidal anti-inflammatory medication may ease local inflammation. Surgical excision may be contemplated for isolated arthritis of either the medial or the lateral sesamoid. After sesamoidectomy, metatarsophalangeal joint motion often fails to improve, although pain may be significantly relieved. When both sesamoids are involved, a combined medial and lateral sesamoidectomy is counterindicated because it will destroy the intrinsic insertion of the flexor digitorum brevis and may lead to clawing of the hallux.[1,2] A Keller resection arthroplasty is another alternative, although this, too, may lead to postoperative clawing of the toe.[36] A metatarsophalangeal joint arthrodesis may be necessary to alleviate pain.

Infection

Although uncommon, several cases of infection have been reported in the orthopaedic literature.[19-25] Osteomyelitis can occur after a puncture wound, trauma, or the breakdown of the plantar skin with chronic neuropathic ulceration. Often this leads to a gram-negative bacterial infection. Typically the joint becomes swollen and erythematous; pain is elicited with manipulation of the toe. Frequently diagnosis is delayed because of the unusual and indolent nature of the infection. Delayed radiographic changes may also slow diagnosis.

In patients whose feet are insensitive because of myelodysplasia, diabetic neuropathy, sciatic nerve injury, peripheral neuropathy, or other causes, callus formation beneath the sesamoid may lead to increased pressure distribution. Skin breakdown and ulceration may occur with subsequent osteomyelitis. Pressure beneath the sesamoids may be reduced by using a molded insole or metatarsal pad, or by trimming abundant callus, if present.

Where localized infection is refractory to medical management or where there is osteomyelitis of the sesamoid, surgical excision may be necessary. Excision of either or both sesamoids is determined by the extent of the infection. Irrigation, extensive debridement, and aggressive localized wound care are often necessary to manage an open wound (Fig. 7). Typically, a double sesamoidectomy should be avoided, but osteomyelitis may necessitate their removal. A localized subperiosteal resection, combined with preservation of the tendons of the abductor and adductor hallucis, may maintain toe function. Typically, restricted range of motion and decreased strength are noted, but the scar tissue that forms with infection may prevent the cock-up deformity that generally occurs after bilateral sesamoid resection.

Nerve Compression

The digital nerves lie adjacent to the medial and lateral sesamoids. Helfet[37] noted impingement of the plantar lateral cutaneous branch to the hallux on the border of the lateral sesamoid. Similarly, the plantar medial digital nerve may be compressed by the medial sesamoid. Pain secondary to nerve compression may be difficult to differentiate from localized sesamoid pain. Occasionally a positive Tinel's sign will be present at the

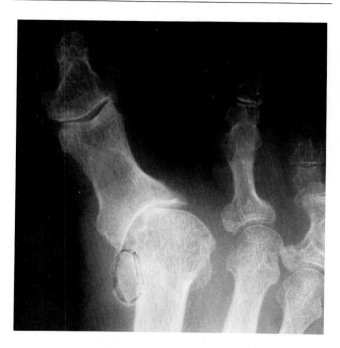

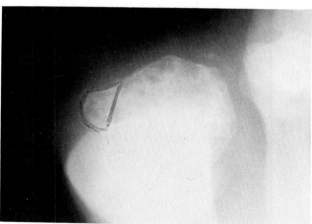

Fig. 5 Top, Dorsal plantar radiograph demonstrating hallux varus with dislocation of medial sesamoid. **Bottom,** Axial radiograph demonstrating medial dislocation of medial sesamoid.

site of the nerve compression. Decreased sensation may also be noted.

Surgical excision may relieve compression symptoms, but care must be taken to avoid injury to either of these nerves. Subsequent neuroma formation can be as symptomatic as the original complaint.

Bipartite Sesamoids and Fracture

The frequency and cause of divided or partite sesamoids are subjects of some controversy in the literature. Dobas and Silvers,[38] who examined radiographs of 1,000 feet (Table 1), found a 19% incidence of bipartite sesamoid. Kewenter[4] examined 800 feet and found a 31% incidence. Rowe,[20] who reported an in-

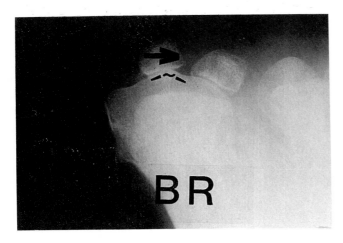

Fig. 6 Arthritis of the medial sesamoid associated with hallux valgus.

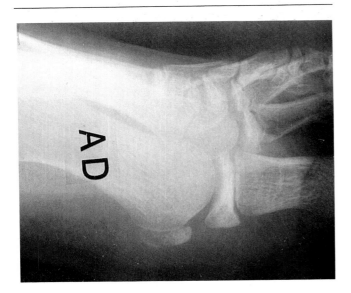

Fig. 7 Osteomyelitis of the medial sesamoid in a skeletally immature individual.

cidence of 6% to 8%, stressed that 90% of the bipartite sesamoids were medial sesamoids.

Dobas and Silvers concluded that, of 193 bipartite sesamoids, 87% were tibial sesamoids. One fourth of the patients with a divided tibial sesamoid had an identical contralateral tibial sesamoid. Although Giannestras[39] stated that bipartite sesamoids are symmetric, this is obviously not the case. A medial sesamoid may frequently be divided into two, three, or four parts; a lateral sesamoid is rarely divided into more than two parts. Inge and Ferguson[1] found that 85% of the bilateral sesamoids had asymmetric divisions. They further noted that the incidence of division decreased with

Table 1
Proportion of tibial and fibular division in representative series of cases

Authors	No. of Cases	Tibial Division (%)	Fibular Division (%)
Kewenter[4]	800	30.6	1.3
Dobas and Silvers[38]	1,000	16.8	2.5
Burman and Lapidus[13]	1,000	7.2	0.6

time, thus implying a gradual osseous union in the divided sesamoid. They noted that with bipartite sesamoids, the articular cartilage tended to dip down between the two osseous fragments, which may predispose a bipartite sesamoid to fracture with minimal injury. As to why the medial sesamoid is more frequently bipartite than the lateral sesamoid, they speculated that the medial sesamoid is more frequently traumatized because of its greater weightbearing.[1] It is not known whether continued trauma with ambulation prevents the union of divided segments or whether some of these partite sesamoids are actually nonunions.

Although fracture of a sesamoid is relatively rare, numerous cases have been reported in the orthopaedic literature.[1–4,7–15,32] Severe trauma with dislocation of the metatarsophalangeal joint and simultaneous fracture of both sesamoids has been noted,[11] but, in general, sudden violence or jumping or falling onto the forefoot is the most frequent mechanism of injury. Kewenter[4] examined 529 sesamoids in 130 cadavers and concluded that congenitally divided or partite sesamoids were more easily fractured by trauma than were normal sesamoids.

It is frequently difficult to distinguish between a symptomatic bipartite sesamoid and a fractured sesamoid. With a fractured sesamoid, the major symptom is pain localized to the region of the sesamoid bones. Symptoms are reduced with rest and exacerbated with ambulation. A patient typically walks on the outside of the foot to avoid loading of the sesamoid complex. Passive dorsiflexion can also cause discomfort. Nonspecific swelling of the plantar surface of the sesamoid may also be observed. The development of pain from minimal trauma in the presence of a bipartite sesamoid should make the clinician highly suspicious of a superimposed fracture of a bipartite sesamoid.

An acute fracture may be characterized by a relatively sharp radiolucent line, but Inge and Ferguson[1] cautioned that a fracture should not be diagnosed unless callus is present. Delay in diagnosis of fracture[7,9] is common because of the difficulty of establishing radiographic confirmation of fracture.

Hobart[15] recommended casting and nonweightbearing until the fracture heals, usually after six to eight weeks. Usually arch supports or metatarsal pads just proximal to the sesamoid region can relieve discomfort. If symptoms persist, surgical excision may be necessary.

Osteochondritis

Osteochondritis typically is characterized by pain, tenderness to palpation, and osseous mottling or fragmentation (Fig. 8) on radiographic examination.[26,29] First described by Renander[31] in 1924, osteochondritis occurs infrequently.[29] Its cause is unclear. Helal[3] speculated that osteochondritis developed after crush injuries or trauma. Kliman and associates[26] postulated that a stress fracture and a subsequent reparative process caused osteochondritis. Although trauma is probably the most frequent cause, Jahss[2] associated osteonecrosis with aseptic necrosis. Diagnosis is usually made by an axial radiograph, which depicts the sesamoids in profile. Conservative care includes padding or molded shoe inserts and nonsteroidal anti-inflammatory medications. Conservative care can be used for a time, but the appearance of fragmentation usually indicates that surgical resection of the involved sesamoid will be necessary if symptoms persist.

Sesamoiditis

Sesamoiditis is a diagnosis of exclusion. It frequently occurs in teenagers and young adults, is often associated with some type of trauma, and is characterized by pain on weightbearing. There is local tenderness to palpation over the sesamoids, often accompanied by inflammation or a thickening of the bursa on the plantar aspect of the sesamoid mechanism. Radiographic examination is typically normal. Dobas and Silvers[38] defined sesamoiditis as inflammation and swelling of the peritendinous structures of the sesamoids.

Degeneration of the articular cartilage of the sesamoid has been noted by many clinicians.[3,10,26,27,29–31] Apley[27] dissected the medial sesamoid of the first metatarsophalangeal joint and found remarkable similarities with the articular cartilage degeneration seen with chondromalacia of the patellofemoral joint. A decrease in ambulatory activities and use of orthotics, pads, and decreased heel height to reduce weightbearing on the involved sesamoid may alleviate symptoms. If symptoms persist, surgical excision usually provides excellent relief of pain.

Intractable Plantar Keratoses

A cavus foot deformity with or without an associated plantar-flexed first ray must be considered when evaluating a callus formation beneath the first metatarsal head. A more diffuse callosity beneath the entire metatarsal head is usually associated with this condition. A more localized keratotic lesion is usually associated with a prominent sesamoid (Fig. 9). Often a keratotic lesion can be treated with a molded metatarsal insert, or a metatarsal pad placed just proximal to the lesion. Intermittent paring of the callus may alleviate discomfort. Sesamoid shaving may alleviate symptoms without impairing joint function. Occasionally sesamoidectomy is necessary for intractable lesions. Sesamoid resection

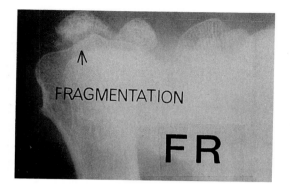

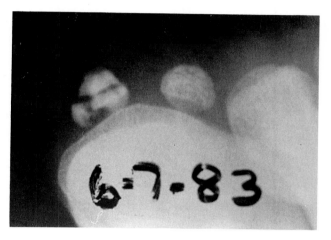

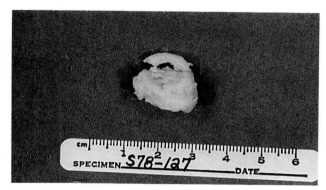

Fig. 8 Top, Osteochondritis is characterized by fragmentation of the involved sesamoid. **Center,** Osseous fragmentation of medial sesamoid seen on axial radiograph. **Bottom,** Pathologic specimen demonstrating fragmentation of sesamoid.

for a plantar-flexed first ray is associated with recurrence of the plantar keratoses. A dorsiflexion metatarsal osteotomy is preferable in this situation.

Conservative Care

Most sesamoid problems can be treated effectively with nonsurgical management. A decrease in activity, both in sedentary patients and in athletes, may play a

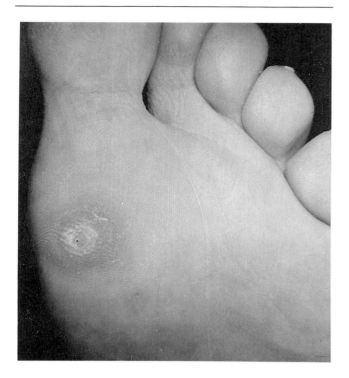

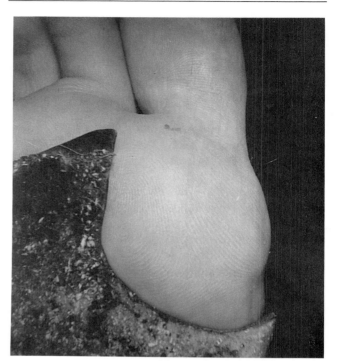

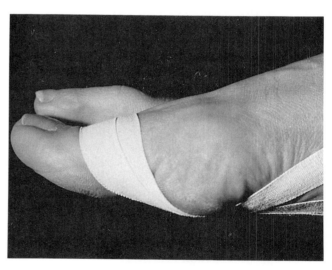

Fig. 9   Intractable plantar keratotic lesion directly beneath the tibial sesamoid.

Fig. 10   **Top,** A molded insert may help to decrease weightbearing on the sesamoids. **Bottom,** Taping of the hallux to reduce dorsiflexion may decrease symptoms.

major role in diminishing symptoms. Wearing low-heeled shoes will decrease pressure on the sesamoids and may relieve discomfort. Where a fracture has occurred, a wooden-soled shoe or a short leg walking cast may be used to decrease stress on the sesamoid and the metatarsophalangeal joint. A metatarsal arch support or a molded insole (Fig. 10, *top*) may help decrease pressure in the sesamoid region caused by fracture, sesamoiditis, or other localized inflammation, or an intractable plantar keratotic lesion. Taping the hallux in a neutral position (Fig. 10, *bottom*) to prevent dorsiflexion may reduce localized inflammation in the metatarsophalangeal joint. The use of nonsteroidal anti-inflammatory medications may augment splinting and taping. The infrequent judicious use of an intra-articular steroid injection may relieve localized inflammation or sesamoiditis, but an injection in the presence of a fracture or osteonecrosis is contraindicated.

Surgical Excision

Surgical excision of the chronically painful sesamoid is advocated when conservative treatment has failed.[1-3,7,9,10,15,19-27,29-31,40,41] Dual sesamoidectomy may be necessary with infection, but it may lead to a clawtoe deformity and should be avoided if possible.[1,3] Scranton and Rutkowski,[5] in reporting on dual sesamoid exci-

sion, recommended a reapproximation of the surgically induced defect to minimize disability. Jahss[2] likened reestablishment of the defect in the flexor hallucis brevis to a repair of the quadriceps mechanism after patellectomy.

The choice of the surgical approach for sesamoid excision depends on which sesamoid is to be resected. The medial sesamoid is approached by either a medial[1,2,26,30] or a plantar medial incision.[3,9] The plantar approach was avoided by Kliman and associates[26] because of the proximity of the plantar digital nerves and by Mann and associates[42] because of the possibility of a painful plantar scar developing.

The fibular sesamoid is approached from either a dorsal or a plantar incision. Mann and Coughlin[35] used a dorsal lateral approach to resect the fibular sesamoid in cases of hallux valgus and advocated this approach for isolated fibular sesamoidectomy as well.[42]

Jahss,[2] Helal,[3] and Van Hal and associates[9] all recommend a longitudinal plantar incision adjacent to the fibular sesamoid. Jahss found the dorsal approach for sesamoidectomy "almost impossible."

Technique of Surgical Excision of the Tibial Sesamoid

The tibial sesamoid is approached through a plantar-medial incision. This longitudinal approach is extensile and the medial plantar cutaneous nerve can easily be identified and retracted with the plantar skin flap so that injury can be avoided (Fig. 11). The sesamoid is identified on the plantar border of the abductor hallucis tendon. Care is taken not to interrupt the tendinous insertion of the abductor hallucis into the base of the proximal phalanx. The sesamoid is dissected sharply on its borders and is removed by incising the intersesamoidal ligament. The tendon of the flexor hallucis longus should be inspected to make sure that it has not been violated by the dissection. The defect created by the dissection is approximated if adequate tissue is present,[2,5] although complete closure of the defect is often difficult.

Tibial sesamoidectomy may predispose the first ray to a progressive hallux valgus deformity. Nayfa and Sorto[43] noted a 42% incidence of hallux valgus after tibial sesamoidectomy. Medial capsular reefing or medial reefing with a lateral capsular release may be combined with tibial sesamoidectomy when mild valgus deviation is present. When an increased intermetatarsal angle is present, a proximal osteotomy of the first metatarsal may be used to augment the first metatarsophalangeal realignment.

After surgery, the foot is wrapped in a compression dressing and the patient is allowed to walk, wearing a wooden-soled shoe. If medial or lateral drifting of the great toe occurs, taping may be used for six to eight weeks to align the hallux.

Technique for Shaving a Prominent Tibial Sesamoid

Surgical excision of a prominent tibial sesamoid may be used to treat an intractable keratotic lesion, but an alternative is to shave the tibial sesamoid. Removing the plantar half of the tibial sesamoid and beveling it flat can reduce a prominent tibial sesamoid enough to relieve a keratotic lesion.

A longitudinal plantar-medial incision is made, like that used for a medial sesamoidectomy. The sesamoid is exposed by reflecting the plantar fat pad. A sagittal saw is used to resect the plantar surface of the tibial

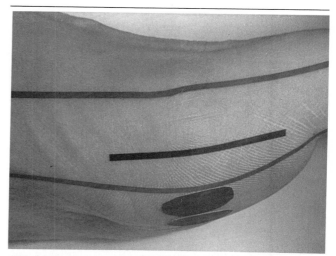

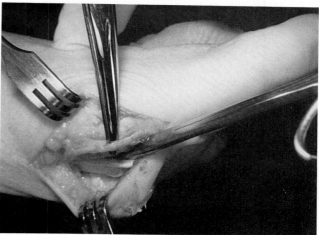

Fig. 11 **Top,** A medial plantar incision is used to expose the medial sesamoid. The location of the dorsal and plantar medial sensory nerves should be appreciated. **Bottom,** Surgical dissection demonstrating the plantar medial sensory nerve just dorsal to the medial sesamoid.

sesamoid (Fig. 12). Care is taken to protect the flexor digitorum longus tendon, which lies immediately lateral to the tibial sesamoid. Once the tibial sesamoid has been shaved, sharp edges are beveled with a rongeur. For six weeks the patient wears a wooden-soled shoe for walking. Because the metatarsophalangeal joint has not been disturbed, motion usually returns fairly rapidly.

Technique of Excising the Fibular Sesamoid

The fibular sesamoid is approached through a dorsal incision in the first interspace. A Weitlander retractor is used to spread the first and second metatarsals and subluxate the fibular sesamoid. Using the tendon of the adductor hallucis as a guide, the surgeon then opens the interval between the adductor and the joint capsule. The tendon of the adductor hallucis is reflected from the lateral sesamoid. The intersesamoidal ligament is severed, and the remaining resection is completed. With this approach, no repair of the capsular tissue is

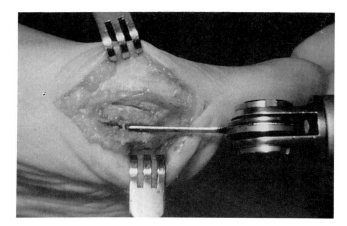

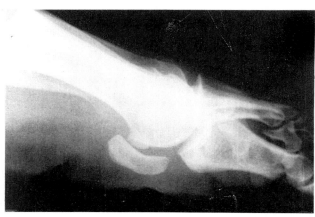

Fig. 12   Top, The technique for shaving of a prominent tibial sesamoid. **Bottom,** Lateral radiograph demonstrating postoperative view of shaved medial sesamoid.

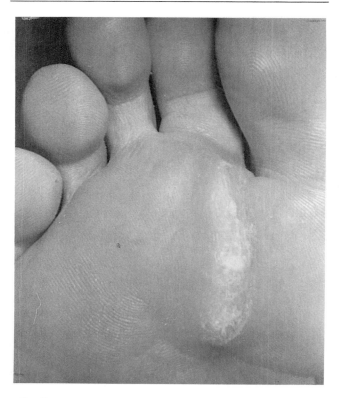

Fig. 13   Painful plantar scar after sesamoid excision through plantar approach.

possible. The wound must be inspected to ensure continuity of both the flexor hallucis longus and the adductor hallucis.

A soft compression dressing is used after surgery, and the patient is allowed to walk wearing a wooden-soled shoe. If necessary, the toe can be taped into alignment for six to eight weeks.

If a plantar incision is used to approach the fibular sesamoid, an intermetatarsal incision is preferable to placing an incision directly beneath the first metatarsal head. Postoperative scarring and/or keloid formation directly under the metatarsal can cause intractable pain (Fig. 13).

A plantar longitudinal 2-cm incision is made in the first interspace. Care is taken to isolate and protect the plantar digital nerve on the lateral aspect of the hallux. The sesamoid is identified directly beneath the soft-tissue fat pad. With sharp dissection, the capsular fibers of the flexor hallucis brevis are released. The sesamoid is detached laterally, distally, and proximally, and, finally, the intersesamoidal ligament is severed. The tendon of the flexor hallucis longus is inspected to make

sure it has not been transected. A repair of the defect by suturing of capsular structures should be performed if sufficient tissue is present. After closure, a soft compression dressing is used. The patient is allowed to walk, wearing a wooden-soled shoe, and the toe is taped in position for six to eight weeks following surgery.

Postoperative Results

Migration of the Hallux

Isolated excision of a sesamoid can create a muscular imbalance at the metatarsophalangeal joint. The potential for a hallux varus deformity after fibular sesamoidectomy was noted by Mann and Coughlin[35] who, in a review of the McBride procedure, reported an 8% incidence. Nayfa and Sorto[43] reported a 6.2-degree valgus drift of the hallux and a 2.2-degree increase in the intermetatarsal angle after tibial sesamoidectomy. Jahss[2] noted that a wide medial excision of a tibial sesamoid could disrupt the medial mechanism and lead to a hallux valgus deformity. A wide lateral excision can lead to a hallux varus deformity.

Mann and associates,[42] reporting on a series of sesamoidectomies, noted a varus or valgus drift in 10% of patients (Fig. 14). Maintenance of the integrity of the adductor hallucis and lateral capsule, when the fibular

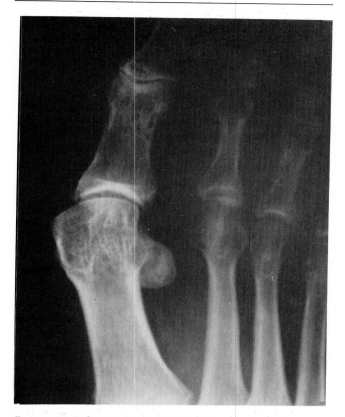

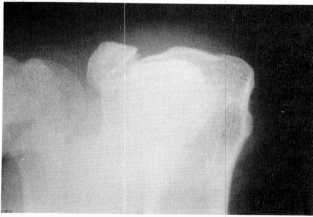

Fig. 14 **Top,** Valgus drift of the hallux after tibial sesamoidectomy. **Bottom,** Axial radiograph of the same patient with fibular sesamoid subluxation after tibial sesamoidectomy.

sesamoid has been excised, and maintenance of the medial capsule and abductor hallucis, when a tibial sesamoid has been excised, is important in diminishing postoperative migration of the hallux. When possible, surgical repair of the defect left by sesamoid excision is advantageous. Augmenting a tibial sesamoidectomy with a lateral capsular release, medial capsular reefing, and even metatarsal osteotomy may be considered if there appears to be an increased risk of hallux valgus after excision of the tibial sesamoid.

Relief of Pain

Surgical excision of a diseased sesamoid is frequently recommended[1-3,7,9,10,15,19-27,29-31,34,40,41] when conservative care proves unsuccessful, but little information is available regarding postoperative results. Some reports[7,9,30] noted complete relief of pain and resumption of normal activities, but Inge and Ferguson[1] noted this result in only 41% of patients. Mann and associates[42] reported complete pain relief in only 50% of patients.

Motion and Strength

Several series suggest that surgical excision can lead to stiffness.[2,21,22,26,30,42] In one series,[42] restricted range of motion was noted in a third of the cases. Of those 14 patients with a full range of motion, ten had had tibial and four fibular sesamoidectomies. In seven patients with restricted range of motion, four tibial sesamoidectomies and three fibular sesamoidectomies had been carried out.

Van Hal and associates[9] noted no diminution in great-toe flexor power and no cock-up deformity, but Inge and Ferguson[1] found a 17% incidence of clawing of the hallux. Furthermore, 58% of the patients in their series had postoperative restricted motion, clawing, and/or continued pain. Mann and associates[42] noted plantar-flexion weakness in 60% of cases. No predilection for weakness followed either a tibial or fibular sesamoidectomy.

Discussion

In 1933, Inge and Ferguson[1] reported on sesamoidectomy in 31 patients. Of the patients, 77% were women; their average age was 25 years. Of 41 feet involved, 25 had both sesamoids excised, 15 had the medial sesamoid excised, and in one the fibular sesamoid was excised. Only 41.5% of patients reported normal function and complete relief of pain after surgery. There was a 17% incidence of clawtoe deformity. This was probably related to the fact that in many cases both sesamoids were excised (Fig. 15). Various complaints, including impaired range of motion, mild to severe pain, and a clawtoe deformity, were noted by 59.5% of the patients.

In 1985, Mann and associates[42] reported on surgical excision of sesamoids in 21 patients. Of these patients, 66% were women; their average age was 41 years. Eight fibular sesamoids and 13 tibial sesamoids were removed. Postoperatively only 50% of patients noted complete relief of pain. Of the 50% in whom discomfort was still present, 75% noted only occasional or mild pain. Twelve patients (60%) noted plantar-flexion weak-

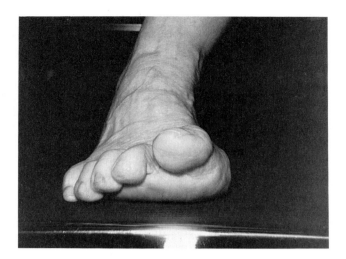

Fig. 15 Clawing of the hallux after combined medial and lateral sesamoidectomy.

ness. One third of the patients noted restricted range of motion. There appeared to be no significant difference between excision of a tibial sesamoid and excision of a fibular sesamoid. In 10% of the cases, there was mild drift of the hallux after excision. In one case, there was a mild varus inclination after fibular sesamoid resection. In another, in which the tibial sesamoid was resected, there was mild valgus deviation. Although the subjective level of patient satisfaction was high, the objective postoperative limitations noted were of a significant nature.

Conclusion

The sesamoids of the first metatarsophalangeal joint play an integral part in the dynamic function of the first metatarsophalangeal joint. Disruption of normal function through fracture, inflammation, trauma, or through iatrogenic causes can lead to significant disability. Surgical intervention may be necessary in the case of the chronically painful sesamoid, but the sesamoid complex should be preserved whenever possible. Where conservative care is ineffective and a sesamoidectomy is necessary, care should be taken to maintain the integrity of the remaining intrinsic complex in order to maintain the stability and function of the first metatarsophalangeal joint.

A single diseased sesamoid can be removed with acceptable results, but this does not guarantee relief of symptoms, normal range of motion, or normal strength. Resecting both sesamoids should be avoided unless absolutely necessary.

Acknowledgment

Figures 3 through 15 were reproduced with permission from Michael J. Coughlin, MD.

References

1. Inge GAL, Ferguson AB: Surgery of the sesamoid bones of the great toe: An anatomic and clinical study, with a report of forty-one cases. *Arch Surg* 1933;27:466–489.
2. Jahss MH: The sesamoids of the hallux. *Clin Orthop* 1981;157:88–97.
3. Helal B: The great toe sesamoid bones: The lus or lost souls of Ushaia. *Clin Orthop* 1981;157:82–87.
4. Kewenter Y: Die Sesambeine des I. Metatarsophalangealgelenks des Menschen: Eine röntgenobgische, klinische und pathologisch-histologische studie. *Acta Orthop Scand* 1936;2(suppl):1–113.
5. Scranton PE Jr, Rutkowski R: Anatomic variations in the first ray: Part II. Disorders of the sesamoids. *Clin Orthop* 1980;151:256–264.
6. Resnick D, Niwayama G, Feingold ML: The sesamoid bones of the hands and feet: Participators in arthritis. *Radiology* 1977;123:57–62.
7. Zinman H, Keret D, Reis ND: Fracture of the medial sesamoid bone of the hallux. *J Trauma* 1981;21:581–582.
8. Brown TI: Avulsion fracture of the fibular sesamoid in association with dorsal dislocation of the metatarsophalangeal joint of the hallux: Report of a case and review of the literature. *Clin Orthop* 1980;149:229–231.
9. Van Hal ME, Keene JS, Lange TA, et al: Stress fractures of the great toe sesamoids. *Am J Sports Med* 1982;10:122–128.
10. DuVries HL (ed): *Surgery of the Foot*, ed 2. St. Louis, CV Mosby, 1965, pp 259–278.
11. DeLuca FN, Kenmore PI: Bilateral dorsal dislocations of the metatarsophalangeal joints of the great toes with a loose body in one of the metatarsophalangeal joints. *J Trauma* 1975;15:737–739.
12. Bizarro AH: On the traumatology of the sesamoid structures. *Ann Surg* 1921;74:783–791.
13. Burman MS, Lapidus PW: The functional disturbances caused by the inconstant bones and sesamoids of the foot. *Arch Surg* 1931;22:936–975.
14. Parra G: Stress fractures of the sesamoids of the foot. *Clin Orthop* 1960;18:281–285.
15. Hobart MH: Fracture of sesamoid bones of the foot: With report of a case. *J Bone Joint Surg* 1929;11:298–302.
16. Salamon PB, Gelberman RH, Huffer JM: Dorsal dislocation of the metatarsophalangeal joint of the great toe: A case report. *J Bone Joint Surg* 1974;56A:1073–1075.
17. Giannikas AC, Papachristou G, Papavasiliou N, et al: Dorsal dislocation of the first metatarso-phalangeal joint: Report of four cases. *J Bone Joint Surg* 1975;57B:384–386.
18. Konkel KF, Muehlstein JH: Unusual fracture-dislocation of the great toe: Case report. *J Trauma* 1975;15:733–736.
19. Smith R: Osteitis of the metatarsal sesamoid including a report of a case of acute pyogenic osteomyelitis. *Br J Surg* 1941–42;29:19–22.
20. Rowe MM: Osteomyelitis of metatarsal sesamoid. *Br Med J* 1963;1:1071–1072.
21. Colwill M: Osteomyelitis of the metatarsal sesamoids. *J Bone Joint Surg* 1969;51B:464–468.
22. Torgerson WR, Hammond G: Osteomyelitis of the sesamoid bones of the first metatarsophalangeal joint. *J Bone Joint Surg* 1969;51A:1420–1422.
23. Gordon SL, Evans C, Greer RB III: *Pseudomonas* osteomyelitis

of the metatarsal sesamoid of the great toe. *Clin Orthop* 1974;99:188–189.

24. Enna CD: Observations of the hallucal sesamoids in trauma to the denervated foot. *Int Surg* 1970;53:97–107.

25. Cartlidge IJ, Gillespie WJ: Haematogenous osteomyelitis of the metatarsal sesamoid. *Br J Surg* 1979;66:214–216.

26. Kliman ME, Gross AE, Pritzker KP, et al: Osteochondritis of the hallux sesamoid bones. *Foot Ankle* 1983;3:220–223.

27. Apley AG: Open sesamoid: A re-appraisal of the medial sesamoid of the hallux. *Proc R Soc Med* 1966;59:120–121.

28. Salvi V, Tos L: L'osteochondrosi dei sesamoidi. *Arch Orthop* 1962;75:1294–1304.

29. Ilfeld FW, Rosen V: Osteochondritis of the first metatarsal sesamoid: Report of three cases. *Clin Orthop* 1972;85:38–41.

30. Scranton PE: Pathologic anatomic variations in the sesamoids. *Foot Ankle* 1981;1:321–326.

31. Renander A: Two cases of typical osteochondropathy of the medial sesamoid bone of the first metatarsal. *Acta Radiol* 1924;3:521–527.

32. Orr TG: Fracture of great toe sesamoid bones. *Ann Surg* 1918;67:609–612.

33. Richardson EG: Injuries to the hallucal sesamoids in the athlete. *Foot Ankle* 1987;7:229–244.

34. Leonard MH: The sesamoids of the great toe: The pedal polemic. Report of 3 cases. *Clin Orthop* 1960;16:295–301.

35. Mann RA, Coughlin MJ: Hallux valgus: Etiology, anatomy, treatment and surgical considerations. *Clin Orthop* 1981;157:31–41.

36. Coughlin MJ, Mann RA: Arthrodesis of the first metatarsophalangeal joint as salvage for the failed Keller procedure. *J Bone Joint Sug* 1987;69A:68–75.

37. Helfet AJ: A neurological cause of pain under the head of the metatarsal bone of the big toe. *Lancet* 1954;2:846.

38. Dobas DC, Silvers MD: The frequency of partite sesamoids of the first metatarsophalangeal joint. *J Am Podiatry Assoc* 1977;67:880–882.

39. Giannestras NJ: *Foot Disorders: Medical and Surgical Management*, ed 2. Philadelphia, Lea & Febiger, 1973, p 426.

40. Golding C: Museum pages: V. The sesamoids of the hallux. *J Bone Joint Surg* 1960;42B:840–843.

41. Speed K: Injuries of the great toe sesamoids. *Ann Surg* 1914;60:478–480.

42. Mann RA, Coughlin MJ, Baxter D, et al: Sesamoidectomy of the great toe. Presented at the 15th Annual Meeting of the American Orthopaedic Foot and Ankle Society, Las Vegas, Jan 24, 1985.

43. Nayfa TM, Sorto LA Jr: The incidence of hallus abductus following tibial sesamoidectomy. *J Am Podiatry Assoc* 1982;72:617–620.

Etiology and Treatment of the Bunionette Deformity

Michael J. Coughlin, MD

Introduction

The fifth toe typically deviates medially at the metatarsophalangeal joint. The magnitude of this deviation is calculated as the metatarsophalangeal-5 angle (Fig. 1). A bunionette is characterized by a prominence of the lateral condyle of the fifth metatarsal head. Chronic irritation of the overlying bursa caused by friction between the underlying bony abnormality and constricting footwear can cause a thickened callus to develop on the lateral or plantar-lateral aspect of the metatarsal head.[1-5]

While Kelikian[6] stated that the prominent lateral condyle of the fifth metatarsal is "analogous to the medial eminence of the first metatarsal head in hallux valgus," it appears that several anatomic variations in the fifth metatarsal may lead to a symptomatic bunionette.[2,5,7,8] The deformity may occur in the metatarsal head region, the metatarsal diaphysis, or along the entire axis of the metatarsal. The location of the abnormality influences the choice of treatment.

Divergence of the fourth and fifth metatarsals may result in a prominent fifth metatarsal head (Fig. 2).[2,9-11] The intermetatarsal angle between the fourth and fifth

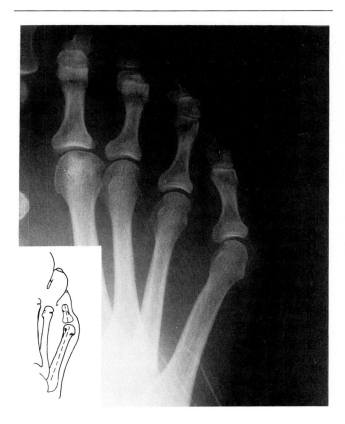

Fig. 2 Abnormally wide 4–5 intermetatarsal angle.

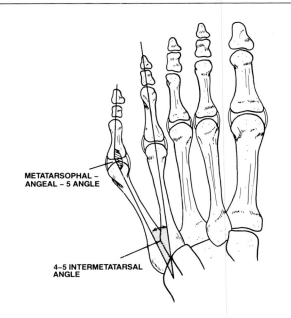

Fig. 1 The fifth metatarsophalangeal and 4–5 intermetatarsal angle.

metatarsals is measured at the intersection of lines bisecting the surgical neck and base of the fourth and fifth metatarsals.[12] Fallat and Buckholz[7] reported that in normal feet, this angle averaged 6.2 degrees, with a range of 3 to 11 degrees. In patients with a symptomatic bunionette, the angle averaged 9.6 degrees and had a range of 5 to 14 degrees. Others[9,12-14] have stated that an angle of more than 8 degrees is abnormal. Even with an intermetatarsal angle of more than 8 degrees, if the concurrent bunionette deformity causes no symptoms, the patient does not require treatment.

Lateral bowing in the diaphysis of the fifth metatarsal (Fig. 3) may also cause a prominence of the fibular condyle of the fifth metatarsal head.[5,7,8,14,15] In this situation the 4–5 intermetatarsal angle[7] usually is normal, but a lateral curvature occurs in the diaphysis of the fifth metatarsal.[7,8,14,15]

An enlargement of the fifth metatarsal head (Fig. 4)

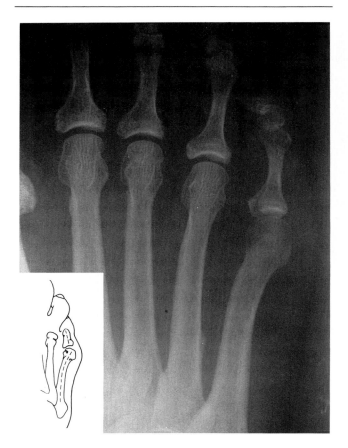

Fig. 3   Lateral bowing of the fifth metatarsal.

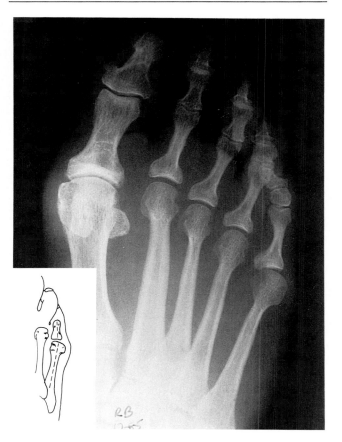

Fig. 4   Enlarged fifth metatarsal head.

may cause bunionette formation.[5,7,16] While hypertrophy of the lateral condyle may occur, Fallat and Buckholz[7] and Throckmorton and Bradlee[17] found that pronation of the foot causes the lateral plantar tubercle of the metatarsal to rotate to a more lateral position. Fallat and Buckholz suggested that with a pronated fifth ray, the radiographic appearance is comparable to that of a hypertrophied fifth metatarsal head. The association of pes planus[3,4,7,17,18] with bunionette formation supports this concept. Fallat and Buckholz also reported that the angle between the fourth and fifth metatarsals increased by 3 degrees with pronation. Whether it is caused by fifth metatarsal pronation or by hypertrophy of the fifth metatarsal head, a prominent fifth metatarsal lateral condyle can become symptomatic without divergence or deviation of the fifth metatarsal.

Kitaoka and associates[19] noted that in patients with symptomatic bunionettes, an increase in the 4–5 intermetatarsal angle was the most commonly associated metatarsal abnormality. Lateral fifth metatarsal deviation and an enlarged fifth metatarsal head together occurred in less than 10% of these patients.

No matter what the underlying metatarsal anatomy and metatarsophalangeal joint orientation, increased pressure can develop over the fifth metatarsal head if constricting footwear is worn.[5,20] The high frequency of occurrence of a bunionette deformity among women[2] is probably the result of wearing fashionable shoes that constrict the forepart of the foot. In time, a thickened bursa and hypertrophic keratoses may develop, leading to a progressively symptomatic deformity.

Physical Findings

On physical examination, an inflamed bursa[4,16,17] may accompany a plantar,[2,4,18] a lateral,[18] or combined plantar-lateral keratotic lesion.[3,18] Diebold and Bejjani[18] found that 50% of their patients had a pure lateral callus, while 33% had a pure plantar lesion. The location of the keratotic lesion plays a major role in the surgical decision-making process.

A bunionette may occur as an isolated deformity,[18] but pes planus is an associated deformity in two thirds of the patients. A splayfoot deformity that combines hallux valgus with an increased angle between the first and second metatarsals and bunionette formation with an increased angle between the fourth and fifth metatarsals has also been reported.[1,4,9,11,13,20]

Conservative Care

Shoes that place pressure on a prominent fifth metatarsal head frequently aggravate symptoms. Davies[1] noted that "rarely do these cases require active treatment other than provision of well fitting shoes." The exacerbation of pain and swelling over a bunionette that results from constricting footwear has led to the recommendation of well-fitted shoes as a primary means to relieve discomfort.[1,2,6,11,15,16] To relieve symptoms, Leach and Igou[2] and Mann[15] also advocated padding the metatarsal prominence, and Leach and Igou recommended trimming of any prominent callus.

Although conservative treatment is effective in a large number of patients,[1,2,6,11,15,16,21] the development of chronic soft-tissue thickening and keratoses may call for surgical intervention.

Surgical Treatment

Various surgical procedures have been used to correct a bunionette deformity. These include lateral condylectomy,[5,11,15,16,22-24] metatarsal head resection,[6,21] ray resection,[25] distal metatarsal osteotomy,[2-4,9,20,26,27] diaphyseal metatarsal osteotomy,[15,28-30] and proximal metatarsal osteotomy.[3,7,13,18,31,32] Correction of the underlying abnormality is mandatory to prevent recurrence, but preservation of function of the fifth metatarsophalangeal joint may also prevent postoperative complications such as dislocation,[15] subluxation,[15] transfer lesion formation,[9] and recurrence.[6]

Lateral Condylectomy

Where isolated prominence of the lateral condyle occurs without either a significant increase in the angle between the fourth and fifth metatarsals or lateral deviation of the distal fifth metatarsal shaft, a lateral condylectomy may effectively treat the deformity.[15] The presence of pes planus or a pronated fifth ray may not be a contraindication to a lateral condylectomy if the prominent metatarsal head is the only deformity present.

Technique A longitudinal incision is made directly over the lateral eminence. Care must be taken to protect the dorsal cutaneous nerve to the fifth toe. Although various capsular incisions have been advocated with this technique, an inverted L-shaped capsular incision allows excellent exposure (Fig. 5, *left*). The capsule is detached along the proximal and dorsal aspect of the metatarsal head. The lateral condyle is resected with a sagittal saw. The metatarsophalangeal joint is distracted with distal traction on the fifth toe and the medial capsule is released. The fifth toe is realigned by reefing the lateral capsule to the fifth metatarsal metaphyseal periosteum and the abductor digiti quinti (Fig. 5, *right*). When there is insufficient tissue to reattach the capsule, interrupted sutures placed through drill holes in the fifth metatarsal metaphysis will achieve a stable repair.

After surgery, the fifth toe is held in proper alignment by a gauze-and-tape dressing that is maintained for six weeks. For walking, the patient wears a wooden-soled shoe at first, later replacing it with a sandal.

Discussion Although this procedure has been recommended frequently,[1,5,11,15,16,21,23,24] only anecdotal follow-up has been published for lateral condylectomy. Reported complications after surgery include poor weightbearing with excessive resection,[2] subluxation of the metatarsophalangeal joint,[3,15,20] and recurrence of the bunionette deformity.[2,4,6,8,21,23]

Meticulous capsular repair[15,20] may prevent subluxation and recurrence of the deformity. Attention to repair of the abductor digiti quinti tendonous insertion, as recommended by Kaplan and associates,[3] may prevent later dislocation of the metatarsophalangeal joint.

Radiographic evaluation of the bunionette deformity before surgery is important. A condylectomy will not effectively reduce the prominence when divergence of the fifth metatarsal shaft occurs either because of an increased angle between the fourth and fifth metatarsals or lateral deviation of the distal fifth metatarsal shaft. In this situation, a fifth metatarsal osteotomy is necessary to reduce the intermetatarsal angle.[32] The significant recurrent rate of deformity following lateral condylectomy is due to the use of a condylectomy when a metatarsal osteotomy is indicated.

Metatarsal Head Excision

The failure of lateral condylectomy to correct bunionette deformity has led to the recommendation of more extensive resection procedures. Resection of the fifth metatarsal head[33] and resection of the fifth metatarsal head with resection of the lateral base of the proximal phalanx[10] have been advocated. McKeever[21] excised the fifth metatarsal head and from one half to two thirds of the metatarsal shaft. Brown[25] resected almost the entire ray, and also amputated the fifth toe. Kelikian[6] modified McKeever's technique by syndactylizing the flail fifth toe to the fourth toe.

Technique A longitudinal incision is made directly over the lateral eminence. When a plantar ulceration makes it necessary to excise the fifth metatarsal head, a dorsal incision may be used. In rheumatoid arthritis, when multiple metatarsal heads are resected, a longitudinal intermetatarsal incision may be placed in the fourth interspace. The capsular structures are released and the fifth metatarsal head is delivered into the surgical wound. The metatarsal head is transected in the metaphyseal region with a bone-cutting forceps, and any

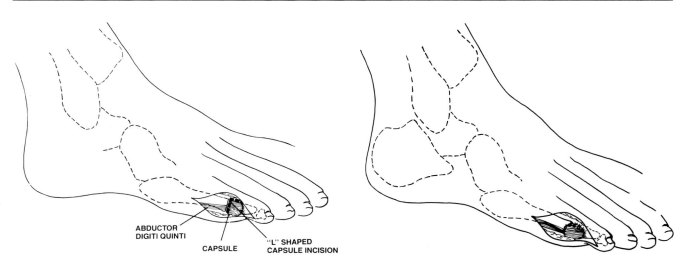

Fig. 5 **Left,** Inverted L-shaped capsular incision. **Right,** Reefing of the lateral capsule.

irregular areas are beveled with a rongeur. In the absence of infection, the fifth toe and metatarsal diaphysis are aligned with a 0.045-inch Kirschner wire, which is left in place for approximately three to four weeks. The capsular structures and skin are closed loosely and a compression gauze-and-tape dressing is applied. A wooden-soled shoe is worn for walking. After removal of the Kirschner wire, tape is used for four to six weeks to hold the toe in appropriate alignment.

Discussion Extensive metatarsal resection can lead to retraction of the fifth toe,[2] subluxation of the fifth toe,[3] and development of a transfer keratotic lesion beneath the fourth metatarsal.[2] In general, ray resection and extensive fifth metatarsal excision should be considered a salvage procedure indicated for infection, intractable ulceration, severe deformity, in treating rheumatoid arthritis, when multiple metatarsal head resections are performed, and in cases in which recurrence is complicated by significant soft-tissue contracture. Less radical procedures that preserve function are generally preferred to resection arthroplasty.

Osteotomy

Osteotomy of the fifth metatarsal may be used to correct angulation of the fifth metatarsal. While Davies[1] found it "unnecessary and unsatisfactory" to perform a fifth metatarsal osteotomy, LeLievre[32] suggested that the goal of surgery should be to reduce a "high intermetatarsal angle." Although Kelikian[6] reported delayed healing with fifth metatarsal osteotomies, the location and technique of osteotomy has a significant effect on successful healing. Proximal, diaphyseal, and distal osteotomies have been recommended for treating a bun-

ionette deformity. The rationale for a proximal fifth metatarsal osteotomy is that it achieves correction at the site of the deformity. However, recent information[34] regarding the arterial supply to the proximal fifth metatarsal may make this choice less desirable. Various types of distal fifth metatarsal osteotomies have also been performed. Although it reduces the angle between the fourth and fifth metatarsals less than would a more proximal osteotomy, a distal metatarsal osteotomy achieves decidedly more correction than does a lateral condylectomy. The difficulty of maintaining alignment with a relatively unstable distal osteotomy has created concern regarding loss of alignment,[3] the possibility of transfer lesion,[9] and recurrence[9] of deformity.

Diaphyseal metatarsal osteotomy allows greater correction than distal metatarsal osteotomy and does not appear to threaten the proximal metatarsal vascular supply. When internally fixed, it allows correction without significant risk of a transfer lesion.

Proximal Metatarsal Osteotomy

A proximal metatarsal osteotomy has been advocated as a way of correcting a large intermetatarsal angle.[3,7,18] This procedure has been successful in treating metatarsus primus varus of the first ray, but controversy surrounds proximal osteotomy in the fifth ray. Le-Lievre[32] advocated a transverse osteotomy at the styloid process, but Diebold and Bejjani[18] noted "the risk of disruption of the tarsal-metatarsal joint is not negligible" (Fig. 6, *top left* and *top right*).

Bishop and associates,[13] working with 72 patients, and Estersohn and associates,[14] with four, performed opening wedge osteotomies of the proximal fifth metatarsal to reduce the intermetatarsal angle. For these

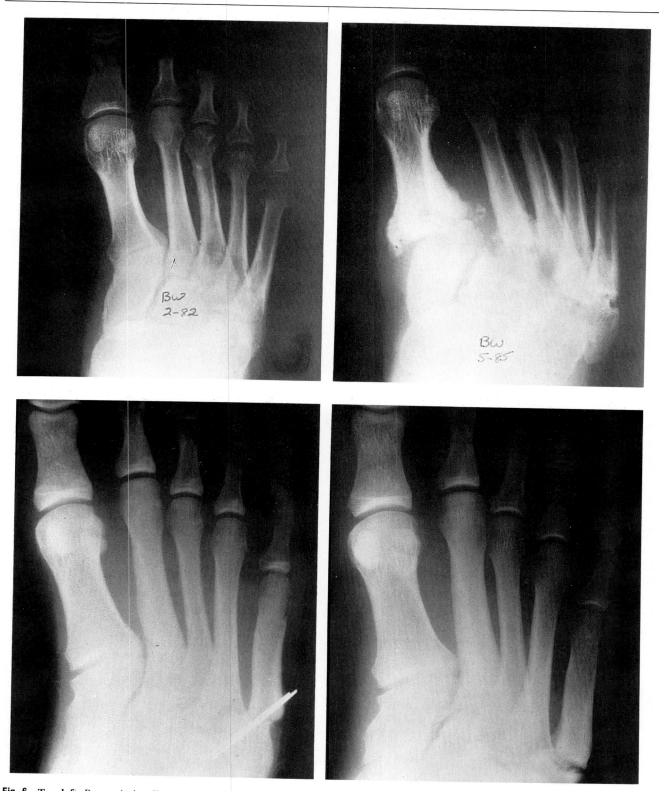

Fig. 6   Top left, Presurgical radiograph prior to proximal fifth metatarsal osteotomy. **Top right,** Same patient with postoperative desta-bilization of the tarsal-metatarsal joint following proximal fifth metatarsal osteotomy. **Bottom left,** Presurgical radiograph prior to proximal fifth metatarsal osteotomy. **Bottom right,** Delayed union following proximal fifth metatarsal osteotomy.

series, no long-term results were reported regarding the intermetatarsal angle, development of transfer lesions, or delayed union. Regnauld[31] reported on a technique that used a closing wedge osteotomy and employed a distal cerclage wire for fixation. No results were reported.

In the only published series on proximal fifth metatarsal osteotomy that had significant followup, Diebold and Bejjani[18] performed a horizontal chevron osteotomy 1 cm distal to the fifth metatarsal base. In 12 patients, they reported excellent results in 90% of cases. Biplanar immobilization was achieved using Steinmann pin fixation between the fourth and fifth metatarsals for four to six weeks.

Although Kaplan and associates[3] and Hohmann[26] stated that proximal and distal osteotomies heal well because of their rich vascular supply, Diebold and Bejjani[18] noted the poor healing potential of fractures in this region (Fig. 6, *bottom right*). Gerbert and associates[29] noted that a proximal metatarsal osteotomy makes the anastomosing arterial branches of the fourth interspace vulnerable to injury. Delayed healing of fractures of the proximal 2 cm of the fifth metatarsal region has been reported.[35–43] Carp[35] stated that the main cause of delayed healing was the poor vascular supply in this region. The nutrient branch to the proximal fifth metatarsal described by both Estersohn and associates[14] and Carp[35] enters on the medial aspect of the fifth metatarsal. Estersohn and associates cautioned that damage to this vascular supply should be avoided.

Shereff and associates[34] analyzed the extraosseous and intraosseous vascular anatomy of the fifth metatarsal. The extraosseous supply originates from the dorsal metatarsal artery and several branches of the lateral plantar artery (Fig. 7). The interosseous supply is maintained by a periosteal plexus, the nutrient artery, and by metaphyseal and epiphyseal vessels. Shereff and associates noted that fracture or osteotomy in the proximal 1 to 2 cm may disrupt the extraosseous and intraosseous vascular supply and, in certain cases, can lead to impaired healing capacity (Fig. 7). Although a proximal metatarsal osteotomy appears to be a straightforward means of correcting a bunionette deformity when an increased intermetatarsal angle is present, the potential for delayed union, nonunion, or metatarsaltarsal instability makes this alternative less desirable.

Distal Metatarsal Osteotomy

Osteotomy of the distal fifth metatarsal has also been used to correct a bunionette deformity. Hohmann[26] described a transverse osteotomy of the metatarsal neck. Kaplan and associates[3] reported a closing wedge osteotomy fixed with a 2-mm K-wire. They commented that internal fixation was necessary, because an unstable distal osteotomy can rotate and lose correction. Haber and Kraft,[4] describing a distal crescent-shaped oste-

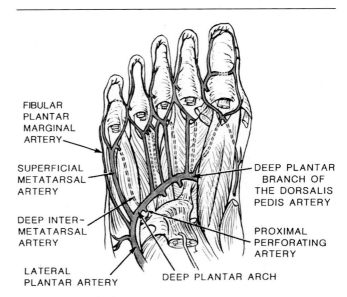

Fig. 7 The plantar circulation is provided by the deep plantar arch which is the source of several smaller arteries—the superficial metatarsal artery, the deep plantar metatarsal artery, the deep plantar intermetatarsal artery, and the fibular plantar marginal artery. From these vessels, numerous discrete branches supply the proximal fifth metatarsal. An area of convergence of these vessels in the proximal 1 to 2 cm of the proximal fifth metatarsal appears to be vulnerable to delayed union with interruption of the arterial circulation at this level. (Courtesy Michael J. Shereff, MD, Hospital for Joint Diseases, Orthopaedic Institute, New York, NY.)

otomy without internal fixation, reported delayed healing and excessive callus formation.

Throckmorton and Bradlee[17] performed a transverse chevron osteotomy without fixation, relying on the intrinsic stability of the chevron osteotomy to maintain alignment. They noted that this procedure did not allow for correction of a plantar keratotic lesion.

Sponsel[20] performed an oblique distal osteotomy, allowing the fragment to "float" without fixation. An 11% rate of delayed union was reported.

Keating and associates[9] also performed a distal oblique osteotomy without fixation. A 76% rate of transfer lesion, a 12% recurrence rate, and a 56% success rate were reported. Keating and associates noted that transfer lesions and recurrent lesions may be attributable to the amount of dorsiflexion and medial displacement of the capital fragment that occurs with healing of this osteotomy. Diebold and Bejjani[18] also found a distal fifth metatarsal osteotomy to be unsatisfactory because of the difficulty of achieving fixation in the narrow fifth metatarsal neck.

Sponsel[20] attempted a distal osteotomy of the Mitchell type without success. Leach and Igou,[2] who performed a "reverse Mitchell" procedure on 11 feet, reported that an average presurgical intermetatarsal angle of 11.7 degrees was reduced after surgery to an average of 4.9 degrees. No nonunions were reported.

Leventen and Kitaoka[27] performed a modified distal

oblique osteotomy for symptomatic bunionette deformities both with and without intractable plantar keratotic formation. Twenty-three feet in 16 patients were treated surgically. The intermetatarsal angle was decreased from 13 degrees to 8 degrees and the forefoot width was decreased by approximately 4 mm. Good results were reported in 88% of the cases. One nonunion was noted.

Technique of Distal Oblique Osteotomy A longitudinal incision is made directly over the lateral eminence. The proximal and dorsal capsule is detached through an L-shaped capsular incision that allows exposure of the lateral condylar process (Fig. 5, *left*). The abductor digiti quinti is divided. The lateral eminence is resected with a sagittal saw, and using a double-action bone cutter, an oblique osteotomy of the neck of the metatarsal is performed (Fig. 8, *top*) in a distal lateral to proximal medial direction. The neck portion of the distal fragment is removed and the distal fragment is displaced medially and impacted upon the proximal fragment (Fig. 8, *bottom*). No fixation or cast immobilization is used. The foot is dressed in a soft gauze bandage. The patient is allowed to walk, but must wear a special shoe. Following removal of the bandage, the toe is taped in a corrected position for four weeks.

Technique of Distal Chevron Procedure An alternative procedure is resection of the prominent lateral condyle in combination with a distal chevron osteotomy. A midlateral skin incision down to the capsule allows protection of the superficial neurovascular bundles on the dorsal and plantar aspect. An inverted L-shaped capsular incision is used to release the dorsal and proximal margins (Fig. 5, *left*). Care must be taken to minimize soft-tissue stripping, so that the distal metatarsal fragment does not suffer vascular compromise and possible osteonecrosis. The lateral eminence is resected with a sagittal saw (Fig. 5, *right*). Approximately 2 mm of bone is removed. A 0.045-inch K-wire is then used to drill a hole in the midportion of the metatarsal head to mark the apex of the osteotomy. Then, a sagittal saw is used to create a proximally based horizontal chevron osteotomy oriented in a lateral to medial direction with an angle of 60 degrees (Fig. 9, *left*). The fifth metatarsophalangeal medial capsular structures are not disrupted. The distal fragment is then displaced approximately 3 mm in a medial direction and impacted into the proximal fragment (Fig. 9, *right*). K-wire fixation is optional, but should be used if there is any tendency toward angulation or redisplacement at the osteotomy site.

Any prominent metaphyseal bone is removed and the lateral capsule is attached either to the abductor digiti quinti or to holes drilled in the metaphysis, depending on the adequacy of the metaphyseal capsule.

Discussion The distal oblique osteotomy or the chev-

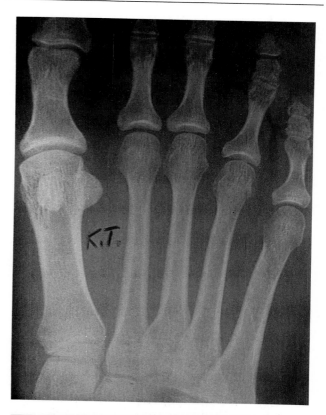

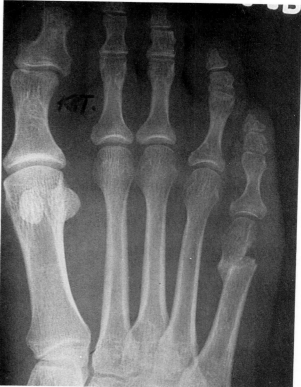

Fig. 8 Top, Preoperative anteroposterior radiograph of distal oblique osteotomy. **Bottom,** Anteroposterior radiograph following displacement of distal oblique osteotomy.

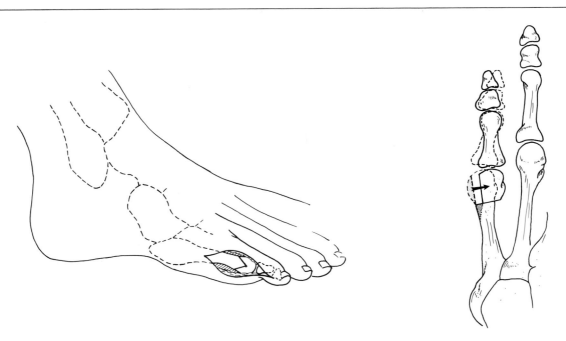

Fig. 9   **Left,** Lateral view of distal chevron osteotomy. **Right,** Anteroposterior view of distal Chevron osteotomy.

ron osteotomy appears to afford more correction than the condylar resection alone, and a distal osteotomy can effectively reduce a bulbous fifth metatarsal head or an enlarged lateral condyle.

The potential for displacement, malunion, or development of a transfer lesion makes the use of internal fixation or the creation of a stable osteotomy preferable to a floating-type osteotomy as described by Hohmann,[26] Sponsel,[20] or Keating and associates.[9] When a pure lateral keratosis is present, either osteotomy will suffice. However, because a chevron-type osteotomy does not allow dorsal translation of the distal fragment, it is contraindicated when a plantar or plantar-lateral keratosis has occurred.

Midshaft Osteotomy

Transverse osteotomy in the diaphyseal region is rarely used to correct a bunionette deformity because of problems with rotation, angulation, and pseudarthrosis. In 1986, Mann[15] described an oblique fifth metatarsal diaphyseal osteotomy for the treatment of large, diffuse keratotic lesions on the plantar and plantar-lateral aspect of the fifth metatarsal head. The oblique nature of the osteotomy allows a dorsal-medial translation of the metatarsal as the distal fragment is rotated. Mann advocated fixation with a small fragment screw, K-wire, or a wire loop. He did not realign the fifth metatarsophalangeal joint in this procedure. No series was presented although he did report one case of nonunion. In 1987, Coughlin[30] reported on a modification of Mann's oblique diaphyseal osteotomy, in which a

fifth metatarsophalangeal realignment was performed as well. Eleven patients (16 feet) underwent surgical correction and all healed successfully. The intermetatarsal angle was reduced from 9.13 degrees to −0.04 degrees postoperatively. The metatarsophalangeal-5 angle, which averaged 17.6 degrees before surgery, was reduced to an average of 0 degrees postoperatively. No transfer lesions were reported.

Technique   A midlateral longitudinal incision, made on the dorsal aspect of the fifth metatarsal, extends from the base of the fifth metatarsal to the middle of the proximal phalanx. The dorsolateral cutaneous nerve is isolated and protected. The abductor digiti minimi is reflected plantarward to expose the fifth metatarsal diaphysis. The metatarsophalangeal joint capsule is incised along the dorsal and proximal aspect, using an L-shaped incision, and the lateral eminence is exposed (Fig. 5, *left*). The fibular condyle of the metatarsal head is excised using a sagittal saw to perform an osteotomy parallel with the metatarsal shaft. The medial capsule of the fifth metatarsophalangeal joint is released so that the metatarsophalangeal joint can be realigned at the conclusion of the procedure.

A sagittal saw is used for the diaphyseal osteotomy of the fifth metatarsal. When only a lateral keratosis is present, the osteotomy is directed in a dorsal proximal to plantar distal direction (Fig. 10). The distal fragment is rotated medially, and the osteotomy site is fixed with a small fragment screw or multiple K-wires. Any prominent bone at the osteotomy site is resected with the

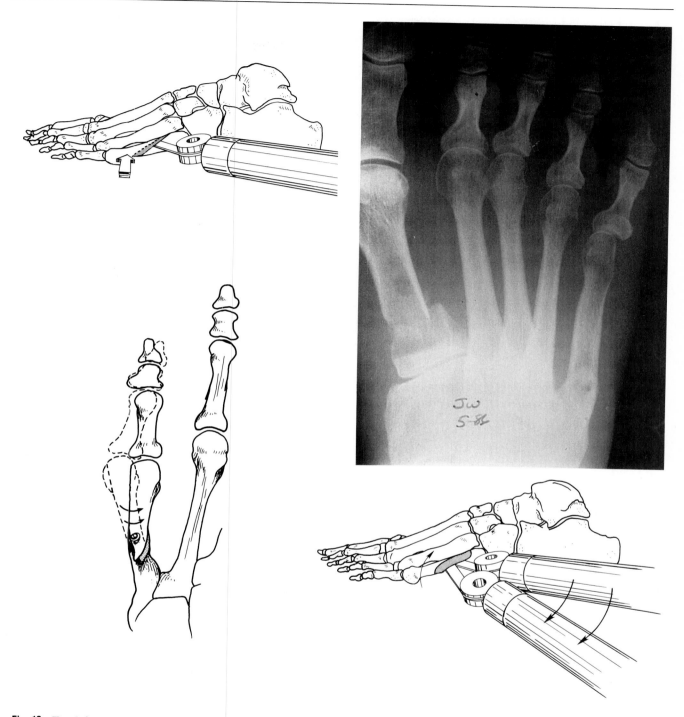

Fig. 10   Top left, Orientation of the diaphyseal horizontal oblique osteotomy. **Bottom left**, Rotation of the diaphyseal osteotomy fixation with small fragment screw. Lateral eminence resection with lateral capsular reefing may be included. **Top right**, Anteroposterior radiograph demonstrating correction with diaphyseal osteotomy. **Bottom right**, Where intractable plantar keratotis is present, the saw blade is directed in a cephalad direction (where osteotomy site is rotated, the fifth metatarsal head will elevate).

sagittal saw (Fig. 10, *bottom left*). The capsule is repaired, and the fifth toe is realigned using the repair as described for a lateral condylectomy (Fig. 5, *right*).

A soft compression dressing is applied and changed

weekly for six weeks. The patient wears a wooden-soled shoe for walking. Casting is recommended for an unreliable patient or if a patient is unsteady when walking.

When a combined lateral and plantar lateral keratosis

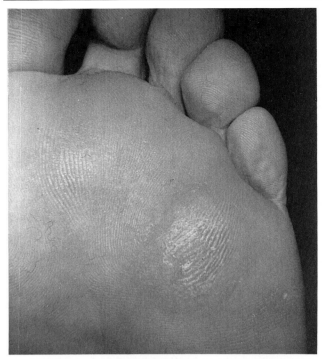

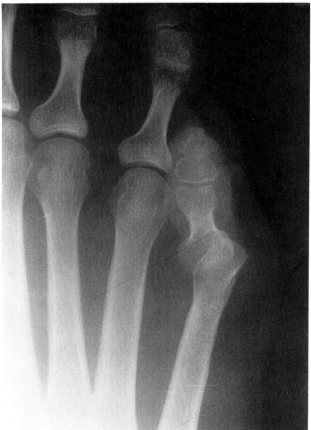

Fig. 11 Top, Complication-transfer lesion beneath fourth metatarsal head following distal fifth metatarsal osteotomy. **Bottom,** Dislocation of fifth metatarsophalangeal joint following lateral condylectomy.

is present, the oblique osteotomy is still oriented in a dorsal proximal to plantar distal direction. In this situation, however, the saw blade is directed in a slightly cephalad direction in order to have an elevating effect on the distal fragment as this fragment is rotated (Fig. 10, *bottom right*). The fifth metatarsophalangeal joint is realigned and closure is carried out as before. K-wires are removed with the patient under local anesthesia six to eight weeks after surgery. Screws are removed only if they cause problems.

The indications for an osteotomy in the diaphyseal region is a bunionette deformity associated with either an increased intermetatarsal angle or with lateral metatarsal deviation or bowing. Concurrent metatarsophalangeal joint realignment with a lateral eminence resection to correct the deviated fifth toe can be performed simultaneously if necessary.

Discussion More than 20 different procedures used to treat bunionette deformity have been described. Lateral condylar excision, metatarsal head resection, and fifth ray resection, as well as distal, diaphyseal, and proximal metatarsal osteotomies, either with or without metatarsophalangeal arthroplasties, have been performed. The paucity of follow-up on most of these procedures and the anecdotal reports of success with various techniques raise questions as to their long-term results. Because bunionette deformities are associated with a wide range of anatomic variations, the choice of surgical correction is complicated.

An enlarged or bulbous fifth metatarsal head (with or without a pronated fifth ray) may be treated with either a lateral condylectomy and metatarsophalangeal joint realignment or with a distal metatarsal osteotomy. The presence of a pure lateral keratotic lesion makes a chevron osteotomy preferable because of its inherent stability. K-wire fixation may be used to insure a stable osteotomy site. When a plantar or a plantar-lateral keratotic lesion is present without lateral metatarsal deviation or an increased intermetatarsal 4–5 angle, a distal oblique osteotomy as described by Leventen and Kitaoka[27] is preferable to the chevron procedure. A diaphyseal biplane osteotomy may also be used in this situation.

While there is disagreement regarding the need for internal fixation for a fifth metatarsal osteotomy, malunion, nonunion, delayed union, and intractable plantar keratotic lesions have developed in cases in which floating osteotomies (Fig. 11) have been performed. This indicates a need for either an inherently stable osteotomy or the use of rigid internal fixation. The principles of osteotomy with internal fixation applied elsewhere in the musculoskeletal system also apply to the foot.

When a bunionette is associated with an abnormally wide angle between the fourth and fifth metatarsals or the less common laterally deviated fifth metatarsal shaft, a diaphyseal osteotomy with distal soft-tissue re-alignment affords an excellent means of correction.

Recent reports on the circulatory patterns of the proximal fifth metatarsal have caused concern regarding the possibility of vascular compromise with proximal metatarsal osteotomy. It appears that a diaphyseal osteotomy offers a less vulnerable location for metatarsal correctional osteotomy.

Conclusion

Evaluation of the radiographic abnormalities associated with a bunionette is important in analyzing the nature of the deformity. Correlation with physical findings and the location of keratotic lesions will help in defining the appropriate treatment.

A clear understanding of the underlying abnormality will help in determining whether a condylectomy with distal soft-tissue repair, a distal metatarsal osteotomy, or a diaphyseal osteotomy will offer the best solution for the painful bunionette deformity.

Acknowledgment

Figures 1 through 6 and 8 through 11 were reproduced with permission from Michael J. Coughlin, MD.

References

1. Davies H: Metatarsus quintus valgus. *Br Med J* 1949;1:664–665.
2. Leach RE, Igou R: Metatarsal osteotomy for bunionette deformity. *Clin Orthop* 1974;100:171–175.
3. Kaplan EG, Kaplan G, Jacobs AM: Management of fifth metatarsal head lesions by biplane osteotomy. *J Foot Surg* 1976;15:1–8.
4. Haber JH, Kraft J: Crescentic osteotomy for fifth metatarsal head lesions. *J Foot Surg* 1980;19:66–67.
5. DuVries HL: *Surgery of the Foot*, ed 2. St. Louis, CV Mosby, 1965, pp 456–462.
6. Kelikian H: Deformities of the lesser toe, in Kelikian H (ed): *Hallux Valgus: Allied Deformities of the Forefoot and Metatarsalgia.* Philadelphia, WB Saunders, 1965, pp 327–330.
7. Fallat LM, Buckholz J: An analysis of the tailor's bunion by radiographic and anatomical display. *J Am Podiatr Assoc* 1980;70:597–603.
8. Yancey HA Jr: Congenital lateral bowing of the fifth metatarsal: Report of 2 cases and operative treatment. *Clin Orthop* 1969;62:203–205.
9. Keating SE, DeVincentis A, Goller WL: Oblique fifth metatarsal osteotomy: A follow-up study. *J Foot Surg* 1982;21:104–107.
10. Weinstein F (ed): *Principles and Practice of Podiatry.* Philadelphia, Lea & Febiger, 1968, pp 167–169.
11. Dickson FD, Diveley RL: *Functional Disorders of the Foot*, ed 3. Philadelphia, JB Lippincott, 1953, p 230.
12. Schoenhaus H, Rotman S, Meshon AL: A review of normal intermetatarsal angles. *J Am Podiatr Assoc* 1973;63:88–95.
13. Bishop J, Kahn A III, Turba JE: Surgical correction of the splayfoot: The Giannestras procedure. *Clin Orthop* 1980;146:234–238.
14. Estersohn H, Scherer P, Bogdan R: A preliminary report on opening wedge osteotomy of the fifth metatarsal. *Arch Podiatr Med Foot Surg* 1974;1:317–327.
15. Mann RA: Keratotic disorders of the plantar skin, in Mann RA (ed): *Surgery of the Foot*, ed 5. St. Louis, CV Mosby, 1986, pp 194–198.
16. Stewart M: Miscellaneous affections of the foot, in Edmonson AS, Crenshaw AH (eds): *Campbell's Operative Orthopedics*, ed 6. St. Louis, CV Mosby, 1980, p 1733.
17. Throckmorton JK, Bradlee N: Transverse v sliding osteotomy: A new surgical procedure for the correction of tailor's bunion deformity. *J Foot Surg* 1978;18:117–121.
18. Diebold PF, Bejjani FJ: Basal osteotomy of the fifth metatarsal with intermetatarsal pinning: A new approach to tailor's bunion. *Foot Ankle* 1987;8:40–45.
19. Kitaoka HB, Nestor BJ, Bergmann AD: Radiologic anatomy of the painful bunionette. Presented at the Fourth Annual Summer Meeting of the American Orthopaedic Foot and Ankle Society, Minneapolis, July 1988.
20. Sponsel KH: Bunionette correction by metatarsal osteotomy: Preliminary report. *Orthop Clin North Am* 1976;7:809–819.
21. McKeever DC: Excision of the fifth metatarsal head. *Clin Orthop* 1959;13:321–322.
22. McGlamry ED, Butlin WE, Kitting RW: Metatarsal shortening: Osteoplasty of head or osteotomy of shaft. *J Am Podiatr Assoc* 1969;59:394–398.
23. LeLievre J: Exostosis of the head of the 5th metatarsal bone, tailor's bunion. *LeConcours Med* 1956;78:4815–4816.
24. Giannestras NJ: Other problems of the forepart of the foot, in Giannestras NJ (ed): *Foot Disorders: Medical and Surgical Management*, ed 2. Philadelphia, Lea & Febiger, 1973, pp 420–421.
25. Brown JE: Functional and cosmetic correction of metatarsus latus (splay foot). *Clin Orthop* 1959;14:166–170.
26. Hohmann G: *Fuss und Bein.* Munich, JF Bergman, 1951, pp 172–173.
27. Leventen E, Kitaoka HB: Medial displacement metatarsal osteotomy for the treatment of the painful bunionette. *Clin Orthop* 1989;243:172–179.
28. Voutey H: *Manueal de chirurgie orthopaedique et de reeducation du pied.* Paris, Masson et Cie, 1978, pp 149–151.
29. Gerbert J, Sgarlato TE, Subotnick SI: Preliminary study of a closing wedge osteotomy of the fifth metatarsal for correction of a tailor's bunion deformity. *J Am Podiatr Assoc* 1972;62:212–218.
30. Coughlin MJ: Correction of the bunionette with midshaft oblique osteotomy. *Orthop Trans* 1988;12:30.
31. Regnauld B: *Technique chirurgicales du pied.* Paris, Masson et Cie, 1974, p 23.
32. LeLievre J: *Pathologie du pied*, ed 5. Paris, Masson et Cie, 1971, pp 526–528.
33. Weisberg MH: Resection of the fifth metatarsal head in lateral segment problems. *J Am Podiatr Assoc* 1967;57:374–376.
34. Shereff MJ, Yang QM, Krummer FJ, et al: The vascular anatomy of the fifth metatarsal. *Orthop Trans* 1988;12:30.
35. Carp L: Fracture of the fifth metatarsal bone: With special reference to delayed union. *Ann Surg* 1927;86:308–320.
36. Kavanaugh JH, Brower TD, Mann RV: The Jones fracture revisited. *J Bone Joint Surg* 1978;60A:776–782.
37. Acker JH, Drez D Jr: Nonoperative treatment of stress fractures of the proximal shaft of the fifth metatarsal (Jones' fracture). *Foot Ankle* 1986;7:152–155.
38. Lehman RC, Torg JS, Pavlov H, et al: Fractures of the base of the fifth metatarsal distal to the tuberosity: A review. *Foot Ankle* 1987;7:245–252.
39. Torg JS, Balduini FC, Zelko RR, et al: Fractures of the base of the fifth metatarsal distal to the tuberosity: Classification and guidelines for non-surgical and surgical management. *J Bone Joint Surg* 1984;66A:209–214.
40. Dameron TB Jr: Fractures and anatomical variations of the prox-

imal portion of the fifth metatarsal. *J Bone Joint Surg* 1975;57A: 788–792.

41. Zelko RR, Torg JS, Rachun A: Proximal diaphyseal fractures of the fifth metatarsal: Treatment of the fractures and their complications in athletes. *Am J Sports Med* 1979;7:95–101.

42. DeLee JC, Evans JP, Julian J: Stress fracture of the fifth metatarsal. *Am J Sports Med* 1983;11:349–353.

43. Lichtblau S: Painful nonunion of a fracture of the 5th metatarsal. *Clin Orthop* 1968;59:171–175.

Surgical Arthrodesis Techniques for Foot and Ankle Pathology

Andrea Cracchiolo III, MD

Introduction

In the adult foot and ankle, arthrodesis can be considered a reconstructive procedure rather than a salvage operation. If the patient's joint abnormality is localized to the foot or ankle, a successful arthrodesis may result in pain-free, relatively normal ambulation. However, even an excellent result still limits certain activities, such as jogging or running, and may limit the patient's selection of footwear.

All arthrodesis techniques have a number of features in common. Each of the procedures is demanding and must be done with considerable precision. Soft tissues must be handled carefully, because wound-healing problems can be quite serious. Bony surfaces require optimal preparation. Most arthrodesis procedures require some form of internal or external fixation. Because an arthrodesis is usually done under tourniquet control, a careful assessment of the neurovascular supply before surgery is essential. This is particularly important in patients who have a history of trauma to the joint that is to be fused, in older patients, or in patients who have any disease in which there may be vascular compromise.

The use of autogenous bone grafts is important in achieving an arthrodesis in some cases. Whenever there is any possibility of a graft being needed, the appropriate donor site, usually an iliac crest, should be prepared and surgically draped before the arthrodesis procedure is begun.

Arthrodesis of the Hallux Joints

The Hallux Interphalangeal Joint

Indications One indication for arthrodesis of the hallux interphalangeal joint is an arthritic joint, as a result either of trauma or of inflammatory arthritis. Arthrodesis is also indicated as part of a surgical procedure that transfers the extensor hallucis longus or when the joint must be stabilized because of a nonfunctioning long extensor or flexor tendon.

Techniques The hallux interphalangeal joint can be exposed through a dorsal incision that is transverse across the joint and extends proximally along the fibular side of the hallux. If a large plantar bursa is to be excised, the same incision on the plantar surface of the foot may be indicated. Care must be taken to avoid damaging the digital nerve.

A narrow-blade oscillating saw is used to resect the joint surfaces so that planar bony surfaces can be opposed. Some method of internal fixation is needed to enhance the rate of fusion. A 4-mm cancellous bone screw can be placed across the joint as follows. A second transverse incision is made through the pulp of the tip of the hallux beneath the nail. Using a 2-mm drill bit, a hole is drilled through the distal phalanx from proximal to distal, exiting through the second incision. The drill bit is removed and passed manually from distal to proximal through the predrilled hole in the distal phalanx. The two prepared bony surfaces are reduced and the drill is advanced into the proximal phalanx. A 4-mm cancellous bone screw of appropriate length is used to fix the two bones securely. This method works best when the bone quality of the proximal phalanx is excellent, allowing good purchase for the cancellous screw.

Pneumatically driven titanium staples, either 10 × 10 mm or 10 × 7 mm, can also be used to fix the cut surfaces securely. Before placing the staples, a 0.062-inch Kirschner wire is used temporarily to hold the two bones together. After the first two staples have been placed, the wire is removed, and an additional one or two staples are inserted. The dorsally placed staples act as a tension band against an intact flexor tendon and provide good internal fixation.

The Metatarsophalangeal Joint

Indications Indications for arthrodesis of the metatarsophalangeal joint include inflammatory, septic, or traumatic arthritis; failure of a previous reconstructive procedure to the hallux metatarsophalangeal joint, such as a Keller arthroplasty; degenerative arthritis following a previous bunion surgery; or a failed hallux implant.

Positioning the Arthrodesis It is critical to select and achieve the optimum position for the arthrodesis because it cannot be corrected after surgery. Over the years the angle of arthrodesis has generally been reduced, but this should be discussed with the patient. This is especially important if the patient is a woman who is used to wearing a particular type of shoe. It also important to remember that the first metatarsal normally is angled 15 degrees plantarward to the floor. Thus, if the joint is fused in the plantigrade position, there will be insufficient dorsiflexion to permit efficient rollover as the foot passes from the foot-flat position to the toe-off position during gait. At least another 10 to 15 degrees of dorsiflexion should be added. Therefore, referenced from the ground, the amount of dorsiflexion would be about 15 degrees, or about 30 degrees if referenced from the inclination of the first metatarsal. It may be necessary to add a few more degrees of dorsiflexion for women who prefer to wear a shoe with a higher heel. Valgus should be no less than 10 degrees and no more than 20 degrees. The hallux should remain in neutral rotation. In the presurgical planning, Wilson[1] believes, it is generally helpful to hold the sole of the foot at a 90-degree angle to the leg and then place the pulp of the hallux in line with the sole of the foot in the lateral plane and comfortably next to the second toe in the dorsoplantar plane. Neutral rotation is judged by the position of the nail.

Techniques A dorsal medial longitudinal incision gives good exposure. The joint capsule should also be opened through a longitudinal incision, and a medial and lateral flap of all the capsular soft tissues should be fashioned. This flap will later be sutured over the fusion site. After the metatarsal head and the base of the proximal phalanx have been exposed, one should evaluate the overall alignment of the hallux and the position of the sesamoids. If the sesamoids are laterally displaced, it may be necessary to perform a lateral release of the capsule, adductor tendon, and transverse metatarsal ligament. Usually the arthrodesis properly aligns the hallux metatarsal; however, a significant fixed metatarsus primus varus may require correction by a concomitant proximal first metatarsal osteotomy.

The proximal phalanx and metatarsal head surfaces should be carefully prepared for the arthrodesis. Two planar surfaces provide the optimal stability for a surgical fusion.[2] The joint surfaces can be transected with an oscillating saw. Any method of fixation that holds these flat bone surfaces together can be used. In patients whose bone is of poor quality and in patients with a previous Keller procedure or a silicone implant, two double-tipped Steinmann pins drilled retrograde across the joint are an effective method.[3,4] An assistant holds the bony surfaces together tightly and at the proper angle. The Steinmann pins are threaded and typically the ones used are 3.6-mm and 3.2-mm pins (Fig. 1). Although the pins cross the hallux interphalangeal joint, no decrease in motion of the joint after they are removed has been reported.[4]

Screws are also effective in holding the bony surfaces together. This method has the advantage of not crossing the interphalangeal joint, but requires bone of better quality. If possible, two screws should be placed across the joint.

After the joint surfaces are prepared, a 0.062-inch K-wire is passed from the dorsal distal base of the proximal phalanx into the metatarsal head (Fig. 2). This temporarily stabilizes the joint and holds the proper angle for arthrodesis. The first screw is placed from the medial flare of the base of the proximal phalanx into the metatarsal head. The K-wire is removed and the wire hole drilled with the appropriate drill bit and fitted with a second screw (Fig. 3). Alternatively, two screws can be placed from the medial side of the metatarsal head obliquely into or across the proximal phalanx.[5]

Two types of screws can be used. If the bone, especially the cancellous bone, is of good quality, a 4-mm cancellous bone screw can be used. A 2-mm drill bit is used to make the holes across the arthrodesis site. In bone that is somewhat osteoporotic, a 3.5-mm cortical screw is preferred. A 2-mm drill hole is made across the arthrodesis site, and a 3.5-mm tap is inserted across both cortices. The first cortex is then overdrilled with a 3.5-mm drill bit to act as a guiding hole. Adequate fixation of the arthrodesis site can be achieved by the screw head holding one cortex and the screw threads holding the opposite cortex. If there is any doubt about screw fixation, the screws should be removed and Steinmann pins used instead.

Postoperative Care A wooden-soled shoe is usually worn for six to ten weeks. The Steinmann pins can be removed when clinical and radiographic signs of union have appeared, which usually occurs by three months. Screws are removed only if they cause discomfort.

Arthrodesis of the Hindfoot

Initially, triple arthrodesis was performed in patients with a flail foot secondary to polio deformity. Arthrodesis of one or more hindfoot joints is now used for patients with rheumatoid or traumatic arthritis and, selectively, for patients with posterior tibial tendon dysfunction, neurologic deformities, and congenital abnormalities. The primary indication for this arthrodesis is pain or instability of the hindfoot that has not responded to conservative care.

Various techniques are used to perform hindfoot arthrodesis in adults. These include a technique using a bone graft, such as the rotated-dowel technique,[6] or an inlay-graft method, which is probably best suited for the subtalar joint but which can be used for all three joints. Internal fixation, using cancellous bone screws or power-driven titanium staples, is another effective way of obtaining solid fusion. For patients who do not have a hindfoot deformity, either technique may be suitable. However, in feet with a deformity some method of internal fixation is preferable.

Physical Examination of the Hindfoot

Patients with hindfoot abnormality should be examined while they are seated and again while standing. It is important to determine the extent of any fixed deformity, particularly a planovalgus deformity. The forefoot should also be evaluated for abnormality and

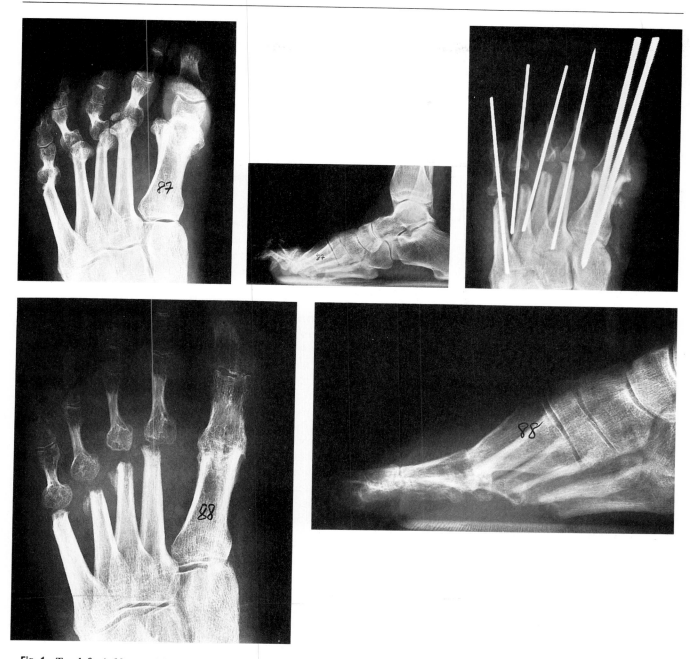

Fig. 1   **Top left**, A 60-year-old woman with advanced rheumatoid arthritis and forefoot pain. Ten years previously, she had a resection of all her metatarsal heads through a plantar approach. She was asymptomatic for about eight years until these deformities recurred. **Top center**, Lateral weightbearing radiograph showing recurrence of the dorsal dislocation of the toes. **Top right**, Anteroposterior radiograph following re-excision of the residual bone growth at the end of the metatarsals and 0.062-inch K-wire temporary fixation to maintain alignment. Arthrodesis was performed on the hallux metatarsophalangeal joint, using 3.2-mm double-pointed Steinmann pins. **Bottom left**, An anteroposterior weightbearing radiograph six months postoperatively; the hallux metatarsophalangeal joint shows a solid arthrodesis. **Bottom right**, A lateral weightbearing radiograph also showing a solid arthrodesis of the hallux metatarsophalangeal joint with 30 degrees of extension.

to determine whether it will be plantigrade if a fixed hindfoot deformity is corrected. The hindfoot angle is measured by placing one arm of a goniometer along the posterior portion of the middle of the lower leg and the other arm along the middle of the calcaneus. This is done with the patient standing and with the patient in the prone position. These measurements will indicate the amount of fixed or flexible deformity. All muscles that cross the ankle and hindfoot should be assessed. Because of its known frequency of dysfunction, the posterior tibialis should be specifically evaluated. Both feet and both ankles must be assessed, be-

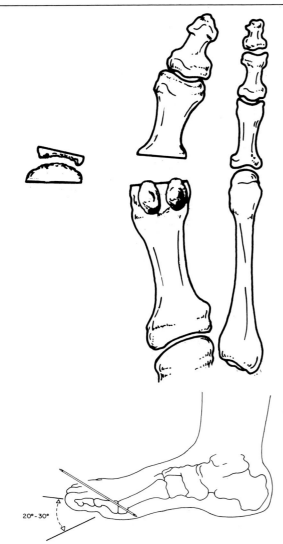

20°-30°

Fig. 2 **Top**, If there are no significant deformities of the lateral toes, then only a small amount of bone needs to be resected for arthrodesis of the hallux metatarsal phalangeal joint. Planar surfaces are created that provide good stability and facilitate the use of internal fixation. **Bottom**, Thirty degrees of extension as measured from the metatarsal is a satisfactory position for arthrodesis of the hallux metatarsophalangeal joint in most patients. A 0.062-mm K-wire is passed from distal dorsal across the base of the proximal phalanx to temporarily hold the joint securely. This wire should avoid the route of the first screw, which is usually from the medial side of the flare of the proximal phalanx across the arthrodesis site to the lateral side of the metatarsal head.

cause in unilateral involvement a comparison with the normal side is helpful. On the lateral side, palpation of the sinus tarsi and the distal fibula may reveal considerable tenderness, especially in valgus deformity. Abutment of the calcaneus against the distal fibula also causes lateral pain and tenderness and may result in a stress fracture of the distal fibula. Passive motion may distinguish hindfoot abnormality from ankle abnormality. Classically, patients with an arthritic hindfoot have pain during inversion and eversion when the ankle

is held in neutral. Crepitation will also be felt. Patients with planovalgus deformity may have considerable lateral hindfoot pain on even gentle forced eversion.

Presurgical Radiographic Evaluation of the Hindfoot and Ankle

The biomechanics of the ankle and the hindfoot are closely correlated. For this reason, it is essential to evaluate both areas with weightbearing radiographs to determine whether some or all of the deformity is in the tibiotalar or subtalar joint. Anteroposterior views of the foot and ankle permit evaluation of the talonavicular and calcaneocuboid joints, as well as the overall alignment of the metatarsals and forefoot. The ankle view evaluates the tibiotalar joint and gives some indication of the alignment of the calcaneus. In a severe hindfoot valgus, the calcaneus can be seen abutting the distal fibula. Lateral weightbearing views of both feet are used to evaluate the subtalar joint and the degree of cavus or planus that may be present. A helpful measurement is the lateral talar-first metatarsal angle, which is normally zero. Fifteen degrees or more in either direction distinguishes a significant cavus or planovalgus deformity. Because it is impossible to isolate and measure ankle motion on the clinical examination, the only way to measure ankle movement accurately is by weightbearing lateral views, while the patient either shifts the body weight forward and backward or elevates first the forefoot and then the heel on blocks. There is no way to isolate the dorsiflexion and plantar flexion that occur only at the tibiotalar joint. Although stress views of the ankle are usually not helpful if an arthrodesis of that joint is being planned, they may be considered if a triple arthrodesis is to be performed in a patient with ankle instability.

Exposure of the Hindfoot Joints

The patient is positioned with a towel under the ipsilateral buttock so that the foot to be operated on and the lower extremity are in neutral or slight internal rotation. A lateral and a medial incision should be used to expose the hindfoot joints. The lateral incision, performed first, is a longitudinal incision centered over the sinus tarsi. Distally the incision curves somewhat anteriorly just in front of the peroneal tendons. Care should be taken to avoid injury to the sural nerve. The incision can be extended proximally to avoid tension on the wound edges. The fat pad within the sinus tarsi should be sharply incised and carefully retracted so that some subcutaneous tissue remains to aid wound closure. Care should be taken not to enter the ankle joint. The medial incision is centered over the dorsal medial aspect of the talonavicular joint. All the joints must be freed so that any significant deformity can be corrected and the hindfoot placed in a good weightbearing position. If there is no fixed forefoot deformity, the calcaneus should be in about 6 degrees of valgus and the talus should be in a line with the first metatarsal. This

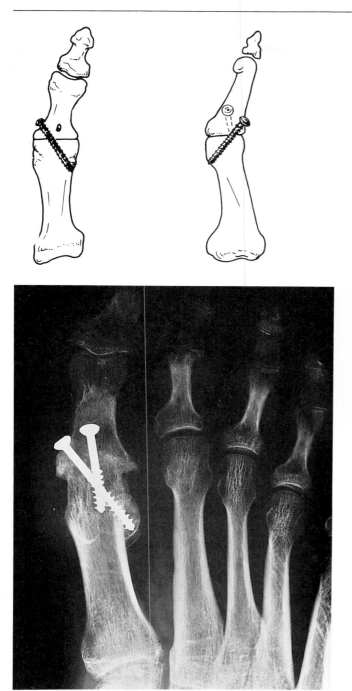

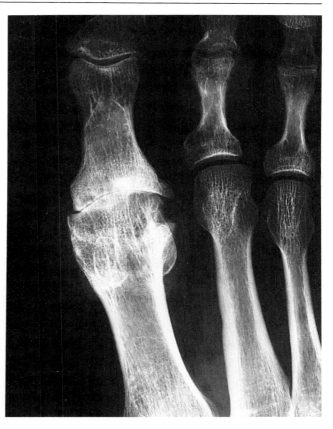

Fig. 3 Top left, Following placement of the first screw, the K-wire is removed and a second screw can then be placed at the site of the K-wire. Note the 10 degrees of valgus at the arthrodesis site. **Top center**, A lateral view with the dorsal screw in place as well as the medial screw. **Top right**, An anteroposterior view of a 55-year-old man who does heavy labor. He wished a definitive procedure for his painful hallux rigidus. **Bottom left**, Using 4.0-mm cancellous screws, the hallux metatarsophalangeal joint was successfully fused.

position must be modified if there is a fixed deformity of the forefoot, because after surgery the foot must be plantigrade. A small lamina spreader is frequently helpful and can be placed in the sinus tarsi to help judge the amount of correction needed, particularly if there is a valgus deformity.

Dowel-Fusion Technique

The dowel-fusion technique consists of rotating a dowel graft across the joint to be fused, placing a dowel of bone from the iliac crest into a joint (usually the subtalar joint), or using the dowel-graft technique supplemented with staples (Fig. 4).[6]

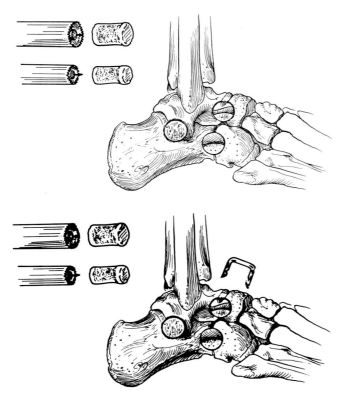

Fig. 4 Dowels of bone can easily be rotated across the talonavicular and calcaneocuboid joint. **Top,** The dowel is composed of one half of each adjacent joint surface. Rotating the dowel surfaces 90 degrees places a bony bridge across the joint, allowing bony fusion. Usually a 12-mm or 14-mm dowel is a sufficient size. Because of the surface of the subtalar joint, especially if there has been some bone loss, it is preferable to drill out a 12-mm hole and replace this with a dowel the same size or one size larger obtained from the iliac crest. **Bottom,** Hand-driven staples have been used to secure the dowels. Some form of internal fixation is helpful in holding the corrected position, because the patient will require a few cast changes before solid fusion occurs.

Cancellous Bone Screw Fixation for Hindfoot Arthrodesis

Solid internal fixation for arthrodesis of the hindfoot joints may be achieved with 6.5-mm cancellous bone screws.[7] This technique can be performed either with or without bone grafting of the subtalar joint. However, bone grafting of the talonavicular or calcaneocuboid joint is usually unnecessary. Before arthrodesis, it is essential first to restore normal or near-normal alignment of the hindfoot. The position gained at the time of the operation will be maintained by the screws during the time needed for the fusion. Once solid internal fixation has been achieved, it is no longer possible to change the position of the arthrodesis. Thus, a patient with no significant hindfoot deformity is an ideal subject for this technique. The adjacent joint surfaces are removed with flat and curved sharp periosteal elevators similar to those used in spinal surgery. If possible, a small gouge is used to further roughen the surfaces and expose some cancellous bone. When correcting a

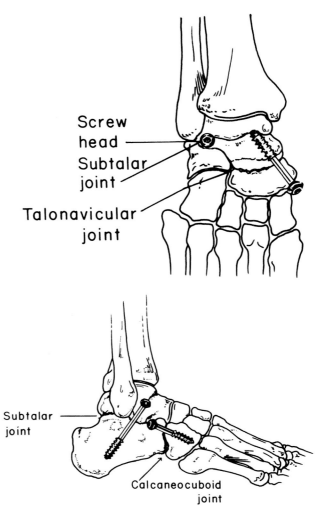

Fig. 5 Top, Following satisfactory preparation of the joint surfaces, a 6.5-mm cancellous screw can be used to hold the subtalar joint and the talonavicular joint. The subtalar joint is usually stabilized first. **Bottom,** Lateral view showing the placement of a 65-mm-long, 6.5-mm screw across the subtalar joint. Although it is more difficult, it is also possible to place a shorter screw across the calcaneocuboid joint.

severely deformed hindfoot, it is most helpful to fix the subtalar joint and talonavicular joint temporarily with 0.062-inch K-wires and to obtain an intraoperative radiograph to confirm proper positioning of the hindfoot joints. This avoids overcorrection or undercorrection of the deformity. The first screw is usually placed across the posterior facet of the subtalar joint. To do this, the anterior neck of the talus is exposed, usually through the longitudinal anterolateral incision or occasionally through a very small stab incision. It is necessary to place the drill hole for the screw near the anterior capsule of the ankle joint (Fig. 5). A 3.2-mm drill is directed inferiorly and posteriorly, aiming toward the posterior tuberosity of the calcaneus. Frequently, the drill can be seen as it crosses the posterior facet of the subtalar joint. If necessary, this position can be checked with an intraoperative lateral radiograph. A 6.5-mm cancellous bone screw that is approximately 65 mm long and is fitted with a washer is passed across the subtalar joint to gain solid purchase in the calcaneus. The 3.2-mm drill is inserted across the tuberosity of the navicular into the body of the talus, using the medial incision. Stabilization of this joint usually requires a 50-mm cancellous bone screw. A washer is used if the bone is osteoporotic (Fig. 6). A shorter screw (35 mm long) can also be placed across the calcaneocuboid joint, working through the distal portion of the lateral incision. The drill is directed distally and inferiorly from the anterior process of the calcaneus into the body of the cuboid.

After successful arthrodesis, it is simple, using local anesthesia, to remove the screw across the talonavicular joint. It is usually removed if it bothers the patient. Frequently, the screw across the posterior facet of the subtalar joint lies close to the ankle joint and should be removed after successful fusion (Fig. 6). It may be necessary to use small retractors to find the screw head, and patients generally find this procedure uncomfortable.

Some form of internal fixation is particularly helpful if only selected hindfoot joints require fusion. This is most common in rheumatoid patients who have selective involvement of the talonavicular joint (Fig. 7). Some patients require only arthrodesis of the transverse tarsal joints.

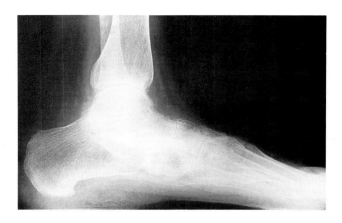

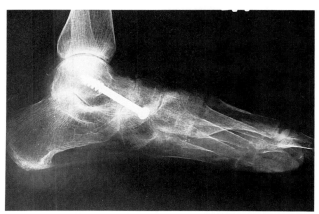

Fig. 7 **Top**, A lateral weightbearing radiograph of a 35-year-old rheumatoid patient with symptomatic involvement of only the talonavicular joint. **Bottom**, A lateral radiograph of the same patient with a 55-mm-long, 6.5-mm cancellous screw, which achieved a solid arthrodesis at the talonavicular joint.

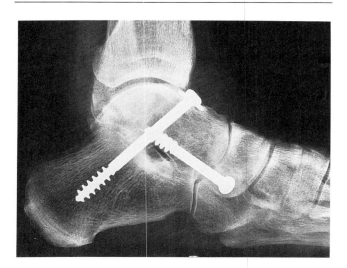

Fig. 6 A 55-year-old woman with rheumatoid arthritis who required a hindfoot arthrodesis. Her calcaneocuboid joint was uninvolved. A 6.5-mm cancellous screw was used with 16-mm threads. A washer was also required as the talus was somewhat osteoporotic. No washer was needed for the screw across the talonavicular joint. The position of the screw across the subtalar joint required its subsequent removal following solid arthrodesis.

Power-Driven Titanium Staple Fixation for Hindfoot Arthrodesis

Another method of internal fixation used to stabilize the talonavicular and calcaneocuboid joints in adults is the powered metaphyseal stapler system, which drives titanium staples into cancellous bone (Fig. 8).[8] These staples come in various widths and lengths sufficient to bridge the joints. The sizes most often used are 16 × 20 mm and 16 × 25 mm. Each cartridge contains five staples, and at least three or four should be used to secure each joint (Fig. 9). These staples are wide enough to bridge the subtalar joint in adults and children. If an inlay graft is used, especially in adults, the staple may not be wide enough to bridge the graft and both bones, but staples can still be used to stabilize the graft. This is done by placing one leg of a staple into the graft and the other leg into the calcaneus. A second staple is placed into the graft and the talus in the same way.

The joints are approached and the joint surfaces prepared as previously described. The subtalar joint is stabilized first, using one of the methods previously de-

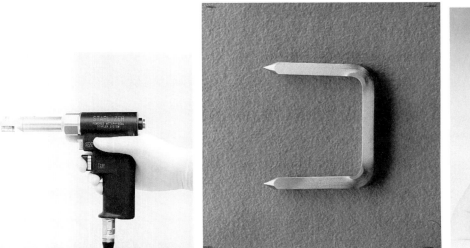
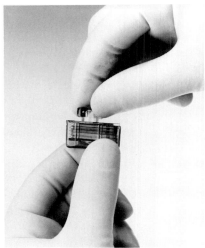

Fig. 8 **Left,** The power metaphyseal stapler system with the staple cartridge in the staplizer gun. The first trigger loads the staple into position, and the gun is fired by depressing the second trigger. **Center** and **Right,** A titanium staple and the staple cartridge, which contains five staples.

scribed. A 0.062-inch K-wire passed across the talonavicular joint provides temporary stability. A cartridge of staples is inserted into the gun, and the gun is tested to ensure that 100 to 110 mm Hg of nitrogen pressure is used to drive the staple. Optimally, four staples are placed across the talonavicular joint beginning medially and putting staples on the plantar and dorsal side of the joint. Similarly, staples of the same size are used to secure the calcaneocuboid joint. This method of internal fixation should not require supplemental fixation.

Subtalar Joint Bone Grafting

At times it is necessary to use a bone graft for subtalar joint arthrodesis. A bone graft is also used to help correct a valgus hindfoot deformity. Bone grafting may be needed if there is erosion of the joint, sometimes seen in rheumatoid arthritis, or if there is bone loss after a calcaneal fracture that involves the subtalar joint.

Three methods can be used to bone graft the subtalar joint. In the first method, the dowel method, a 12-mm Cloward drill is passed from lateral to medial across about 80% of the posterior facet of the subtalar joint.[6,7] A dowel cutter is then used to obtain a graft of the same diameter or a wider diameter from the iliac crest. The graft is impacted into the hole created by the drill.

In the second grafting procedure, a bicortical or tricortical graft is obtained from the iliac crest and impacted into a slot cut across the subtalar joint. This is similar to a Grice procedure. A 0.062-inch K-wire, or power-driven titanium staples, can be used to add stability to either graft. The wire, which passes across the neck of the talus and the graft and into the calcaneus, should be removed after about three weeks.

In the third procedure, the posterior facet of the subtalar joint is excised and the defect filled with a mass of bone graft. This technique requires internal fixation with either a large Steinmann pin or a 6.5-mm cancellous bone screw across the subtalar joint. Its use has been reported in an isolated talocalcaneal arthrodesis.[9]

Wound Closure and Postoperative Care

The wounds are carefully closed and skin staples are routinely used. Frequently, the lateral incision requires the use of interrupted mattress sutures, particularly in the midportion of the wound. Skin closure there may be difficult, particularly after correction of a significant valgus deformity. Two flat silicone drains are used in the lateral incision, and one is used in the medial incision. A soft dressing supplemented with a posterior plaster splint is used for the first two days. The foot and leg are elevated in a sling and the patient is instructed in nonweightbearing ambulation using bilateral upper-extremity support. Before leaving the hospital, the patient is placed in a short leg nonweightbearing cast. After a valgus deformity has been corrected, the ankle may be in equinus. The equinus, caused by a tight heel cord, is seen after the normal relationship among the talus, calcaneus, and navicular has been reestablished. The cast is usually changed approximately two weeks after the surgery, at which time the sutures are usually removed and the equinus position reduced if possible.

In general, a short leg nonweightbearing cast is used for six weeks. By this time the equinus contracture has been relieved and the foot is plantigrade. A short leg walking cast is then worn until the patient is fully weightbearing without hindfoot pain and the arthrodesis appears to be solid. This usually takes another five to six weeks.

Selection of Arthrodesis Technique for Hindfoot Joints

All three techniques described here are effective in achieving a solid hindfoot arthrodesis. Therefore, the selection of one of the procedures depends on the following variables. The surgeon must be familiar with a specific technique and the equipment used to perform the operation. Any hindfoot deformity present should be corrected, if possible. This requires freeing all three joints and keeping the forefoot plantigrade. In such cases a bone graft is usually necessary to supplement the subtalar joint. Stability across these arthrodesis sites can be best achieved using power-driven staples for the talonavicular and calcaneocuboid joints, 6.5-mm cancellous bone screws for the talonavicular and subtalar joints, a smooth Steinmann pin for the subtalar joint, and screws, staples, or a combination of the two for the transtarsal joints.

Techniques of Ankle Arthrodesis

Methods

Many methods for surgically fusing the ankle have been described over the years. Arthrodesis of the ankle gained importance about ten years ago when it became clear that cemented ankle implant arthroplasties had a high failure rate. Surgical techniques for ankle arthrodesis focus on two basic types of procedures, external fixation and, more recently, bone screws, used to fix the tibia and talus.

The use of external fixators was popularized by the Charnley device. As other fixator systems, including the Wagner, Hoffman, Day, and Calandruccio devices, were introduced for fixation of fractures or osteotomies, they were adapted and used for ankle fusion. These fixators vary in complexity but provide good stability to the ankle arthrodesis site. The main disadvantage of this method is the daily nursing care that the fixation pins require. Also, the fixator is bulky and may hamper ambulation, especially in a patient who has other musculoskeletal deformities.

The use of cancellous bone screws eliminates the need for external fixation pins. After this surgery, the ankle is usually placed in a short leg cast, which is generally well tolerated by the patient. However, there are some drawbacks to this method of arthrodesis. Bone quality must be good because the screws do not hold well in osteoporotic bone. The technique leaves no room for error and so the method must be precise. Once the screws are placed, the position of the arthrodesis is fixed and can be changed only by removing all the screws. Because the amount of talus for fixation of the screws is limited and the 6.5-mm cancellous bone screws create rather large holes, it may not be possible

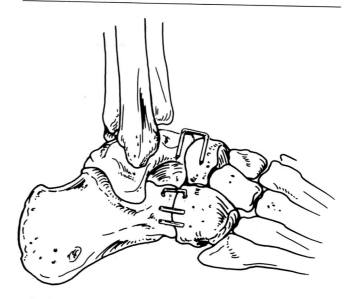

Fig. 9 A drawing of the staples in place across the calcaneocuboid joint and talonavicular joint. At least three or four staples should be used for each joint.

to insert enough screws a second time to gain solid fixation.

The Position of Ankle Arthrodesis

As important as a solid arthrodesis is the position in which the foot is placed.[10-12] It is generally accepted that in the best position the foot is plantigrade and at 90 degrees to the leg when viewed laterally, the heel is between neutral and about 7 degrees of valgus, and the foot should be in about 5 to 10 degrees of external rotation. If the patient has no other lower-extremity deformities or if only the subtalar joint is stiff, this is the position to select. In addition, the foot should be positioned well posterior to and beneath the leg. If the ankle is fused with the foot too far forward, gait will be abnormal because the patient will have to vault over the long lever of the foot. Another guideline used in ankle fusion is the position of the contralateral ankle, especially if it is normal. Its position may aid in determining the degree of external rotation in which the ankle is to be placed.

The ankle arthrodesis must not produce a varus of the hindfoot because this position abnormally loads the lateral side of the foot and because any varus of the hindfoot, especially the calcaneus, will lock the transtarsal joints—the talonavicular and calcaneocuboid joints—and thus inhibit the plantar-flexion motion these joints provide. Mazur and associates[11] measured 16 degrees ± 8 degrees of plantar flexion in these joints after ankle arthrodesis. When this motion exists before surgery, it is essential to maintain it. By positioning the talus in neutral or in 5 degrees of dorsiflexion, this amount of plantar flexion can compensate for some of

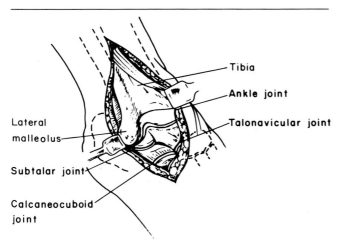

Tibia

Ankle joint

Talonavicular joint

Lateral malleolus

Subtalar joint

Calcaneocuboid joint

Fig. 10 The anterolateral exposure of the ankle joint, which can also be extended to expose the subtalar joint and the calcaneocuboid joint. (Reproduced with permission from Helal B, Wilson D (eds): *The Foot.* New York, Churchill Livingstone, 1988 pp 1205–1244.)

the plantar flexion and dorsiflexion lost by the ankle fusion. Therefore, properly positioning of the talus and the calcaneus maintains the existing transverse tarsal motion, giving the patient a better postoperative gait.

The ipsilateral knee may also be affected by the position of ankle arthrodesis. Patients with 5 to 10 degrees of fixed equinus develop knee recurvatum, although this can be compensated for by the heel height of the shoe.[11,12] Conversely, patients who have 10 to 20 degrees of flexion contracture of the knee should have the ankle fused in a position of neutral to 10 degrees of dorsiflexion. Patients with severe knee flexion contractures, such as are seen in rheumatoid arthritis, usually require knee arthroplasty, and this should be done before the ankle surgery.

When there is no motion of the hindfoot, as in patients with a previous triple arthrodesis, the result after ankle fusion will be a pantalar arthrodesis. Such ankles should be fused in 5 to 10 degrees of dorsiflexion. This position allows the patient to rise more easily from a chair and may allow such shoe modification as a rocker sole to be more effective.

Surgical Approaches for Ankle Arthrodesis

Anterior access to the ankle can be gained through a longitudinal skin incision. The joint is opened by an incision either through the bed of the anterior tibialis tendon or between the anterior tibialis tendon and the extensor hallucis longus. Alternatively, the deep dissection may proceed between the extensor hallucis longus and the extensor digitorum communis. When either of the latter two longitudinal incisions is used, care must be taken to avoid injuring the neurovascular bundle. The choice of anterior approach may be dictated by the abnormality or by previous incisions.

The traditional anterolateral approach to the ankle joint also gives excellent exposure (Fig. 10). The incision is longitudinal and parallels either the peroneus tertius or the most lateral extensor digitorum longus tendon. This incision is particularly useful if the subtalar joint is abnormal and if other surgical procedures to the hindfoot are contemplated.[7] If there is significant deformity medially, a short longitudinal medial incision on either side of the anterior tibialis tendon can be used for access to the medial side of the ankle joint.

If the distal fibula is to be used as a strut graft, the incision is placed closer to the fibula. The dissection must free the anterior 7 to 9 cm of the distal fibula. An oblique osteotomy of the proximal exposed fibula is performed from a distal lateral to proximal medial direction. The fibula can be retracted laterally, which aids in exposing the ankle joint.

A posterior approach is also a good alternative procedure for ankle arthrodesis.[13] With the patient in the prone position, the incision is made longitudinally just medial to the Achilles tendon. Care should be taken to avoid injury to the sural nerve. The ankle joint is approached after dividing the Achilles tendon, usually in a Z-fashion. The tibiotalar joint is exposed easily, and it is also possible to visualize the posterior facet of the subtalar joint. In the prone position, the patient's posterior iliac crest is available as an autogenous bone graft donor site. Additionally, the muscle bellies of the flexor hallucis longus and flexor digitorum communis overlie the fusion site and provide a suitable covering for the bone graft.

Preparation of the Articular Surfaces

If the height of the dome of the talus is satisfactory, a thin portion of the articular cartilage down through the subchondral bone can be removed with an oscillating saw. The cut surface should be at a right angle to the long axis of the tibia. Transecting the talus first facilitates exposure of the distal tibia. In a similar fashion, the distal tibial articular surface is removed with an oscillating saw with an appropriate blade width. If adhesions between the posterior tibia and the surrounding soft tissues make it difficult to remove the posterior portion of the distal tibial cut, the bone can be sectioned longitudinally and removed with rongeurs.

A narrower oscillating saw or narrow, flat osteotome can be used to remove articular cartilage from the inner surface of the medial malleolus and the corresponding medial side of the talus. These extra surfaces on the inside of the medial malleolus and the corresponding talus provide useful surfaces for arthrodesis. It is important not to displace the calcaneus medially beyond the weightbearing line of the lower extremity, a situation that might occur in a patient with a varus deformity. However, in a patient with a neutral foot or a valgus deformity, this small amount of medial displacement may help restore overall lower-extremity alignment. The resected surfaces are then further exposed by using an appropriate gouge to raise small amounts of subchondral cancellous bone. This procedure brings a wider surface of bone into apposition for the arthrodesis.

Conversely, it also possible to use a high-speed power burr to remove the articular cartilage on the dome of the talus and the tibia down to and through the subchondral bone until normal-appearing bleeding surfaces can be apposed. This method retains the curved surfaces of both the distal tibia and the talus. This procedure may be difficult to perform if an anterior or posterior incision is used, but is easy when a proximal fibula osteotomy allows this bone to be reflected posteriorly, thus allowing wide exposure of the ankle joint from the lateral side.

Bone Grafting Techniques for Ankle Arthrodesis

Routine use of a bone graft to achieve solid tibiotalar arthrodesis is unnecessary if satisfactory bone is present. However, if there is deficiency of either the distal tibia or the talus, an autogenous bone graft is used to supplement the arthrodesis site. In the past, the most common reason for extensive bone grafting was to salvage a failed total ankle replacement, which usually left a large rectangular defect on both sides of the joint. The best bone graft is autogenous iliac crest graft removed from either the anterior or the posterior iliac crest. With a wide defect, it is frequently necessary to section the iliac crest and then sandwich these grafts across the defect. Appropriately fashioned bone grafts are intrinsically stable initially, and their width provides enough distraction of the bony surfaces to give some temporary stability.

Supplemental bone can be used as needed, and autogenous iliac grafting in the form of corticocancellous chips is also helpful. With the posterior approach, it has been reported, processing the graft through a bone mill and then placing the composite along the posterior portion of the tibia and onto the calcaneus leads to a satisfactory tibiocalcaneal arthrodesis.[13]

It has also been reported that excision of the joint surfaces as a block and then replacing this block with a corresponding block of iliac graft provides an excellent ankle arthrodesis.[14]

Most ankle-fusion techniques also require the removal of some bone on either side of the joint. An interpositional bone graft can be used to make up this space. However, unless significant amounts of the talus or tibia are missing—as in a failed ankle implant—it is best to appose the prepared tibial surface to the talar surface because, in adults, the use of interpositional bone grafts delays the time to a secure arthrodesis.

The Effect of the Malleoli on Ankle Arthrodesis

Although some limb shortening is acceptable, a fused ankle that is too wide will prove bothersome. The malleoli, the main cause of this extra width, frequently rub against the counters of the shoe, which causes pain and makes shoe fitting difficult. Therefore, in planning an ankle arthrodesis, the final contour of the malleoli must be considered. The malleoli can be excised if necessary or, which may be preferable, they can be used as supplemental bone graft. Stewart and associates[15] described an arthrodesis technique that uses the medial and lateral malleoli as grafts while narrowing the ankle joint. The use of the distal fibula as a strut graft also narrows the joint area.[16] The medial malleolus can be partially excised, as described by Scranton,[17] leaving only the posterior third to protect the neurovascular bundle and the tendons.

External Fixator for Ankle Fusion

Clinical Considerations

An ankle arthrodesis of almost any type can be performed by means of an external fixator. An external fixator is recommended for a surgical procedure that requires extensive bone grafting because internal fixation is difficult with large bone grafts. In patients with bone of poor quality, such as those with osteoporosis, screws or other forms of internal fixation may be unstable, and only a fixator can give proper stability to the arthrodesis site. The use of a fixator requires cooperation from the patient as well as additional nursing care to keep fixation pins clean and avoid infection.

Surgical Technique

In stabilizing the ankle arthrodesis site with an external fixator, the pins usually traverse either the talus or the calcaneus in a mediolateral direction. Placement of the fixation pins distally and proximally is determined by surface landmarks and whatever instrument guides are available for the individual fixator. Therefore, the major incision to expose the joint is best placed either anterior or posterior.

An anterior incision through the bed of the anterior tibialis tendon sheath may be best if there is significant anteromedial deformity. Conversely, the anterolateral incision is preferable if there is lateral deformity or if the distal fibula is to be used as a supplemental graft. The posterior approach should be considered if the anterior skin is suboptimal, if there are previous scars that might affect healing, or if a tibiocalcaneal arthrodesis is to be performed. Whatever incision is used, the exposure must give a wide access to the joint so that the bony surfaces can be well prepared and bone grafts added if necessary.

After preparation of the bone surfaces, the fixator pins are placed. I find that the Calandruccio clamp[13] is easy to use and provides an effective system of external fixation for ankle arthrodesis. The 5-mm centrally threaded Steinmann pins are most effective and are drilled through the talus or the calcaneus from a medial to lateral direction, as previously described.[6] Care must be taken to avoid injury to the posterior tibial neurovascular bundle. If the most posterior pin is going to pass through the lateral malleolus, this part of the malleolus must be removed to allow effective compression of the posterior arthrodesis site. The tibial pins can be passed from medial to lateral so that the central, threaded part of the pin does not traverse the muscle bellies of the lateral compartment. After the fixator has been attached to the pins, a compressive force is applied to hold the bony surfaces rigidly together. Although it is difficult to calculate the exact amount of compression force, a good rule is to compress the site until it is stable enough to resist any mediolateral, anteroposterior, or rotary forces that are applied manually. Another guide is to watch the fixation pins as compression is applied. When the ends begin to bend toward each other, there is probably sufficient compressive force. Further compression will only continue to bend the pins. To minimize bulkiness, the fixator must be close to the leg, but sufficient room must remain between the skin and fixator to allow wound and pin care. Any compression or stretching of the skin around the pin must be released to avoid local skin necrosis, which might lead to bacterial contamination.

Wound closure is usually not a significant problem because in most cases the tibiotalar area is somewhat shortened by the arthrodesis. However, it is essential to have good wound closure. Because there is rarely sufficient room to use a suction drain effectively, flat silicone drains are used. A sterile dressing covers the wound and the pins. For a few days after surgery, the foot and leg can also be wrapped in a bulky cotton compression dressing. It is necessary to instruct the patient and usually some family member in pin care, which usually requires daily cleansing of each fixation pin. To provide a splint between the skin and the external compression apparatus, it may be best to wrap the pin with a sterile gauze. Follow-up at regular intervals is necessary to assess pin care and to note any difficulties with the wounds. If a pin tract becomes inflamed or infected, it must be treated with local debridement and oral antibiotics. If the local inflammation or infection continues, the pin should be removed. This usually occurs only if there has been some breakdown in care after surgery.

Removal of the External Fixator

Ankle arthrodeses vary regarding how long the external fixator remains in place. If the arthrodesis is done on a patient with good bone, if there are no postoperative complications, and if the fixator remains stable, the fixator can usually be removed approximately six weeks after surgery. Radiographs at that time typically indicate that the bony surfaces are well apposed, but they usually show no sign of fusion. In some cases it may be necessary to leave the fixator in place longer, particularly if there has been extensive bone grafting. It is difficult to state how long a fixator can remain in place, but usually there is little value to leaving a standard fixator in place much beyond eight to ten weeks after surgery. It is possible to add compression to the arthrodesis site by slowly tightening the fixator during the first few weeks after surgery. Another factor to consider is soft-tissue healing. If there is a wound problem or if a skin graft or other wound procedure has been used, it may be helpful to leave the fixator in place for a longer period.

Removal of the fixator is usually uncomfortable for the patient, but a local anesthetic injected about the pins is helpful. A 22-gauge needle is passed along the pin until it touches the junction of the pin and bone. Next, a small amount of local anesthetic without epinephrine is injected to anesthetize the soft tissues and the periosteum. Although this gives relief, some pain and the sensation of a large pin being removed will remain. A sedative given intravenously will allow a smooth and nontraumatic removal of large pins.

After removal of the pins, the wounds are dressed and the leg is placed in a walking cast. Typically, the pins are removed at six weeks and a walking cast worn for an additional six weeks. While in the walking cast, the patient is encouraged to use crutches or a walker. As soon as the ankle site is painless or has minimal pain with weightbearing, the patient can start using a cane. One sign of adequate healing that permits removal of the cast is the patient's ability to bear full weight and walk comfortably in the cast. On removal of the cast, radiographs are made to check the arthrodesis site. These should show some bony trabeculae crossing the arthrodesis site. If there is some question, the patient can try to walk without a cast, using either crutches or a walker. If pain returns, the cast should be reapplied for at least another three weeks.

Internal Fixation for Ankle Arthrodesis With Bone Screws

Clinical Considerations

This method can be used for ankle arthrodesis in most patients[18] as long as the bone quality permits the screws to hold the arthrodesis site securely. Severe osteoporosis or bone loss requiring extensive grafts can pose a problem in using screws for internal fixation. Internal fixation may make postoperative ambulation easier for certain patients, particularly if they have arthritic deformities of the hip or knee and an abnormal gait. Such patients may find it difficult to walk while wearing a bulky external fixator.

Surgical Technique

The anterolateral approach gives excellent exposure to the ankle joint. Placing the screws usually requires a short longitudinal incision just above the medial malleolus to expose that portion of the tibia for insertion of a screw. If a screw is to be placed through the posterior malleolus, a posterior incision is also required.

Selection and Placement of Screws For use across the tibiotalar joint,[7] the 6.5-mm cancellous bone screws are ideal for strength because the talus and calcaneus are mostly cancellous bone. In general, the screws usually pass from the tibia into the talus (Fig. 11). Depending on the size of the talus, screws with either the 16-mm thread or the 32-mm thread can be used. It is essential that these screws be long enough so that the thread does not cross the arthrodesis site. For this reason, the screw with the 16-mm thread is commonly used. A 3.2-mm drill bit is used to make the preliminary hole. If the cortex of the tibia is particularly thick, then tapping the entry hole may facilitate placement of the screw. If the cortex has been weakened, a metal washer should be used.

After the proper position for ankle arthrodesis has been achieved, it is frequently helpful to stabilize that position while the screws are being placed. This stability can be achieved by placing a smooth Steinmann pin through a small stab incision on the plantar surface of the heel and passing it through the calcaneus and the posterior talus up into the tibia. This pin temporarily transfixes the arthrodesis site while the first screw is placed. Another method uses 3.2-mm drills as temporary fixation devices. After the surfaces are positioned, a 3.2-mm drill is passed from the dorsomedial aspect of the tibia across the arthrodesis site and into the talus. A second 3.2-mm drill is then passed from the lateral aspect of the tibia approximately 2 to 3 inches above the arthrodesis site, placed to avoid the first drill bit. If the bone quality is satisfactory, these two drill bits

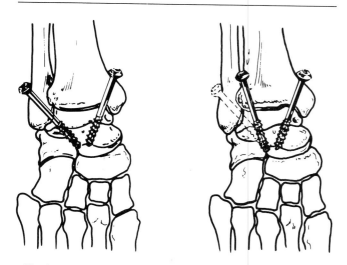

Fig. 11 Ankle arthrodesis using 6.5-mm cancellous screws across the tibiotalar joint. (Reproduced with permission from Helal B, Wilson D (eds): *The Foot.* New York, Churchill Livingstone, 1988 pp 1205–1244.)

afford temporary fixation. At this point it is a good idea to check the position of the ankle and the drills radiographically. This is particularly helpful in preventing the placement of screws across the posterior facet of the subtalar joint. If the radiographic assessment shows that all is satisfactory, the first drill bit is removed and a 6.5-mm cancellous bone screw of the appropriate length is inserted. Before final tightening of that screw, the second drill bit is removed and the second screw inserted in that hole. These two screws may be sufficient to hold the arthrodesis site[18] (Fig. 11), but other factors will determine whether further fixation is necessary. A third screw, usually shorter than the others, can be placed from the anterior tibia into the talus.

Fibular Strut-Graft Technique Additional fixation can be achieved by using a fibular strut graft (Fig. 12). Using an oscillating saw, the fibula is transected obliquely from distal lateral to proximal medial, approximately 7 to 9 cm above the tip of the lateral malleolus. The fibula can then be placed against the bony surface of the lateral talus as well as the tibia. In this position, the fibula can be transfixed as a strut graft. The lateral malleolus and the lateral side of the talus are cleared of their articular surfaces. A short 16-mm thread screw is then placed across the distal lateral malleolus into the talus, and the proximal portion of the strut graft is transfixed to the tibia using a 3.5-mm or a standard 4.5-mm cortical screw. The cortical screw is useful proximally because the cancellous bone of the distal tibia is frequently insufficient to hold the 6.5-mm cancellous screw. Therefore, passing the cortical screw through the medial cortex of the tibia, much as one would do in holding a plate to the bone, may provide greater stability. It may be preferable to insert the proximal screw first, then, while compressing the talus against the tibia, insert the distal screw.

Alternative Methods of Screw Placement Another method uses a 6.5-mm cancellous bone screw placed through the posterior malleolus and into the neck of the talus (S.T. Hansen, personal communication, 1986). Although the patient must be positioned prone or laterally to allow surgical access to the posterior lateral ankle, this disadvantage is offset by the good quality of the bone of the posterior tibia. The screw is directed into the lateral side of the neck of the talus, where the cancellous bone is usually of the best quality. Of equal importance, this screw also properly positions the talus in its anteroposterior alignment and prevents it from being placed too far anteriorly. Again, it is important to remember that the position achieved at the conclusion of this procedure will be the final position for the arthrodesis.

The screws may also be placed through the lateral incision alone. In some patients a screw can be placed through the talus, beginning at the sinus tarsi, and directed medially and superiorly into the tibia (Fig. 13).

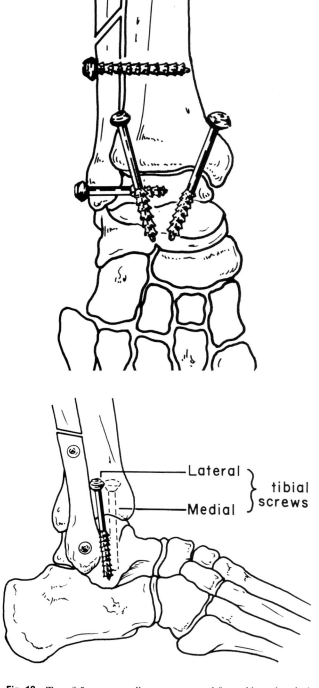

Fig. 12 **Top,** 6.5-mm cancellous screws used for ankle arthrodesis also utilizing a fibular strut graft. The proximal screw in the fibular strut is a cortical screw and should traverse both cortices of the tibia. The fibula should be displaced as close to the tibia and talus as possible to narrow the ankle joint area postoperatively. **Bottom,** A lateral view of the fibular strut used to supplement the ankle arthrodesis.

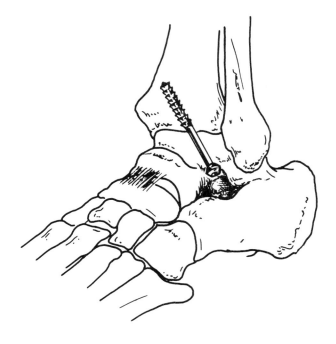

Fig. 13 Placement of a 6.5-mm cancellous screw from the talus into the tibia beginning in the area of the sinus tarsi. Additional screws necessary for internal fixation can be placed laterally from the tibia into the talus. A fibular strut graft can also be employed if needed.

Other screws are then placed across the ankle joint from the lateral side of the tibia and the fibula as required to gain solid internal fixation.

Postoperative Care

Patients should be instructed that after the cast is removed some swelling will occur about the foot and ankle. An elastic ankle support or some other form of external support should be prescribed: this is replaced later by a support-type stocking. The swelling usually begins to recede after a few weeks, especially after the patient is able to walk more. Because of this swelling, it is unwise to prescribe any type of special shoe immediately after the cast is removed. Meanwhile, the patient can protect the foot by wearing a wide athletic-type shoe. Support, by crutches or a cane, will assist in ambulation. These problems in walking after the cast is removed should be explained to the patient.

Many patients prefer to wear their own shoes after surgery. If they have minimal other deformities or if only the tibiotalar joint was arthritic, they may do well. However, during the first six to 12 months after the fusion many patients have difficulty wearing shoes. Several factors should be considered when assessing the patient after surgery. Leg length should be measured with the patient standing to determine the degree of functional shortening. Usually 1 to 1.5 cm of shortening will not affect the patient's gait. Shortening beyond this may require use of a lift. The patient should be examined to determine if there is any transverse tarsal motion. If there is between 10 and 20 degrees of motion, the patient will probably do well in any standard shoe. If there is significant loss of the dome of the talus, so that the malleoli impinge on the shoe counters, this may require a shoe modification. The most helpful shoe modifications are a modified solid-ankle, cushion heel (S.A.C.H.) and a rocker-bottom sole. A full solid-ankle, cushion heel is usually too unstable, but a wedge of material inserted into the body of the heel will cushion heel strike. The rocker sole aids the patient in the stance phase of gait. However, in most cases in which ankle arthrodesis was successful and the patient has no other significant deformity, the patient within one year will be able to use a standard shoe that he or she finds acceptable.

References

1. Wilson DW: Hallux valgus and rigidus, in Helal B, Wilson D (eds): *The Foot.* New York, Churchill Livingstone, 1988, vol 1, pp 411–483.
2. Sykes A, Hughes AW: A biomechanical study using cadaveric toes to test the stability of fixation techniques employed in arthrodesis of the first metatarsophalangeal joint. *Foot Ankle* 1986;7:18–25.
3. Coughlin MJ, Mann RA: Arthrodesis of the first metatarsophalangeal joint as salvage for the failed Keller procedure. *J Bone Joint Surg* 1987;69A:68–75.
4. Mann RA, Thompson FM: Arthrodesis of the first metatarsophalangeal joint for hallux valgus in rheumatoid arthritis. *J Bone Joint Surg* 1984;66A:687–692.
5. Turan I, Lindgren U: Compression-screw arthrodesis of the first metatarsophalangeal joint of the foot. *Clin Orthop* 1987;221:292–295.
6. Cracchiolo A III: Surgery for rheumatoid disease: Part I. Foot abnormalities in rheumatoid arthritis, in Murray JA (ed): American Academy of Orthopaedic Surgeons *Instructional Course Lectures, XXXIII.* St. Louis, CV Mosby, 1984, pp 386–404.
7. Cracchiolo A: Operative technique of the ankle and hindfoot, in Helal B, Wilson D (eds): *The Foot.* New York, Churchill Livingstone, 1988, vol 2, pp 1205–1244.
8. Östgaard H-C, Herberts P: Evaluation of the 3M staplizer: A new internal fixation system. *Injury* 1988;19:28–30.
9. Russotti GM, Cass JR, Johnson KA: Isolated talocalcaneal arthrodesis: A technique using moldable bone graft. *J Bone Joint Surg* 1988;70A:1472–1478.
10. Buck P, Morrey BF, Chao EY: The optimum position of arthrodesis of the ankle: A gait study of the knee and ankle. *J Bone Joint Surg* 1987;69A:1052–1062.
11. Mazur JM, Schwartz E, Simon SR: Ankle arthrodesis: Long-term follow-up with gait analysis. *J Bone Joint Surg* 1979;61A:964–975.
12. King HA, Watkins TB Jr, Samuelson KM: Analysis of foot position in ankle arthrodesis and its influence on gait. *Foot Ankle* 1980;1:44–49.
13. Russotti GM, Johnson KA, Cass JR: Tibiotalocalcaneal arthrodesis for arthritis and deformity of the hind part of the foot. *J Bone Joint Surg* 1988;70A:1304–1307.
14. Campbell CJ, Rinehart WT, Kalenak A: Arthrodesis of the ankle: Deep autogenous inlay grafts with maximum cancellous-bone apposition. *J Bone Joint Surg* 1974;56A:63–70.
15. Stewart MJ, Beeler TC, McConnell JC: Compression arthrodesis of the ankle: Evaluation of a cosmetic modification. *J Bone Joint Surg* 1983;65A:219–225.
16. Wilson HJ Jr: Arthrodesis of the ankle: A technique using bilateral hemimalleolar onlay grafts with screw fixation. *J Bone Joint Surg* 1969;51A:775–777.
17. Scranton PE Jr: Use of internal compression in arthrodesis of the ankle. *J Bone Joint Surg* 1985;67A:550–555.
18. Morgan CD, Henke JA, Bailey RW, et al: Long-term results of tibiotalar arthrodesis. *J Bone Joint Surg* 1985;67A:546–550.

Hindfoot Arthrodeses

Kenneth A. Johnson, MD

Introduction

In my experience, when an orthopaedic surgeon sees a patient who may require arthrodesis of the hindfoot, three questions will be discussed in detail. These have to do with when the surgery should be done, if it is to be done; the extent of the arthrodesis, if indicated; and which procedure would be best for this patient.

Indications

Pain is the primary indication for a surgical procedure of this type. In this situation, the relevant question is whether or not the pain significantly affects the person's lifestyle. The answer must take into account personality, occupation, and recreational factors. Furthermore, if the pain is described by the patient as significant, but physical examination and radiographic study provide no correlating objective findings, then surgery should be deferred.

Finally, there should be no contraindications. Vascular, metabolic, and infection problems may militate against surgical treatment. Age, on the other hand, is a minor consideration. Although it is true that a hindfoot arthrodesis necessitates about three months of cast immobilization, an older patient in good health might well be a good candidate for surgery.

Extent

In the past, the triple arthrodesis was the most common procedure. The theory of triple arthrodesis was based on the functional interrelationship of the talo-

calcaneal, calcaneocuboid, and talonavicular joints. For a long time, it was thought that if one of the triad underwent arthrodesis, the others would soon become painful and a further procedure would have to be done. Indeed, if the technique of arthrodesis caused malalignment of the other joints of the triad, then such subsequent fusions were likely. Trying to appose bone surfaces after resecting joints invariably led to such malalignments. An alternative method of arthrodesis, which involves insertion of bone graft to make up for the resected surfaces, does not lead to adjacent joint malalignments. This chapter presents such a technique.

The concept of fusing only the degenerated or deformed joint of the hindfoot seems to be increasingly more accepted.[1] The talocalcaneal (subtalar), calcaneocuboid, or talonavicular joints may be individually treated, or a combination of any two of the three may be used.

In my practice, the single talocalcaneal arthrodesis is the procedure most frequently used. Indications for this arthrodesis include conditions such as posttraumatic talocalcaneal joint arthrosis, acquired adult flatfoot attributed to dysfunction of the posterior tibial muscle, nonunion after an unsuccessful arthrodesis attempt, talocalcaneal coalition, rheumatoid arthritis, cerebral palsy, and residual talipes equinovarus.

Occasionally, the talonavicular joint or, less frequently, the calcaneocuboid joint undergoes individual arthrodesis for localized arthrosis. It should be noted that when the talonavicular alone is fused, motion at the other two joints is markedly restricted. This is probably because motion of the three joints is closely coupled, and restriction of one affects all three.

Less frequently, a formal triple arthrodesis will be

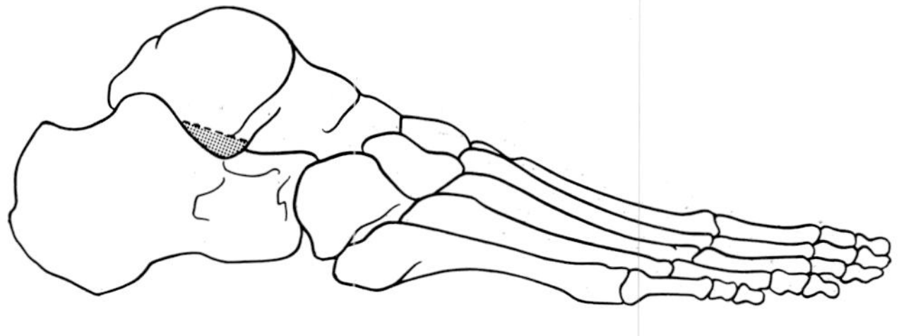

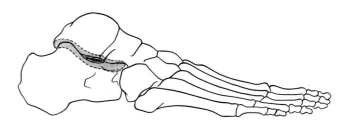

Fig. 1 Excision of the anterior process of the posterior talus facet allows access for posterior facet resection.

Fig. 2 Cortical and articular surface is removed from the subtalar region. Removal begins just posterior to the calcaneocuboid joint and extends through the funnel-shaped sinus tarsi back into the posterior facet.

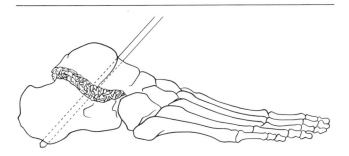

Fig. 3   With the ankle in dorsiflexion, a Steinmann pin is inserted across the neck of the talus into the calcaneus.

used. The indication is usually a very late severe pes planus of unknown cause. In such a condition, degeneration involves all three joints and the deformity is so severe that a triple procedure is necessary. This chapter gives surgical techniques for arthrodesis of the talocalcaneal (subtalar) arthrodesis as well as the triple, or combined talocalcaneal-calcaneocuboid-talonavicular, arthrodesis.

Procedure

In older textbooks that include techniques for an isolated subtalar or a triple arthrodesis, the diagrams show neat and straight bone surface resections. A final fixation diagram usually shows everything fitting together in an anatomic corrected position. In my experience, using the textbook diagram as a guideline usually gave a result that was disappointing. As the technique of the moldable bone graft evolved, surgeons discovered the advantages of this method of arthro-

desis. Using it, the union rate for the isolated subtalar arthrodesis is 98%.[1] I feel that the triple arthrodesis will also have a good union rate. The moldable bone graft technique is applicable to either a varus or a valgus hindfoot deformity. It is no longer necessary to attempt to take a medially based wedge resection of the subtalar joint through a lateral incision for a hindfoot valgus deformity. The moldable technique is particularly helpful for the triple, where it allows sequential correction of a deformed hindfoot. Each aspect of the hindfoot abnormality is corrected through a separate joint rather than at a single arthrodesis site. Fixation is easy. The stout Steinmann pins used are subsequently removed, and no metal that might cause problems for the patient remains in the foot.

Talocalcaneal, or Subtalar, Arthrodesis Technique

The patient is placed in the supine position with a sandbag under the ipsilateral hip and a pneumatic tourniquet on the ipsilateral thigh. A 6-cm slightly oblique incision is directed along the lateral aspect of the hindfoot over the region of the sinus tarsi. The sural nerve and peroneal tendons, lying posteroinferiorly to the

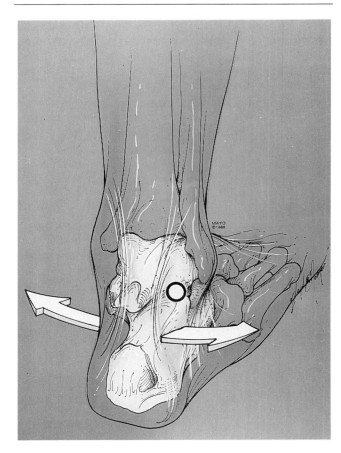

Fig. 5   The arthrodesis of the talocalcaneal joint establishes hindfoot varus-valgus position. (Reproduced with permission from the Mayo Foundation.)

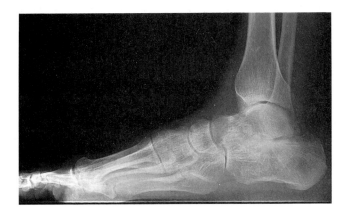

Fig. 4   A completed subtalar arthrodesis is seen on radiograph. Only the posterior portion of the posterior talocalcaneal facet remains ununited.

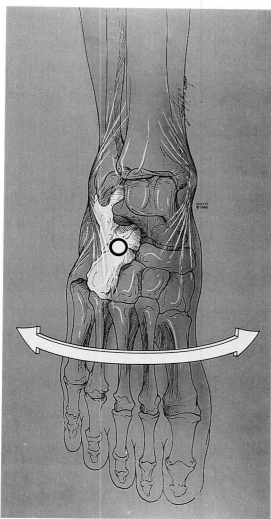

Fig. 6 Positioning of the calcaneocuboid joint arthrodesis determines forefoot abduction-adduction. (Reproduced with permission from the Mayo Foundation.)

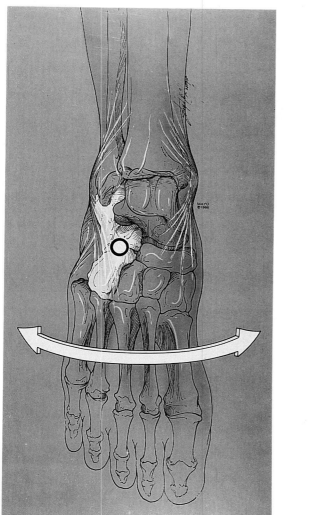

Fig. 7 Rotation at the talonavicular joint establishes the metatarsal heads in a transverse position. (Reproduced with permission from the Mayo Foundation.)

incision, are protected. The extensor digitorum brevis origin is reflected from the calcaneus and retracted distally. The sinus tarsi is then visualized and cleared of soft tissue.

The anteroinferior process of the posterior facet of the talus is identified and excised (Fig. 1). The talocalcaneal joint surfaces are denuded of articular cartilage and cortical bone, beginning adjacent to the surfaces of the calcaneocuboid and talonavicular joints and extending into the posterior subtalar facet (Fig. 2). Removal of the articular cartilage and subchondral bone creates a gap approximately 5 mm in height between the talus and the calcaneus.

A unicortical autogenous bone graft is taken from the outer aspect of the ipsilateral anterior iliac crest and is morsellized, using a bone mill. The resultant

bone morsels are packed into the prepared host bed between the talus and the calcaneus. If there has been adequate resection of cortical bone and cartilage from the talocalcaneal joint surfaces, the surgeon can position the calcaneus beneath the talus in the position desired. Thorough resection of the joint surfaces is also important to encourage union at the arthrodesis site. The correct alignment of the hindfoot in regard to varus or valgus depends on the surgeons's judgment. Any varus or valgus deformity of the hindfoot present before surgery can be corrected at this time.

When the surgeon is satisfied with the position of the hindfoot, a longitudinal 1-cm incision is made slightly lateral to the anterior tibialis tendon just above the neck of the talus. A 0.4-cm smooth Steinmann pin or a 6.5-mm cancellous bone screw of appropriate

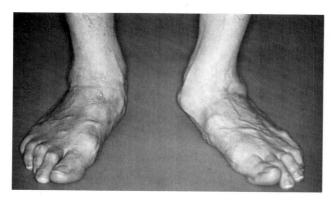

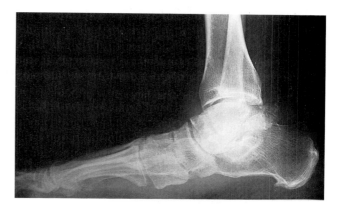

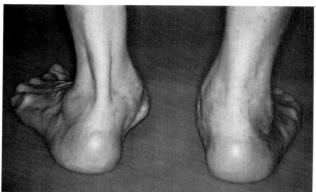

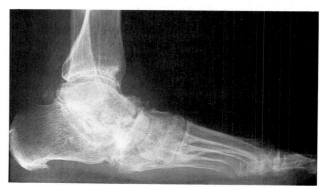

Fig. 8   Top, This 70-year-old man had a symmetric deformity of his feet with incapacitating pain. This photograph was taken six months after his right triple arthrodesis and before his left triple arthrodesis. **Bottom**, A posterior view of the same man shows realignment of the right foot after surgery. The left foot shows the position that, before surgery, was also present in the right foot.

Fig. 9   Top, A lateral radiograph shows the left hindfoot position before triple arthrodesis. **Bottom**, After triple arthrodesis, the radiograph shows the foot in a plantigrade position.

length is directed through the neck of the talus and into the calcaneus (Fig. 3). It is recommended that the hindfoot be stabilized in approximately 5 degrees of valgus if the forefoot is mobile. If the forefoot is rigid, the correct position of the hindfoot is one that places the metatarsal heads parallel to the floor in the plantigrade position.

Final packing of the bone graft into the host bed between the talus and the calcaneus is now completed. Excessive bone graft should not be placed laterally, as this may subsequently cause symptoms by impinging on the distal fibula. The wound is closed in standard fashion. If a Steinmann pin is used, it is cut off beneath the skin on the dorsum of the foot but is left accessible to palpation for subsequent extraction. A bulky compression dressing with a stirrup plaster splint that immobilizes the hindfoot is applied.

On about the third day after surgery, the compression dressing is replaced by a below-knee, nonweightbearing cast. At approximately six weeks, the Steinmann pin or cancellous bone screw is removed under local anesthesia, and a below-knee walking cast is ap-

plied for an additional four weeks. After the cast is removed, ten weeks after surgery (Fig. 4), an elastic compression stocking is worn with a stiff-soled shoe, and the patient is allowed to walk with gradually increasing weightbearing. No formal physical therapy is required.

Talocalcaneal-Talonavicular-Calcaneocuboid, or Triple, Arthrodesis Technique

For this arthrodesis, the same moldable bone graft technique is used as for the talocalcaneal arthrodesis. The lateral incision over the sinus tarsi is slightly less oblique so that the calcaneocuboid joint is easily exposed along with the talocalcaneal joint. The subtalar joint is cleared of cortical and articular surface in the same way used for the subtalar arthrodesis. In addition, the surfaces of the calcaneocuboid joint are also resected down to cancellous bone. Enough of the calcaneocuboid surface is removed so that any forefoot adduction deformity can be straightened by shortening the lateral column of the foot.

For the talonavicular joint, a second incision is made dorsally in the safe interval between the tibialis anterior and extensor hallucis longus tendons. Because the talonavicular is a deeply convex-concave joint, it is necessary to remove the talar dome at the level of the dorsal joint line and to perform the osteotomy on the navicular beyond the depth of its concave joint apex in order to obtain good bone apposition.

With all three joints adequately removed, the hindfoot will be pliable and ready for sequential repositioning. The bone graft is prepared in a morsellated slurry just as it was for the talocalcaneal arthrodesis. Some bone graft is placed in the posterior facet region of the subtalar joint. With the surgeons's attention focused on the subtalar varus-valgus position, the talocalcaneal arthrodesis site is placed in about 5 degrees of valgus (Fig. 5). The 0.4-cm Steinmann pin is inserted through the neck of the talus into the calcaneus to fix this joint.

Next the calcaneocuboid joint is positioned. Through this joint the forefoot abduction-adduction is realigned (Fig. 6). With the lateral border of the foot straight, another 0.4-cm Steinmann pin is inserted through the cuboid into the calcaneus.

Finally, the forefoot rotation is aligned through the resected talonavicular joint (Fig. 7). The forefoot rotation is adjusted so that the line of metatarsal weightbearing is transverse to the tibia, and this joint area is stabilized with a third Steinmann pin.

The foot has now been sequentially positioned with proper alignment of hindfoot varus-valgus through the talonavicular joint, forefoot abduction-adduction at the calcaneocuboid region, and forefoot rotation determined by positioning of the talonavicular arthrodesis site. I find this technique easier (Fig. 8) than trying to resect the surfaces and collapse the hindfoot into the proper position.

When the foot is correctly repositioned, bone graft is packed into each resection area with finger pressure, and the three Steinmann pins are cut off just beneath the skin (Fig. 9). Postoperative care is the same as for the talocalcaneal arthrodesis described above.

Summary

In summary then, pain is the primary indication for a hindfoot arthrodesis procedure. Arthrodesis is performed only on those joints that show degeneration or significant deformity. Finally, the technique described uses a moldable bone graft. This technique is applicable both for an isolated talocalcaneal joint arthrodesis and for triple arthrodeses.

Reference

1. Russotti GM, Cass JR, Johnson KA: Isolated talocalcaneal arthrodesis: A technique using moldable bone graft. *J Bone Joint Surg* 1988;70A:1472–1478.

Ankle Fractures

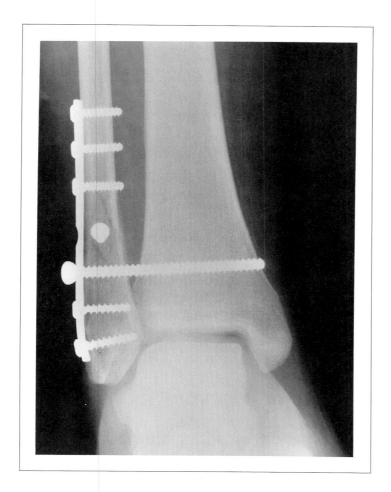

The Pathogenesis and Treatment of Ankle Fractures: Historical Studies

Frank C. Wilson, MD

"Our ancestors deserve our best thanks for the assistance they have given us; where we find them to be right we are obliged to embrace their opinions as truths; but implicit faith is not required from man to man, and our reverence for our predecessors must not prevent us from making our own judgements," Percivall Pott,[1] 1768.

Before the 1900s, knowledge of ankle injuries was based on clinical observation and cadaver experimentation, although the significance of these early observations is clouded by ambiguous terminology and by the failure of the authors to distinguish experimental findings from clinical impressions. Considering that these investigators had neither radiography nor the opportunity for direct observation (except at autopsy), their work is often remarkably insightful; however, it was not until the 20th century that radiography, open treatment, and the science of biomechanics allowed a more complete understanding of the pathomechanics of ankle injuries.

Although scattered reports may be found before the work of Sir Percivall Pott,[1] his *Some Few General Remarks on Fractures and Dislocations*, published in 1768, was the first to relate clinical findings to pathology. Even then it was almost an afterthought, because Pott was primarily concerned with promulgating his concept of relieving muscle spasm by immobilization in the flexed position. Only in his discussion of that topic did he mention a fracture of the fibula, which he described as occurring "within two or three inches of its lower extremity"and accompanied by a tear of the deltoid ligament and lateral subluxation of the talus (Fig. 1). As he ascribed the injury only to "leaping or jumping," no statement can be made as to the direction of the force that produced it; and by failing to include the syndesmotic injury that must accompany such a lesion, Pott actually described a fracture that does not exist. Following this description, the name "Pott's fracture" has been applied to bimalleolar fractures—an unfortunate usage because, in Pott's case, neither malleolus was broken. Because of these inaccuracies, Pott's eminence in the field of ankle fractures is probably undeserved, although he was the first to describe the clinical findings in what we now recognize as a classic injury pattern.

From Pott's work until the study of Ashhurst and Bromer[2] in 1922, most studies on the production of ankle injuries were carried out by the French, beginning with Jean-Pierre David,[3] who in 1771 provided the

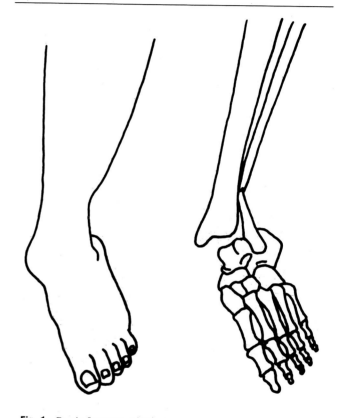

Fig. 1 Pott's fracture, 1768.

first description of the production of fractures by indirect (*contre-coup*) forces.

Although he failed to acknowledge the influence of Boyer, Guillaume Dupuytren,[4] in 1816, using cadaver experiments for the first time, produced ankle fractures by abduction and adduction. Concentrating his studies on "outward movement" (abduction) of the foot, Dupuytren reproduced, at a slightly higher level, the fibular fracture observed by Pott. Although he did not comment generally on the relationship of such a fibular fracture to damage of the syndesmotic structures, he did cite one case in which the talus was dislocated outward and upward, which "left no doubt that the ligaments connecting the tibia and fibula were torn through." He found this lesion to be extremely rare, occurring only once in some 200 cases. The French speak of the "high Dupuytren" lesion, referring to a transverse or short oblique fracture at the junction of the middle and distal thirds of the fibula accompanied by disruption of the syndesmosis, and a "low Dupuytren" fracture, which refers to a mediolaterally directed short oblique fracture of the lateral malleolus either just above the attachments of torn tibiofibular ligaments or just below the attachment of intact ligaments. It is thus legitimate to credit Dupuytren for emphasizing the role of abduction in the production of ankle injuries, although most of the "high Dupuytren" lesions are undoubtedly accompanied by an element of external rotation. As suggested by Nélaton's[5] illustration in 1844 of the Dupuytren fracture (Fig. 2), it is the high lesion, with or without intercrural dislocation of the talus, that most deserves designation as the Du-

puytren fracture, although because of the confusion it is probably wiser to avoid the eponym altogether.

Maisonneuve,[6] a pupil of Dupuytren, was the first, and almost only, writer before the 20th century to recognize the importance of external rotation in the production of ankle fractures and to characterize both the ligamentous and bony lesions that accompany this mechanism. In the 1840s he clarified the relationship between ligamentous injury and fracture pattern, organized fracture patterns into groups, and suggested that treatment be based on mechanism of injury. In cadaver experiments, he showed that the level of the fibular fracture was determined by the strength of the syndesmosis. He felt that the forces developed were usually resisted by the anterior tibiofibular ligament, producing an oblique fracture of the fibula beginning anteriorly just below the (intact) ligament and extending posterosuperiorly to just above the attachment of the posterior tibiofibular ligament (Fig. 3). (Because this fracture begins below and ends above the level of the tibial plafond, it has been labeled the "mixed oblique" fracture.) Maisonneuve demonstrated that if

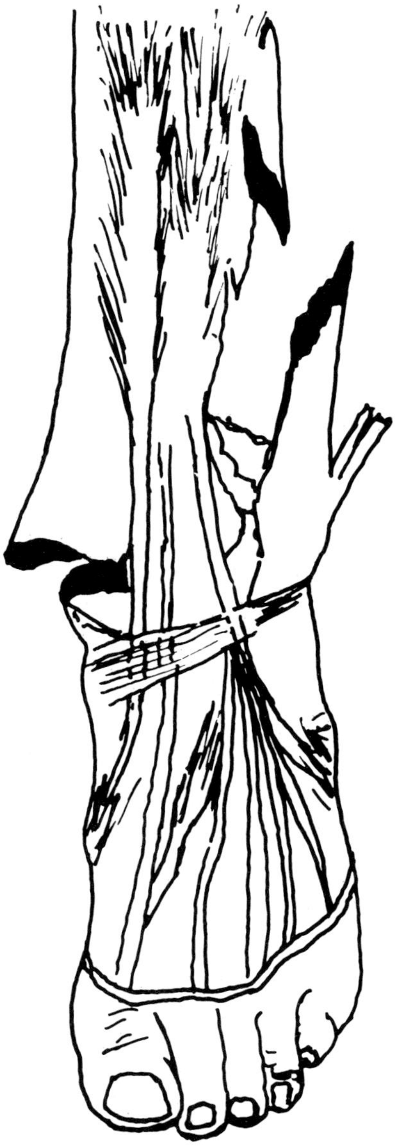

Fig. 2 Dupuytren's fracture, illustrated by Nélaton, 1844.

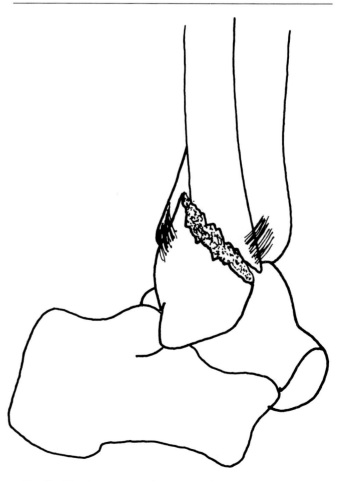

Fig. 3 The low external rotation fracture, described by Maisonneuve.

the anterior tibiofibular ligament yields first, the fibular fracture can occur as high as the proximal third of the fibula, producing the fracture that bears his name (Fig. 4). He failed to comment upon the likelihood of an associated tear of the interosseous membrane, perhaps because he considered that rupture of the anterior inferior tibiofibular ligament alone was sufficient to permit the proximal fibular fracture. Although overshadowed in reputation by Dupuytren, Maisonneuve made the single most important contribution to understanding the pathogenesis of ankle injuries.

Huguier[7] reproduced Maisonneuve's external rotation experiments in 1848, noting rupture of the interosseous membrane as far proximally as the fibular neck fracture.

Almost 30 years later, Hönigschmied,[8] who carried out the largest series (125) of cadaver experiments, studied the effect of external rotation in 22 specimens. He found that the fibula can fracture without ligamentous rupture, and that diastasis can occur without fracture or rupture of the posterior tibiofibular ligament. Among six cases with fibular fracture, two fractures occurred in the upper third, but in no case was the interosseous membrane ruptured higher than "the middle of the leg." Pankovich[9] found that rupture of the interosseous membrane invariably accompanied the Maisonneuve fracture, although he did not specify the proximal extent of the rupture.

To Tillaux[10] (1848) must go credit for describing the fracture fragment avulsed from the inferolateral corner of the tibia by the tibiofibular ligament, although he did not state whether this *"fragment troisième"* was anterolateral or posterolateral. His drawings show both, and it may be presumed that either the anterior or posterior tibial tubercles could be the source of Tillaux's third fragment. It is noteworthy that this third (anterior) fragment was depicted, without comment, in Astley Cooper's[11] 1822 treatise on fractures (Fig. 5).

Wagstaffe,[12] in 1875, reported the rarely encountered fibular counterpart of the Tillaux fracture, although he did not comment on the mechanism of its production. Le Fort[13] described this lesion more fully in 1886, and the injury was confirmed experimentally by his pupil, LeRoy.[14] Both LeRoy and Le Fort interpreted the mechanism as supination and adduction rather than the more probable external rotation.

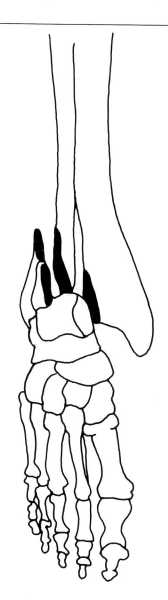

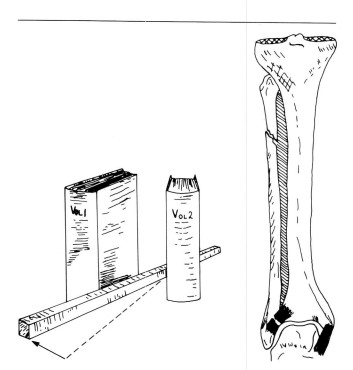

Fig. 4 The (high) Maisonneuve fracture, 1840.

Fig. 5 The Tillaux fracture (avulsion fracture) from the inferolateral corner of the tibia.

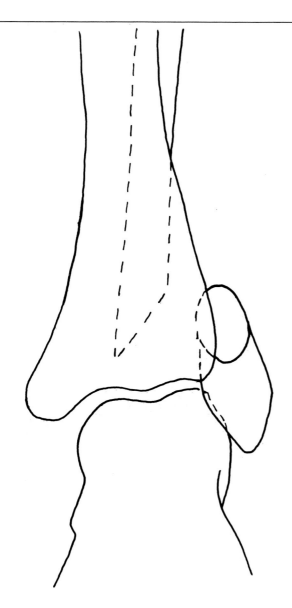

Fig. 6   Bosworth fracture, 1947.

Sir Astley Cooper[11] was the first to call attention to articular fractures of the posterior tibia by including in his treatise an illustration of one that had healed with posterior talar subluxation. Earle,[15] in 1829, reported a fresh posterior lip fracture encountered at autopsy, which he considered "perfectly novel." Lucas-Championnière[16] theorized that this lesion was produced by vertical compression, a mechanism that was later documented by Rochet,[17] who produced a fracture of the posterior articular lip of the tibia by dropping a weight on the upper end of the tibia with the ankle held in plantar flexion. In 1912, Cotton[18] delivered a paper to the American Medical Association entitled "A New Type of Ankle Fracture," calling attention to a fracture of the posterior articular margin of

the tibia as a previously undescribed injury and suggesting that this fracture, when associated with fractures of the medial and lateral malleoli, be termed "Cotton's fracture."

Fracture of the anterior articular margin of the distal tibia was recorded first in 1874 by Nélaton[19] in a young patient who fell from a great height. Although reported more often after radiography became available, it is a rare lesion, occurring in less than 0.5% of all ankle fractures.

Bosworth,[20] in 1947, provided the first description of a low external rotation fracture of the fibula in which the proximal fragment became locked in a displaced position against the posterior tibia, where it was held firmly by the intact interosseous membrane (Fig. 6). Irreducible posterior dislocation of the intact fibula had been reported earlier by Woods,[21] in 1942. This dislocation, as has usually been the case with the Bosworth lesion, required open reduction.

Finally, tribute should be made to the work of Bonnin,[22] whose exceptional 1950 monograph not only summarizes and relates historical milestones, mechanisms of injury, fracture patterns, classification, and treatment, but also offers fresh insights. Bonnin was the first to distinguish anterior and posterior collicular fractures of the medial malleolus and to provide an extensive classification of ankle injuries based on progression in severity of the lesions.

References

1. Pott P: *Some Few General Remarks on Fractures and Dislocations.* London, Hawes, Clarke, Collins, 1768.
2. Ashhurst APC, Bromer RS: Classification and mechanism of fractures of the leg bones involving the ankle: Based on a study of three hundred cases from the Episcopal Hospital. *Arch Surg* 1922;4:51–129.
3. David J-P: Mémoire sur les contre-coups dans les differentes parties du corps autre que la tête. *Pris Acad R Chir,* 1771.
4. Dupuytren G: Of fractures of the lower extremity of the fibula, and luxations of the foot. [Reprinted in] *Med Classics* 1939;4:151–172.
5. Nélaton A: *Elemens de Pathologie Chirurgicale.* Paris, 1844, vol 1, preface.
6. Maisonneuve JG: Recherches sur la fracture du perone. *Arch Gen Med* 1840;7:165–187,433–473.
7. Huguier P-C: Mémoire sur les luxations du pied considerées en géneral. *Union Med* (Paris) 1848;2:120.
8. Hönigschmied J: Leichen experimente über die zerrissungen der bänder im sprunggelenk, mit rucksicht auf die entstehung der indirecten knockelfracturen. *Dtsch Z Chir* 1887;8:239.
9. Pankovich AM: Maisonneuve fracture of the fibula. *J Bone Joint Surg* 1976;58A:337–342.
10. Tillaux P: *Traité de Chirurgie Clinique.* Paris, Asselin et Houzeau, 1848, vol 2, p 842.
11. Cooper AP: On dislocation of the ankle joints, in *A Treatise on Dislocations and on Fractures of the Joints.* London, Longman, Hurst, Reese, Orme and Brown and E Cox and Son, 1822.
12. Wagstaffe WW: An unusual form of fracture of the fibula. *St Thomas Hosp Rep* 1875;6:43.
13. Le Fort L: Note sur une variété non décrite de fracture verticale

de la malléole externe par arrachement. *Bull Gen Therap* 1886; 110:193–199.

14. LeRoy L: *De la fracture marginale anterieure de la malleole externe.* Paris, 1887.

15. Earle H: Simple, succeeded by compound dislocations forwards, of the inferior extremity of the tibia, with fracture of its posterior edge: Comminuted fracture of the fibula, amputation of the leg, and death. *Lancet* 1828–1829;2:346–348.

16. Lucas-Championnière J: *Bull Soc Anat Paris* 1870;45:212.

17. Rochet V: Du mécanisme des luxations doubles de l'astragale (énucléation). *Rev Orthop* 1890;1:296.

18. Cotton FJ: A new type of ankle fracture. *JAMA* 1915;64:318–321.

19. Nélaton A: *Elémens de Pathologie Chirurgicale*, ed 2. Paris, Germer-Bailliere, 1874, vol 3, p 296.

20. Bosworth DM: Fracture-dislocation of the ankle with fixed displacement of the fibula behind the tibia. *J Bone Joint Surg* 1947; 29:130–135.

21. Woods RS: Irreducible dislocation of the ankle-joint. *Br J Surg* 1942;29:359–360.

22. Bonnin JG: *Injuries to the Ankle.* New York, Grune & Stratton, 1950.

The Pathogenesis and Treatment of Ankle Fractures: Classification

Frank C. Wilson, MD

The classification of ankle injuries has challenged investigators for almost 200 years. More than an intellectual exercise, classification promotes ordered thought, a rational approach to management, and a means for comparing results.

The first necessity for classification is a comprehensive knowledge and understanding of the lesions that may be encountered, knowledge that was unavailable before the development of radiography. Before this era, classifications emphasized each new concept rather than an inclusive schema that embraced and organized all concepts.

The earliest classifications were, like the latest, based on mechanisms of injury. The classifications of Boyer,[1] in 1790, and Dupuytren,[2] in 1847, were limited to abduction and adduction violence. With Maisonneuve's[3] work in 1840, which defined the external rotation fracture, a meaningful mechanistic classification became possible. Although not fully developed, Maisonneuve's description of fibular fractures was based on their production by *arrachement*, divulsion, or diastasis, which correspond roughly to adduction, external rotation, and abduction mechanisms. By his more complete description of the divulsion or external rotation injury, Maisonneuve corrected Dupuytren's perception that medial injury always preceded fibular fracture.

Because it was not vigorously propounded, Maisonneuve's work was largely overlooked by his contemporaries, and the anatomic classification of fractures as unimalleolar, bimalleolar, and trimalleolar held sway during the 19th century, even though such classifications failed to emphasize the importance of associated ligamentous injury. The anatomic systems were unable, for example, to encompass the fractures described by Maisonneuve.

Hönigschmied's[4] studies on cadavers in 1887 renewed interest in the mechanisms of ankle injury; and the advent of radiography stimulated a new burst of organizational activity, beginning with the classifications of Chaput[5] in 1908 and Destot[6] in 1911. Chaput's classification contained both mechanistic and anatomic headings, incorporating fractures produced by abduction, diastasis, and adduction with supramalleolar and marginal fractures. Other than the inclusion of Maisonneuve's fracture in the diastasis category, this schema added little to previous mechanistic classifications. Destot made the valuable distinction between "tibial pilon" (supramalleolar) and "mortise" (malleo-

lar) fractures, but, by incorporating more types of fractures, his system became clumsy and unworkable.

Quénu's[7] 1912 classification, with the addition of terms to identify the extent of injury to the plafond, was even more overwhelmed by detail.

Tanton,[8] in 1916, emphasized the role of the talus in defining five major anatomic categories of fractures. His five categories were: (1) talocrural ligaments (sprain or rupture), (2) tibiofibular ligaments (diastasis), (3) malleoli (isolated fractures), (4) tibial pilon (rarely seen as isolated fractures), and (5) malleoli and tibial pilon (frequent). Malleolar and pilon fractures were extensively subdivided, but the subcategories bore no sequential relationship to one another, and therefore lacked utility and defied recall.

In 1910, Lane,[9] who also pioneered open reduction, stripped away much of this unwieldy complexity and returned in his classification to abduction and adduction fractures, which he subdivided by degrees according to the sequence of injury. Had he included external rotation injuries, his system would undoubtedly have gained wider and more enduring recognition.

The most detailed analysis of ankle injuries to that point was produced in 1922 by Ashhurst and Bromer,[10] who organized the radiographs of 300 ankle fractures into an extensive but easily recalled system of classification based on the direction of talar displacement. They described first-, second-, and third-degree fractures under the categories of external rotation, abduction, adduction, and (vertical) compression, noting that 61% of the injuries were caused by external rotation, 21% by abduction, 13.3% by adduction, and 2.7% by compression. (The remainder were caused by direct injuries.) First- and second-degree fractures in each category accurately reflected the sequential development of uni- and bimalleolar fractures; however, third-degree injuries were stated to be supramalleolar fractures, which are not final stages of external rotation, abduction, or adduction injury. Further, the system failed to emphasize appropriately the role of ligamentous injury and diastasis or to describe the more frequent occurrence of fractures caused by a combination of mechanisms, as, for example, abduction and external rotation. (It should also be noted that transverse fractures of the medial and lateral malleoli, listed as second-degree adduction injuries, may also occur from abduction.)

Bonnin,[11] in 1950, recognized that mechanism was the most satisfactory basis for classification and proceeded, under the general headings of external rotation, abduction, adduction, and compression forces, to define subheadings according to progression in the severity of lesions. This classification has the values of symmetry and recognition that treatment and prognosis parallel severity of injury. The major difference between his classification and that of Ashhurst and Bromer is Bonnin's substitution of trimalleolar for supramalleolar fractures as the third degree of injury. He added categories of supramalleolar fractures and injuries by direct violence.

While taking into account the importance of ligamentous injury, Bonnin, too, failed to stress the importance of mixed injuries; nor did he go far enough in clarifying third-degree injuries. Fractures, for example, involving a significant portion of the posterior articular surface of the tibia are commonly produced by vertical compression of the plantarflexed talus, whereas nonarticular fractures of the posterior tubercle result from shear or avulsion, which may or may not occur as the last stage in the development of the full fracture pattern.

The most detailed and precise classification of ankle fractures was provided by Lauge-Hansen,[12-16] who, from a combination of cadaver experiments and surgical observations, distinguished four mechanisms of injury: external rotation, adduction, abduction, and dorsiflexion. Ingeniously, he then described the sequence of injury in each according to whether the foot was supinated or pronated at the time the injury occurred. The first word in each category of injury refers to the position of the foot and the second to the direction of the force. This dual nomenclature is confusing unless one understands that Lauge-Hansen used the terms "eversion" for external rotation and "inversion" for internal rotation. The five types of ankle fractures described by Lauge-Hansen, and the stages in each, are illustrated in Figure 1 and outlined in the following paragraphs.

The Lauge-Hansen Classification System

A. Supination-Adduction Injuries (10–20%)

Stage I In stage I there is transverse fracture of the lateral malleolus at varying heights or tear of the lateral collateral ligaments.

Stage II Stage II is the same as stage I with the addition of fracture of the medial malleolus.

B. Supination-Eversion (External Rotation) Injuries (40–75%)

Stage I In stage I there is rupture of the anterior inferior tibiofibular ligament, occasionally by avulsion of a bone fragment from the tibia or fibula. Whether rupture of this ligament always precedes stage II is debated.

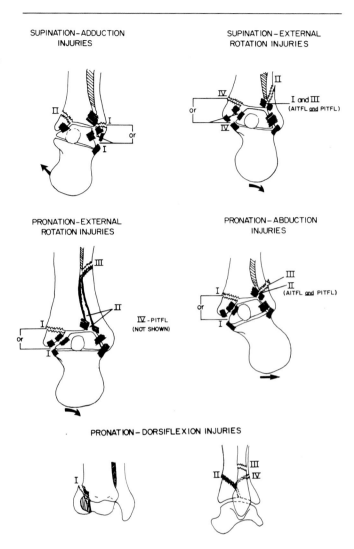

Fig. 1 The Lauge-Hansen classification of ankle fractures. The stages (sequence in which the injuries occur) are indicated by the Roman numerals.

Stage II Stage II is the same injury as stage I with the addition of a spiral-oblique fracture of the lateral malleolus. The fracture line is directed from anteroinferior to posterosuperior and does not involve the interosseous membrane. The fibular fracture is frequently comminuted posteriorly.

Stage III Stage III is the same as stage II with the addition of a fracture of the posterior lip of the tibia, which usually involves little or none of the articular surface.

Stage IV Stage IV adds to stage III a fracture of the medial malleolus or tear of the deltoid ligament.

C. Pronation-Abduction Injuries (5–21%)

Stage I Stage I involves fracture of the medial malleolus (slightly oblique or transverse) or tear of the deltoid ligament.

Stage II Stage II adds to stage I a rupture of the anterior and posterior inferior tibiofibular ligaments and transverse ligament, often with a nonarticular fracture of the posterior lip of the tibia.

Stage III Stage III adds to stage II a supramalleolar fracture of the fibula directed from inferomedial to superolateral. Typically, only the anterior and posterior tibiofibular ligaments tear, but in some cases the tear extends into the interosseous membrane, with the fibular fracture occurring at the proximal extent of the interosseous tear. The fibular fracture is frequently comminuted laterally.

D. Pronation-Eversion (external Rotation) Injuries (7–19%)

Stage I This is the same as stage I of pronation-abduction injuries.

Stage II Stage II adds to stage I a tear of the anterior inferior tibiofibular and interosseous ligaments.

Stage III Stage III adds to stage II an interosseous membrane tear and spiral fracture of the fibular 7 to 8 cm proximal to the tip of the lateral malleolus. (This is likely the most common mechanism for production of the lesion that Pott and Dupuytren described; the higher Maisonneuve fracture is probably a variant.)

Stage IV Stage IV adds to stage III a nonarticular fracture of the posterior lip of the tibia. (This fracture can be produced by traction from the posterior inferior tibiofibular ligaments, but, perhaps more commonly, is produced by compression of the rotating fibula prior to tearing of the interosseous ligament.)

E. Pronation-Dorsiflexion (with axial loading) (1%)

Stage I Stage I involves fracture of the medial malleolus.

Stage II In stage II there is a larger anterior tibial lip fracture, with major involvement of the articular surface.

Stage III In stage III there is a supramalleolar fracture of the fibula.

Stage IV In stage IV the posterior articular surface of the tibia is fractured. This injury, with comminution of the tibial plafond, has been termed a *pilon* (pestle) fracture by European surgeons.

Lauge-Hansen did not produce the pronation-dorsiflexion injury in cadavers; rather, his description was based on a single postmortem dissection and the study of radiographs. Whether he simply did not or could not produce this fracture in cadaver specimens is unclear.

By placing the foot in different positions before delivering the force of injury, Lauge-Hansen was able to simulate combination injuries experimentally. For example, external rotation of the pronated foot approaches the external rotation-abduction pattern seen clinically, in which the obliquity of the fibular fracture lies between the anteroposterior plane of external rotation fractures and the mediolateral plane of abduction fractures. Unfortunately, Lauge-Hansen did not distinguish clearly in his categories between nonarticular posterior lip fractures and fractures that involve the articular surface, which require the addition of axial loading.

Another difficulty with this classification lies with the artificial distinction between supination and pronation-external rotation injuries, which is based on Lauge-Hansen's observation that external rotation produced extensive damage to the syndesmotic ligaments only when the foot was pronated, thus producing a higher fibular lesion than that encountered when the foot was supinated; however, Pankovich[17] found syndesmotic injury also following external rotation of the supinated foot, thereby invalidating any such distinction.

Lauge-Hansen based "pathogenetic reduction" on reversal of the injuring forces in inverse order to that in which they occurred, which he thought essential to obtain anatomic reduction. These descriptions are detailed, cumbersome, and probably unnecessary, because it has not been documented that reversing the injuring forces in precisely the inverse order of occurrence produces a more anatomic reduction than reversal in more random order. Thus, while its therapeutic practicality may be questioned, Lauge-Hansen's work advanced the study of ankle injuries significantly, by more closely simulating clinical events experimentally, by defining clearly the relationship of ligamentous injury to fracture pattern, and by providing a detailed and precise means for comparing modes of treatment and prognosis.

The Danis-Weber Classification System

The Danis-Weber[18] classification, which points out that the higher the fibular injury, the greater the syndesmotic injury and likelihood of displacement, is based even more completely on the location and appearance of the fibular fracture. In this classification, three types of fibular fracture are recognized (Fig. 2). Type A, caused by internal rotation and adduction, is a transverse (tension) fracture at or below the joint line, with a possible oblique (compression) fracture of the medial malleolus. Type B, resulting from external rotation, produces a fracture rising obliquely from the joint line in an anteroposterior plane, with or without rupture of the anterior inferior tibiofibular ligament and associated medial injuries. Type C (abduction) fractures have been subdivided into those resulting from abduction alone (C-1), which causes a mediolaterally oblique fibular break above a ruptured tibiofibular ligament, and those

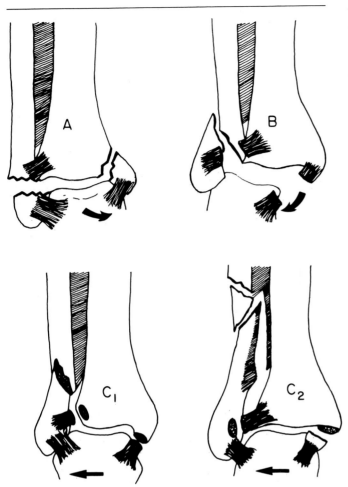

Fig. 2   The Danis-Weber classification. The external rotation fracture (**B**) is incorrect, because this fibular fracture normally runs from anteroinferior to posterosuperior.

resulting from a combination of abduction and external rotation (C-2), which produce more extensive interosseous rupture and a higher fibular fracture. (The implication that the fracture does not occur below an intact ligament is untrue.) Either C-type injury can be associated with a tear of the deltoid ligament or a transverse medial malleolar fracture, and all types can have associated posterior lip fractures. In this classification system, type A lesions correspond to the supination-adduction injuries of Lauge-Hansen, type B lesions to supination-external rotation injuries, and type C-1 lesions to the pronation-abduction mechanism of Lauge-Hansen. Type C-2 lesions have no Lauge-Hansen counterpart. Illustrations of the Danis-Weber classification may be misleading in that the obliquity of the fibular fractures shown for type B (external rotation) injuries is usually shown as directed mediolaterally rather than anteroposteriorly.[19] The advantages of this classification sys-

tem lie in its simplicity and in the fact that it includes (in C-2 fractures) combination injuries.

Conclusion

The most practical value of any classification system lies in its applicability to treatment. By recalling that almost all fractures are produced by abnormal motion of the talus, which either pushes off, or, by means of ligamentous attachments, pulls off, a malleolus, and understanding that bending fractures are usually oblique in the direction of the injuring force, while traction fractures are transverse, malleolar fractures can easily be analyzed to determine whether a given fracture was the result of one of the primary movements (external rotation, abduction, adduction, and vertical compression) or whether, as more often happens, it resulted from a combination of these forces. While it is necessary to appreciate all the forces involved to reduce the fracture, it is less clear that the order in which the reducing forces are applied makes any real difference.

References

1. Boyer AB: *Traite des Maladies Chirurgicales, et des Operations qui leur Conviennent*, ed 5. Paris, 1814, vol 3, pp 884–914.
2. Dupuytren G: Diseases and injuries of bones. *Trans Sydenham Soc* London, F le Gros Clarke, 1847.
3. Maisonneuve JG: Recherches sur la fracture du perone. *Arch Gen Med* 1840;7:165–187,433–473.
4. Hönigschmied J: Leichen experimente über die zerrissungen der bänder im sprunggelenk, mit rucksicht auf die entstehung der indirecten knockelfracturen. *Deutsch Zeit f Chir* 1887;8:239.
5. Chaput V: *Les Fractures Malléolaires du Cou-de-pied, et les Accidents du Travail*. Paris, Masson et Cie, 1908.
6. Destot E: *Traumatismes du Pied et Rayons X*. Paris, Masson et Cie, 1911.
7. Quénu E: Étude critique sur les fractures du cou-de-pied. *Rev de Chir* 1912;45:1,211,416,560.
8. Tanton J: Fractures du membre inferior, in *Nouveau Traité de Chirurgie*. 1916, vol 7, p 79.
9. Lane WA: *The Operative Treatment of Fractures*. London, Medical Publishing Company, 1910.
10. Ashhurst APC, Bromer RS: Classification and mechanism of fractures of the leg bones involving the ankle: Based on a study of three hundred cases from the Episcopal Hospital. *Arch Surg* 1922;4:51–129.
11. Bonnin JG: *Injuries to the Ankle*. New York, Grune & Stratton, 1950.
12. Lauge N: Fractures of the ankle: Analytic historic survey as the basis of new experimental, roentgenologic and clinical investigations. *Arch Surg* 1948;56:259–317.
13. Lauge-Hansen N: Fractures of the ankle: II. Combined experimental-surgical and experimental-roentgenologic investigations. *Arch Surg* 1950;60:957–985.
14. Lauge-Hansen N: Fractures of the ankle: IV. Clinical use of the genetic roentgen diagnosis and genetic reduction. *AMA Arch Surg* 1952;64:488–500.
15. Lauge-Hansen N: Fractures of the ankle: V. Pronation-dorsiflexion fracture. *AMA Arch Surg* 1953;67:813–820.
16. Lauge-Hansen N: Fractures of the ankle: III. Genetic roentgen-

ologic diagnosis of fractures of the ankle. *Am J Roentgenol* 1954; 71:456–471.

17. Pankovich AM: Maisonneuve fracture of the fibula. *J Bone Joint Surg* 1976;58A:337–342.

18. Weber BG: Die verletzungen des oberen sprunggelenkes, in *Aktuelle Probleme in der Chirurgie*. Bern, Verlag Hans Huber, 1966.

19. Müller ME, Allgöwer M, Willenegger H: *Manual of Internal Fixation*. New York, Springer-Verlag, 1970.

The Pathogenesis and Treatment of Bimalleolar Ankle Fractures

Laurence E. Dahners, MD

Biomechanics

Before discussing treatment of bimalleolar fractures, it is helpful to review briefly the biomechanics of bone failure and internal fixation, especially as they apply to the ankle.

Tension

Bone loaded in tension fails with a fracture line that is transverse to the direction of pull, that is, not necessarily transverse to the shaft of the bone but perpendicular to the lines of tension (Fig. 1, *left*). A similar type of failure is seen when a rope under tension is ruptured. In the ankle, fractures of this type are frequently seen in the malleolus when the ligament attached to the malleolus pulls the bone apart (Fig. 1, *center*). Open reduction and internal fixation of bone that has failed in tension is relatively easy because comminution is infrequent. Either a lag screw, which applies compression across the fracture, or a plate, which similarly applies compression across the fracture, will provide excellent internal fixation for this problem (Fig. 1, *right*).

Bending

As bone that is loaded in bending begins to fracture, it develops compressive forces along one surface and tensile forces along the other. As described above, the side of the bone that is loaded in tension fails with a simple transverse break (Fig. 2, *left*). The other side of the bone is loaded in compression. Bone is extremely strong in compression. Thus, instead of being compressed to a smaller size, it fails along shear lines, usually oriented 45 degrees to the axis of the compressive load (Fig. 2, *left*). Depending on the violence of this compressive load, there can be a simple butterfly, at two 45-degree shear angles, or there can be comminution as many shear planes develop.

Bending fractures in the ankle commonly involve a fracture of the fibula. The talus, thrust laterally by an abduction force, produces a transverse fracture of the medial portion of the fibula with lateral comminution

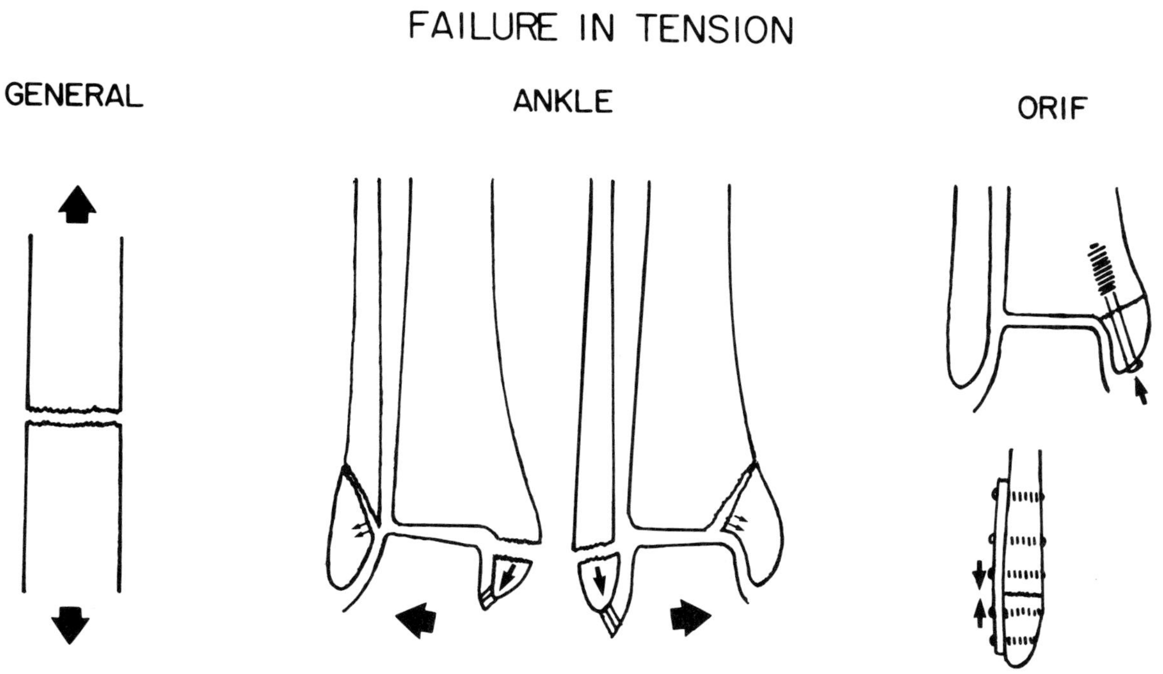

FAILURE IN TENSION

GENERAL   ANKLE   ORIF

Fig. 1 The mechanics of bone failure in tension with types of tension ankle fractures and means for internal fixation.

FAILURE IN BENDING

GENERAL   ANKLE   ORIF

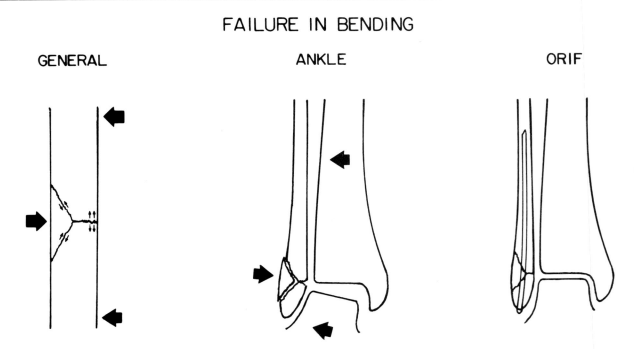

Fig. 2   The mechanics of bone failure in bending with a bending fibular fracture and means of internal fixation.

FAILURE IN TORSION

GENERAL   ANKLE   ORIF

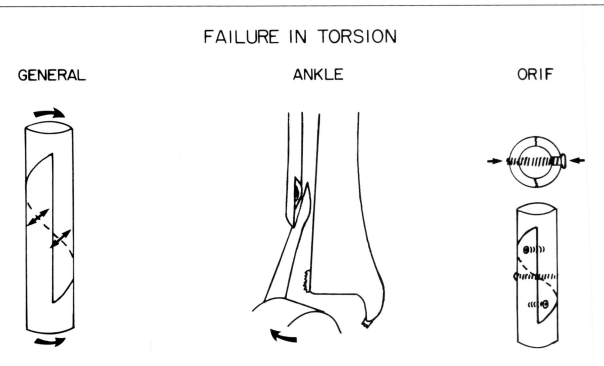

Fig. 3   The mechanics of bone failure in torsion with a torsion fibular fracture and means of internal fixation.

(Fig. 2, *center*). The best internal fixation device for treatment of a fracture caused by bending is an intramedullary rod (Fig. 2, *right*). A rod is strong when loaded in bending, as opposed to a plate, which is relatively weak. Lag screws provide less fixation and are not capable of holding comminuted fractures together.

Torsion

When bone is loaded in torsion, the classic spiral fracture is produced. A perfect spiral fracture consists of a vertical-longitudinal portion in continuity with a portion of the fracture that spirals around the bone (Fig. 3, *left*). In most spiral fractures, however, the longitudinal portion also tends to spiral somewhat. In the ankle, the most common torsional injury is the spiral fracture of the fibula. This injury classically occurs above the plafond when an external rotational force is applied to the ankle. The fibula is twisted externally by the talus after failure of the medial side of the ankle (Fig. 3, *center*). This fracture is particularly amenable to interfragmentary lag screw fixation if the spiral is long and there is minimal comminution (Fig. 3, *right*). If the spiral is short, or there is comminution, it is wise to reinforce this with a plate.

Surgical vs Closed Treatment

The debate about the merits of open reduction and internal fixation of displaced ankle fractures still continues. There is no doubt that even a 20- to 30-year follow-up of nonsurgically treated ankle fractures will show that good results can be obtained.[1,2] Recent articles have claimed that open reduction and internal fixation has no advantage over closed reduction for patients in whom an excellent reduction is achieved by closed means.[3–5] Other recent articles claim that internal fixation achieves a better result.[6] Some of these reports have even been prospective, randomized studies.[3,4,6] However, I suspect that the truth is to be found in the words of Tunturi and associates,[7] who believed that the clinical end result correlated with the radiologic result (reduction) at the end of the treatment and not with the type of injury or the type of treatment. This is not to say, however, that an anatomic reduction guarantees a good result.

I believe that most ankle fractures deserve at least an attempt at obtaining a closed reduction. Those in whom an anatomic reduction cannot be achieved should be treated by open reduction and internal fixation. Closed reductions should not be attempted in patients who do not have a shoulder of malleolus against which the talus can be reduced, or in patients who have open fractures. I believe that open fractures of the ankle should be treated with immediate irrigation, debridement, reduction, and rigid internal fixation. I believe that rigid immobilization of the fracture

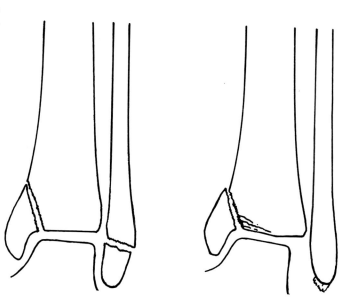

ADDUCTION INJURIES

Fig. 4   Typical types of adduction ankle fractures. Specifically note the high frequency of impaction of the medial tibial plafond shown on the right.

fragments lowers the incidence of uncontrollable infection, and this belief is supported by a study from the University of Washington.[8]

Specific Injuries

Adduction Injuries

The adduction injury is caused by inversion of the foot with medial displacement of the talus (Fig. 4). Adduction commonly causes failure of the lateral ligaments, resulting in the typical and extremely common lateral sprain. Fractures produced by adduction are relatively rare even though inversion sprains occur frequently. In the typical inversion injury, the foot is slightly plantar flexed. This results in rupture of the anterior talofibular and/or the calcaneofibular ligament, while protecting the posterior talofibular ligament. The talus then tends to roll under the tip of the medial malleolus without causing a fracture or deltoid ligament disruption. Injuries that do result in a fracture frequently involve considerable axial loading in association with the adduction. This increased axial loading keeps the talus from simply rolling over the tip of the malleolus and instead tends to force it vigorously against the malleolus, shearing off the malleolus. The lateral malleolus fails in tension, and the medial malleolus fails in shear. This produces a nearly vertical fracture of the medial malleolus and a transverse dis-

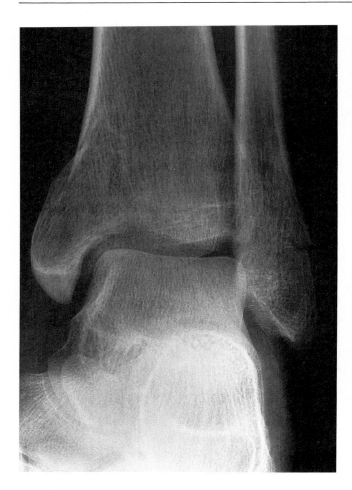 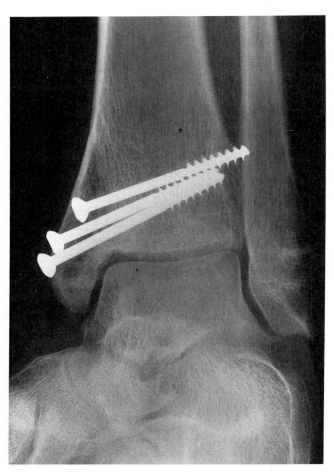

Fig. 5 **Left**, An adduction ankle fracture with an avulsion fracture of the fibula in tension. Also note a vertical fracture of the medial malleolus in shear and impaction of the anterior medial plafond. **Right**, Internal fixation of the ankle fracture. An instrument was used to push the articular surface back down into a reduced position. Cancellous graft was packed into the defect and the medial malleolus was held with three lag screws.

ruption of the lateral malleolus or lateral ankle ligaments (Fig. 4, *right*). Because of compressive loading, there is a high association of impaction of the medial tibial plafond.

Closed Reduction In theory, closed reduction is easily accomplished by simple abduction of the ankle and application of a cast. However, there are frequently intra-articular fragments from the comminution resulting from compression on the medial side, and these should be removed. In addition, if the medial plafond has a large area that is depressed, it should be elevated. Thus, the indication for closed reduction is a simple fracture without comminution and preferably one in which the fibular fragment has been avulsed below the level of the plafond so that the talus cannot be overreduced.

Open Reduction and Internal Fixation Open reduction and internal fixation is commonly required. In Figure 5,

left, the patient had an avulsion of the fibular malleolus with a vertical fracture of the medial malleolus, accompanied by depression of the anterior medial tibial plafond. This depressed fragment, which constitutes a substantial portion of the articular surface, is a strong indication for open reduction and internal fixation. The medial malleolus was swung away like a door, allowing placement of an instrument into the compressed cancellous bone and leverage of the underlying articular cartilage into a reduced position. Cancellous bone was then packed into the defect above the compressed articular surface. The malleolus was reduced and held with lag screws as shown in Figure 5, *right*.

Complications and Prognosis This particular patient was a marathon runner before being injured and has since resumed the sport with only mild aching after long runs. However, the prognosis for this fracture is not generally as good as with other ankle fractures because

ABDUCTION INJURIES

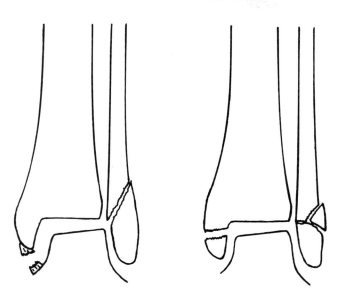

Fig. 6   Typical forms of abduction ankle fractures.

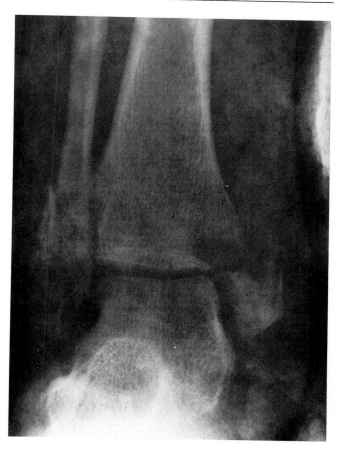

Fig. 7   An attempted closed reduction of an abduction ankle fracture with no remaining shoulder of medial malleolus. Without this shoulder, the adduction used to reduce the fracture has overreduced the talus, pushing it past its anatomic location beneath the plafond.

comminution and compression of the plafond is more difficult to restore and predisposes the ankle to traumatic arthritis.

Abduction Injuries

Abduction injuries are less common than adduction injuries but are more apt to result in fractures than in ligamentous sprain. Thus, the abduction fracture is more common than the adduction fracture and is recognized by avulsion of the medial malleolus or by rupture of the deltoid ligament, as denoted by widening of the medial joint space in excess of 4 mm. Typically, an oblique fracture of the distal fibula starts at the plafond and shears upward and laterally (Fig. 6, *left*). There may be comminution of the lateral cortex if the fibula is loaded in bending rather than shear (Fig. 6, *right*). Comminution of the articular surface, resulting in intra-articular fragments, is less common.

Closed Reduction   Closed reduction and casting can be successful in treating this fracture. Indications include rupture of the deltoid ligament or avulsion of the medial malleolus at a level that leaves enough medial shoulder of the plafond to prevent overreduction of the talus (Fig. 7). The cast is applied with the ankle adducted. The reduction should be judged by the same criteria used to judge an open reduction. The most important factor is that the talus be completely reduced underneath the plafond in all planes and firmly seated against the remaining medial malleolus. There is, however, evidence that even as little as 2 to 4 mm of fibular short-

ening and 15 degrees of rotation can increase articular contact pressures by 37% to 102%.[9] Confirmation of reduction requires an excellent mortise radiograph. These radiographs are repeated frequently for the first two weeks after fracture to confirm maintenance of this reduction. Loss of reduction in the first two weeks occurs with moderate frequency, but after the first two weeks, loss of reduction is uncommon.

Open Reduction and Internal Fixation   Open reduction and internal fixation of this fracture is indicated when there is no shoulder of medial malleolus, when there are fragments within the joint, or when closed reduction fails to obtain and maintain anatomic reduction of the ankle mortise. I prefer to expose both the medial and lateral malleoli, debride both fractures, and irrigate the joint. In all ankle fractures, I initially apply internal fixation to the fracture that is least comminuted. This reduces the ankle joint, holds the more comminuted fracture in a relatively reduced position, and allows the internal fixation of that more difficult fracture to proceed more easily. In abduction fractures, the least comminuted

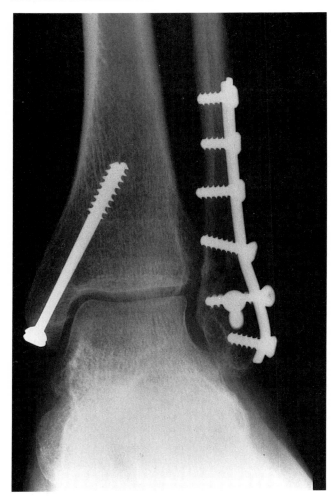

Fig. 8 Open reduction and internal fixation of the fracture shown in Figure 7. Two lag screws were used in the medial malleolus and a plate on the fibula.

fracture is usually the medial side, as it failed in tension. Thus, I will fix it, using two 4.0-mm cancellous lag screws if possible (Fig. 8), although on occasion only one can be inserted. The lateral side is then fixed with an intramedullary device such as a Rush rod or one of the nails[10] recently proposed for the distal fibula. It can also be repaired with a lag screw reinforced with a plate (Fig. 8). Even though biomechanically a rod provides stronger fixation, I prefer to use a plate because obtaining an anatomic reduction with an intramedullary device is technically difficult, if not impossible, with this fracture.

After surgery, I place the ankle in a bivalved fiberglass cast with Velcro straps. This is removed several times a day to allow range of motion of the ankle. After four to six weeks, I place the patient in a short leg walking cast and allow weightbearing ambulation for an additional four weeks, at which time healing is usually complete.

Complications and Prognosis Complications of closed reduction usually involve incomplete reduction, loss of reduction related to compression of the lateral plafond, or loose bodies within the joint. A serious complication of open reduction can arise from massive swelling, resulting in a wound that is very difficult to close. This is best avoided by operating either within the first 24 hours after injury or at least five days after injury, after the swelling has subsided. If, at the end of surgery, swelling is so severe that the wounds are difficult to close, it is wise to dress them open and complete wound closure three or four days later.

Open fractures are more common with abduction injuries, but the infection rate is relatively low if they are treated early with irrigation, debridement, internal fixation, and delayed closure. In general, the prognosis for abduction fractures is relatively good, assuming that they do not have any of the complicating factors mentioned above.

External Rotational Injuries

External rotational injuries are usually caused by rotating the body about a planted foot or by sudden deceleration of the externally rotated forefoot. As the talus rotates externally, it produces an avulsion of the anterior portion of the medial malleolus or a rupture of the deltoid ligament (Fig. 9). As rotation proceeds, the fibula is twisted externally and is frequently pushed posteriorly by the talus, which is now anterior to the fibula. If the thrust is mostly posterior, the fibula fractures obliquely in a posterosuperior to anteroinferior direction (Fig. 9, *left*). If the force produces more twisting, it results in a spiral fracture of the fibula (Fig. 9, *right*). This spiral fracture frequently occurs far up the fibula after tearing of the syndesmotic ligaments between the tibia and fibula to the level of the fibula fracture.

Closed Reduction Closed reduction by internal rotation of the ankle and application of a long leg cast frequently succeeds in achieving reduction (Fig. 10). An important factor in achieving this reduction is dorsiflexion of the foot to diminish tension on the anterior aspect of the deltoid ligament. Otherwise, the avulsed anterior portion of the medial malleolus will be maintained in a displaced position (Fig. 11). Obtaining a good mortise and lateral radiograph in plaster is very important to make certain that the talus is adequately reduced. Displacement is an indication for open reduction and internal fixation. It may be necessary to delay weightbearing for up to three months to prevent widening of a torn syndesmosis.

Open Reduction and Internal Fixation Surgical treatment of these fractures involves exposing both the medial and lateral sides of the joints before undertaking internal fixation of either one. The medial side is explored and debrided of clots to ensure that no obstructions to re-

EXTERNAL ROTATION INJURIES

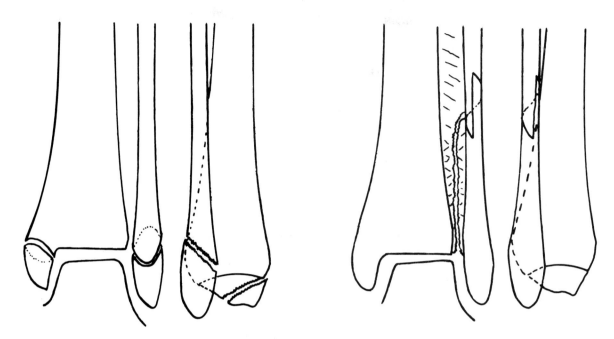

Fig. 9   A diagram of typical external rotation fractures. Note especially that the obliquity of the fractures may make them difficult to see on the anteroposterior view (as displayed on the left pair of diagrams). High fibular fractures are associated with tearing of the interosseous membrane to the level of the fracture.

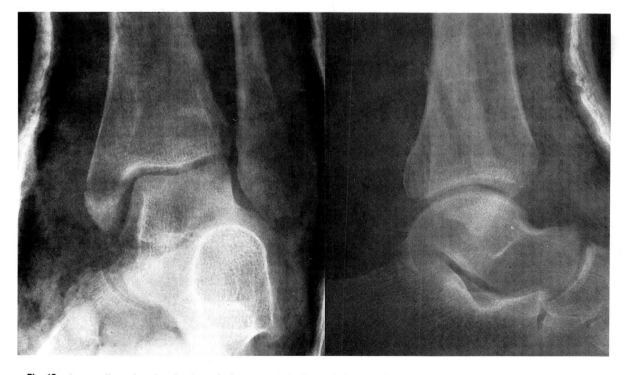

Fig. 10   An excellent closed reduction of what was originally a relatively widely displaced external rotational fracture with an anterior medial malleolar avulsion and an oblique anterior-inferior to posterior-superior fibular fracture.

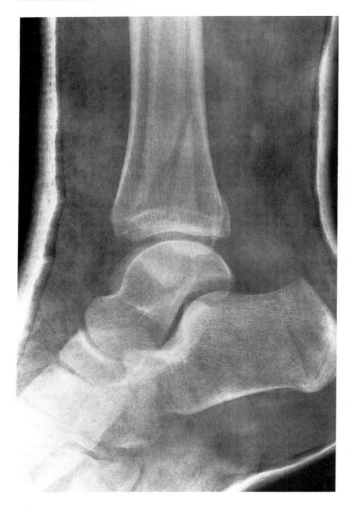

Fig. 11 An external rotational fracture reduced by internal rotation; however, insufficient dorsiflexion of the ankle was applied. This resulted in wide distraction of the medial malleolus by pull from the anterior fibers of the deltoid ligament.

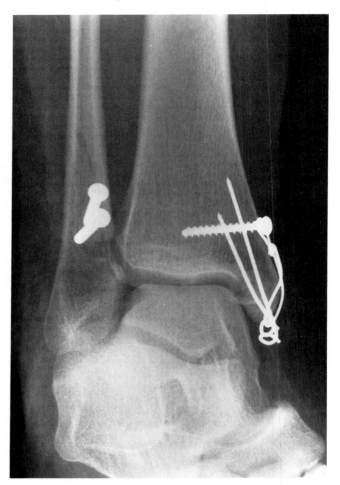

Fig. 12 The small and comminuted fracture of the anterior medial malleolus was fixed with two Kirschner wires that were subsequently looped around the tension band wire to prevent backing out. The tension band wire has been attached to a screw proximally rather than drill holes. The oblique fracture of the distal fibula has been fixed with two interfragmentary screws.

duction, such as an infolded deltoid ligament or a displaced posterior tibial tendon, have slipped into the joint. The medial malleolar fracture fragment is frequently small and will be found anteriorly. Screws used to reduce it should be inserted transversely to the fracture site, which means they are directed not only superiorly but posteriorly. When the medial malleolus is comminuted, which sometimes occurs from the injury and occasionally happens during screw insertion, the best treatment is to insert two or three Kirschner wires and secure them with a figure-of-eight tension band wire (Fig. 12). On the lateral side, an oblique or spiral distal fracture may be amenable to fixation with two or three interfragmentary lag screws. If there is comminution, it may be necessary to reinforce this fixation with a plate. I believe that an intramedullary device is contraindicated for these fractures, because such a device is not good at preventing malrotation of these

obliquely directed fragments. When the fracture occurs above the syndesmotic ligaments, I prefer to maintain reduction of this joint with a screw. When the fibular fracture is very proximal, I sometimes apply a screw to the syndesmosis and ignore the more proximal fracture (Fig. 13). However, if the fracture is distal and is thus easily accessible, I prefer to start by obtaining an accurate reduction of the fibula fracture with interfragmentary screws. Once I am certain that the rotation and length of the fibula are correct (Fig. 14), I manually reduce the fibula into its recess on the lateral surface of the tibia and hold it there while an assistant drills a 3.2-mm hole from the fibula across the tibia to its medial cortex. It is important that this screw be directed posterolaterally to anteromedially. If the screw is oriented too much in the medial-to-lateral direction, it will pass posterior to the tibia. The ankle is held in dorsiflexion while the hole is drilled and tapped. A 4.5-mm

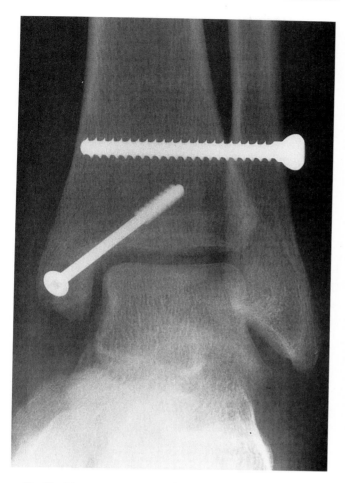

Fig. 13 This external rotational fracture had an extremely high fibular fracture and so was treated without internal fixation of the fracture of the fibula. This was done by obtaining a manual reduction of the syndesmosis and internally fixing it with a single 4.5-mm cortical screw with threads in both the fibula and tibia.

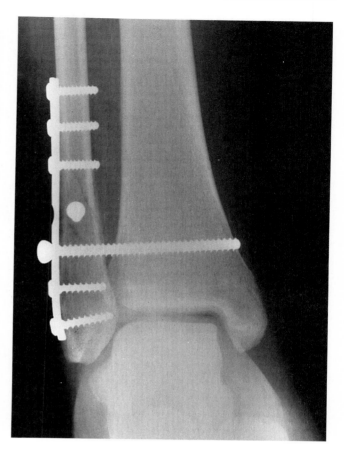

Fig. 14 This spiral fibular fracture was initially reduced with a single lag screw that was then reinforced with the one-third tubular plate. The syndesmosis was then manually reduced (correct rotation and length of the fibula having been ensured with open reduction and internal fixation) and fixed with a 4.5-mm cortical screw (which will indeed fit through the one-third tubular plate, making it prominent and easy to remove).

cortical screw, long enough to fix both cortices of the fibula and tibia, is inserted. Do not overdrill the fibula, because it is easy to depress the fibula, overcompress the syndesmosis, and excessively narrow the ankle joint (or tilt the distal fragment if the screw is proximal). It is also important that the screw protrude through the medial cortex of the tibia so that if it fractures within the syndesmosis, the tip of the screw can be used to remove the screw from the medial side of the ankle. I avoid using syndesmotic bolts, which I believe are easily capable of overcompressing the syndesmosis. Care after surgery is similar to that described previously. Weight-bearing is begun at six weeks, and syndesmotic screws should be removed after three to six months. Some surgeons delay weightbearing until after screw removal to prevent syndesmotic screw breakage.

Complications and Prognosis The prognosis for pure external rotational injuries is relatively good because there is usually less damage of the articular cartilage. When the lateral fracture is far above the syndesmosis, closed treatment can be complicated by late widening of the syndesmosis and shift of the talus. There can also be problems with malrotation of the fibular fragment and nonunion of a wide gap in the medial malleolus. In addition to the complications common to all ankle surgery, surgical treatment can be complicated by failure of the syndesmotic screw or by overreduction of the syndesmosis.

Combination Injuries

Probably the most frequent injury to the ankle involves a combination of abduction and external rotation. The fractures will appear as intermediates between the abduction-type fractures and the external rotation-type fractures that have already been described.

Closed reduction requires a long leg cast applied with both internal rotation and adduction of the ankle. There must be sufficient medial malleolus remaining to buttress the talus and prevent overreduction. As in the other fractures, the cast must remain in place for four to six weeks with frequent radiographic examination of the ankle during the first two weeks. The patient then wears a short leg walking cast unless the fibular fracture is above the syndesmosis, in which case the patient should probably continue touch-down weightbearing for three months. After eight to 12 weeks of immobilization, the patient is allowed to bear weight and, if the syndesmosis was ruptured, a close watch should be kept to make sure it is not widening. Open reduction is necessary when there is no medial buttress, when an anatomic reduction cannot be obtained closed, or when there are intra-articular fragments. The surgical technique is the same as that described before. I emphasize once again the importance of exploring both sides and then achieving fixation of the side that can be most solidly and anatomically fixed before undertaking reduction and internal fixation of the more comminuted side.

References

1. Bauer M, Jonsson K, Nilsson B: Thirty-year follow-up of ankle fractures. *Acta Orthop Scand* 1985;56:103–106.

2. Kristensen KD, Hansen T: Closed treatment of ankle fractures: Stage II supination-eversion fractures followed for 20 years. *Acta Orthop Scand* 1985;56:107–109.

3. Bauer M, Bergström B, Hemborg A, et al: Malleolar fractures: Nonoperative versus operative treatment. A controlled study. *Clin Orthop* 1985;199:17–27.

4. Rowley DI, Norris SH, Duckworth T: A prospective trial comparing operative and manipulative treatment of ankle fractures. *J Bone Joint Surg* 1986;68B:610–613.

5. Wilson FC Jr, Skilbred LA: Long-term results in the treatment of displaced bimalleolar fractures. *J Bone Joint Surg* 1966;48A:1065–1078.

6. Phillips WA, Schwartz HS, Keller CS, et al: A prospective, randomized study of the management of severe ankle fractures. *J Bone Joint Surg* 1985;67A:67–78.

7. Tunturi T, Kemppainen K, Pätiälä H, et al: Importance of anatomical reduction for subjective recovery after ankle fracture. *Acta Orthop Scand* 1983;54:641–647.

8. Franklin JL, Johnson KD, Hansen ST Jr: Immediate internal fixation of open ankle fractures: Report of thirty-eight cases treated with a standard protocol. *J Bone Joint Surg* 1984;66A:1349–1356.

9. Zindrick MR, Knight GS, Gogan WJ, et al: The effect of fibular shortening and rotation on the biomechanics of the talocrural joint during various stages of stance phase. *Trans Orthop Res Soc* 1984;9:136.

10. McLennan JG, Ungersma JA: A new approach to the treatment of ankle fractures: The Inyo nail. *Clin Orthop* 1986;213:125–136.

Ankle Fractures With Diastasis

James B. Stiehl, MD

Introduction

Fractures of the ankle involving the distal tibiofibular joint have been recognized since the early 19th century. Diastasis, from the Greek word meaning "to separate," in this instance implies significant loss of continuity of the tibia and fibula. Several authors, in studying this injury, noted that there must be significant stretching or rupture of the distal tibiofibular syndesmosis in addition to fracture of the distal fibula.[1,2] Rarely, this ligamentous disruption may take place without fracture.[3,4]

Because of the strong ligamentous attachment of the distal fibula to the tibia, one can assume that great force is required to cause this injury. Attempts to create this injury in the laboratory showed that an axial loading force of at least three times body weight, with concomitant external rotation, is required to cause this injury (D.A. Skrade and J.B. Stiehl, unpublished data). Many authors have defined this injury as the most severe and unstable of ankle fractures that do not involve the distal tibial plafond.[5-7]

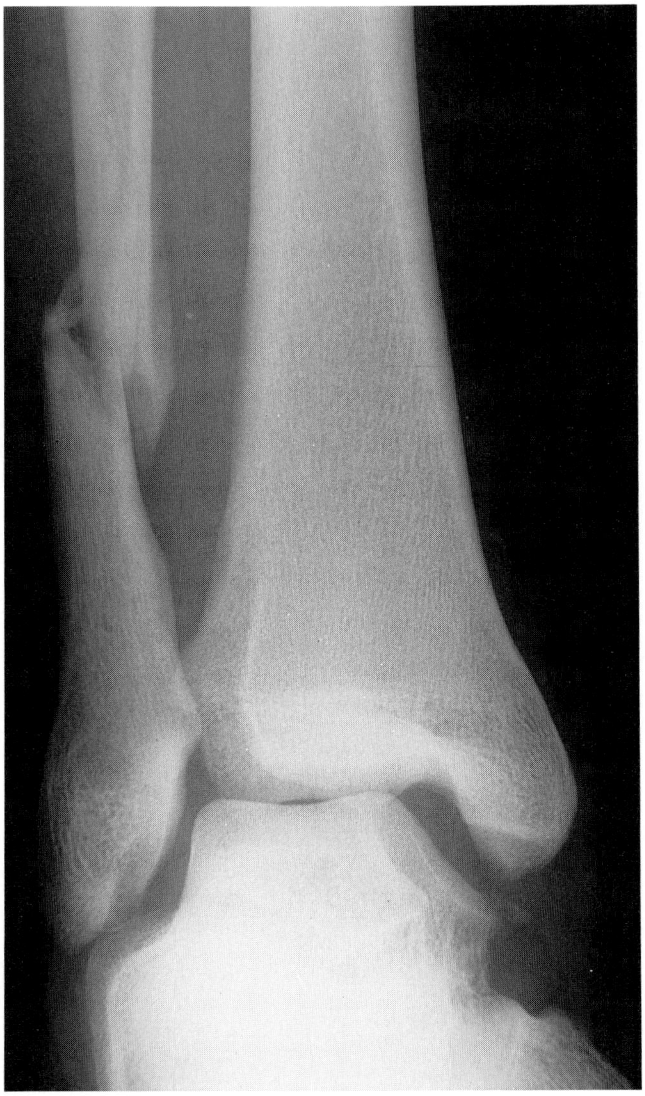

Fig. 1 Fracture-dislocation of right ankle with diastasis, anteroposterior radiograph. (Weber type C or pronation, external rotation type IV)

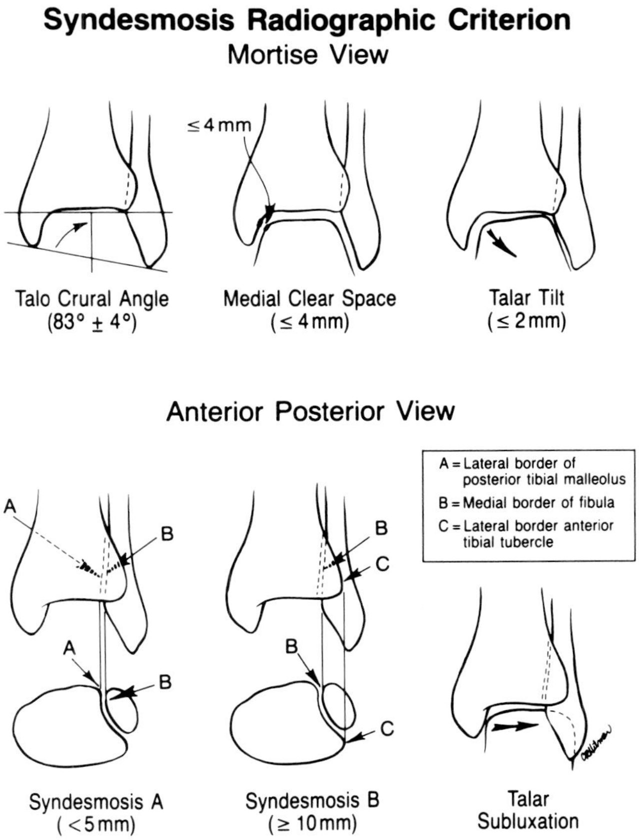

Syndesmosis Radiographic Criterion
Mortise View

Talo Crural Angle (83° ± 4°) Medial Clear Space (≤ 4 mm) Talar Tilt (≤ 2 mm)

Anterior Posterior View

A = Lateral border of posterior tibial malleolus
B = Medial border of fibula
C = Lateral border anterior tibial tubercle

Syndesmosis A (< 5 mm) Syndesmosis B (≥ 10 mm) Talar Subluxation

Fig. 2 Radiologic criteria for evaluation of the syndesmosis.

The classifications of Ashhurst and Bromer[8] and Lauge-Hansen[9] attempted to define both the fracture and ligamentous injury. One author felt that the mixed oblique fracture of the distal fibula was never associated with distal tibiofibular diastasis.[2] More recently, it has been recognized that variants of this fracture pattern (supination-external rotation IV) may occur above the syndesmosis and must by necessity involve the structures of the syndesmosis.[1] Thus, any fracture with a primary force of external rotation or abduction may include diastasis of the distal tibiofibular joint (Fig. 1). The Weber classification takes a more simplistic viewpoint by defining fractures of the fibula above the joint line that involve the structures of the syndesmosis as type C. All diastasis injuries by definition would fall into this category.[10]

Anatomic Considerations

The distal fibula is stabilized in a longitudinal groove on the lateral surface of the tibia, a groove known as the fibular notch. At the distal tibiofibular joint, the articular surface of the tibia faces posteriorly and laterally, so that the axis of the fibula and the fibular notch are directed anteriorly about 30 degrees.[11] The anterior tubercle of the tibia is more prominent than the posterior one and provides an easier landmark for reduction of this joint.

The fibula is held in the joint by four ligaments[12]: (1) The tibiofibular interosseous ligament is a massive ligament that anchors the fibula to the tibia with oblique fibers that run laterally in a distal direction. In the distal segment the fibers are nearly transverse, and a few fi-

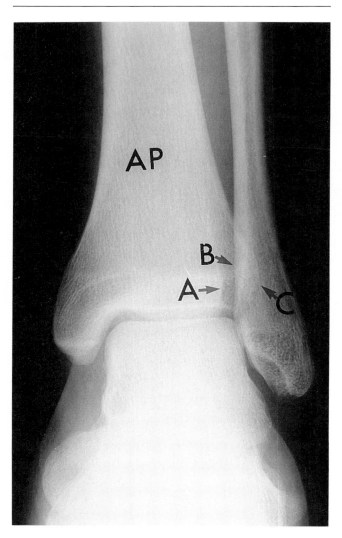

Fig. 3 Normal anteroposterior radiograph. Point A, posterior tibial tubercle: point B, medial border of fibula: point C, anterior tibial tubercle.

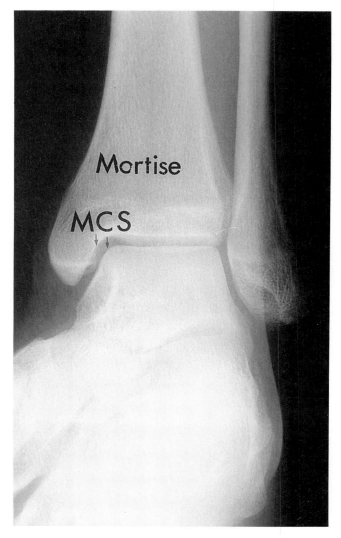

Fig. 4 Normal mortise radiograph demonstrating medial clear space (MCS).

bers run from the tibia in a proximal direction. (2) The anterior inferior tibiofibular ligament arises from the anterior tubercle of the tibia and passes obliquely distally and laterally to the anterior lateral malleolus. (3) The posterior inferior tibiofibular ligament arises from a broad origin on the posterior tubercle of the tibia and passes obliquely distally and laterally to the posterior lateral malleolus. (4) The transverse tibiofibular ligament is separate from the posterior inferior tibiofibular ligament and passes from the posterior tibial margin to the osteochondral junction on the posterior and medial margins of the distal fibula.

Biomechanical Considerations

From the work of Close[13] and Inman,[14] we know that normal articular motion in the ankle joint depends on a precise relationship determined by the syndesmosis. Most importantly, the talus normally articulates with the ankle mortise throughout the range of motion. To accommodate the varying width of the talus, the intermalleolar distance increases approximately 1.5 mm as the ankle goes from plantar flexion to dorsiflexion, and

the fibula demonstrates motion in all planes. Close[13] estimated the rotation of the fibula to be 5 to 6 degrees, but, at this time, the actual amount of anterior-posterior or proximal-distal motion has not been quantified.

Using cineradiography, Weinert and associates[15] showed that the fibula moves distally on stance-phase weightbearing. This would seem logical because the mortise deepens to provide the greatest stability at the moment of greatest loading or impact; however, no experimental model to date has documented this finding.

Sammarco and associates[16] demonstrated that the instant centers of rotation created by ankle motion constantly change in a reproducible fashion. This clearly indicates that the ankle joint is not a hinge joint. Rotation normally occurs with the tibia rotating internally on the fixed talus during dorsiflexion and externally during plantar flexion.[14]

Studies have been made regarding the individual function of each ligament of the syndesmosis. Close[13] sectioned all the ligaments of the syndesmosis and found minimal widening of the mortise of 2 mm. However, when the deep horizontal section of the deltoid ligament was cut, this diastasis increased to 3.7 mm.

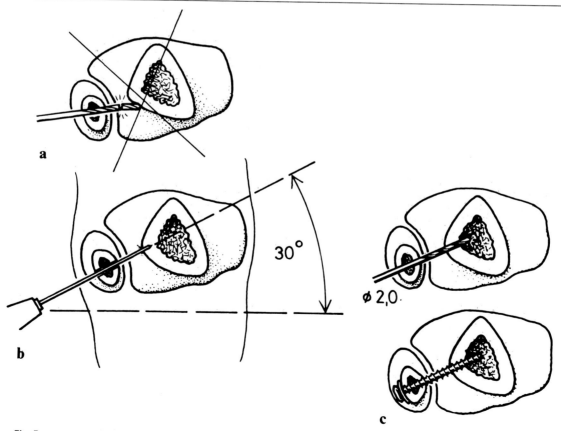

Fig. 5 Insertion of transverse position screw must be angled 30 degrees anteriorly. (Reproduced with permission from Heim U, Pfeiffer KM: *Small Fragment Set Manual.* Berlin, Springer-Verlag, 1982.)

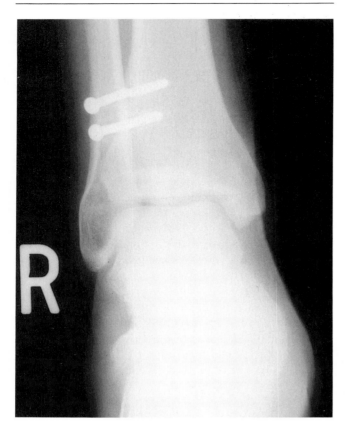

Fig. 6 Broken syndesmotic screw, also showing lucencies about the screws.

Close found that the deltoid ligament stretches only about 2 mm at its greatest dimension. Thus, for gross diastasis of the ankle to occur, the deltoid ligament or medial malleolus must be disrupted.

In an experimental study on the effect of a syndesmosis screw, Olerud[17] found that dorsiflexion was limited by 0.1 degrees for every degree of plantar flexion at the time of insertion of the syndesmosis screw. He recommended that syndesmosis screws be set with the ankle in maximal dorsiflexion. However, this potential anatomic constraint was felt to be negligible as an explanation for potential ankle stiffness. An investigation of the effect of the syndesmosis screw on other parameters, including talar tilt, anterior posterior drawer, and rotation, showed that external rotation is the only motion significantly limited in the loaded specimen.[18] Theoretically, the screw should be removed before resuming normal weightbearing, to allow for physiologic movement of the fibula. Clinical opinions differ widely on this subject.

Clinical Assessment

In addition to pain, swelling, and inability to bear weight, certain objective findings can be elicited from clinical evaluation. Tenderness may be present along the lateral border of the leg to the level of the fibular fracture. I recommend assessing distal stability by using the Cotton test. This test, described by Cotton[19] in 1910, involves stabilizing the distal lower leg with one hand and grasping each side of the foot at the talus with the thumb and forefinger of the other hand. By applying a mediolateral force, crepitus and instability can be assessed from mortise widening. Instability of less than 3 to 4 mm can be treated without surgery, but greater amounts imply damage to both the fibula and/or syndesmosis and the medial structures. Unstable ankle fractures are best treated with internal fixation.

Radiographic Considerations

For planning before surgery and assessment afterwards, a knowledge of the radiographic criteria of normal ankle anatomy is essential. The following infor-

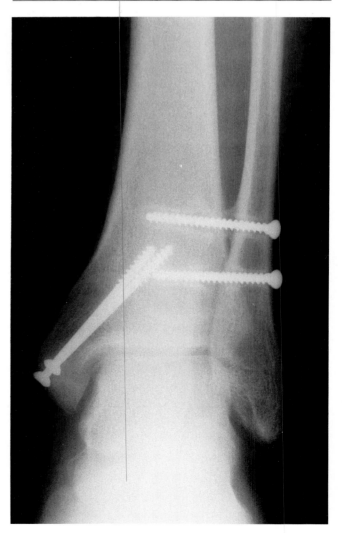

Fig. 7 Syndesmotic screws with lucencies from micromovement.

mation is derived from review of the literature (Figs. 2 to 4).[20,21]

Talocrural Angle This angle is formed by a line perpendicular to the distal tibial articular surface and a line joining the tips of both malleoli on the mortise view. The normal adult talocrural angle is 83 ± 4 degrees. There is normally less than 2 degrees of difference between sides, and any difference greater than 5 degrees is abnormal.[22]

Medial Clear Space This is the distance from the lateral border of the medial malleolus to the medial border of the talus at the level of the talar dome on the mortise radiograph. A space greater than 4 mm is abnormal.[23]

Talar Tilt This is any difference in the widths of the joint space proximal to the medial and lateral talar ridges on the mortise radiograph. A difference of 2 mm is considered the upper limit of normal.[8]

Syndesmosis A This is a measurement of the tibiofibular clear space from the lateral border of the posterior tibial malleolus (point A) to the medial border of the fibula (point B) on the anteroposterior radiograph. It is normally less than 5 mm and, if abnormal, represents syndesmosis disruption.[20]

Syndesmosis B This is a measurement of the overlap from the medial border to the fibula (point B) to the lateral border of the anterior tibial prominence (point C) on the anterior posterior radiograph. This is abnormal if less than 10 mm.[20]

Talar Subluxation This is a subjective assessment of congruity of the tibial articular surface and talar dome on the anterior radiograph. Any incongruity is abnormal.

Surgical Treatment

Because of the severity and instability of these injuries, swelling is marked. Surgical reduction within 12 hours is mandatory to avoid wound-healing problems from compromised soft tissues. The most dangerous time is after three to four days have passed and fracture blisters as well as contused skin increase the risk of infection by several-fold. In these instances, it is best to perform an adequate closed reduction and to wait two to three weeks. Infection of the ankle joint is a serious problem that can result in fusion or may even require amputation.

Internal fixation of the ankle has been described elsewhere and follows the principles of the AO method.[10] The primary goal is anatomic restoration, including temporary stabilization of the syndesmosis until early ligament healing is present.

In order to restore the normal mortise, the fibula must be brought to length and fixed with a contoured semitubular plate. Contour is important, because if no bend is placed, a painful ankle can result from the straightened distal fibula. Comminution can be spanned by a plate, and appropriate length can usually be determined by assembling major fragments.[24] Nonunion is uncommon in the distal fibula, and bone graft can fill small defects. Fractures of the fibula located more proximally should be plated if there is shortening or displacement. Attempts to maintain proper length of the fibula by closed means will fail because of the amount of tension from the surrounding soft tissues.

If total syndesmosis disruption has occurred and the posterior tubercle of the distal tibia is fractured, the fibula drifts posteriorly and reduction by closed methods is nearly impossible to maintain. A transverse position or syndesmosis screw is used to hold the fibula in reduction. Before it can be inserted, all other bony

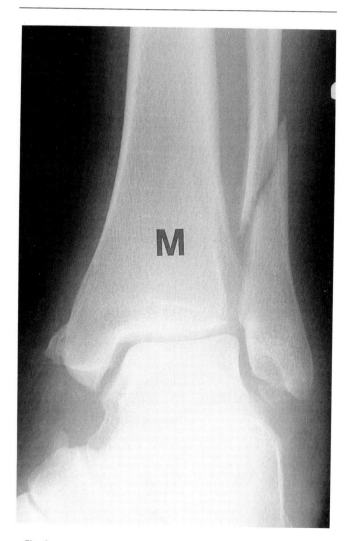

Fig. 8   Case 1. Mortise radiograph.

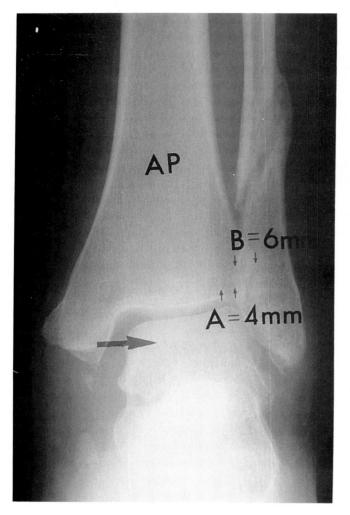

Fig. 9 Case 1. Anteroposterior radiograph at six-month follow-up showing talar subluxation and abnormal syndesmosis B.

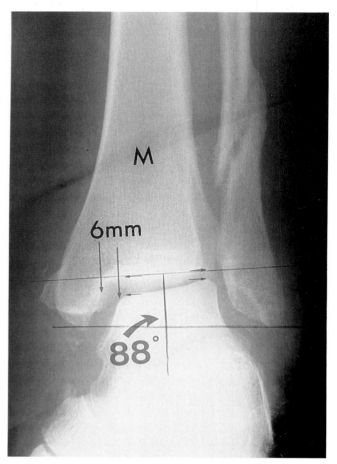

Fig. 10 Case 1. Mortise radiograph showing abnormal talocrural angle, medial clear space, and talar tilt.

structures must be stabilized and the joint reduced. I believe the posterior tubercle and malleolar fragment should be fixed if it is large enough to have articular cartilage present. Important weightbearing surface may be gained and stability is enhanced because the posterior and transverse tibiofibular ligaments are attached to this fragment. The posterior malleolus is best fixed directly through a posterolateral approach.

Before inserting the syndesmosis screw, the Cotton sign is assessed. It will usually be 5 mm or more, but it must revert to zero after screw placement. The screw is usually inserted 2 cm above the joint and may be placed through the plate. It must be directed anteriorly about 30 degrees from the coronal plane of the lower leg to center the screw (Fig. 5) or the screw may skive off the posterior surface of the tibia. Reduction of the tibiofibular joint is done by reversing the mechanism of injury with internal rotation and firm thumb pressure holding the fibula firmly in a slightly anterior di-

rection against the anterior tubercle of the distal tibia. All four cortices of the fibula and tibia are carefully drilled and tapped while reduction is held. I recommend a 4.5-mm AO screw or the new, stronger 3.5-mm cortical screw, placed through four cortices. The older types of 3.5-mm cortical screws are too weak and will break with weightbearing. Also, the three-cortex, elastic-type fixation described by the AO group is suspect and can lead to screw failure (Figs. 6 and 7).

Before the wound is closed, anteroposterior and mortise radiographs must be carefully assessed to make certain all parameters described above are anatomic. The wound is closed over suction drains, and the foot is splinted in the neutral position.

Postoperative Management

To allow syndesmosis and fracture healing, the patient should be kept nonweightbearing for six weeks. However, early active range of motion is started at five to seven days after surgery, as soon as wound healing is assured. The leg may be protected by a short leg orthosis. I believe that all syndesmosis screws should be removed at six to eight weeks to allow for return of normal fibular motion. Following screw removal, full weightbearing can be initiated, but the short leg orthosis should be worn for at least another four to six weeks. At final release to normal activity, no tenderness should be present about the ankle, and the Cotton sign should be physiologic. Stretching and strengthening exercises are recommended until normal function is achieved. Plate removal may be considered in younger patients at 12 to 18 months following injury.

Case Studies

Case 1 A 52-year-old woman who fell at home sustained a Weber type C fracture-dislocation of the left ankle (Fig. 8). Surgical treatment was refused and a cast was applied. Reduction of the distal fibula was inadequate. The patient developed significant ankle pain over ensuing months and was noted at one year to have painful ambulation requiring anti-inflammatory medication (Figs. 9 and 10).

Case 2 A 25-year-old man who injured his right ankle playing softball sustained a Weber type C (pronation, external rotation type IV) fracture-dislocation (Fig. 11). Immediate open reduction and internal fixation was done, plating the fibula and placing a transverse position screw at the ankle to stabilize the syndesmosis (Fig. 12). The syndesmosis screw was removed at 55 days and the plate removed at 12 months. Final follow-up at 83 months revealed an asymptomatic ankle with perfect anatomic result (Fig. 13).

Case 3 A 43-year-old man injured his right ankle playing soccer and sustained a Weber type C (supination, external rotation type 4) fracture-dislocation. Initial closed reduction proved inadequate and subsequent open reduction and internal fixation was done. A 4.5-mm cortical AO screw stabilized the syndesmosis and was removed at 43 days. Follow-up at 86 months revealed anatomic reduction with slight radiographic ar-

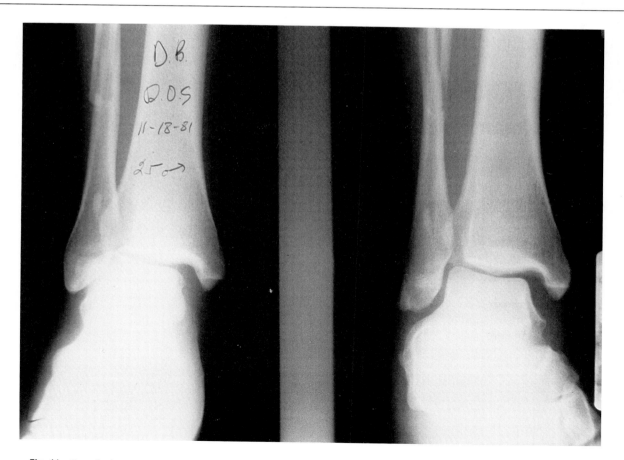

Fig. 11 Case 2. Anteroposterior and mortise view of pronation, external rotation type IV ankle fracture.

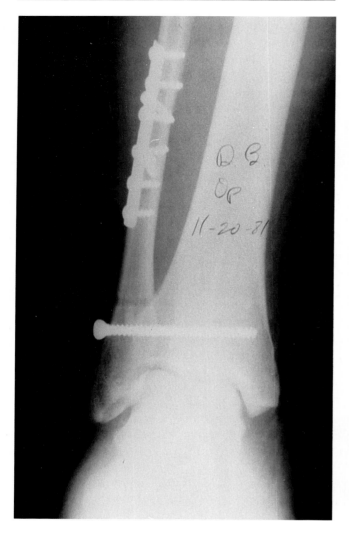

Fig. 12 Case 2. Postoperative radiograph.

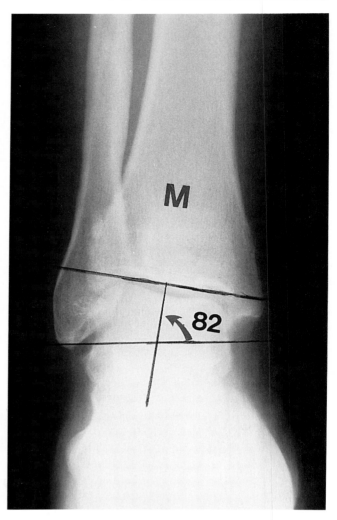

Fig. 13 Follow-up mortise view at 83 months with normal talo-crural angle.

thritic changes associated with minimal symptoms after prolonged activity.

Conclusions

Any approach to these most difficult fractures requires a thorough understanding of the anatomy in order to restore damaged structures accurately. Experience has shown that anything less than perfect anatomic restoration will lead to early degenerative arthritis. The use of a transverse position screw has been widely affirmed in these fractures, but opinion differs as to which technique should be used and when the screw is to be removed. My approach is based on experimental work and 12 years of clinical experience.

References

1. Pankovich AM: Fractures of the fibula proximal to the distal tibiofibular syndesmosis. *J Bone Joint Surg* 1978;60A:221–229.
2. Colton CL: Fracture-diastasis of the inferior tibio-fibular joint. *J Bone Joint Surg* 1968;50B:830–835.
3. Bosworth DM: Fracture-dislocation of the ankle with fixed displacement of the fibula behind the tibia. *J Bone Joint Surg* 1947;29:130–135.
4. Woods RS: Irreducible dislocation of the ankle-joint. *Br J Surg* 1942;29:359–360.
5. Pankovich AM: Fractures of the fibula at the distal tibiofibular syndesmosis. *Clin Orthop* 1979;143:138–147.
6. Hughes JL, Weber H, Willenegger H, et al: Evaluation of ankle fractures: Non-operative and operative treatment. *Clin Orthop* 1979;138:111–119.
7. de Souza LJ, Gustilo RB, Meyer TJ: Results of operative treatment of displaced external rotation-abduction fractures of the ankle. *J Bone Joint Surg* 1985;67A:1066–1074.
8. Ashhurst APC, Bromer RS: Classification and mechanism of frac-

tures of the leg bones involving the ankle: Based on a study of three hundred cases from the Episcopal Hospital. *Arch Surg* 1922;4:51–129.

9. Lauge-Hansen N: Fractures of the ankle: II. Combined experimental-surgical and experimental-roentgenologic investigations. *Arch Surg* 1950;60:957–985.

10. Heim U, Pfeiffer KM: *Small Fragment Set Manual.* Berlin, Springer- Verlag, 1982.

11. Heim U: Malleolarfrakturen. *Unfallheilkunde* 1983;86:248–258.

12. Grath GB: Widening of the ankle mortise: A clinical and experimental study. *Acta Chir Scand* 1960;263(suppl):1–88.

13. Close JR: Some applications of the functional anatomy of the ankle joint. *J Bone Joint Surg* 1956;38A:761–781.

14. Inman VT: *The Joints of the Ankle.* Baltimore, Williams & Wilkins, 1976.

15. Weinert CR Jr, McMaster JH, Ferguson RJ: Dynamic function of the human fibula. *Am J Anat* 1973;138:145–149.

16. Sammarco GJ, Burstein AH, Frankel VH: Biomechanics of the ankle: A kinematic study. *Orthop Clin North Am* 1973;4:75–96.

17. Olerud C: The effect of the syndesmotic screw on the extension

18. Needleman RL, Skrade DA, Stiehl JB: The effect of the syndesmotic screw on ankle motion. *Foot Ankle,* in press.

19. Cotton FJ: *Fractures and Joint-Dislocations.* Philadelphia, WB Saunders, 1910, p 549.

20. Pettrone FA, Gail M, Pee D, et al: Quantitative criteria for prediction of the results after displaced fracture of the ankle. *J Bone Joint Surg* 1983;65A:66–77.

21. Phillips WA, Schwartz HS, Keller CS, et al: A prospective, randomized study of the management of severe ankle fractures. *J Bone Joint Surg* 1985;67A:67–78.

22. Sarkisian JS, Cody GW: Closed treatment of ankle fractures: A new criterion for evaluation—a review of 250 cases. *J Trauma* 1976;16:323–326.

23. Joy G, Patzakis MJ, Harvey JP Jr: Precise evaluation of the reduction of severe ankle fractures: Technique and correlation with end results. *J Bone Joint Surg* 1974;56A:979–993.

24. Limbird RS, Aaron RK: Laterally comminuted fracture-dislocation of the ankle. *J Bone Joint Surg* 1987;69A:881–885.

capacity of the ankle joint. *Arch Orthop Trauma Surg* 1985;104:299–302.

Trimalleolar Ankle Fractures and Open Ankle Fractures

S. Ashby Grantham, MD

Fractures of the Posterior Lip of the Tibia

As he was with so many other skeletal injuries, Sir Astley Cooper in 1822 was probably the first to recognize a posterior tibial lip fracture, which he depicted in association with posterior talar subluxation. Earle wrote in 1829 of a similar novel finding at autopsy. Lucas-Championnière's 1870 theory that vertical compression was important in causing the fracture was documented experimentally in 1890 by Rochet. Destot named the posterior lip of the tibia "the third malleolus" in 1912, and, in the same year, Frederick Jay Cotton in Boston described this ankle fracture as "a new type of ankle fracture." Henderson in 1932 applied the clear and descriptive term, trimalleolar, to this injury. The word malleolus, as used by Vesalius, means "little hammer."[1]

Understanding the biomechanics of an ankle fracture is important, particularly for closed treatment. Over the years several classifications have been developed to provide pathomechanical insight, notably those of Ashhurst and Bromer in 1922, Lauge-Hansen in 1950, and Danis and Weber (AO) in 1970. The Lauge-Hansen system is the most widely used, although it is clinically cumbersome. It consists of four major types of injury: supination-adduction, supination-eversion, pronation-abduction, and pronation-eversion, with two to four

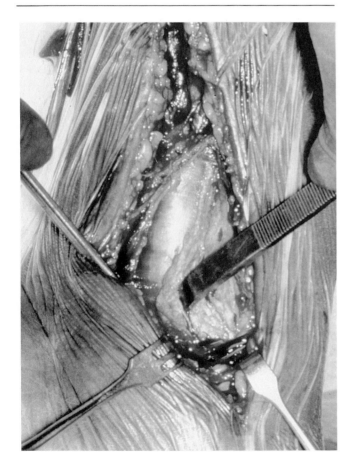

Fig. 1 Shelton technique. Left ankle, medial incision with foot at bottom and knee at top. Shows the medial malleolar fracture and start of posterior tibial sheath elevation from the proximal posterior tibia.

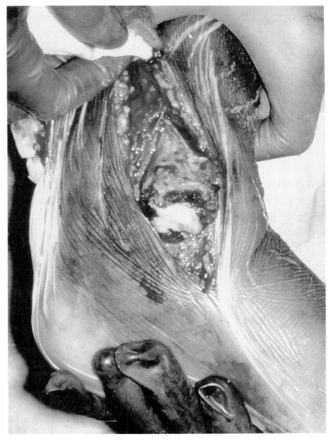

Fig. 2 The foot is being subluxed laterally through the non-visualized fibular malleolar fracture—the tibial plafond is being presented into the wound.

stages for each type. If external rotation is substituted for eversion, Lauge-Hansen's intent becomes somewhat clearer. A posterior lip fracture may be produced by a continuation of the traumatic force in each type except the supination-adduction group.

Analysis of posterior lip fracture size is sometimes difficult, although large ones are obvious and small ones clinically irrelevant. Interpretation is best done after relocation of marked displacement. In a large series over 20 years, McLaughlin[2] concluded that displacement of a posterior fragment involving less than 10% of the plafond can be safely ignored, whereas fragments involving more than 25% require surgical repair. With 10% to 25% of the surface involved, posttraumatic arthritis develops in 20% of the ankles within two years. Two problems should be considered, however. First, the fracture line of the posterior lip may be somewhat oblique instead of transverse, which can make assessment difficult. Second, an intermediate or intercalary fracture segment is commonly present. Part of the posterior tibial articular overhang may be compressed and fractured by the talus before a small posterior lip breaks off, which leads to an underestimation of the degree

of damage, to inadequate treatment, and to tibiotalar joint incongruity and posterior talar subluxation with late arthritic changes.

Closed treatment of a displaced large trimalleolar fracture is usually ineffective and inappropriate.[3] Reduction of the bimalleolar component may be lost by the strong dorsiflexion of the ankle necessary to reduce the posterior lip, as well as by the anterior force needed to resist posterior talar subluxation. Dorsiflexion of the great toe has been reported to aid the maneuver. This therapeutic dilemma leads to poor position of one or both components of the injury and predictably poor results.

The principles of surgery include prompt reduction of gross displacement, but carrying out the surgery only when the soft tissues permit. A tourniquet is usually unnecessary and careful attention and protection must be given to the soft tissues and wound margins at surgery. Anatomic reduction and secure fixation must be achieved so that motion can be begun early. Weight-bearing is deferred for at least eight weeks. Minimal displacements produce remarkable alterations in tibiotalar contact pressures. A 1-mm lateral displacement, for example, produces 42% loss of contact[4] and a step-

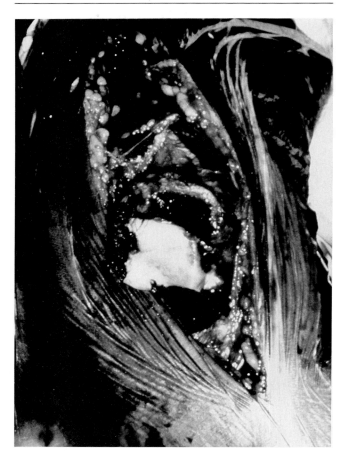

Fig. 3 Further presentation of the tibial plafond with visualization of the fracture bed of the posterior lip and medial malleolus.

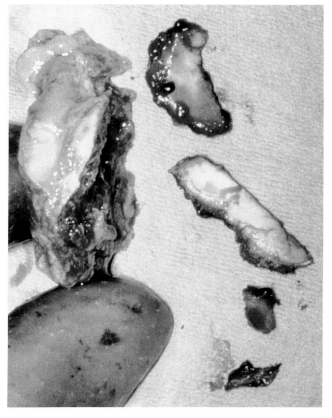

Fig. 4 The posterior lip fragment has been dissected from the depths of the surgical exposure by release of the posterior fibulotalar ligament. Some intercalary fracture fragments are also seen here.

off of more than 2 mm produces predictable arthritic wear.

Most fracture authorities recommend surgery for the large posterior lip fracture, but differ on how best to achieve reduction and stabilization. The ideal fracture treatment suggested by Clay Ray Murray would have us "wish the fragments into place, hold them there by moral suasion, and send the patient on about his business while the fracture heals."[2]

Key and Conwell[5] made the following recommendations. If the fragment is more than 25%, try manipulation, by applying distal traction and anterior force on the foot, and immobilize the ankle in a neutral cast. If a radiograph taken one or two days later shows loss of reduction, surgery will be necessary. Make a posterolateral incision, push the fragment into place and hold it with two screws or nails. Then fix the lateral fracture and, finally, the medial malleolar fracture.

Wilson[1] stated that if the fragment involves more than 25% of the joint surface, open reduction is indicated, using two-screw fixation of the posterior lip followed by a treatment of the residual bimalleolar fracture.

Yablon and Segal[6] recommended stabilization of the medial or lateral malleolus, a posterolateral approach to the posterior lip, manipulation of the fragment into place, insertion of a K-wire from front to back, and, if reduction is confirmed radiographically, insertion of a lag screw from front to back.

Sisk[7] suggested an anteromedial incision for the medial malleolus and a posterolateral incision for the posterior lip and fibula, or a separate posteromedial incision for the posterior lip with retraction of the flexor hallucis longus medially and Achilles tendon laterally, followed by reduction of the fragment and stabilization with one or two screws inserted from back to front.

Werner and Farber used a posterolateral incision, with turn-down of the fibula as in the Gatellier and Chastang approach, followed by reduction and fixation of the posterior lip with two lag screws from the front and repair of the malleoli.[7]

Harper and Hardin[8] recently offered a different approach. Their premise is that anatomic reduction and fixation of the lateral malleolus automatically ensures reduction of the posterior lip via the posterior fibulotalar ligament. This is exactly what Denham[9] advocated 25 years ago, and he credited Gissane (personal communication, 1955). Harper and Hardin reported on 38 patients, comparing trimalleolar fixation in 15 with bimalleolar fixation in 23. Results at two years were comparable and no posterior subluxation was seen in any patient. This approach does not achieve exact and stable reconstruction, does not allow early motion, nor does it address the issue of comminution.

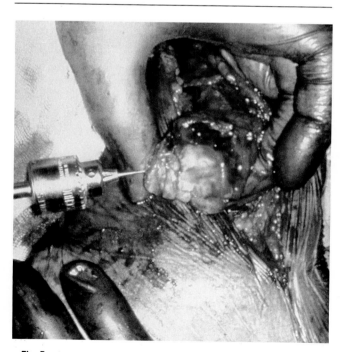

Fig. 5 Accurate reassembly of the plafond can be done with supportive bone grafting as necessary.

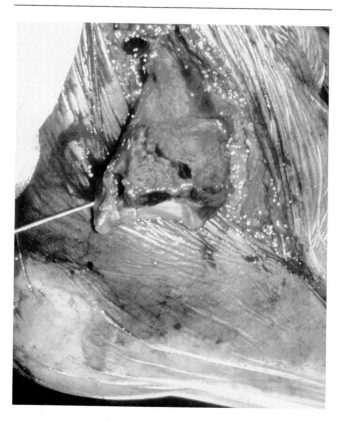

Fig. 6 View of the reconstructed arc of the distal tibia. Temporary pinning is replaced by screws or buttress plate. After the tibia is relocated, the fibular fracture is repaired, and then the medial malleolar fracture is repaired.

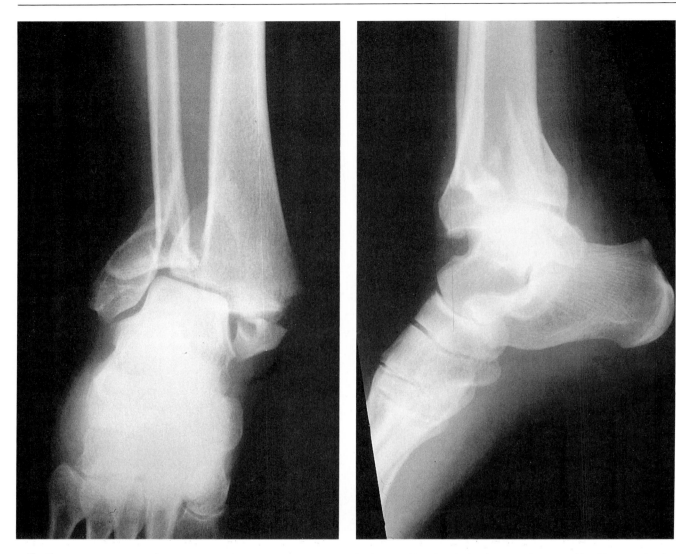

Fig. 7   Anteroposterior (**left**) and lateral (**right**) initial radiographs of a right ankle trimalleolar fracture show considerable comminution and displacement. The lateral radiograph shows a large posterior lip fracture with some comminution in addition to posterior talar displacement.

For many trimalleolar fractures that require surgery, I prefer the procedure devised by Shelton.[10] Shelton (Rosenwasser and associates, unpublished data) reviewed 394 ankle fractures over a seven-year period and found 118 trimalleolar ankle fractures. Of these, 45 were repaired by his technique. Average patient age was 48 years, average amount of joint involvement was 32%, and average follow-up was 43 months. Of the patients, 83% were women. Results were good and complications were few, with only one infection and one case of phlebitis. No osteonecrosis was seen and none of the cases required subsequent fusion.

Shelton advised using a 6- to 7-inch oblique medial incision from the posterior tibial margin proximally to anterior and below the medial malleolus distally (Fig.

1). Release of the superficial fascia and a 3- inch elevation of the posterior tibial tendon and sheath distally allows excellent visualization of the tibial plafond into the wound by dislocation of the talus and foot laterally (Figs. 2 and 3). The posterior marginal fragment is completely freed by releasing the posterior fibulotalar ligament (Fig. 4). The joint surface is then comfortably and accurately reconstructed (Figs. 5 and 6). Intercalary comminution or a depressed segment can be fully corrected, rather like a tibial plateau fracture. The foot is reduced and a "bimalleolar" fracture repair carried out. Radiographs of an injured ankle (Fig. 7), the same ankle after surgery (Fig. 8), and two-year follow-up radiographs (Fig. 9), show the effectiveness of this technique.

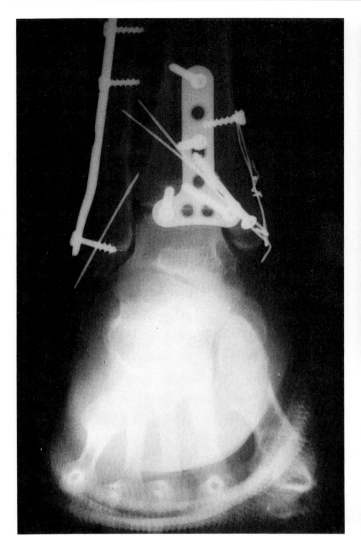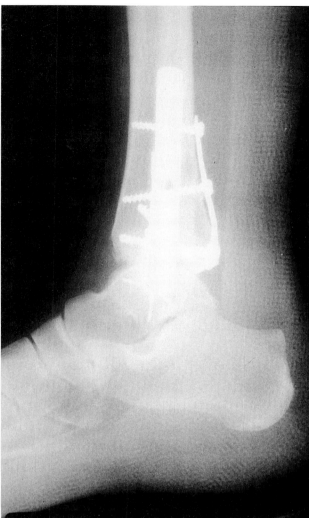

Fig. 8 Anteroposterior (**left**) and lateral (**right**) radiographs taken shortly after surgery.

Fractures of the Anterior Lip of the Tibia

Anterior lip fractures are much less common than fractures of the posterior lip.[11] Most anterior lip fractures are caused by vertical loading with dorsiflexion of the foot, but some of the small marginal fractures can be caused by severe plantar flexion with capsular avulsion of bone. These fractures respond well to treatment as outlined for the posterior lip fracture unless the anterior lip fracture is part of a pilon or talar neck fracture or the anterior tibial vessels are damaged.

Reconstruction of a large anterior lip fracture through an anterolateral exposure is easier than reconstruction of the posterior counterpart. Intercalary fragments are common, however, and should be dealt with as in posterior lip fractures.

Open Fractures of the Ankle

Open fractures in general and open ankle fractures in particular present special problems. Most open fractures should be treated in the operating room where adequate debridement under satisfactory anesthesia can be carried out. The first priority is prevention of infection. Tetanus prophylaxis and prophylactic antibiotics are used. For both wound and fracture, the sooner surgery is carried out, the better. The wound is usually cultured in the emergency room or before debridement in the operating room.

Gustilo and Anderson[12] made it possible to communicate better about open fractures. Most ankle fractures are type I or II injuries and can be converted to a clean surgical wound. Adequate internal fixation sta-

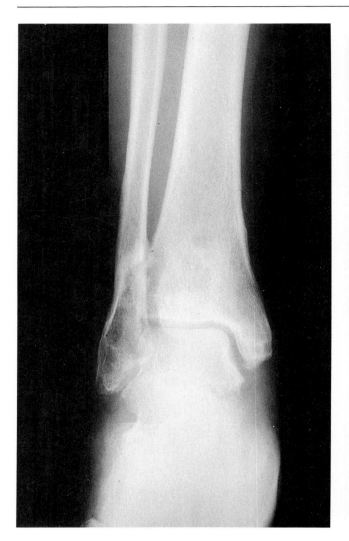
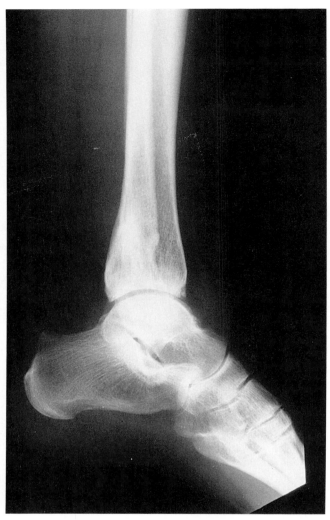

Fig. 9   Radiographs of the same ankle two years after surgery. The anteroposterior radiograph (**left**) shows the ankle to be well healed, with good joint space and excellent function. The lateral radiograph (**right**) shows no arthritis or subluxation.

bilizes and rests the injured tissues, provides easier access for wound care, and allows precise restoration of joint surfaces. Thorough cleansing is paramount. The 10-L irrigation rule precludes abbreviation of this tedious part of the procedure.

Type III injuries are not usually associated with uncomplicated bimalleolar or trimalleolar fractures. These injuries need expert care to avoid amputation, and in many cases multiple operations will be necessary. The external fixator, free flaps, and microvascular repairs have significantly improved results in certain of these injuries.

References

1. Wilson FC: Fractures and dislocations of the ankle, in Rockwood CA Jr, Green DP (eds): *Fractures in Adults*, ed 2. Philadelphia, JB Lippincott, 1984, vol 2, pp 1665–1701.

2. McLaughlin HL: Injuries of the ankle, in McLaughlin HL (ed): *Trauma*. Philadelphia, WB Saunders, 1959, pp 357–360.

3. McDaniel WJ, Wilson FC: Trimalleolar fractures of the ankle: An end result study. *Clin Orthop* 1977;122:37–45.

4. Ramsey PL, Hamilton W: Changes in tibiotalar area of contact caused by lateral talar shift. *J Bone Joint Surg* 1976;58A:356–357.

5. Key JA, Conwell HE: *The Management of Fractures, Dislocations, and Sprains*, ed 5. St. Louis, CV Mosby, 1951, pp 1116–1120.

6. Yablon IG, Segal D: Ankle fractures, in Evarts CM (ed): *Surgery of the Musculoskeletal System*. New York, Churchill Livingstone, 1983, vol 3, pp 8:87–8:114.

7. Sisk TD: Fractures, in Edmonson AS, Crenshaw AH (eds): *Campbell's Operative Orthopaedics*, ed 6. St. Louis, CV Mosby, 1980, vol 1, pp 508–713.

8. Harper MC, Hardin G: Posterior malleolar fractures of the ankle associated with external rotation-abduction injuries: Results with and without internal fixation. *J Bone Joint Surg* 1988;70A:1348–1356.

9. Denham RA: Internal fixation for unstable ankle fractures. *J Bone Joint Surg* 1964;46B:206–211.

10. Shelton ML, Anderson RL Jr: Complications of fractures and dislocations of the ankle, in Epps CH Jr (ed): *Complications in Orthopaedic Surgery*, ed 2. Philadelphia, JB Lippincott, 1986, vol 1, pp 599–648.

11. Hamilton WC: Fractures of the posterior and anterior tibial margins, in Hamilton WC (ed): *Traumatic Disorders of the Ankle*. New York, Springer-Verlag, 1984, pp 187–196.

12. Gustilo RB, Anderson JT: Prevention of infection in the treatment of one thousand and twenty-five open fractures of long bones: Retrospective and prospective analyses. *J Bone Joint Surg* 1976;58A:453–458.

CHAPTER 12

Open Fractures of the Ankle Joint

James B. Stiehl, MD

Introduction

In recent years, the treatment of open joint injuries has focused on the use of internal fixation to restore articular congruity, and, at the same time, to allow treatment of soft-tissue injury. Improved implants, prophylactic antibiotics, and good surgical techniques have greatly reduced the incidence of infection.

Franklin and associates[1] reported 38 open ankle fractures treated with initial wound debridement, immediate rigid anatomic internal fixation, and delayed wound closure at five days. At follow-up, there were no nonunions and only one possible deep infection in the group, which included 16 grade III open fractures (Outline 1).

Bray,[2] in a similar series, compared surgical debridement and immediate internal fixation with debridement and delayed open reduction. There was one infection in each group, but the immediate fixation group had statistically better motion. Also, hospitalization, which averaged nine days in the delayed fixation group, was shortened to an average of six days. This chapter reviews current thinking on open ankle fractures.

Emergency Management

Management of the open fracture starts at the scene of the accident. It is appropriate for the emergency medical team to return the foot to the neutral position by applying gentle axial traction. This enhances stability and improves vascular flow to the foot. The wound should be dressed with sterile, saline-soaked gauze. A splint is applied, but tight circumferential wrapping, which could further compromise the distal circulation, is to be avoided.

When the patient reaches the emergency room, evaluation includes checking neurovascular status, defining fracture stability by examination, and obtaining anteroposterior, mortise, and lateral radiographs. Wounds should remain untouched or at least minimally and sterilely exposed until the patient reaches the operating room. Tscherne and Gotzen[3] found a significantly higher infection rate when the wound was exposed in the emergency room.

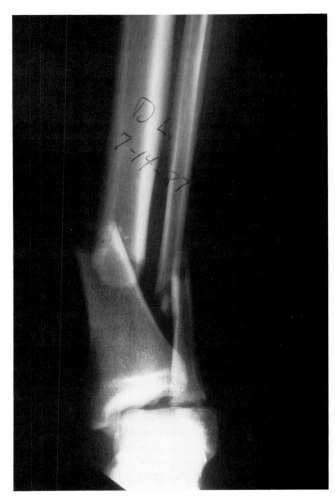

Fig. 1 Fracture of the distal tibia and fibula with displaced fracture-dislocation of the ankle.

Outline 1
Classification of Open Fractures

Type 1   An open fracture with a clean wound less than 1 cm long.

Type 2   An open fracture with a laceration more than 1 cm long without extensive soft-tissue damage, flaps, or avulsons.

Type 3   An open fracture with massive soft-tissue damage; compromised vascularity; severe wound contamination; and marked fracture instability.
  - A. Adequate soft-tissue coverage of a fractured bone despite extensive soft-tissue laceration or flaps, or high-energy trauma irrespective of the size of the wound.
  - B. Extensive soft-tissue injury loss with periosteal stripping and bone exposure, usually associated with massive contamination.
  - C. Open fracture associated with arterial injury requiring repair.

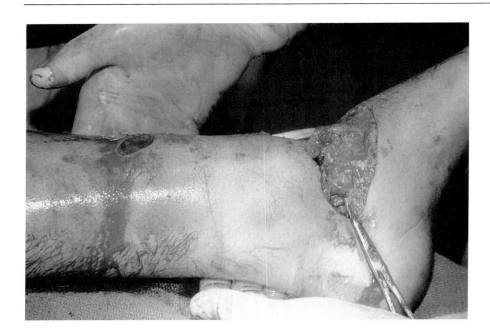

Fig. 2 Grade II open wound of distal tibia with grade IIIC fracture-dislocation of the ankle. Hemostat demonstrates lacerated posterior tibial artery.

Prophylactic antibiotics are started early and continued for 48 hours. For grades I and II injuries, a broad-spectrum, first-generation cephalosporin is satisfactory. With grade III wounds, a cephalosporin plus an aminoglycoside is used. For severe grade III, farm-type injuries, intravenous penicillin is added.[4,5] Tetanus toxoid should be given alone or in combination with hyperimmune globulin, if indicated.

Presurgical Planning

For any surgical procedure, a satisfactory outcome depends on careful consideration of all potential problems. Important considerations in open ankle fractures include assessing the soft-tissue injury (Outline 1), determining subsequent fracture management, and being prepared to handle any other exigencies. A surgeon capable of repairing small vessels must be on hand to treat injury to the anterior and posterior tibial artery. Proper instruments, drills, and implant sets should be selected in advance. External fixation devices should be available as indicated.

A detailed plan for fracture reduction and anticipated implants should be made on tracing paper along with a step-by-step outline of the procedure. With experience, this approach facilitates technique, avoids errors, and shortens the time required for surgery.

Surgical Management

In the operating room, the wound is handled sterilely and the debridement starts while the patient is being prepared for surgery. All dirt, grease, or other particulate matter must be removed. Minimal shaving is needed. The ankle is held carefully while the nurse scrubs it. It may not be appropriate to let the leg hang on a legholder. Debridement is done by incising the skin edges and then systematically debriding to deeper layers. All questionable tissue must be removed to avoid having it be a nidus for future infection. Pulsed mechanical lavage is then done, using 12 L of saline with antibiotic solution. Deep cultures can be made after debridement is complete. The leg is redraped, the surgeons regown and glove, and clean instruments are put on the table. A vascular injury, which does not require bone stability, can be repaired at this point.

The soft-tissue wound determines the type of fracture stabilization to use. For grades I and II fractures, and some grade III fractures, standard internal fixation techniques may be used. I use the AO method, which has been well described elsewhere.[6] Anatomic restoration and rigid stable internal fixation to allow early active range of motion are the goals.

A transverse medial wound, caused by laceration of the skin as the foot displaces laterally, is common. Minimal internal fixation using screws or Kirschner wires is done, to allow closure over the joint and implants. Primary closure of the skin can be delayed for three to five days. Skin graft is used for skin defects. A separate lateral incision, made for lateral internal fixation, can be closed in the usual fashion. Similarly, most incisions made to expose open ankle fractures can be safely closed. Closed suction drainage is employed in all wounds closed primarily.

For severely contaminated wounds (grade IIIB), internal fixation may not be indicated. In these situations,

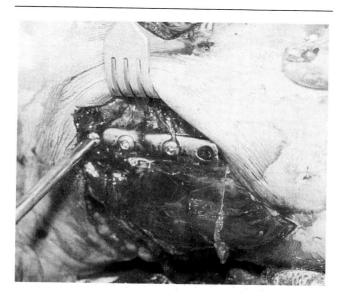

Fig. 3 Distal fibula is repaired with semitubular plate. Soft tissue covered the plate primarily.

external fixation should be used. A triangular frame is satisfactory for this purpose. Three-point fixation is obtained by placing two pins in the distal tibia, two pins in the calcaneus, at a safe distance from the neurovascular bundle, and adding an extension to include the first metatarsal. The fixation device can maintain fracture reduction for eight to ten weeks, or it can be removed after soft tissues have healed. External fixation devices maintain length when there is severe bone loss or comminution. They are also used to control joint position for later arthrodesis.

Soft-tissue management is important to prevent deep osteomyelitis. Because vital structures, including bone, tendon, and nerve, can be left exposed for only a limited period, soft-tissue flap coverage must be planned within five to seven days.[7] Microvascular flap coverage, either immediate or done within 48 hours, carries an excellent prognosis for flap survival if the wound is appropriate. It is important to anticipate from the outset the need for a flap and to have appropriate personnel on hand to carry out the procedure.

Postoperative Management

The leg must be splinted and elevated for at least 48 hours after surgery. In grades I or II injuries, closure can be delayed until the fifth day. For grade III injuries, the patient is returned to the operating room within 48 hours for redebridement and dressing change. When the wound is well vascularized and free of infection, flap coverage is considered. This may be done with a local transposition flap—either a fasciocutaneous flap or a muscle flap covered with split-thickness graft—

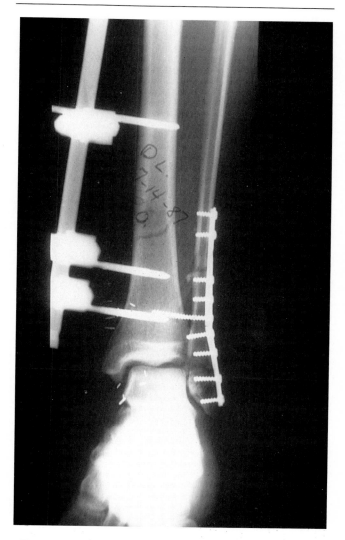

Fig. 4 Initial postoperative radiographs show anatomic reduction of the tibia and ankle joint.

or a free flap transfer may be used. The goal is adequate uninfected coverage within seven days.[7]

Case Studies

Case 1

A 26-year-old man involved in a motorcycle accident had a grade II open fracture of the left tibia and a grade IIIC open fracture of the left ankle (Fig. 1). The ankle wound was extensive with complete avulsion of the deltoid ligament as well as disruption of the posterior tibial artery at the level of the medial malleolus. The fibula sustained an open segmental fracture at the level of the joint line and 3 inches above the joint (Fig. 2). Primary treatment included thorough surgical debridement, followed by repair of the posterior tibial artery. A unilateral double-bar external fixator was ap-

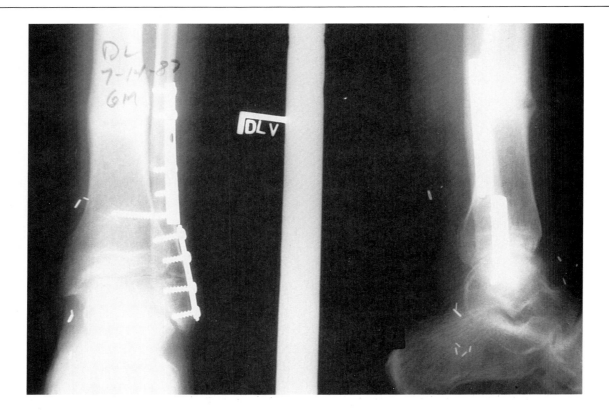

Fig. 5   Final radiographs at six months show all fractures healed and anatomic restoration of the joint.

plied to the tibia, and the fibula was repaired through a separate incision, using two semitubular plates (Figs. 3 and 4). Delayed wound closure was done five days later, using a split-thickness skin graft over the ankle wounds. The ankle was splinted for six weeks, and full weightbearing with a dynamized frame was then allowed for six weeks. A short leg orthosis was worn for an additional month. The fracture was healed at four months, and, at one-year follow-up, excellent pain-free range of motion had returned (Fig. 5).

Case 2

A 48-year-old man involved in a motor-vehicle accident sustained a grade IIIB intra-articular distal pilon fracture of the tibia. Initial debridement and irrigation was done and the fracture stabilized with a triangular frame. After one subsequent debridement, a split-thickness skin graft was applied seven days after injury. The wound and fracture healed without complication, and the external frame was removed 12 weeks after the injury. A short leg orthosis was worn for two additional months. At one-year follow-up, the patient had excellent range of motion and had returned to work.

Conclusions

Open ankle fractures are serious injuries that require aggressive management to prevent infection. Soft-tissue care takes priority, and initial internal fixation is helpful in grades I or II injuries. In grade III open fractures, minimal internal fixation or external fixation may be needed, together with sophisticated soft-tissue flap techniques to achieve a wound that is clean, closed, and dry early in the treatment course.

References

1. Franklin JL, Johnson KD, Hansen ST Jr: Immediate internal fixation of open ankle fractures: Report of thirty-eight cases treated with a standard protocol. *J Bone Joint Surg* 1984;66A:1349–1356.
2. Bray TJ: Soft-tissue techniques in the management of open ankle fractures. *Techn Orthop* 1987;2:20–28.
3. Tscherne H, Gotzen L (eds): *Fractures With Soft Tissue Injuries.* Berlin, Springer-Verlag, 1984, p 11.
4. Gustilo RB, Mendoza RM, Williams DN: Problems in the management of type III (severe) open fractures: A new classification of type III open fractures. *J Trauma* 1984;24:742–746.

5. Patzakis MJ, Wilkins J, Moore TM: Use of antibiotics in open tibial fractures. *Clin Orthop* 1983;178:31–35.
6. Heim U, Pfeiffer KM: *Internal Fixation of Small Fractures*. Berlin, Springer-Verlag, 1987.
7. Cierny G III, Byrd HS, Jones RE: Primary versus delayed soft tissue coverage for severe open tibial fractures: A comparison of results. *Clin Orthop* 1983;178:54–63.

Injury of the Foot

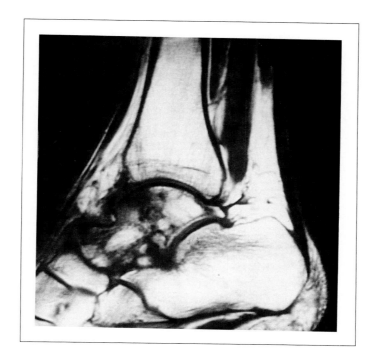

Management of Soft-Tissue Loss on the Plantar Aspect of the Foot

John S. Gould, MD

Introduction

Soft-tissue defects secondary to trauma can occur anywhere on the body. Several guiding principles are used in managing these defects. If skin alone is missing and a subcutaneous base remains, healing can take place by second intention, or simple split-thickness or full-thickness skin grafts can be applied. Although simple grafting is a possibility, flap-tissue coverage should be considered if muscle, fascia, joint capsule, or bone is exposed in the wound (Fig. 1). Flap coverage is required if the base's blood supply is questionable. Flaps are also desirable if future surgery beneath the covering tissue is anticipated, or when durability or appearance of the surface is important.

The foot and ankle make special demands on coverage tissues. The tissue must not contract, because contraction can cause such deformities as an elevated or depressed toe. It is also important that coverage tissue not restrict normal ankle motion or normal pronation and reformation of the arch with gait. The tissue must be durable enough to withstand shear forces. In various areas, especially on the plantar surface, it must be either sensate or capable of neoneurotization. It must be stable, and it must allow the person to wear reasonable footwear after recovery.

Each area of the foot and ankle has special requirements. Areas to consider include the malleoli, the anterior ankle, the Achilles tendon, the dorsum of the foot, heel, and other plantar areas. The malleoli need thin coverage. The Achilles tendon and the dorsum of the foot need ultrathin tissue. The anterior ankle and areas behind the malleoli need thicker filler tissue. These problems have been discussed in earlier publications.[1] The plantar areas, which have even more demanding requirements, are the subject of this chapter.

One option for flap coverage is to use local tissue. A local-tissue flap can be skin, subcutaneous tissue, and fascia, or it can be muscle or musculocutaneous tissue. Transpositional flaps or island pedicle flaps are used. Flaps from a distance are usually free flaps made up of skin and subcutaneous tissue, skin and muscle, muscle covered by split-thickness skin graft, or fascial flaps. At present, most difficulties with free-tissue transfers of the foot and ankle stem from damaged recipient vessels. If the damaged area, or zone of injury, extends too far proximally, the prolonged pedicle is at risk of compression or kinking by passage across joints or through scarred tissue. A superiorly based cross-leg flap

is used when the recipient foot has inaccessible major vessels. In choosing a donor site, the surgeon should first look for good local options. If these are unacceptable, then the distant flaps will be considered as indicated by damage to the local area or special requirements of the site.

To improve the result, adjuncts to basic surgery include secondary surgical measures, such as defatting, debulking, revision of marginal scars, use of nerve grafts to increase sensibility, additional nerve-island flaps, and judicious use of shoe inserts and modifications.

Specific Requirements of Plantar Areas

Replacement of plantar skin presents special difficulties because this durable, highly sensitive, glabrous skin is found only on the soles of the feet and the palms of the hand. Because the palm is an inappropriate donor site, matching tissue must come from one of the soles, or a compromise tissue must be used.

Tissue transfers to the foot must be able to tolerate the shear forces produced during walking and running. This is especially true of the heel pad, which must be stable and durable with heel strike. Weightbearing continues along the lateral plantar surface, across the metatarsal heads, and ends with toe off. Cutaneous ligaments limit movement of the skin over metatarsal heads; the plantar aspects of the toes, particularly the hallux; and the heel pad. When this tissue cannot be duplicated, shear problems and gait disturbances occur. This tissue must have a sensory nerve or at least sensory end organs to allow neural connection with adjacent skin. Finally, it must be thick enough to pad bony prominences, but thin enough to fit into shoes. These weightbearing areas, particularly the metatarsal heads, require durable tissue. The longitudinal arch skin must be flexible enough to stretch to allow normal pronation, which decreases the shock effect on the foot and leg. Because the arch skin need not be as thick and durable as the weightbearing areas, other donor options can be used here.

Options for Coverage

Unfortunately, there is no perfect substitute for the highly specialized heel pad. The best option, when avail-

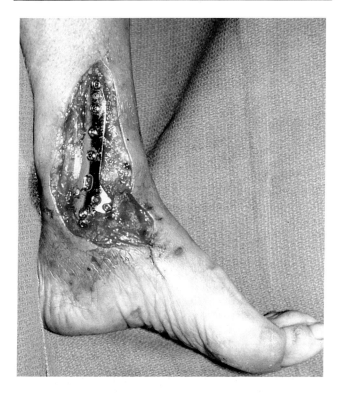

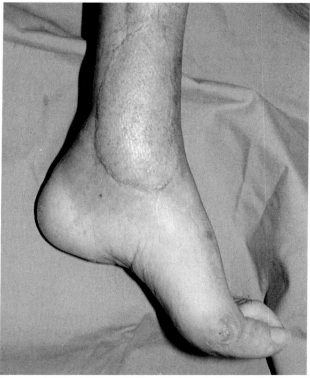

Fig. 1 **Top,** Exposed bone and metal fixation over the distal medial tibia. **Bottom,** Well-contoured coverage provided by a free muscle flap covered with split-thickness skin.

able, is the arch skin (instep flap),[2] which may be shifted posteriorly with its medial plantar vessel pedicle or taken as a free flap from the contralateral foot. Although swivel will still occur because of the lack of cutaneous septa, the other requirements for the flap are satisfied. Partial innervation may be preserved from the cutaneous branches of the metatarsal nerves if the flap is mobilized on the ipsilateral side, or the flap can be spontaneously innervated if the surrounding skin is reasonably intact. Another local option is the flexor digitorum brevis muscle,[3] which can be mobilized and covered with a skin graft. Although this tissue lacks sensory reinnervation, it is able to detect deep pressure. The origin and insertions of the flexor digitorum brevis can be fully mobilized and, when it is safe to do so, the distal lateral plantar vessel can be divided to allow more proximal coverage, but this transfer is limited by the size of the lesion and by its proximal extent. When overlying skin is taken with the flexor brevis, as a musculocutaneous flap, innervation is preserved.[4] Small, deep defects may be covered by abductor hallucis and abductor digiti minimi flaps.[5] Small, shallow defects have the option of free skin-graft coverage from the longitudinal arch of either foot.

Many options for distant flaps have been described for the heel. I believe that the best choices are either cutaneous flaps (with or without nerve supply, depending on the potential for spontaneous reinnervation) or a muscle flap covered with split-thickness skin (0.018 inch meshed 1.5 to 1, but not spread). For the muscle donor site, I usually use a tailored latissimus dorsi, but the rectus abdominus and gracilis are also excellent. Muscle attaches well to the os calcis and minimizes swivel as a fibrous shear plane develops between the graft and flap and between the muscle and bone.[6] The skin graft over muscle hypertrophies and is very durable, especially with good orthotics. Sensibility, however, is limited.

Choosing a cutaneous flap depends on the potential for spontaneous reinnervation. The scapular flap[7,8] allows good reinnervation and has thick skin, but it does have some swivel problems (Fig. 2). Lateral arm-flap skin is softer, but the flap can be neurocutaneous, as can the forearm radial artery flap, which is even softer and more pliable (Fig. 3). I usually choose the scapular flap.

The longitudinal arch is a nonweightbearing area in normal and cavus type feet, but it may bear some weight in the patient with a flatfoot. If the foot is flexible, minimal shear occurs in this area and coverage need only be pliable. Here, full-thickness (groin) or thick split-thickness skin (0.018 inch) is satisfactory. While not a requirement in a nonweightbearing area, full-thickness skin can be reinnervated. It is also more pliable and does not hyperpigment as deeply as split skin. When deep tissues have also been lost, especially if the loss extends beyond the arch, a free flap may be re-

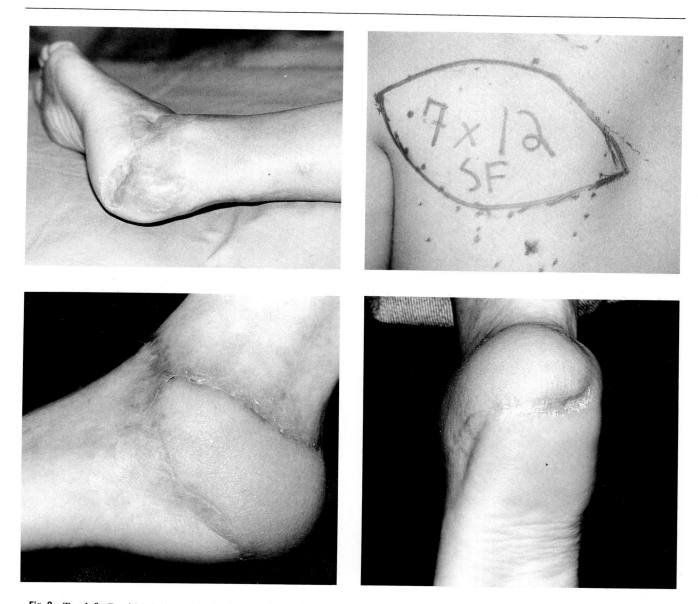

Fig. 2   Top left, Crushing injury to the heel covered primarily with an unstable split-thickness skin graft. **Top right**, Donor site from scapular area. **Bottom left**, Scapular flap to heel, vascularized by anterior tibial vessels. **Bottom right**, Plantar view of scapular flap. Debulkings were required. (Reproduced with permission from Gould JS: Reconstruction of soft tissue injuries of the foot and ankle with microsurgical techniques. *Orthopedics* 1987;10:151–157.)

quired. The needs of the weightbearing area determine the best approach. Neurovascular reconstruction under the arch may also demand flap coverage. Tissue with a durable surface is needed under the metatarsal heads. Here, too, I prefer the scapular flap or muscle covered with skin graft (Fig. 4). Swivel is less with muscle; sensibility is better with cutaneous flaps. Neurocutaneous flaps are used occasionally, and the deltoid flap[9] is one such choice. For coverage of toe pads, cross-toe flaps from the dorsum of an adjacent digit came into common use when the great toe was used as a donor for the thumb "wrap-around" flap.[10] Compared

to cross-finger flaps, the cross-toe technique has a higher failure rate, and simple skin grafting remains the primary coverage method when the toe is otherwise viable. This simple technique can result in painful hyperkeratotic lesions, and toe shortening may be indicated to provide primary skin closure. The use of adjuncts, described below, has obviated the need for sophisticated surgery on the plantar aspects of the toes.

Adjunctive Maneuvers

Tailoring of initial flaps can minimize the need for revisions, but debulking and defatting of oversized flaps

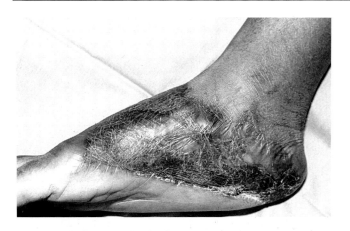

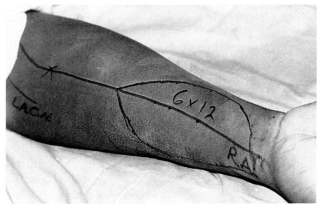

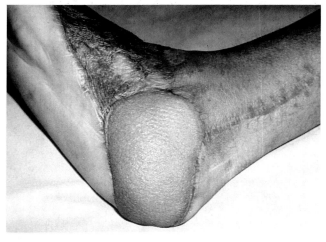

Fig. 3 Top left, Heel injury covered with unstable split-thickness skin. Patient also complained of neuromatous pain from calcaneal branches of tibial nerve. **Top right**, Forearm donor site for radial artery flap. **Bottom**, Radial artery forearm flap to heel. The calcaneal branches were sutured to the lateral antebrachial cutaneous nerve of the flap, which eliminated neuromatous pain and provided sensibility. (Reproduced with permission from Gould JS: Reconstruction of soft tissue injuries of the foot and ankle with microsurgical techniques. *Orthopedics* 1987;10:151–157.)

will still be required (Fig. 2, *bottom right*). Muscle flap bulk may decrease spontaneously after denervation and hence may not be a problem. Conversely, such flaps may not retain their desired bulk, although this is rare. Muscle flaps, however, can be narrowed or shaved thinner with regrafting.

Cutaneous flaps may increase their fat layer as an individual gains weight. Cutaneous flaps may be defatted mechanically; usually half the flap on either side of the pedicle axis is thinned, with a three-month interval between procedures. The timing is empirical. Suction lipectomy, a technique that has come into widespread use in cosmetic surgery, has also been used.

Hypertrophic marginal scars remain a problem because they may not be improved with surgical revision. Elastic garments, used in burn reconstruction, should be tried initially. The various techniques devised to improve sensibility include suturing a sensory nerve to the motor nerve of a muscle in hope of improving deep pressure or proprioception. Other efforts include placing the end of sensory nerve (or the prolonged grafted end) under insensate skin.[11,12] Lister[13] described the use of an innervated full-thickness skin graft when an ad-

equate pad remains. Neurovascular island flaps from areas that are innervated by digital nerves and supplied by the digital vessel, such as toe webs, or toe sides and pulp, have been recessed on their pedicles to improve and provide protective sensibility to key insensate areas.[11,12]

Shoe inserts and modifications are used to support irregular and insensitive areas. Total-contact orthotics are fabricated by using wax, plaster, or other conforming material to make a mold of the foot. Plaster of paris poured into the mold duplicates the surface of the foot. Troublesome areas are marked for special attention. Using a vacuum-forming process, an insert is made out of yielding materials, such as polyethylene foam, to defuse stress and to protect high contact areas. To decrease shear, closed micropore rubber material is added to the insert. The various materials used are bonded to each other, and more durable materials are used at deeper layers. A viscoelastic gel material has proven effective in diffusing stress in troublesome areas (Fig. 5). At the heel, the orthosis has a heel cup to contain the soft tissues and to protect against swivel. The arch area is filled in to allow the arch to share weightbearing

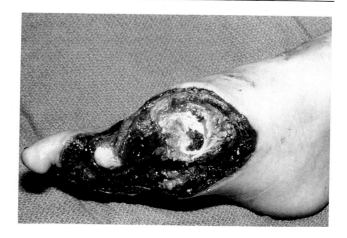

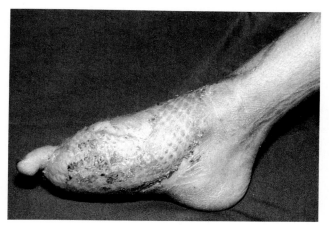

Fig. 4 **Top**, Avulsion injury of the medial and distal plantar area of the foot. **Bottom**, Medial and plantar coverage provided by a well tailored latissimus dorsi flap covered with split-thickness skin graft.

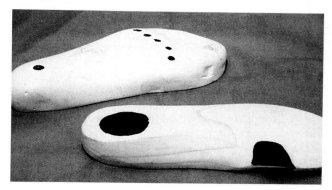

Fig. 5 The plaster-of-paris model noted above is made from a cast of the foot and is marked in problem areas. The insert, shown upside down, has wells created in the basic polyethylene foam material. These are filled with viscoelastic polymer.

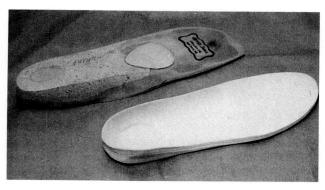

Fig. 6 Full-length, total-contact orthotics showing both the surface contacting the foot and the undersurface with a built-in metatarsal pad.

to decrease stress in the metatarsals or lateral border areas. When only the heel or proximal surface is involved, a three-quarter-length orthotic is used, and the toe box of the shoe can be of standard depth. When the distal tissues also need protection, a full-length orthotic is fabricated, with a deeper toe box (Fig. 6).

The sides of the shoe, the counter, or the entire interior of the shoe upper may be lined with special moldable material. Even the leather of the shoe may be made of deerskin or some other malleable material. To increase hindfoot stability, the heel may be broadened with medial or lateral flares, or both. Heel strike may be cushioned by adding a wedge of compressive material, like the solid-ankle, cushion-heel material used in prosthetic feet, between the layers of the heel. A rocker sole with a more proximal apex may be used to shift the weightbearing behind the metatarsal heads. To limit joint motion in the foot, the sole can be stiffened with an extended steel shank. The rocker sole is then used to keep the heel from lifting out of the shoe at toe off. Finally, the sole is made of a cushioned crepe

rubber material that further absorbs floor stress. To summarize, numerous pedorthic devices are available to ease potential problems inherent in surgical reconstruction.

Timing of the Reconstruction

Early soft-tissue reconstruction is advantageous for a number of reasons. Delay beyond a few days after injury increases the level of unusable recipient vessels and enlarges the zone of injury. Deeper tissues will desiccate and become necrotic, and the injured areas will become increasingly edematous and stiff. Use of an immediate or acute free flap may be advantageous. Its use obviates the classic technique of split-thickness skin grafting and late reconstruction, and the outcome may be superior.

When wounds are grossly contaminated, however, tissue loss from vascular insufficiency cannot be determined at once, and further debridement may be indicated. Other concomitant injuries may also require more immediate attention. If these factors are present, a delay in primary treatment of as long as two to three weeks may be appropriate.

Summary

Restoration of the plantar surface of the foot demands an appreciation of the unique requirements of this area. Local tissues should be used when available. Otherwise, if recipient vessels are adequate, free-tissue transfer is the treatment of choice. Durable tissues include cutaneous flaps with thicker skin, such as the scapular flap, and muscle flaps covered with split-thickness skin graft. Each method has advantages and deficiencies. Tailoring of the flap can decrease the need for later modifications. Adjunctive procedures, to increase sensibility, and pedorthic devices, to accommodate and moderate imperfect surgical methods, complement the efforts of the reconstructive surgeon to restore maximum function to this critical area.

Acknowledgment

Douglas P. Hanel, MD, provided Figure 4.

References

1. Gould JS: Reconstruction of soft tissue injuries of the foot and ankle with microsurgical techniques. *Orthopedics* 1987;10:151–157.

2. Morrison WA, Crabb DM, O'Brien BM, et al: The instep of the foot as a fasciocutaneous island and as a free flap for heel defects. *Plast Reconstr Surg* 1983;72:56–65.

3. Bostwick J III: Reconstruction of the heel pad by muscle transposition and split skin graft. *Surg Gynecol Obstet* 1976;143:973–974.

4. Hartrampf CR Jr, Scheflan M, Bostwick J III: The flexor digitorum brevis muscle island pedicle flap: A new dimension in heel reconstruction. *Plast Reconstr Surg* 1980;66:264–270.

5. Ger R: The surgical management of ulcers of the heel. *Surg Gynecol Obstet* 1975;140:909–911.

6. May JW Jr, Halls MJ, Simon SR: Free microvascular muscle flaps with skin graft reconstruction of extensive defects of the foot: A clinical and gait analysis study. *Plast Reconstr Surg* 1985;75:627–641.

7. Roth JH, Urbaniak JR, Koman LA, et al: Free flap coverage of deep tissue defects of the foot. *Foot Ankle* 1982;3:150–157.

8. Koman LA: Free flaps for coverage of the foot and ankle. *Orthopedics* 1986;9:857–862.

9. Franklin JB: Deltoid flap anatomy and clinical applications, in Buncke HJ Jr, Furness S (eds): *Symposium on Frontiers in Reconstructive Microsurgery*. St. Louis, CV Mosby, 1983, pp 63–70.

10. Morrison WA, O'Brien BM, MacLeod AM: Thumb reconstruction with a free neurovascular wrap-around flap from the big toe. *J Hand Surg* 1980;5:575–583.

11. Chang KN, Buncke HJ: Sensory reinnervation in reconstruction of the foot. *Foot Ankle* 1986;7:124–132.

12. Chang KN, DeArmond SJ, Buncke HJ Jr: Sensory reinnervation in microsurgical reconstruction of the heel. *Plast Reconstr Surg* 1986;78:652–664.

13. Lister GD: Use of an innervated skin graft to provide sensation to the reconstructed heel. *Plast Reconstr Surg* 1978;62:157–161.

Compartment Syndromes of the Foot

Michael J. Shereff, MD

Introduction

Compartment syndrome of the foot is defined as increased tissue pressure within one or more of the osseofascial compartments of the foot. This pressure compromises the circulation and viability of the structures within that compartment. Although compartment syndrome of the foot is a well-recognized clinical entity,[1,2] the pathogenesis, clinical evaluation, and management of this important injury have only recently been studied in depth. This chapter reviews the anatomic and physiologic basis of this disorder and outlines its clinical evaluation and treatment.

Functional Anatomy: Fascial Compartments of the Foot

Several studies have defined the anatomy of the fascial compartments of the foot.[3-7] Basically, the foot can be divided into four separate compartments, each with distinct boundaries (Fig. 1) and contents.

Medial Compartment

The inferior surface of the first metatarsal shaft forms the roof of the medial compartment of the foot. This osseofascial space is bounded medially by an extension of the plantar aponeurosis and laterally by the medial intermuscular septum.

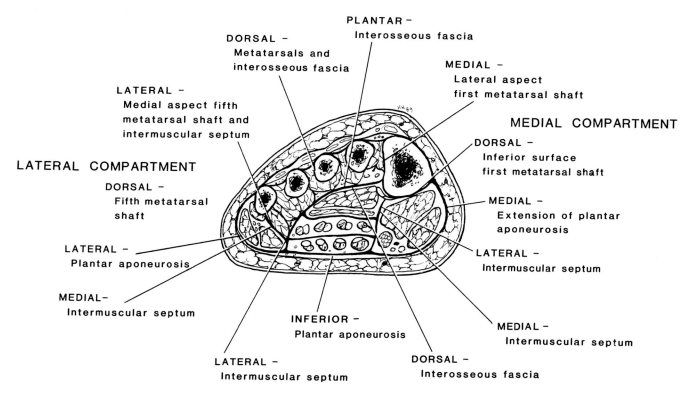

INTEROSSEOUS COMPARTMENT

PLANTAR –
Interosseous fascia

DORSAL –
Metatarsals and
interosseous fascia

MEDIAL –
Lateral aspect
first metatarsal shaft

LATERAL –
Medial aspect fifth
metatarsal shaft and
intermuscular septum

MEDIAL COMPARTMENT

LATERAL COMPARTMENT

DORSAL –
Fifth metatarsal
shaft

DORSAL –
Inferior surface
first metatarsal shaft

MEDIAL –
Extension of plantar
aponeurosis

LATERAL –
Plantar aponeurosis

LATERAL –
Intermuscular septum

MEDIAL–
Intermuscular septum

INFERIOR –
Plantar aponeurosis

MEDIAL –
Intermuscular septum

LATERAL –
Intermuscular septum

DORSAL –
Interosseous fascia

CENTRAL COMPARTMENT

Fig. 1 Artist's illustration indicating the boundaries of the four fascial compartments of the foot.

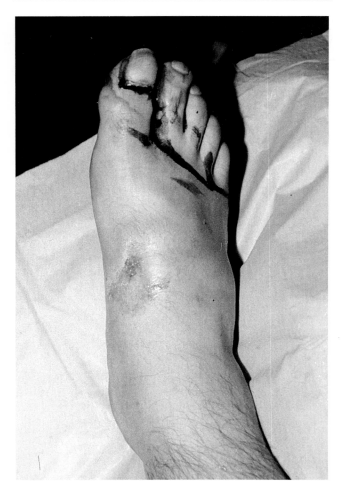

Fig. 2   Clinical photograph of a patient with an acute compartment syndrome of the foot. Note the swelling at the dorsum of the foot as well as the tense overlying skin.

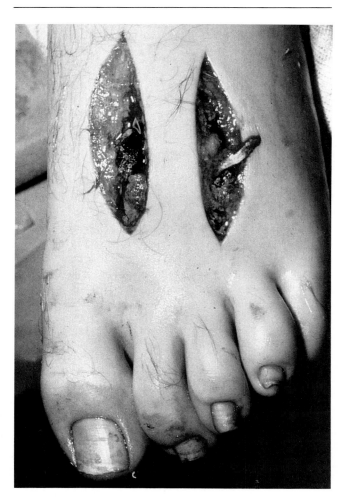

Fig. 3   Postoperative photograph revealing decompression obtained by means of the "double dorsal" fasciotomy.

The muscular and tendinous contents of the medial compartment of the foot include the abductor hallucis muscle, the flexor hallucis brevis muscle, and the flexor hallucis longus tendon. The peroneus longus and posterior tibial tendons traverse both this compartment and the central compartment.

Central Compartment

The floor of the central compartment is formed by the plantar aponeurosis. Two distinct intermuscular septa bound this compartment medially and laterally. The interosseous fascia forms its dorsal boundary. The soft-tissue structures that lie within the central compartment, in order of their appearance from the plantar to the dorsal aspect of the foot, include the flexor digitorum brevis muscle, the flexor digitorum longus tendon, the lumbrical muscles, the quadratus plantae muscle, and the adductor hallucis muscle. The peroneal tendon and the posterior tibial tendon may also be found in this compartment at various levels.

Lateral Compartment

The fifth metatarsal shaft forms the roof of the lateral compartment. The distinct lateral intermuscular septum is the significant limiting structure at its medial aspect. A lateral extension of the plantar aponeurosis forms its lateral boundary.

The three muscles that constitute the contents of the lateral compartment are the abductor digiti quinti muscle, the flexor digitorum brevis muscle to the fifth toe, and the opponens digiti quinti muscle.

Interosseous Compartment

The metatarsals and the dorsal interosseous fascia that lies between them create the dorsal boundary of the interosseous compartment. The lateral aspect of the first metatarsal shaft lies medially, and the medial aspect of the fifth metatarsal shaft and intermuscular septum lies laterally. The plantar interosseous fascia forms the plantar margin of this osseofascial space. Within the interosseous compartment lie the dorsal and plantar interossei muscles.

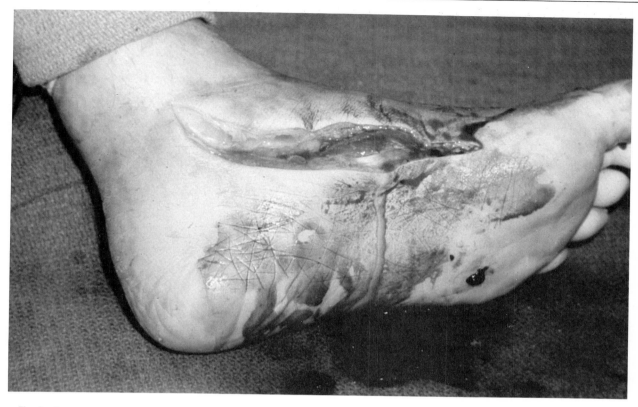

Fig. 4   Postoperative photograph illustrating fasciotomy via a plantar medial approach.

Pathogenesis

Causes

Any significant crush injury to the plantar or dorsal surface of the foot can lead to an acute compartment syndrome. Typical traumatic events involve dropping a heavy object on the dorsum of the foot or a motor-vehicle accident in which the foot is trapped under one of the vehicle's wheels. Crush injuries lead to significant bleeding and edema within the osseofascial spaces and thus cause increased local tissue pressure. Fractures and fracture-dislocations of the forefoot and midfoot can also contribute to increased pressure within the fascial compartments.[8] Even injuries with large open wounds may be associated with a compartment syndrome,[9] and therefore it is wrong to assume that the compartments of the foot have been decompressed by an open injury. Other possible causes include severe twisting or traction injuries to the foot. Postischemic swelling has also been described as a possible causative factor.[10]

Pathophysiology

The actual physiologic events that occur in compartment syndrome have been studied extensively.[10,11] Increased local tissue pressure from whatever cause can increase pressure within the intracompartmental blood vessels. This occurrence will lead to a decreased local arterovenous gradient, resulting in decreased local blood flow evidenced by decreased capillary blood perfusion.

When the local blood flow fails to meet the basic metabolic demands of the structures within that compartment, tissue damage occurs. This sequence of events is manifested by decreased tissue function followed by decreased tissue viability. Myoneural ischemia eventually occurs. The result of an untreated compartment syndrome in the foot is myoneural ischemic necrosis leading to a permanent functional loss associated with contracture, weakness, and sensory disturbance. The end result is typically a severe clawlike deformity of the foot.

Clinical Manifestations

Symptoms

Patients with compartment syndrome of the foot often experience pain that seems out of proportion to the extent of the traumatic injury.[9,11] These patients note that their pain is not decreased by immobilizing the injured part. Some patients describe a feeling of

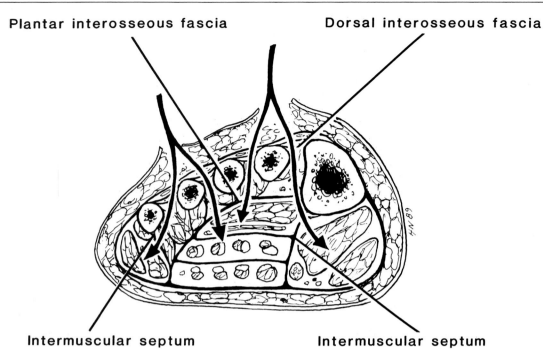

Plantar interosseous fascia   **Dorsal interosseous fascia**

Intermuscular septum   **Intermuscular septum**

Fig. 5 Illustration indicating fascial structures to be incised in the dorsal longitudinal approach.

tautness within the involved compartment. A circumferential dressing or cast may increase symptoms.

Physical Examination

The earliest clinical sign of a compartment syndrome is a swollen and tense foot (Fig. 2). The skin at the dorsal and plantar aspects of the foot may be shiny and warm. Pain may be elicited by means of passive stretch of the muscles in the involved compartment. The most reliable signs are those of sensory deficit secondary to nerve ischemia.[1,2,11] Paresthesias may progress to hypoesthesias and eventually to complete anesthesia of the involved nerves. Neural ischemia is also evidenced by a decrease in light-touch, pin-prick, and two-point discrimination. Peripheral pulses and capillary filling may be intact in patients with acute compartment syndrome of the foot.

Laboratory Evaluation

Intracompartmental Pressure Measurement

The only way to diagnose compartment syndrome of the foot definitively is by measuring the pressure within the involved compartments.[10,11] Pressure measurements may also be used to monitor changes in compartment pressure and to document the adequacy of surgical decompression. Numerous techniques described in the literature include the needle technique, continuous in-

fusion, and measurements using wick and slit catheters.[11-15] Although each of these methods may provide the information required, in my opinion the slit-catheter system is the most accurate and efficient method. Any compartment-tissue pressure measurement above 35 mm Hg is considered to indicate acute compartment syndrome. Hypotension is thought to reduce the tolerance of the limb for increased compartment pressures.

Other Findings

Electromyelographs and nerve-conduction studies may help distinguish a nerve injury from a compartment syndrome. Evaluation of peripheral circulation by means of Doppler studies and arteriography may be required to rule out arterial injuries.

Treatment

Prevention

It is clearly better to prevent acute compartment syndrome of the foot, rather than have to treat it.[9,11] If the mechanism of injury is consistent with the development of increased compartmental pressures, all constrictive dressings should be eliminated. Casts should be bivalved and the cast padding released. Bandages should be loosened. Numerous authorities stress the importance of maintaining systolic blood pressure. The

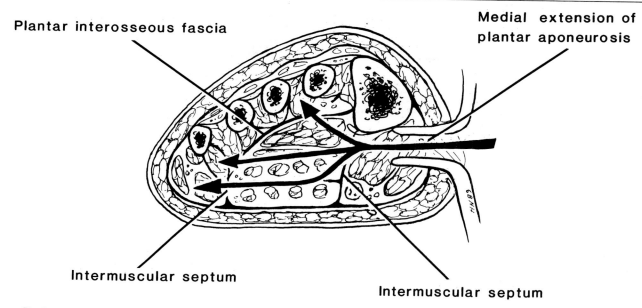

Fig. 6 Fasciotomy by means of a plantar medial approach.

limb is best kept just above the level of the heart, but not excessively elevated, in order to promote arterial blood flow.

Decompressive Fasciotomy

Once increased pressure has developed in the compartments of the foot, the only effective mode of treatment is decompressive fasciotomy. Surgical intervention should be performed in those cases with clinical signs of acute compartment syndrome associated with loss of motor power or sensation to the foot. An increase in tissue pressure to above 30 mm Hg is an absolute indication for fasciotomy.[9,11] The patient's general condition, peripheral perfusion, and blood pressure must also be taken into account. Circumferential full-thickness burns, crush injuries, and multiple fractures and fracture-dislocations of the forefoot and midfoot constitute relative indications for decompressive fasciotomy.

A review of the orthopaedic literature reveals various recommendations regarding the surgical techniques used to decompress the osseofascial compartments of the foot. Mubarak and Hargens[2] recommended two longitudinal dorsal incisions. Hansen,[16] Bonutti and Bell,[17] and Wright and associates[8] suggested a plantar medial incision. Myerson[7,9] compared the use of these two approaches in experimental and clinical studies and found a double dorsal longitudinal approach to be technically easier (Fig. 3). In addition, this approach aids fixation of fractures of the forefoot and midfoot. The plantar medial approach provides more rapid decompression of increased tissue pressure (Fig. 4) and can be extended proximally to allow exploration of the neurovascular bundle and its branches on the medial side of the foot and ankle. Myerson stated that the plantar medial approach is the most effective way to treat compartment syndromes not associated with fractures.

Decompressive Fasciotomy: Double Dorsal Approach

The double dorsal approach (Fig. 5) uses two dorsolongitudinal incisions made over the second and fourth metatarsals from their base to the head and neck junction. The skin and subcutaneous tissues are retracted medially and laterally to visualize the dorsal interosseous fascia overlying the web spaces. The fascia is incised, and dissection is continued on either side of the metatarsal to allow visualization of the plantar interosseous fascia. The interosseous fascia is incised in the first web space, and the dissection is continued medially to allow incision of the intermuscular septum and thus decompression of the medial compartment. The interosseous fascia in the second and third web space is incised to gain entrance to the central compartment. The intermuscular septum plantar to the fifth metatarsal is incised via the fourth web space to decompress the lateral compartment. The skin and fascia are left open and covered with a sterile dressing.

Decompressive Fasciotomy: Plantar Medial Approach

The surgical technique used to decompress the compartments of the foot by means of this approach involves a plantar medial incision (Fig. 6) that follows the length of the plantar surface of the first metatarsal. Subcutaneous tissue is incised along the line of the skin incision to visualize the medial extension of the plantar aponeurosis. The medial extension of the plantar aponeurosis is incised longitudinally to decompress the medial compartment. The abductor hallucis muscle is retracted inferiorly and the interosseous compartment is decompressed by incising the plantar interosseous fascia superior to the quadratus plantae muscle. The dissection between the quadratus plantae muscle and the lumbrical muscles is deepened, and a second incision in the interosseous fascia allows decompression of the interosseous compartment. Dissection between the lumbrical muscles and the flexor digitorum brevis muscle allows incision of the lateral intermuscular septum and decompression of the lateral compartment. The skin and fascia are left open, and the wound is covered with a sterile dressing.

Postoperative Care

Starting on the third day after surgery, sterile saline-soaked dressings are applied and are changed daily. On the seventh or eighth day after surgery, a split-thickness skin graft or secondary wound closure is performed.

Summary

Acute compartment syndrome of the foot is a clinical entity that can cause severe impairment and permanent residual disability. Early diagnosis and prompt intervention are necessary to achieve optimal clinical results.

Acknowledgment

Mark S. Myerson, MD, provided Figures 3 and 4.

References

1. Matsen FA III: Compartmental syndrome: A unified concept. *Clin Orthop* 1975;113:8–14.
2. Mubarak SJ, Hargens AR: *Compartment Syndromes and Volkmann's Contracture*. Philadelphia, WB Saunders, 1981.
3. Kamel R, Sakla FB: Anatomical compartments of the sole of the human foot. *Anat Rec* 1961;140:57–60.
4. Grodinsky M: A study of the fascial spaces of the foot and their bearing on infections. *Surg Gynecol Obstet* 1929;49:737–751.
5. Loeffler RD Jr, Ballard A: Plantar fascial spaces of the foot and a proposed surgical approach. *Foot Ankle* 1980;1:11–14.
6. Sarrafian SK: *Anatomy of the Foot and Ankle*. Philadelphia, JB Lippincott, 1983.
7. Myerson MS: Experimental decompression of the fascial compartments of the foot: The basis for fasciotomy in acute compartment syndromes. *Foot Ankle* 1988;8:308–314.
8. Wright JW, Worlock P, Hunter G, et al: The management of injuries of the midfoot and forefoot in the patient with multiple injuries. *Techn Orthop* 1987;2:71–79.
9. Myerson M: Acute compartment syndromes of the foot. *Bull Hosp Jt Dis Orthop Inst* 1987;47:251–261.
10. Matsen FA III, Mubarak SJ, Rorabeck CH: A practical approach to compartmental syndromes, in Evarts CM (ed): American Academy of Orthopaedic Surgeons *Instructional Course Lectures, XXXII*. St. Louis, CV Mosby, 1983, pp 88–113.
11. Whitesides TE Jr, Harada H, Morimoto K: Compartment syndromes and the role of fasciotomy, its parameters and techniques, in American Academy of Orthopaedic Surgeons *Instructional Course Lectures, XXVI*. St. Louis, CV Mosby, 1977, pp 179–196.
12. Mubarak SJ, Carroll NC: Volkmann's contracture in children: Aetiology and prevention. *J Bone Joint Surg* 1979;61B:285–293.
13. Rorabeck CH, Castle GS, Hardie R, et al: Compartmental pressure measurements: An experimental investigation using the slit catheter. *J Trauma* 1981;21:446–449.
14. Whitesides TE Jr, Haney TC, Morimoto K, et al: Tissue pressure measurements as a determinant for the need of fasciotomy. *Clin Orthop* 1975;113:43–51.
15. Matsen FA III, Winquist RA, Krugmire RB Jr: Diagnosis and management of compartmental syndromes. *J Bone Joint Surg* 1980;62A:286–291.
16. Hansen ST Jr: Complex fractures of the foot, in Meyers MH (ed): *The Multiply Injured Patient With Complex Fractures*. Philadelphia, Lea & Febiger, 1984, pp 313–322.
17. Bonutti PM, Bell GR: Compartment syndrome of the foot: A case report. *J Bone Joint Surg* 1986;68A:1449–1451.

Fractures of the Forefoot

Michael J. Shereff, MD

Introduction

Fractures of the forefoot may lead to prolonged disability and residual dysfunction.[1-3] Such injuries may result in malunion, nonunion, and joint stiffness. Difficulties with ambulation can occur, with abnormalities of load distribution during the stance phase of gait.

This chapter emphasizes the application of fracture management principles to the specific problems of the forefoot. Anatomic reduction and adequate fixation, combined with meticulous soft-tissue management, can lead to optimal clinical results.

Fractures of the Metatarsals

Functional Anatomy

Studies on the load-bearing characteristics of the forefoot during the stance phase of gait indicate that each of the lesser metatarsals supports an equal load, and that the first metatarsal carries twice the load of each of the lateral four metatarsals.[4] Displacement of a metatarsal fracture fragment may lead to a nonplantigrade foot.[5] Plantar displacement of the distal fragment will cause increased loading of that metatarsal and may result in an intractable plantar keratosis at that site (Fig. 1). Dorsal displacement of the distal fragment decreases the load applied to that metatarsal and may transfer greater pressure to the adjacent metatarsals.

Medial and lateral displacement of fracture fragments toward an adjacent metatarsal may lead to mechanical impingement and interdigital neuromas (Fig. 2). Medial displacement of the distal fragment of a first metatarsal fracture and lateral displacement of the distal fragment of a fifth metatarsal fracture may lead to prominent bony eminences that can rub against the toe box of the shoe.

Deforming muscle forces result in typical fracture displacement. The strong flexor tendons will usually force the distal fragment of the metatarsal fracture in a plantar and proximal direction. Thus, the distal fragment is often displaced beneath the distal metaphyses.[6]

Intra-articular fractures at the metatarsophalangeal or tarsometatarsal articulation may lead to decreased motion, early arthrosis, and gait abnormalities at these joints (Fig. 3).

Incidence

Metatarsal fractures are relatively common injuries. A recent review stated that the metatarsal most commonly fractured in industrial injuries was the third.[7] Fractures of the first and second metatarsals occurred with equal frequency, and the fourth metatarsal was the least commonly injured. It should be noted, however, that if one includes the common fracture of the base of the fifth metatarsal caused by inversion injuries to the foot, then the incidence, 23%, makes the fifth the most commonly fractured metatarsal.

Mechanism of Injury

Fractures of the metatarsal may result from either direct or indirect forces.[8] Direct injury, common in industrial accidents, often results from a heavy object falling on the dorsum of the forefoot. Indirect injuries occur when the forefoot is held fixed and the leg or foot is twisted, a situation often seen in athletic injuries to the foot.

Clinical Manifestations

Patients describe pain on active motion of the foot as well as difficulty with ambulation. Physical examination reveals localized tenderness and swelling. Palpable motion may be present at the fracture site. Passive motion of the metatarsal distal to the fracture site may reproduce the patient's symptoms. This maneuver is particularly helpful for the evaluation of stress fractures of the metatarsals. The neurovascular status should be evaluated, because the arterial arch, the dorsalis pedis artery, and the dorsal and plantar metatarsal arteries are particularly susceptible to injury in association with metatarsal fractures.[9]

Radiographic Evaluation

Radiographic evaluation of fractures of the metatarsals should include three standard views. The anteroposterior radiograph will reveal medial or lateral displacement of the fracture fragments. The lateral view allows evaluation of dorsal and plantar displacement. Oblique views and tomograms provide information regarding intra-articular extent and degree of fracture comminution.

Treatment

Open Fractures

Treatment of open fractures of the forefoot should follow the same guidelines used for open injuries elsewhere in the musculoskeletal system.[10,11] Appropriate

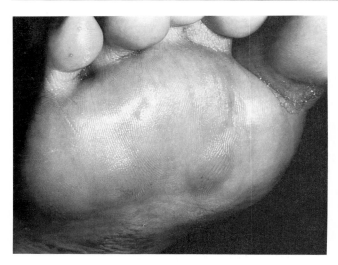
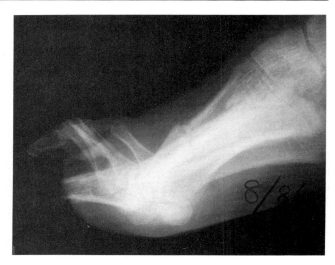

Fig. 1 Left, Clinical photograph of a patient who sustained a fracture of the second metatarsal. **Right**, Lateral radiograph of the same patient. Dorsal angulation at the fracture site and plantar displacement of the distal fragment caused increased weightbearing pressure at the plantar aspect of the second metatarsal head. An intractable plantar keratosis developed at that site.

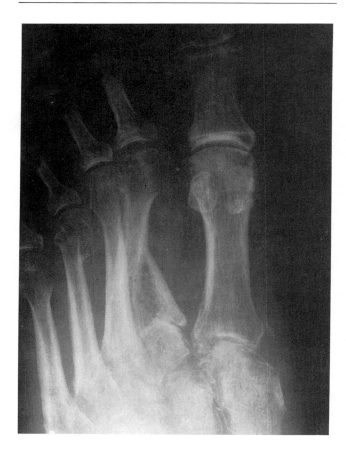
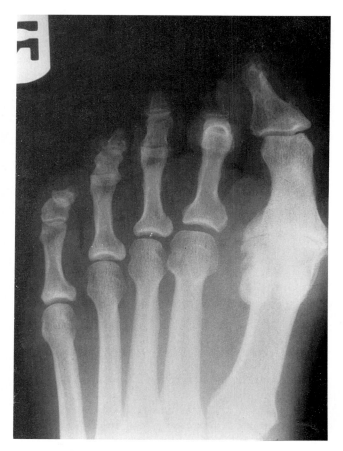

Fig. 2 Lateral displacement of the distal fragment of a second metatarsal fracture in this patient led to mechanical impingement and symptoms indicative of an interdigital neuroma in the second web space.

Fig. 3 This patient sustained an intra-articular fracture at the metatarsophalangeal joint level caused by a stubbing injury. Joint incongruity led to severe arthritis with significant restriction of motion.

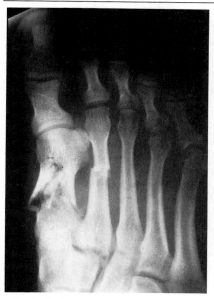
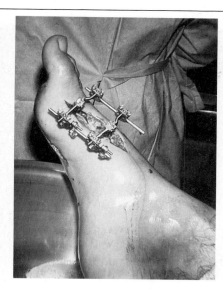
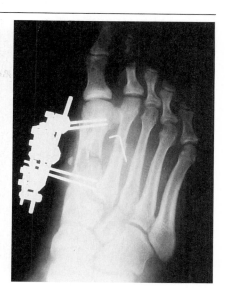

Fig. 4 **Left**, This 23-year-old man sustained a crush injury in association with a motorcycle accident, which caused a grade III open fracture of the forefoot. **Center**, Intraoperative photograph after irrigation of the wounds and debridement of all necrotic and devitalized soft tissues. An external fixator was used to regain length of the first metatarsal and to allow adequate treatment of the soft-tissue injuries. A K-wire was used for internal fixation of the second metatarsal fracture. **Right**, Postoperative radiograph showing external fixation device used for the first metatarsal and internal fixation for the second metatarsal.

prophylaxis for tetanus is given. A wide-spectrum antibiotic is instituted after the wound has been cultured. The patient is then taken to the operating room for irrigation and debridement of the wound and for fracture fixation (Fig. 4). All necrotic and devitalized soft tissues are debrided. Fixation may be external or internal. Adequate fixation is essential to hasten bony union and allow adequate treatment of the soft-tissue injuries. Soft-tissue debridements are performed every 24 to 48 hours, as needed, to ensure optimum wound management. Bone grafting may be required in cases where there is extensive bone loss (Fig. 5). All wounds are left open for delayed primary closure or skin grafting at a later date.

Closed Fractures

Undisplaced Fractures Numerous articles have described various modalities of treatment for undisplaced metatarsal fractures.[1,6,7,12,13] DeLee[1] described the use of adhesive strapping about the forefoot in combination with use of a wooden-soled shoe for a three- to five-week period. Morrissey[13] recommended weightbearing as tolerated using a medial longitudinal arch support with elevation proximal to the metatarsal heads. Johnson[7] recommended initial treatment with a compression dressing followed by a return to weightbearing status as tolerated in a stiff-soled work boot. Giannestras and Sammarco[6] described the use of a short leg walking cast for four to six weeks. Garcia and Parkes[12] described the use of a short leg nonweightbearing cast for three weeks followed by a walking cast for three weeks.

In general, adequate immobilization and avoidance of weightbearing pressure is best achieved by means of a short leg cast, nonweightbearing, for four to six weeks. This is followed by removal of the cast and a slow, gradual return to weightbearing activities as tolerated.

Displaced Fractures Displaced fractures often require reduction and immobilization. Dorsal or plantar displacement and/or angulation of fracture fragments is poorly tolerated. If left unreduced, these fractures may lead to a nonplantigrade foot and difficulties with ambulation. This is particularly true for younger, more active individuals. Medial and lateral displacement may lead to mechanical impingement against adjacent metatarsals. Although specific indications for open reduction of these fractures have not been described in the literature, my recommendation, based on my experience, is that an attempt should probably be made to improve alignment in any metatarsal fracture displaying displacement of greater than 3 to 4 mm or angulation of more than 10 degrees.

Reduction and immobilization can be achieved by various means. The use of Chinese fingertraps applied to the toes with countertraction at the ankle has proved to be most effective in reducing displaced metatarsal fractures (Fig. 6). A short leg cast from the tips of the toes to the tibial tubercle can then be applied while the foot is still in this device. The patient is kept on crutches, nonweightbearing for four to six weeks. After the cast is removed, the patient gradually returns to

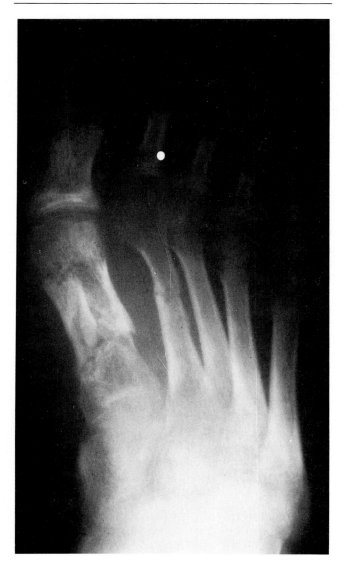

Fig. 5 This patient underwent serial soft-tissue debridement every 24 hours. The wounds were allowed to heal by second intention. Bone grafting was required at 12 weeks. Radiographs at six months after the injury revealed good bony union and satisfactory alignment of the fractures. This patient had an excellent functional recovery.

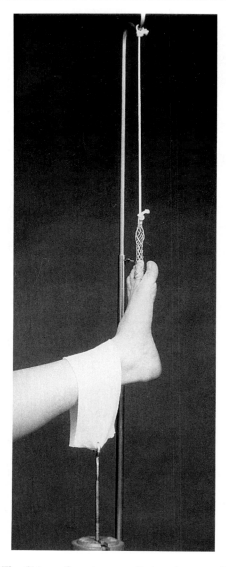

Fig. 6 The Chinese fingertraps applied to the toes with counter traction applied at the ankle have proved an effective means of obtaining reduction of displaced fractures of the metatarsals.

weightbearing activity. If radiographs taken after reduction show that the fracture is unstable, percutaneous pinning can provide excellent fixation of the fracture fragments. For fractures not amenable to closed reduction, open reduction and internal fixation will provide optimum results (Fig. 7). A dorsal longitudinal incision is centered over the involved bone, and the fracture site is exposed subperiosteally. After the fracture ends are cleaned with a curette, the bone is reduced and temporarily held with bone-holding forceps. The choice of fixation method depends on the fracture site and configuration. The type of fixation most commonly used is 0.45-mm smooth Kirschner

wire inserted in a crossed fashion. A short leg cast is applied and the patient is placed on crutches and kept nonweightbearing. If, after six weeks, radiographic union is evident, the pins are removed and a gradual return to weightbearing and ambulation is allowed.

Patients with multiple displaced metatarsal fractures commonly require open reduction and internal fixation (Fig. 8). Intra-articular fractures, especially those at the metatarsophalangeal articulation, require adequate reduction in order to restore articular congruity.

Although transverse fractures are usually amenable to crossed-pin fixation, oblique and spiral fractures may be fixed with interfragmentary lag screws. Multiple K-wire fixation may be helpful in securing long spiral or comminuted metatarsal fractures. The site of the frac-

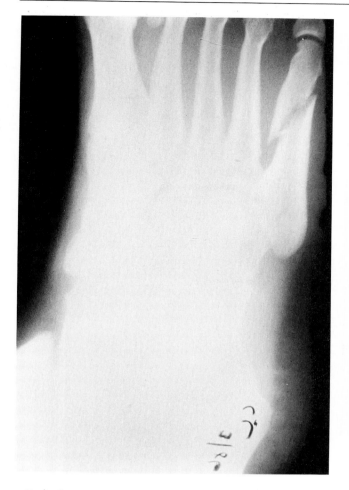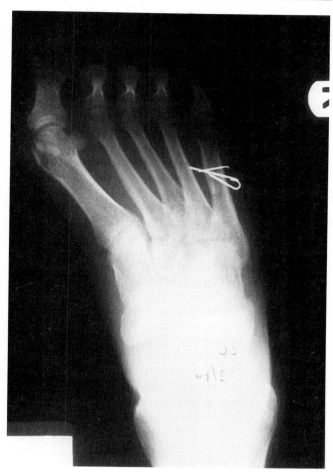

Fig. 7 **Left,** Preoperative radiograph showing displaced fracture of the fifth metatarsal in this 34-year-old man. Note the shortening of the fifth metatarsal caused by overriding of the distal fragment. Note the lateral deviation of the distal fragment. **Right,** Postoperative radiograph revealing the open reduction and internal fixation using multiple K-wire fixation.

ture also determines the type of fixation device used. Small cancellous screws may be used in metaphyseal bone. Interfragmentary cortical lag screws are generally more effective in diaphyseal bone. Intra-articular fractures typically require K-wire fixation, although small plates may be useful for fixing fractures of the metatarsals, especially in the hallux. Intramedullary K-wire fixation may not be advantageous or provide adequate fixation, but small plates may be useful, especially for diaphyseal fractures at the first metatarsal.

Fractures of the Base of the Fifth Metatarsal

This fracture is the subject of much controversy. Numerous orthopaedists[14-16] have recommended a variety of treatments for this common metatarsal fracture. Treatment recommendations are based on the location of the fracture and on whether the injury is acute or chronic. In general, undisplaced fractures may be treated with a short leg nonweightbearing cast for six weeks. Displaced fractures at the junction of

the base and shaft often require open reduction and internal fixation. Displaced fractures of a significant portion of the styloid process often require reduction and fixation. Avulsion of a small fragment of bone by the peroneus brevis may require excision of the fracture fragment and advancement of the tendon into drill holes at the distal aspect of the fifth metatarsal. Symptomatic nonunion of fractures of the fifth metatarsal may require open reduction and internal fixation. Fixation with an intramedullary screw, with or without an inlaid bone graft, has proved quite effective in these cases (Fig. 9).

Fractures of the Phalanges

Fractures of the phalanges are the most common injury in the forefoot.[1] The proximal phalanx of the fifth toe is the one most commonly injured.[8] In either the hallux or the lesser toes, the proximal phalanges

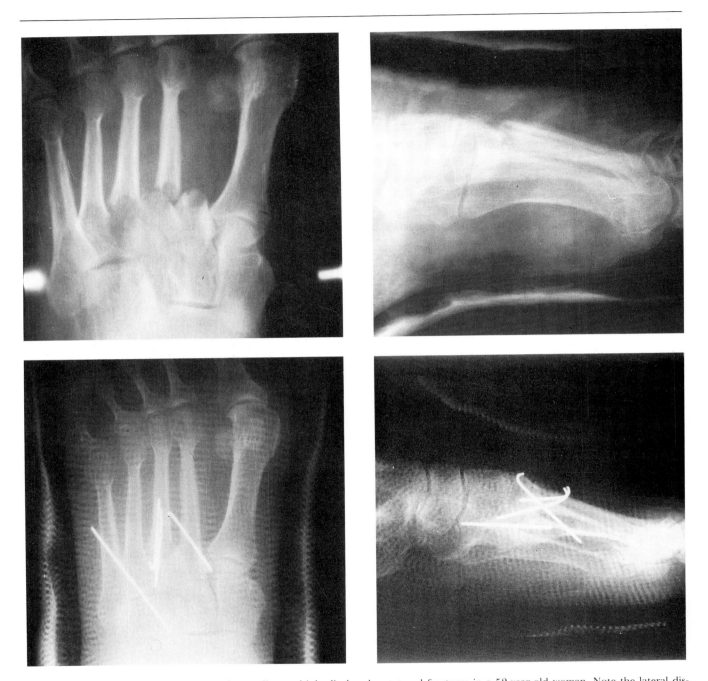

Fig. 8   **Top left**, Preoperative radiograph revealing multiple displaced metatarsal fractures in a 52-year-old woman. Note the lateral displacement of the second and third metatarsals. **Top right**, Lateral radiograph indicating dorsal displacement of the distal fragments. **Bottom, left and right**, Postoperative radiographs after open reduction and internal fixation with multiple K-wires. Note the K-wire crossing the fourth and fifth tarsometatarsal joints to maintain position temporarily in order to allow healing of the interosseous ligaments that had been torn, leading to subluxation at these joints.

are fractured more often than the middle or distal phalanges.[17]

The most common cause of phalangeal fractures in the foot is the application of direct forces either by dropping a heavy object on the foot or by sustaining a stubbing injury. Indirect mechanisms that apply twisting forces to the fixed forefoot are less common.

Patients note pain and swelling of the involved digit. Ecchymosis is quite common. Physical examination reveals localized tenderness and swelling in addition to pain and crepitus on attempted active motion of the toe. A subungual hematoma may be associated with fractures of the distal phalanx.

Anteroposterior, lateral, and oblique views are stan-

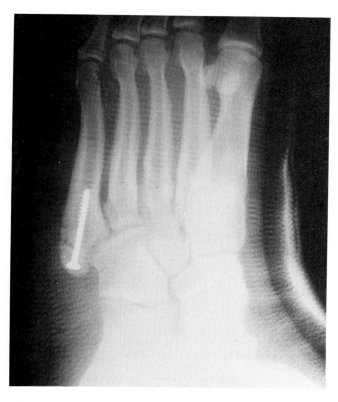

Fig. 9 Postoperative radiograph after open reduction and internal fixation with inlaid bone graft.

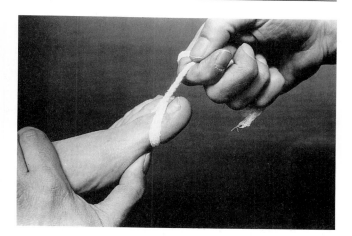

Fig. 10 Clinical photograph revealing a method of closed reduction for displaced fractures of the proximal phalanx of the hallux.

dard in the evaluation of phalangeal fractures. Cone-down views may be very informative.

Treatment

Open fractures of the phalanges receive the same treatment as has been described for the metatarsals. The treatment of closed fractures depends on which phalanx and which digit is involved. Because the hallux bears substantial force during the toe-off phase of gait,

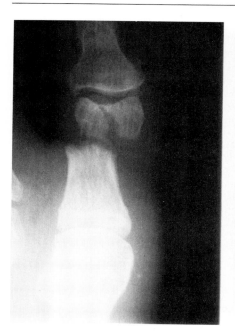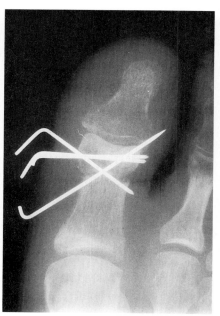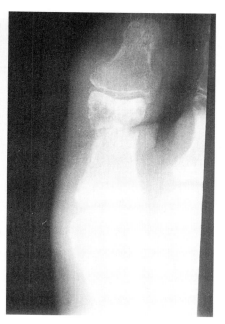

Fig. 11 **Left**, Preoperative radiograph revealing a displaced fracture of the proximal phalanx of the hallux in a 28-year-old man. Note the transverse fracture at the level of the neck of the proximal phalanx and the vertical fracture extending into the interphalangeal joint and splitting condyles of the head of the proximal phalanx. Note the marked medial displacement of the distal fragment. Internal radiograph showed dorsal displacement of the distal fragment. **Center**, Postoperative radiograph showing reduction and fixation. **Right**, Postoperative radiograph after removal of pins reveals radiographic union and satisfactory alignment.

even undisplaced fractures of the proximal phalanx of this digit should be protected. Various means of immobilization have been described.[1,8,17,18] "Buddy taping" of the hallux to the second toe and protected weightbearing with a wooden-soled shoe have been recommended.[17] Immobilization in a short leg walking cast may be appropriate for some patients. Displaced fractures of the proximal phalanx of the hallux may require closed reduction and immobilization in a short leg nonweightbearing cast for four to six weeks (Fig. 10). If the reduction proves to be unstable, consideration should be given to percutaneous pinning. If the fracture is not amenable to closed reduction, then open reduction and internal fixation may be appropriate, particularly in young, active individuals (Fig. 11).

Undisplaced fractures of the distal phalanx of the hallux may be treated with buddy taping to the second toe and protected immobilization in a wooden-soled shoe. Fractures of the distal phalanx of the hallux are rarely displaced. Attempts at closed or even open reduction with immobilization or fixation of these fractures has been described in the literature.[1] This form of treatment is appropriate for intra-articular fractures involving the interphalangeal joint.

Phalangeal Fractures of the Lesser Toes

Undisplaced fractures of the lesser toes may be treated with taping to the adjacent toe and protected mobilization in a wooden-soled shoe. In displaced fractures, closed reduction and buddy taping are often effective. K-wire fixation of proximal phalangeal fractures may be appropriate in severe displacement or angulation not amenable to closed reduction and external fixation. In particular, one should attempt to reduce angulation or displacement leading to gross rotary or other deformities of the digits. Residual bony prominences may lead to interdigital soft corns in areas of mechanical impingement against adjacent toes or to hard corns in areas of pressure from shoewear.

Summary

In conclusion, the principles of fracture management recommended for treatment of musculoskeletal injuries elsewhere should be applied to the forefoot. Anatomic reduction, adequate fixation, and meticulous soft-tissue management will provide optimum functional recovery.

References

1. DeLee JC: Fractures and dislocations of the foot, in Mann RA (ed): *Surgery of the Foot*, ed 5. St. Louis, CV Mosby, 1986, pp 592–808.
2. Lutter LD: Forefoot injuries, in Kiene RH, Johnson KA (eds): *Symposium on the Foot and Ankle*. St. Louis, CV Mosby, 1983, pp 81–88.
3. McKeever FM: Injuries of the forefoot, in Thomson JEM (ed): American Academy of Orthopaedic Surgeons *Instructional Course Lectures, II*. Ann Arbor, JW Edwards, 1944, pp 120–129.
4. Sammarco GJ: Biomechanics of the foot, in Frankel VH, Nordin M (eds): *Basic Biomechanics of the Skeletal System*. Philadelphia, Lea & Febiger, 1980, pp 193–220.
5. Anderson LD: Injuries of the forefoot. *Clin Orthop* 1977;122:18–27.
6. Giannestras NJ, Sammarco GJ: Fractures and dislocations in the foot, in Rockwood CA, Green DP (eds): *Fractures*. Philadelphia, JB Lippincott, 1987, vol 2, pp 1400–1495.
7. Johnson VS: Treatment of fractures of the forefoot in industry, in Bateman JE (ed): *Foot Science*. Philadelphia, WB Saunders, 1976, pp 257–265.
8. Blodgett WH: Injuries of the forefoot and toes, in Jahss MH (ed): *Disorders of the Foot*. Philadelphia, WB Saunders, 1982, vol 2, pp 1449–1462.
9. Shereff MJ, Yang QM, Kummer FJ: Extraosseous and intraosseous arterial supply to the first metatarsal and metatarsophalangeal joint. *Foot Ankle* 1987;8:81–93.
10. Chapman MW: Management of open fractures and complications: Part III. Role of bone stability in open fractures, in Frankel VH (ed): American Academy of Orthopaedic Surgeons *Instructional Course Lectures, XXXI*. St. Louis, CV Mosby, 1982, pp 75–87.
11. Gustilo RB: Principles of the management of open fractures, in Gustilo RB (ed): *Management of Open Fractures and Their Complications*. Philadelphia, WB Saunders, 1982, pp 15–54.
12. Garcia A, Parkes JC: Fractures of the foot, in Giannestras NJ (ed): *Foot Disorders*, ed 2. Philadelphia, Lea & Febiger, 1973, pp 517–564.
13. Morrissey EJ: Metatarsal fractures. *J Bone Joint Surg* 1946;28:594–602.
14. DeLee JC, Evans JP, Julian J: Stress fracture of the fifth metatarsal. *Am J Sports Med* 1983;11:349–353.
15. Stewart IM: Jones's fracture: Fracture of base of fifth metatarsal. *Clin Orthop* 1960;16:190–198.
16. Torg JS, Balduini FC, Zelko RR, et al: Fractures of the base of the fifth metatarsal distal to the tuberosity: Classification and guidelines for non-surgical and surgical management. *J Bone Joint Surg* 1984;66A:209–214.
17. Chapman MW: Fractures and fracture-dislocations of the ankle and foot, in Mann RA (ed): *DuVries' Surgery of the Foot*, ed 4. St. Louis, CV Mosby, 1978, pp 142–204.
18. Jahss MH: Stubbing injuries to the hallux. *Foot Ankle* 1981;1:327–332.

The Treatment of Tarsometatarsal Fracture-Dislocation

Robert S. Adelaar, MD

History

Severe injuries of the forefoot were frequent in the equestrian age when Jacques Lisfranc, one of Napoleon's field surgeons, described an amputation through the tarsometatarsal joint for gangrene. A 0.2% incidence of tarsometatarsal injuries was reported by Gissane[1] in a study from the Royal Infirmary in Edinburgh. Other series by Watson-Jones[2] in 1955, Aitken and Poulson[3] in 1963, Jeffreys[4] in 1963, and English[5] in 1964 have established that these injuries usually result from a low-velocity, longitudinal compression and twisting force on the fixed forefoot. Series of these injuries have been reported.[1-7]

Anatomy

A knowledge of the area's anatomy is critical in understanding the mechanism of injury and the rationale for appropriate treatment. The metatarsal arch, like a Roman arch, has architectural stability because its dorsal surface is wider than the plantar circumference. The second metatarsal, which is inset into the carpal bones, is the keystone of the metatarsal arch and the key to reduction of complex tarsometatarsal dislocations. The interosseous ligament between the medial cuneiform and the second metatarsal, known as Lisfranc's ligament, is well developed. Although there is no interosseous ligament between the base of the first and second metatarsals, there are strong dorsal and even stronger plantar ligaments. In addition, the first metatarsal is stabilized by the anterior tibialis and peroneus longus tendon insertions. The second through fifth metatarsal bones are stabilized by interosseous ligaments as well as the plantar and dorsal ligaments. In injury, a piece of the second metatarsal often remains by the Lisfranc ligament, and its anatomic reduction is critical in analyzing the reduction.[8] Because of the basic intrinsic stability of the bone architecture and the fact that the plantar ligaments are stronger than the dorsal, most dislocations occur in a dorsal direction. The plantar structures are also supported by the plantar fascia, intrinsic musculature, and the peroneus longus.

The critical vascular anatomy is an intermetatarsal branch of the dorsalis pedis that anastomoses with the plantar circulation (Fig. 1).[9] Disruption of the first and second metatarsal base can disrupt the arterial anastomosis, causing significant hemorrhage and morbidity

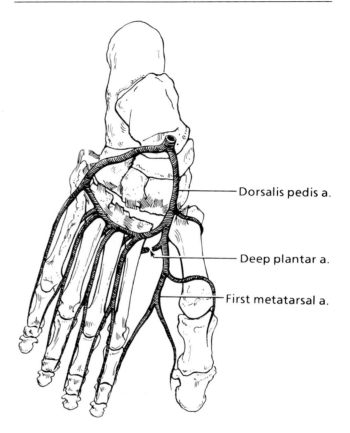

Fig. 1 Disruption of first and second tarsometatarsal complex can cause disruption of the intermetatarsal arterial supply.

— Dorsalis pedis a.

— Deep plantar a.

— First metatarsal a.

in the area. Compartment syndrome can develop in tarsometatarsal disruptions.

Mechanism of Injury

Injury can occur from three different actions. In equestrian warfare, a soldier often was thrown from his horse while his foot remained in the stirrup.[1] These abduction and rotational injuries were characterized by fractures of the base of the second metatarsal, fractures of the cuboid, and fractures of the metatarsal necks.

A second type of injury, common in today's football and rugby competitions, occurs when the plantar-flexed foot is planted on the ground and is struck from a posterior direction by an opposing player. This type of injury can also occur in the performing arts when the loaded foot collapses in the extreme point position. Crushing injuries can cause the rarer plantar dislocations.[8]

In a cadaver experiment, Jeffreys[4] found that certain forces created different types of injury. Pronation of the hindfoot with a fixed forefoot produced a homolateral dislocation of all five metatarsals. Supination of the hindfoot with the forefoot stabilized caused disruption of the first metatarsocuneiform joint. Dislocation or fracture of the second metatarsal base allows further supination, disrupting the lateral complex in a dorsal and lateral direction.

Classification

At the Medical College of Virginia we use the classification system developed by Hardcastle and associates (Fig. 2).[10] Homolateral, or type I, injuries have total incongruity of the metatarsotarsal joints, and the entire metatarsal group shifts in one direction. Only the first metatarsal or the lateral four metatarsals are involved in the isolated, or type II, fracture-dislocation, in which either the first metatarsal is displaced medially or the lateral rays are displaced laterally. In type III, the divergent type, the first metatarsal and lateral four metatarsals diverge in opposite directions. There can be

fractures at the base or at the metatarsal necks of the lateral metatarsals.

Radiologic Criteria

The normal radiographic anatomy is important in the diagnosis of tarsometatarsal injuries. The routine radiographs taken are anteroposterior, lateral, and 30-degree oblique views of the foot. The normal anatomic findings are as follows (Fig. 3): The medial border of the fourth metatarsal is aligned with the medial aspect of the cuboid; the third metatarsal is aligned with the third cuneiform; the medial border of the second metatarsal is aligned with the medial border of the second cuneiform; and the first metatarsal is aligned with the first cuneiform.[6,7,11] A characteristic radiographic finding seen with tarsometatarsal injuries is avulsion fracture of the second metatarsal due to strong attachment of the Lisfranc ligament (Fig. 4). Cuboid fractures suggest abduction-type injuries. Decreased varus of the first metatarsal indicates disruption of the dorsal and plantar ligaments supporting the first metatarsal.

Treatment of Tarsometatarsal Injuries

Treatment of these injuries depends on the nature of the wound and the amount of swelling present. Care

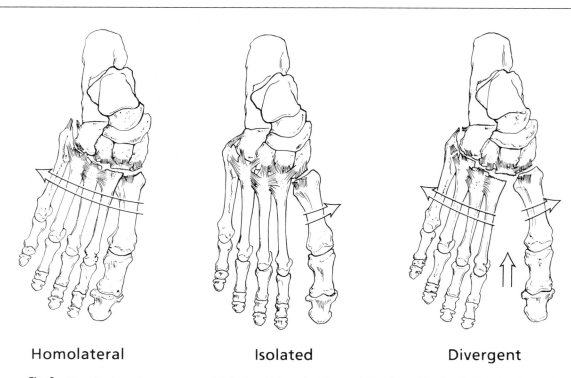

Homolateral Isolated Divergent

Fig. 2 Classification of tarsometatarsal injuries. (Adapted with permission from Hardcastle PH, Reschauer R, Kutscha-Lissberg E, et al: Injuries to the tarsometatarsal joint: Incidence, classification and treatment. *J Bone Joint Surg* 1987;64B:349–356.)

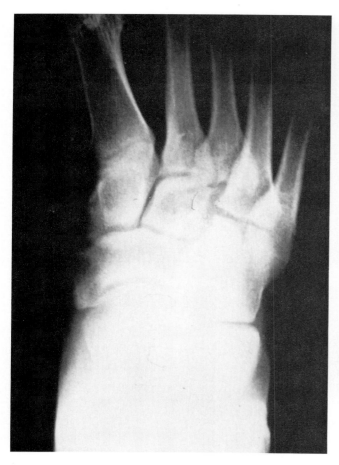

Fig. 3   A normal tarsometatarsal relationship.

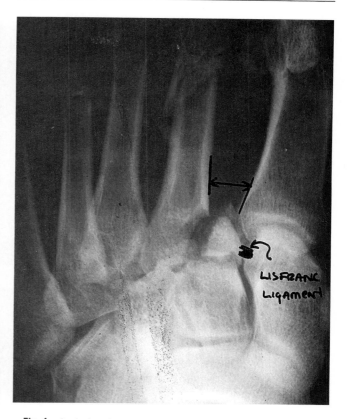

Fig. 4   An isolated tarsometatarsal dislocation with an increase in the standing intermetatarsal space and a large portion of the second metatarsal attached to the Lisfranc ligament.

must be taken to rule out significant arterial injury, and measurements of the forefoot compartments may be indicated.[12] Most tarsometatarsal injuries are closed. In my experience, most injuries can be anatomically reduced by closed methods if they are treated within a few days in an operating room, where adequate anesthesia and radiologic facilities are available.

Closed treatment begins by placing traction on the second metatarsal—the keystone of the foot. As much as 20 lb. of traction may be necessary to reduce the second metatarsal. An image intensifier is used during reduction and pin insertion. After reduction of the second metatarsal complex, the first metatarsal and then the lateral complex are reduced. The metatarsal head usually does not require fixation unless the periosteal cuff is ruptured, in which case pinning is required. The metatarsal heads can be pinned by the plantar percutaneous approach. The plantar pins can cause soft-tissue problems and should not be left in place more than six weeks. At least two 0.062-mm Kirschner wires are inserted from the first metatarsal to the second cuneiforms. The lateral complex also requires two to three

pins (Fig. 5). Final anteroposterior, lateral, and oblique radiographs must be taken to check the final reduction.

Open treatment is necessary for open injuries and when closed reduction cannot be achieved. A dorsal incision is made between the first and second metatarsals. Additional incisions between the fourth and fifth metatarsals may also be required. Care must be taken to preserve the arterial anastomosis between the dorsal and plantar circulations.[8] Reduction criteria call for less than 4 mm of space between the first and second metatarsal; less than a 15-degree angle at the lateral tarsometatarsal axis; no lateral shifting of the third, fourth, and fifth metatarsals; and reasonable reduction of the metatarsal head fractures.[6,7,9] The second metatarsal is treated first because the lateral three metatarsals cannot be aligned until the second metatarsal complex is in place.

Good results have been reported using screw fixation of the base of the metatarsals for acute and chronic dislocations.[13] I have achieved good anatomic results using percutaneous wires, with no loss of reduction if the wires are kept in place for six to eight weeks. Percutaneous pins have been used at the tarsometatarsal junction with no evidence of fusion.

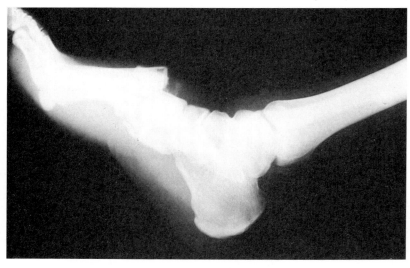

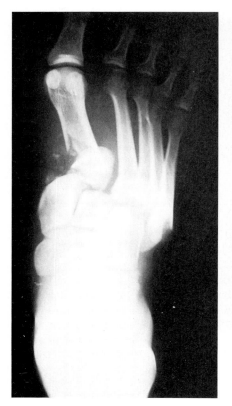 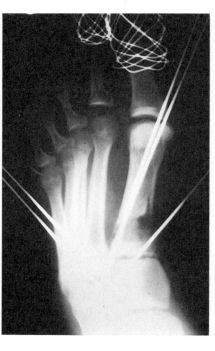 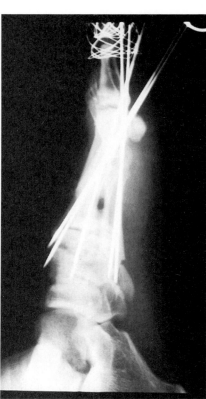

Fig. 5 **Top** and **bottom left**, Severe crush injury with fracture of the first metatarsal base and dislocation of lateral complex. **Bottom center** and **bottom right**, An accurate reduction is obtained by closed techniques. An open decompression of compartments from the dorsal approach was performed. This patient developed a severe sympathetic dystrophy.

After surgery, a nonweightbearing cast is worn for three months, after which a semirigid, full-length orthotic, with metatarsal support, is used for at least one year. Physical therapy has proven helpful in mobilizing the forefoot, midtarsal, and gastrocsoleus complex.

Occasionally, the first metatarsal will not reduce because a portion of the anterior tibialis tendon is entrapped between the first and second metatarsal. This situation requires an open reduction.[14] Cuneiform dislocations, while rare, should be suspected when reduction is difficult.[15]

Results

The results of tarsometatarsal dislocations have been little reported in the literature. Wilson[16] and Wilppula[17] stated that a closed anatomic reduction gives the best long-term results. Their reduction criteria were a slight initial separation between the first and second metatarsals and a reduction of the lateral three metatarsal dislocations. They reported that treatment after a six-week delay did not yield good results. A recent report[8] on tarsometatarsal injuries that included a 4.2-year follow-up stated that anatomic reduction is the key to decreasing long-term morbidity. Of patients who had an anatomic reduction, 81% had a good to excellent result. Only 20% of those who did not have an anatomic reduction had good to excellent results. These investigators also reported that degenerative changes on radiographs did not necessarily correlate with pain at the tarsometatarsal joints.

I have found that although anatomic reduction gives the best results, forefoot stiffness, unequal metatarsal pressure, and intrinsic contractures may still be a problem, particularly when sympathetic dystrophy occurs after severe crush injuries (Fig. 5). Loss of the metatarsal arch and effective plantar pad are best handled by long-term orthotic wear.

Conclusion

In classic treatment of the tarsometatarsal fracture dislocation complex, the main goal is to obtain an anatomic reduction with 4 to 5 mm of space between the first and second metatarsal and an accurate anteroposterior and sagittal reduction of the lateral complex. Attention should be focused on accurate metatarsal-head reduction, particularly if there is plantar deformity. There should be no difficulty in using traction and percutaneous methods to achieve and maintain reduction if treatment is carried out within the first three weeks. Open techniques can be used, but in most cases are not necessary. Results show that an anatomic reduction gives the best long-term results, but that forefoot stiffness, loss of the metatarsal arch, intrinsic con-

tracture, and inequality of metatarsal-head plantar pressure can be problems. Long-term cast and pin treatment are used to maintain the reduction, and long-term orthotics are used to support the longitudinal and metatarsal arch complexes. Compartment syndromes and vascular injuries may be encountered in these injuries, and compartment-pressure techniques should be used if there is any question of this problem. If open treatment is necessary for reduction, it may be appropriate to delay treatment for as much as seven days to allow the soft-tissue reaction to abate. Difficulty with reduction can indicate tendon entrapment, intercuneiform subluxation, or fracture of the cuboid, cuneiform, or navicular. Cast treatment without supplemental fixation has not proven effective.

References

1. Gissane W: A dangerous type of fracture of the foot. *J Bone Joint Surg* 1951;33B:535–538.
2. Watson-Jones R: *Fractures and Joint Injuries*, ed 4. Baltimore, Williams & Wilkins, 1955, vol 2, p 902.
3. Aitken AP, Poulson D: Dislocations of the tarsometatarsal joint. *J Bone Joint Surg* 1963;45A:246–260.
4. Jeffreys TE: Lisfranc's fracture-dislocations. A clinical and experimental study of tarso-metatarsal dislocations and fracture-dislocations. *J Bone Joint Surg* 1963;45B:546–551.
5. English TA: Dislocations of the metatarsal bone and adjacent toe. *J Bone Joint Surg* 1964;46B:700–704.
6. Heckman JD: Fractures and dislocations of the foot: Injuries of the tarsometatarsal (Lisfranc's) joints, in Rockwood CA Jr, Green DP (eds): *Fractures in Adults*, ed 2. Philadelphia, JB Lippincott, 1984, vol 2, pp 1796–1806.
7. DeLee JC: Fractures and dislocations of the foot, in Mann RA (ed): *Surgery of the Foot*, ed 5. St. Louis, CV Mosby, 1986, pp 783–798.
8. Kenzora JE: Morbidity following fracture dislocations of the Lisfranc joint complex. Presented at the American Orthopaedic Foot and Ankle Society, New Orleans, 1986.
9. Shereff MJ, Yang QM, Kummer FJ: Extraosseous and intraosseous arterial supply to the first metatarsal and metatarsophalangeal joint. *Foot Ankle* 1987;8:81–93.
10. Hardcastle PH, Reschauer R, Kutscha-Lissberg E, et al: Injuries to the tarsometatarsal joint: Incidence, classification and treatment. *J Bone Joint Surg* 1987;64B:349–356.
11. Stein RE: Radiological aspects of the tarsometatarsal joints. *Foot Ankle* 1983;3:286–289.
12. Myerson M: Acute compartment syndromes of the foot. *Bull Hosp Joint Dis Orthop Inst* 1987;47:251–261.
13. Arntz CT, Veith RG, Hansen ST Jr: Fractures and fracture-dislocations of the tarsometatarsal joint. *J Bone Joint Surg* 1988;70A:173–181.
14. DeBenedetti MJ, Evanski PM, Waugh TR: The unreducible Lisfranc fracture: Case report and literature review. *Clin Orthop* 1978;136:238–240.
15. Cain PR, Seligson D: Lisfranc's fracture-dislocation with intercuneiform dislocation: Presentation of two cases and a plan for treatment. *Foot Ankle* 1981;2:156–160.
16. Wilson DW: Injuries of the tarso-metatarsal joints: Etiology, classification and results of treatment. *J Bone Joint Surg* 1972;54B:677–686.
17. Wilppula E: Tarsometatarsal fracture-dislocation: Late results in 26 patients. *Acta Orthop Scand* 1973;44:335–345.

Fractures of the Talus

Robert S. Adelaar, MD

Anatomy

The talus has some important anatomic features that are pertinent to the complexity and treatment of its injuries. The talus has seven articular surfaces and no muscular attachments. The anterior width of the talus is larger than the posterior width; therefore, dorsiflexion increases stability.[1-4] With plantar flexion of the ankle there is increased instability, and rotational forces, particularly supination, may cause subluxation or dislocation of the subtalar joint or body. The talar neck deviates in a medial direction and is shortened medially; therefore, biomechanical fixation from the medial side is difficult.[5]

The posterior articular facet maintains the body of the talus in an upright position. The interosseous talocalcaneal ligament is important for maintaining reduction of talar neck fractures. The medial and lateral posterior processes are important because they contain the flexor hallucis longus. The lateral process is usually larger and can be injured or associated as an accessory bone called the os trigonum. The lateral tubercle has many ligamentous attachments[6,7] and can act as a wedge to fracture the os calcis. The weakest area of the talus corresponds to the neck, which is reduced in thickness to allow for dorsiflexion.

Circulation of the Talus

Because approximately 60% of its surface is cartilage, the talus often has problems with circulation. Knowledge of the circulation of the talus is critical to understanding the association of osteonecrosis with talar fractures (Fig. 1).

The extraosseous circulation, with contributions from the anterior tibialis, posterior tibial, and peroneal arteries, forms a vascular ring composed of the tarsal sinus artery and the artery of the tarsal canal. The tarsal sinus artery comes from the dorsalis pedis artery and the lateral malleolar branch of the peroneal artery. These anterolateral vessels traverse the sinus tarsi to the tarsal canal, where they anastomose with the artery of the tarsal canal.[1,8-10] The artery of the tarsal canal consistently arises from the posterior tibial artery about 2 cm below the ankle and passes through the deltoid ligament. The deltoid artery, a branch of the artery of the tarsal canal, supplies the medial fourth of the talar body. The vessels of the sinus tarsi and the tarsal canal provide most of the remaining blood supply to the body of the talus.[9-12]

The talar head has abundant vessels entering from the superior and inferior lateral aspect of the neck with contributions from the anterior tibial artery, the tarsal sinus artery, and the lateral tarsal artery.

History

The first account of an accident to the talus was recorded in 1608 by Fabricius of Hilden, who described a man who had a compound talar dislocation after jumping from a 3-ft fence.[2-4] The first to collect and classify a series of cases was Anderson,[13] a consultant to the Royal Flying Corps of England, who in 1919 described 18 cases of fractured tali associated with aircraft accidents (aviator astragalus). These injuries occurred while the foot was positioned on the rudder bar in extreme plantar flexion. Since then many investigators including Bonnin,[2] Coltart,[14] Dunn and associates,[15] Pennal,[16] Penny and Davis,[17] Gillquist and associates,[18] Mindell and associates,[19] Kenwright and Taylor,[20] and others,[21-25] have reported series of these injuries and described their associated problems. Although severe, these fractures of the talus account for only 6% of all injuries affecting the foot.

Talar Head Fractures

Fractures of the head of the talus constitute approximately 5% to 10% of all injuries to the talus. The mechanism of injury is usually longitudinal compression of a plantar-flexed foot, which results in a compressive load transmitted through the talonavicular joint.[3,4] Because the talar head is well vascularized, the incidence of osteonecrosis is low, only 10%. The key problems with these injuries are malreduction and delayed recognition, with resultant arthrosis and instability.

Physical examination will show midtarsal tenderness and instability. Plain radiographs may show a space in the talonavicular area where the fracture fragment has been displaced. A pronated oblique radiograph as described by Canale and Kelly[21] is helpful in defining the talar head (Fig. 2). Computed tomography may be necessary to define the fracture fragment. The treatment for a nondisplaced talar head fracture is a short

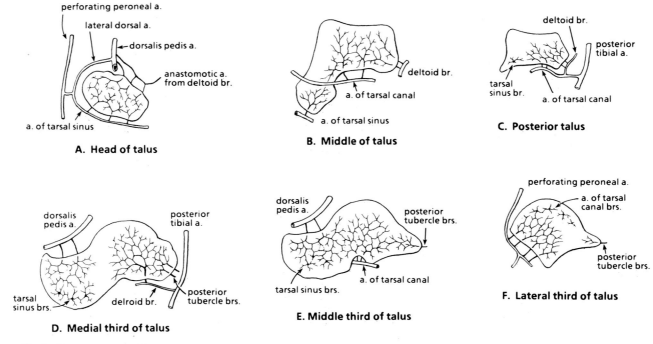

Fig. 1   Extraosseous and intraosseous circulation of talus.

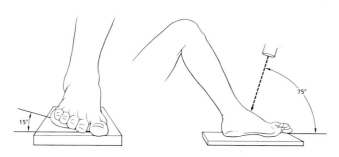

Fig. 2   Positioning the patient for an oblique view of midfoot to obtain a profile of the talar neck. (Adapted with permission from Canale ST, Kelly FB Jr: Fractures of the neck of the talus: Long-term evaluation of seventy-one cases. *J Bone Joint Surg* 1978;60A:143–156.)

leg cast and nonweightbearing activities for approximately eight to 12 weeks. Healing should be confirmed radiographically before weightbearing commences. If the displaced fracture involves more than 50% of the talar head, it usually requires internal fixation (Fig. 3). If the fracture fragment is less than 50% of the talar head and no instability of the talonavicular joint can be demonstrated, excision of the displaced fragments should be considered. These fractures can ultimately cause talonavicular arthritis, which may require arthrodesis.

Talar Neck Fractures

Fractures of the neck of the talus account for 50% of all talus fractures. The mechanism of injury for most talar neck fractures involves an acute dorsiflexion force directed at the midportion of the forefoot. These injuries typically occur during high-energy injuries, such as a fall, motor-vehicle accident, or airplane crash.

The fracture of the neck of the talus usually occurs in the narrowest part of the talar neck, which is the weak area of the talus. The pattern of the fracture is typically in a vertical or slightly oblique plane with the fracture extending between the middle and anterior facets of the calcaneus (Fig. 4). With continued dorsiflexion, the posterior capsule of the ankle and subtalar joint ruptures and the entire foot moves in a dorsal direction. This causes further impingement on the neck of the talus, with subsequent distraction of the body of the talus. If the talocalcaneal ligament ruptures, the body of the talus will dislocate posteriorly, and, typically, this portion of the bone is found at the posterior medial aspect of the Achilles tendon, where it can compromise the adjacent neurovascular structures. When a supination force is added, subluxation of the subtalar joint and ankle can occur.

Fractures of the medial malleolus are associated with talar neck fractures. In some series, medial malleolar fractures have occurred in 19% to 28% of the cases.[3,4] Although less common, lumbar spine injuries are also

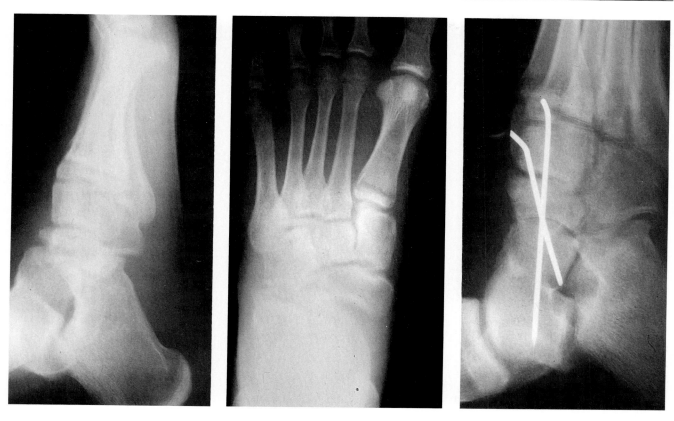

Fig. 3 **Left** and **center**, Lateral view is suggestive of talar head fracture. **Right**, Fracture treated by internal fixation with K-wire.

associated with talar neck fractures. Open injuries are found more frequently when when there is a dislocation or subluxation of the body of the talus.

Treatment

The goal when treating fractures of the talar neck is to recognize those fractures that have a high association with osteonecrosis and osteoarthritis and to develop a treatment protocol that will minimize those risks. The incidence of osteonecrosis increases with the amount of dorsal displacement of the distal talar neck and subluxation of the talar body or subtalar joint. The talocalcaneal ligament, an important structure in obtaining and maintaining reduction by closed means, becomes ruptured when there is significant dorsal displacement of the distal fragment. When this ligament is disrupted, it is difficult to control the dorsal displacement and varus angulation of the distal talus by closed means.

At my institution, we classify these injuries by a modification of the system developed by Hawkins.[22] Class I is a nondisplaced vertical neck fracture with no subluxation. Class II has mild dorsal displacement of the distal talar neck fragment with subluxation of the sub-

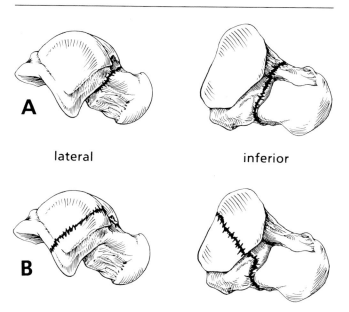

Fig. 4 Fractures of the talar neck (**A**) do not involve the posterior articular facet. Talar body fractures (**B**) do involve the posterior articular facet.

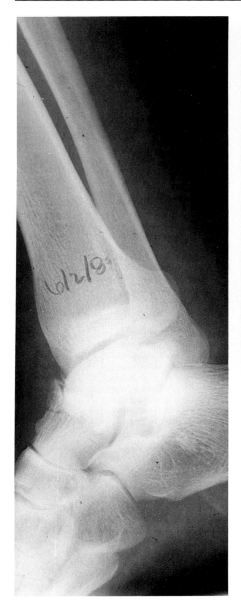

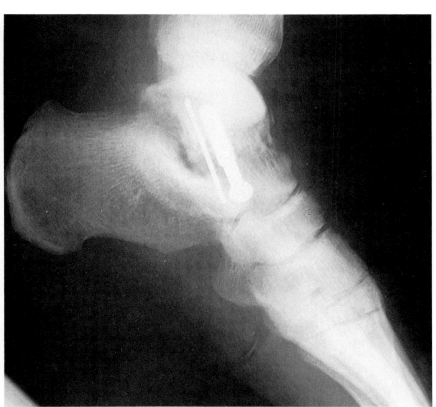

Fig. 5 **Left**, Class II fracture of the talus that required open reduction to reduce the subtalar joint. **Right**, Stabilization by anteromedial approach with cancellous screw and K-wire.

talar joint. Class III involves complete displacement of the talar neck from the body in association with subtalar subluxation. Classifying these injuries helps in planning treatment and satisfying the goals listed above.

Class I injuries can be treated by closed reduction. The key is to make sure that these injuries are indeed nondisplaced and that they maintain acceptable reduction after application of a cast. Because it has been noted that varus deformities can occur in the distal fragment, special views of the talar neck, such as those described by Canale and Kelly,[21] may be useful (Fig. 2). Treatment is a short leg cast, worn for approximately six to eight weeks. Weightbearing is delayed until trabeculation occurs across the fracture site. Early weight-

bearing would increase the shear forces and decrease the potential of osteoblasts to bridge the fracture. Nonunions in class I fractures are rare with this treatment. The circulation typically remains intact, but osteonecrosis does occur in approximately 10% of class I injuries.

In class II injuries it is possible but difficult to obtain anatomic reduction by closed manipulation. Reduction is aided by traction applied to the hindfoot and the foot being positioned in equinus. I advocate open reduction for 3 to 5 mm of dorsal displacement, subtalar malrotation, or 5 degrees of neck rotation. The anteromedial approach in the safe interval between the anterior tibialis and extensor hallucis longus tendon is frequently used (Fig. 5). The problem with the anteromedial approach is that with a shortened and medially deviated neck, the area for screw fixation is less than optimum. Better mechanical fixation can be obtained from screws inserted from a posterior approach that can be made either lateral or medial to the Achilles tendon (Fig. 6).[5,26–28] I do not hesitate to add a limited anteromedial incision, because it is otherwise very difficult to obtain an accurate reduction of neck rotation. Rigid anatomic reduction with AO 6.5-mm cancellous screws, AO malleolar screws, or cannulated screws is recommended. The Kirschner wire in combination with a cannulated screw is helpful in obtaining reduction and maintaining rotational control. An image intensifier is used to check reduction and aid in placement of K-wires, but routine radiographs, including oblique views, are recommended at the end of the each case so that accurate reduction of the varus and dorsal displacement can be confirmed.

The greater displacement seen in these class II injuries requires a longer time for healing. Eight to 12 weeks of nonweightbearing is typically needed in these injuries. Open reduction will speed rehabilitation only if rigid fixation is obtained so that early nonweightbearing motion can be commenced.

For class III injuries, preservation of the remaining compromised blood supply is crucial. If the injury is closed, immediate closed manipulation is used for posterior dislocation of the talar body (Fig. 7). This requires adequate anesthesia, the hindfoot being placed in equinus, and distraction through a pin placed in the os calcis. The subsequent goal is to obtain anatomic reduction and rigid fixation that allows early motion during osseous healing. Osteotomy of the medial malleolus is often used for exposure, with care taken not to injure the deltoid vessels.[29] Less often, a fibular osteotomy may be necessary for exposure.

Because talar neck fractures are relatively uncommon, series describing complications are rare. Some reports from the Scandinavian countries have reported osteonecrosis ranging from 10% in the nondisplaced group to almost 70% in class III injuries.[18,19,25,30,31] Delayed unions and subtalar arthritis occurred primarily in class II and class III injuries. Surgical therapy, however, can be helpful, as patients treated nonsurgically have been reported to have a threefold greater incidence of nonunion and a delay in return to work that was twice as long.

The incidence of osteonecrosis is greatest in those fractures that had the greatest amount of displacement. The Hawkins sign,[22] patchy subchondral osteoporosis seen at six to eight weeks after injury, signifies revascularization and a good prognosis. When examining radiographs in this critical period, it is important to obtain anteroposterior views of the ankle. Other radiographs will not demonstrate the talar body in isolation. Magnetic resonance imaging can demonstrate how

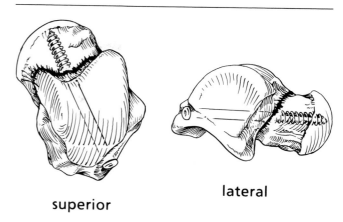

Fig. 6 For proper biomechanical fracture fixation a posterior lateral approach using cancellous screws is best.

superior

lateral

much of the talus is involved with osteonecrosis (Fig. 8).

Revascularization takes from six months to two years, and the rate of fracture healing dictates when controlled weightbearing starts.[20–22,32] Controlled weightbearing can occur as long as varus and valgus stresses are not placed on the talus and as long as the entire talar body is not involved in the revascularization process. If the entire body of the talus is involved, then weightbearing should be limited and angular stresses controlled with a patellar tendon-bearing brace or extended ankle brace.

Talar Body Fracture

Fractures of the body of the talus constitute 13% to 23% of all talus fractures. These fractures include osteochondral fractures, fractures of the body of the talus, posterior tubercle fractures, lateral process fractures, and crush injuries to the talar body. Fortunately, the most common fractures involving the body of the talus are those located in the posterior process and lateral tubercle.[3,4,33–35]

Fractures of the body of the talus without dislocation have approximately a 25% incidence of osteonecrosis, but with dislocation they have an incidence of osteonecrosis of more than 50% and require an average of three to four months to heal. Malunion and osteoarthritis are common in these injuries. These fractures can be classified according to the direction of the fracture—vertical, horizontal, or coronal. Computed tomography, particular in vertical fractures, may be necessary to define the fracture pattern (Fig. 9).

The principles of fixation for talar body fractures are the same as for talar neck fractures and involve temporary fixation with K-wires, followed by cannulated screws or lag-screw fixation to allow rigid fixation and

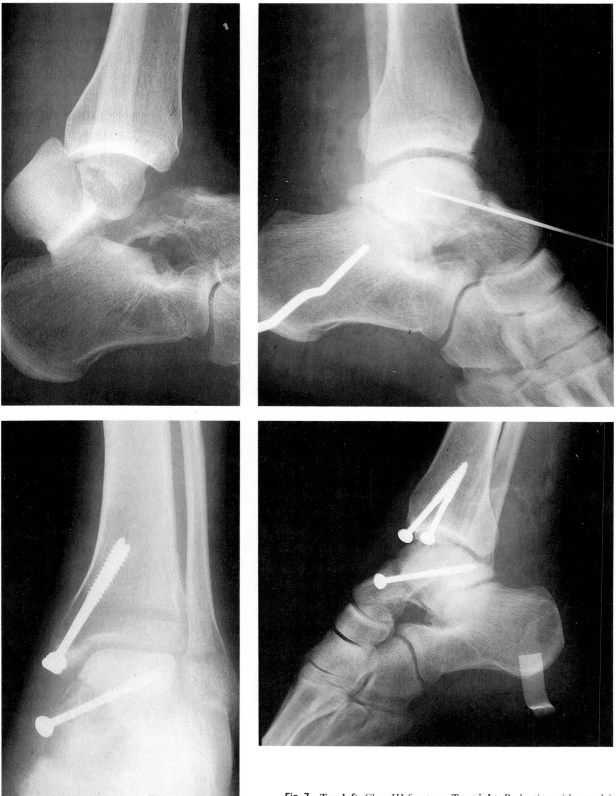

Fig. 7 Top left, Class III fracture. **Top right**, Reduction with os calcis traction and temporary stabilization with K-wire. **Bottom**, Osteotomy of medial malleolus was required to obtain an anteromedial reduction. Sclerosis on anteroposterior ankle view indicates osteonecrosis of the talus.

early motion. Medial or lateral malleolar osteotomy is often required to gain sufficient exposure for fixation.[29]

When the body is significantly comminuted, it is classified as a crush or compression injury. In this injury, computed tomography is often helpful in defining the extent of comminution and in planning the surgery. To obtain even an incomplete reduction may require traction by an external fixation device placed across the ankle. With these injuries, it may be necessary to debride portions of the talar body. A high incidence of subsequent osteoarthritis is associated with these severe injuries.

In treating the severely traumatized and devascularized talus, the goal is to preserve as much motion and length as possible. In my opinion, when the body of the talus is present, the best reconstructive procedure is the Blair tibiotalar arthrodesis.[36] In this procedure, the tibia is fused to the vascularized portion of the head of the talus and the avascular portion of the talar body is removed. Some subtalar joint motion is retained, because the anterior and middle facets of the calcaneus articulate with the remaining portion of the neck. This motion, along with talonavicular joint motion, will allow a functional gait. This is the only salvage procedure that is able to obtain a normal profile of the foot. The

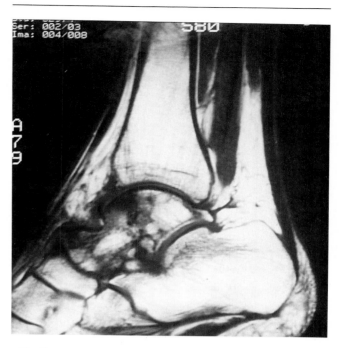

Fig. 8 Magnetic resonance imaging, done three months after a displaced talar neck fracture, demonstrates more than 50% osteonecrosis of the body.

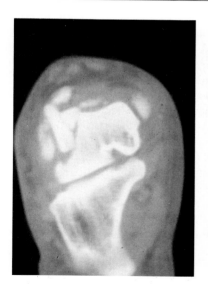
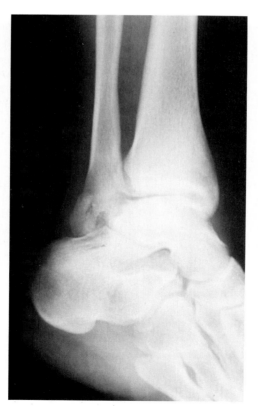
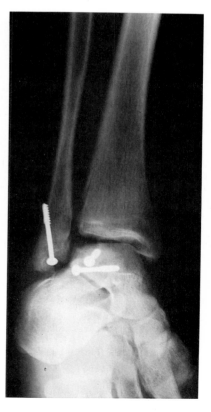

Fig. 9 Vertical talar body fracture. **Left,** Computed tomography. **Center,** Radiograph. **Right,** Postreduction radiograph after fibular osteotomy.

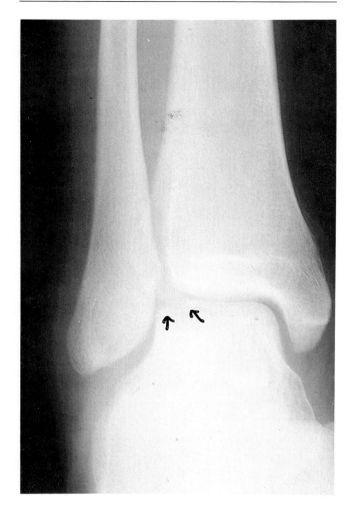

Fig. 10 Lateral osteochondral fracture is often associated with trauma.

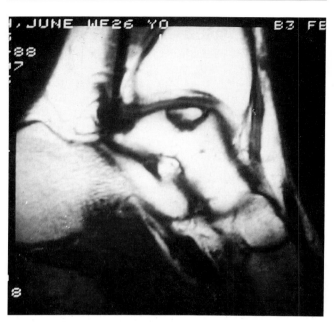

Fig. 11 Magnetic resonance imaging of a medial osteochondral lesion that had existed for ten years.

alignment of the foot in relationship to the ankle and leg is almost normal, and no shortening is produced. However, it is usually best to delay this operation so that the acutely traumatized soft tissues will not compromise healing of the arthrodesis.

If it is not possible to save the body of the talus, then the tibia should be fused to the calcaneus. In my opinion, talectomy is a poor alternative, because it produces severe shortening and instability. For large avascular defects of the body of the talus, bone-grafting techniques have been tried at my institution using large iliac crest autogenous bone grafts to substitute for the avascular talus. It is usually necessary to fuse the talocalcaneal joint when using these techniques, and it is important to use rigid fixation with cancellous or cannulated screws.

Osteochondral lesions of the talus were described as a fracture by Monroe in 1738, Konnig in 1887, and Rendu in 1932.[3,4,34,37-39] Such lesions are often included in the category of osteochondrosis. Joint laxity may coexist with osteochondral fractures.[35,37,40,41] Symptoms are ankle pain, recurrent swelling, and giving way. The symptoms are often slowly progressive and the diagnosis is often delayed. The lesions are either on the medial or lateral aspect of the talus. Lateral lesions[37,42] are often wafer-shaped and are typically located in the anterior portion of the talus (Fig. 10). Medial lesions are typically cup-shaped and are located most often in the posterior portion of the talus. Computed tomography helps in locating the lesion and determining the depth of involvement and attachment. Magnetic resonance imaging also helps by showing the degree of devascularization of the fragment (Fig. 11).

The lateral lesions are probably secondary to a traumatic inversion injury. The medial lesions are more typical of an osteochondrosis and are associated with degenerative cysts. These lesions have been categorized by Berndt and Harty.[37] In their system, stage I has compression of the subchondral bone without a break in the cartilage, stage II is a complete lesion without detachment of the articular cartilage, stage III has a partially detached articular surface, and stage IV has a fragment that is completely detached from the articular surface.[8,37,40]

Long-term results show that few lesions unite when treated surgically, and arthritic changes occur in about 50% regardless of treatment.[35,41] Nonsurgical treatment consists of application of a patellar tendon-bearing cast or brace. Weightbearing is avoided for approximately three months. The surgical approach to these lesions

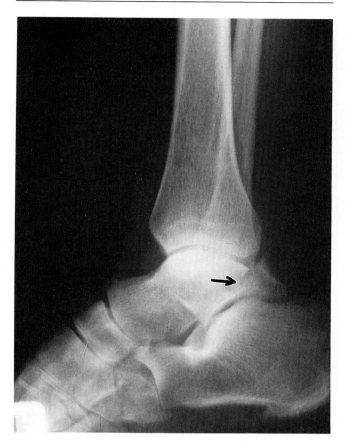

Fig. 12 Fracture of the lateral posterior tubercle.

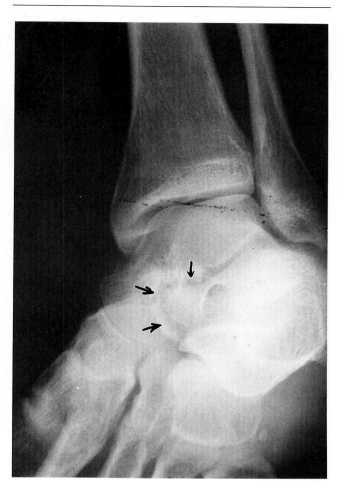

Fig. 13 Fracture of lateral tubercle.

depends on their location. Because the medial osteochondral fractures are typically located posteriorly, they usually require an osteotomy of the medial malleolus, but the anterolateral lesions can be reached by an arthrotomy or arthroscopy. The best treatment for complete lesions is debridement.

Posterior process fractures constitute the largest percentage of fractures involving the body of the talus. A bone scan is used to differentiate a posterior process fracture from an os trigonum, an accessory bone of the lateral posterior process that has a reported incidence of 3% to 30%.[43] The medial and lateral process form a groove for the flexor hallucis longus tendon. Fractures of the posterior tibial tubercle may cause entrapment of the flexor hallucis longus tendon. The lateral posterior process is larger than the medial. The medial tubercle fracture is rare. The lateral process fracture (Fig. 12), if recognized acutely, is treated by casting the foot in mild equinus. If the fracture is chronic in nature, small fragments are excised and larger fragments are internally fixed.

A high index of suspicion should be maintained for lateral tubercle fractures when a prolonged, painful process localizes the symptoms to the lateral aspect of the ankle.[6,7,44] Dorsiflexion and external rotation are the most common mechanisms of injury for these lateral process fractures; however, inversion can cause avulsion of this area and eversion can cause the posterior facet of the talus to be sheared by the lateral malleolus (Fig. 13). Treatment depends on the symptoms and the size of the fragment. If the fragment is small, the patient is placed in a cast in slight equinus and kept nonweightbearing for six weeks. Larger fragments are fixed by open reduction and internal fixation. Debridement may be necessary for large crush injuries.

References

1. Haliburton RA, Sullivan CR, Kelly PJ, et al: The extra-osseous and intra-osseous blood supply of the talus. *J Bone Joint Surg* 1958;40A:1115–1120.
2. Bonnin JG: Dislocations and fracture-dislocations of the talus. *Br J Surg* 1940;28:88–100.
3. Delee JC: Fractures and dislocations of the foot, in Mann RA (ed): *Surgery of the Foot*, ed 5. St. Louis, CV Mosby, 1986, pp 656–715.

4. Heckman JD: Fractures and dislocation of the foot, in Rockwood CA Jr, Green DP (eds): *Fractures in Adults*, ed 2. St. Louis, JB Lippincott, 1984, vol 2, pp 1703–1832.

5. Swanson TV, Bray TJ: Talar neck fractures: A mechanical and histomorphometric study of fixation. Presented at the meeting of the Orthopedic Trauma Association, Dallas, October 1988.

6. Hawkins LG: Fracture of the lateral process of the talus: A review of thirteen cases. *J Bone Joint Surg* 1965;47A:1170–1175.

7. Mukherjee SK, Pringle RM, Baxter AD: Fracture of the lateral process of the talus: A report of thirteen cases. *J Bone Joint Surg* 1974;56B:263–273.

8. Larson RL, Sullivan CR, Janes JM: Trauma, surgery, and circulation of the talus: What are the risks of avascular necrosis? *J Trauma* 1961;1:13–21.

9. Wildenauer E: Die Blutversorgung des Talus. *Z Anat* 1950;115:32–36.

10. Mulfinger GL, Trueta J: The blood supply of the talus. *J Bone Joint Surg* 1970;52B:160–167.

11. Kelly PJ, Sullivan CR: Blood supply of the talus. *Clin Orthop* 1963;37–44.

12. Peterson L, Goldie IF, Irstam L: Fracture of the neck of the talus: A clinical study. *Acta Orthop Scand* 1977;48:696–706.

13. Anderson HG: *The Medical and Surgical Aspects of Aviation*. Oxford Medical Publications, London, 1919.

14. Coltart WD: "Aviator's astragalus." *J Bone Joint Surg* 1952;34B:545–566.

15. Dunn AR, Jacobs B, Campbell RD Jr: Fractures of the talus. *J Trauma* 1966;6:443–468.

16. Pennal GF: Fractures of the talus. *Clin Orthop* 1963;30:53–63.

17. Penny JN, Davis LA: Fractures and fracture-dislocations of the neck of the talus. *J Trauma* 1980;20:1029–1037.

18. Gillquist J, Oretorp N, Stenström A, et al: Late results after vertical fracture of the talus. *Injury* 1974;6:173–179.

19. Mindell ER, Cisek EE, Kartalian G, et al: Late results of injuries to the talus: Analysis of forty cases. *J Bone Joint Surg* 1963;45A:221–245.

20. Kenwright J, Taylor RG: Major injuries of the talus. *J Bone Joint Surg* 1970;52B:36–48.

21. Canale ST, Kelly FB Jr: Fractures of the neck of the talus: Long-term evaluation of seventy-one cases. *J Bone Joint Surg* 1978;60A:143–156.

22. Hawkins LG: Fractures of the neck of the talus. *J Bone Joint Surg* 1970;52A:991–1002.

23. Kleiger B: Fractures of the talus. *J Bone Joint Surg* 1948;30A:735–744.

24. Lorentzen JE, Christensen SB, Krogsoe O, et al: Fracture of the neck of the talus. *Acta Orthop Scand* 1977;48:115–120.

25. Pantazopoulos T, Galanos P, Vayanos E, et al: Fractures of the neck of the talus. *Acta Orthop Scand* 1974;45:296–306.

26. Lemaire RG, Bustin W: Screw fixation of fractures of the neck of the talus using a posterior approach. *J Trauma* 1980;20:669–673.

27. Trillat A, Bousquet G, Lapeyre B: Les fractures-séparations totales du col ou du corps de l'astragale: Intérêt du vissage par voie postérieure. *Rev Chir Orthop* 1970;56:529–536.

28. Gatellier J: The juxtoretroperoneal route in the operative treatment of fracture of the malleolus with posterior marginal fragments. *Surg Gynecol Obstet* 1931;52:67–70.

29. Deyerle WM, Burkhardt B, Comfort T, et al: Displaced fractures of the talus: An aggressive approach. *Orthop Trans* 1981;5:465.

30. Comfort TH, Behrens F, Gaither DW, et al: Long-term results of displaced talar neck fractures. *Clin Orthop* 1985;199:81–87.

31. Fjeldborg O: Fracture of the lateral process of the talus: Supination-dorsal flexion fracture. *Acta Orthop Scand* 1968;39:407–412.

32. Bobechko WP, Harris WR: The radiographic density of avascular bone. *J Bone Joint Surg* 1960;42B:626–632.

33. Sneppen O, Christensen SB, Krogsoe O, et al: Fracture of the body of the talus. *Acta Orthop Scand* 1977;48:317–324.

34. Davidson AM, Steele HD, MacKenzie DA, et al: A review of twenty-one cases of transchondral fracture of the talus. *J Trauma* 1967;7:378–415.

35. Alexander AH, Lichtman DM: Surgical treatment of transchondral talar-dome fractures (osteochondritis dissecans): Long-term follow-up. *J Bone Joint Surg* 1980;62A:646–652.

36. Dennis MD, Tullos HS: Blair tibiotalar arthrodesis for injuries to the talus. *J Bone Joint Surg* 1980;62A:103–107.

37. Berndt AL, Harty M: Transchondral fractures (osteochondritis dissecans) of the talus. *J Bone Joint Surg* 1959;41A:988–1020.

38. O'Farrell TA, Costello BG: Osteochondritis dissecans of the talus: The late results of surgical treatment. *J Bone Joint Surg* 1982;64B:494–497.

39. Yvars MF: Osteochondral fractures of the dome of the talus. *Clin Orthop* 1976;114:185–191.

40. Canale ST, Belding RH: Osteochondral lesions of the talus. *J Bone Joint Surg* 1980;62A:97–102.

41. McCullough CJ, Venugopal V: Osteochondritis dissecans of the talus: The natural history. *Clin Orthop* 1979;144:264–268.

42. Scharling M: Osteochondritis dissecans of the talus. *Acta Orthop Scand* 1978;49:89–94.

43. Dimon JH III: Isolated displaced fracture of the posterior facet of the talus. *J Bone Joint Surg* 1961;43A:275–281.

44. Heckman JD, McLean MR: Fractures of the lateral process of the talus. *Clin Orthop* 1985;199:108–113.

Subtalar Dislocations

Michael J. Brennan, MD

Introduction

Simultaneous dislocation of both the talocalcaneal and talonavicular joints is referred to as a subtalar dislocation. This injury occurs because the weaker talonavicular and talocalcaneal ligaments and capsules rupture, while the strong calcaneonavicular ligament remains intact. This causes the midfoot to displace as a unit. Although this injury is rare enough that few series in the literature have more than ten patients, it is important to recognize the potential problems in treating it.

Most of these injuries occur as a result of high-energy impact, as in a motor-vehicle accident or a fall from a height, but some happen simply as a result of stumbling on the basketball court. About 10% of these injuries are open, and all have some degree of soft-tissue compromise (Fig. 1). However, few cases of neurovascular compromise have been reported. Extensive swelling can mask the deformity. If only ankle radiographs are obtained, the diagnosis can be missed and the appropriate treatment delayed. Figure 2 is part of an ankle series that was interpreted as normal until additional radiographs of the foot, shown in Figure 3, clearly dem-

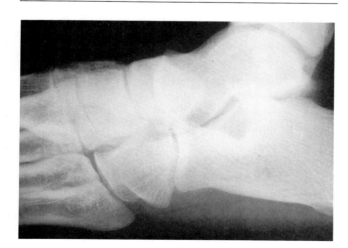

Fig. 1 Soft-tissue damage associated with lateral subtalar dislocation.

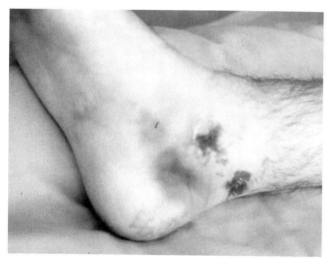

Fig. 2 Medial subtalar dislocation. Note talar head overriding navicular.

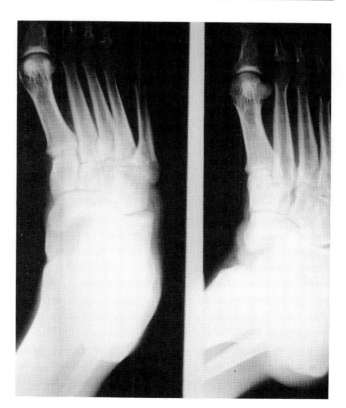

Fig. 3 Anteroposterior and oblique radiographs of foot confirm diagnosis of medial subtalar dislocation.

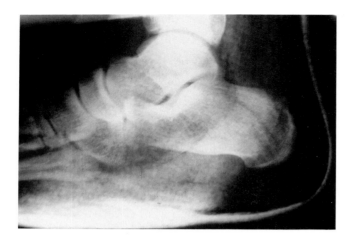

Fig. 4 Post-reduction view.

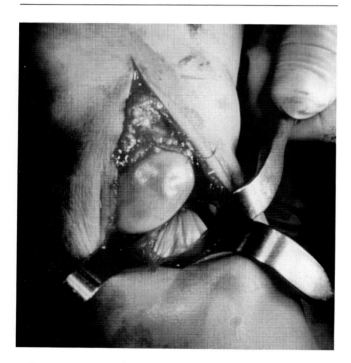

Fig. 5 Extensor tendons block reduction of talar head.

onstrated the medial subtalar dislocation. The post-reduction view (Fig. 4) shows the normal anatomic alignment.

Classifying the dislocation by the displacement of the distal part, 80% of subtalar dislocations are classified as medial and 20% have the foot displaced lateral to the talus. Associated fractures are present in about one half of these injuries. Avulsions from the talar head or body of the calcaneus may block concentric reduction. Impaction of the talar head and navicular may prevent

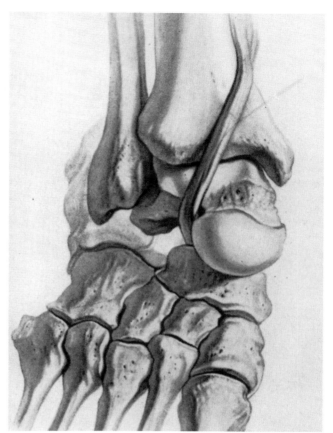

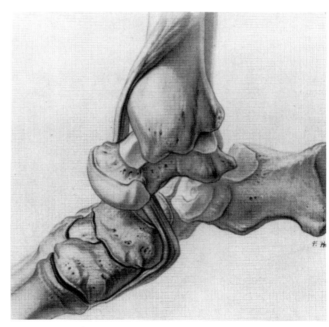

Fig. 6 Posterior tibialis tendon blocks reduction of talar head. (Reproduced with permission from Leitner B: Obstacles to reduction in subtalar dislocations. *J Bone Joint Surg* 1954;36A:304.)

closed reduction. Fractures of the navicular, fibula, or base of the fifth metatarsal may require further care.

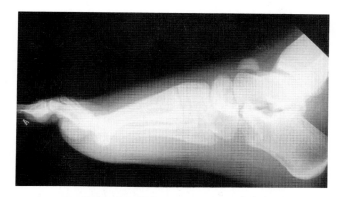

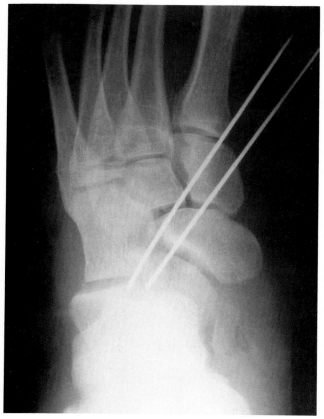

Fig. 7 **Top,** Unstable reduction with osteochondral fragment. **Bottom,** Status after open reduction and internal fixation.

Reduction

Closed reduction is commonly performed with the patient under intravenous sedation, but I prefer to attempt closed reduction with the patient under general anesthesia, because I believe that muscle relaxation decreases the potential of articular cartilage damage and increases the likelihood of a successful closed reduction. If the attempted closed reduction is unsuccessful, I am prepared for immediate open reduction of the dislocation. To perform a closed reduction, use the following maneuver. Flex the knee and the forefoot. Apply

gentle traction. Accentuate and then reverse the deformity, with digital pressure over the talar head. The surgeon can usually feel the dislocated part return to its normal position. The range of motion returns to normal with an intrinsic bony stability, rarely requiring internal fixation.

Irreducible Dislocations

An irreducible subtalar dislocation is usually caused by the talar head being buttonholed through the surrounding longitudinally directed anatomic structures. To achieve reduction, make a longitudinal incision over the protruding talar head, avoiding compromised skin. Subsequent osteonecrosis of the talus is rare, occurring in only 5% to 10% of cases, but the blood supply should be preserved when possible. For this reason, soft tissue should not be stripped from the talar neck. Reduction of medial dislocations may be blocked by the extensor tendons (Fig. 5). In the case of a lateral dislocation, the posterior tibialis tendon can prevent reduction and will require mobilization (Fig. 6). If the tendon must be transected to allow reduction, it should be repaired. Locked impaction fractures may also hinder reduction. Avulsion or osteochondral fragments that can prevent a concentric reduction should be cleared from the joint or, if large enough, reduced and fixed in place (Fig. 7).

Recovery

I immobilize patients in a short leg cast for at least four weeks, increasing this period to six weeks for patients who are young, loose-jointed, or have associated fractures. Historically, the concern has been for loss of subtalar motion after this injury. Some loss of motion is detected in nearly all patients; however, few complain of stiffness. Stiffness may be less functionally impairing than subtalar instability. Zimmer and Johnson[1] reported that five of eight patients treated described problems of instability. These patients tended to be younger and had an average period of immobilization of only 4.4 weeks. Larsen[2] described a patient with recurrent subtalar dislocation. Heppenstall and associates[3] described the loss of reduction of a subtalar dislocation while it was in a cast. For these reasons, the trend to a shorter period of immobilization and early range of motion may be inappropriate for this injury.

References

1. Zimmer TJ, Johnson KA: Subtalar dislocations. *Clin Orthop* 1989;238:190–194.
2. Larsen H-W: Subastragalar dislocation (luxatio pedis sub talo): A follow-up report of eight cases. *Acta Chir Scand* 1957;113:380–392.
3. Heppenstall RB, Farahvar H, Balderston R, et al: Evaluation and management of subtalar dislocations. *J Trauma* 1980;20:494–497.

Surgical Management of Calcaneus Fractures: Indications and Techniques

Michael E. Miller, MD

Introduction

Fractures of the calcaneus are potentially disabling injuries that can disrupt both of the longitudinal arches of the foot, can cause loss of the lever arm for the Achilles tendon, and can lead to incapacitating pain and loss of motion in the subtalar joint. The hindfoot becomes wider and may be unsuitable for standard footwear.[1] Paley and associates,[2] in a study of 44 patients with a minimum follow-up of four years, found that lateral widening of the calcaneus, with subsequent impingement on the peroneal tendons, was a major source of pain and disability. They also found that increased heel width, increased body weight, and occupation as a heavy laborer made a poor outcome more likely. Their studies did not find that calcaneal alignment was a prognostic factor.

The therapeutic view of calcaneal fractures outlined by Trickey[3] in 1975 still persists for many practicing orthopaedic surgeons, that is, that these injuries, when treated by neglect or inadequate closed methods, produce a large percentage of unsatisfactory results, and that they are demanding fractures to treat surgically. The current status of surgical management of the fractured calcaneus is similar to that of acetabular fractures approximately ten years ago. Surgical techniques and skills are only now being disseminated that will finally allow clearer assessment of which fractures should be managed closed, and which should be considered for surgery.

Classification of Fractures

Essex-Lopresti[4] accurately described the two major types of calcaneal fractures more than 35 years ago, and his system has proven both simple and clinically useful. His division of fractures into "tongue type" and "joint-depression type" can be augmented in order to clarify the goals and methods of treatment. I believe that joint-depression fractures should be further subdivided according to the system of Soeur and Remy[5] to include three degrees or grades of what these authors referred to as thalamic fractures. First-degree thalamic, or joint-depression, fractures, which involve only depression of the posterior facet of the calcaneus, are quite rare. These fractures are typically accompanied by a vertical fracture through the bottom of the "V" that is seen on lateral radiographs at the junction of the anterior and posterior facets of the calcaneus. This V shape is actually the thalamus, described by Soeur and Remy as "that part of the bone, formed of a layer of compact bone tissue, which supports the posterior articular facet and continues forward, becoming thinner towards the groove of the sinus tarsi."[5] The second-degree fracture has further comminution of the calcaneus into four major fragments, but no important displacement of this vertical fracture. The third-degree thalamic fracture is marked by greater comminution and displacement of the fracture fragments. This subclassification of joint-depression fractures is summarized in Figure 1.

Preoperative Radiographic Evaluation

Presurgical evaluation of the fractured calcaneus must take into account the complex three-dimensional nature of these injuries. Romash[6] recommended that radiographic evaluation include axial, lateral, anteroposterior, and oblique medial projections. In addition, he believed that computed tomography of the injured hindfoot in two planes should be obtained. The combination of these images gives the surgeon a clear idea of the axial malalignment, shortening, and angulation of the fracture fragments, and computed tomography provides extremely clear images of impaction and splitting of the articular facets of the calcaneus. Because of variations in hindfoot morphology, radiographs of the uninjured side should be obtained as a routine part of the examination. I prefer to use anteroposterior, lateral, Harris, and Brodens' views for preoperative evaluation. With a good conception of the fracture pattern, one can then make an informed decision regarding closed vs surgical treatment.

Results of Closed and Open Treatment

Many reports in the North American and European literature detail the merits of closed management or surgical treatment of the fractured calcaneus,[7-10] but few series compare treatment methods, and none describe randomized, prospective trials. Järvholm and associates[11] compared 20 cases treated closed with 19 managed surgically and examined these patients two to 12 years after injury. These authors found that surgically treated patients retained more subtalar joint mo-

Joint Depression Fractures
(Thalamic Fractures)

First Degree   Second Degree   Third Degree

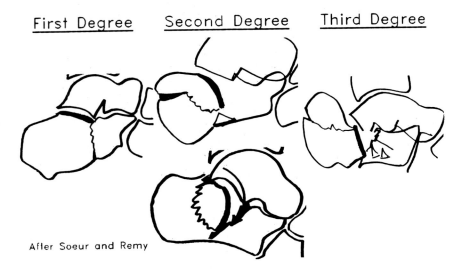

After Soeur and Remy

Fig. 1 Summary of joint-depression-type fractures expanded from Essex-Lopresti's original classification using the three degrees suggested by Soeur and Remy[5] for thalamic fractures.

tion, were better able to run and jump, and could walk longer distances on uneven ground than patients treated closed. Three patients from each group had severe residual symptoms and an equal number had negligible symptoms. Nine of the 20 treated closed and eight of the 19 treated surgically had radiographic signs of posttraumatic arthrosis. The conclusions of many authors are similar. A perfect anatomic reduction combined with stable fixation that allows early motion will produce excellent results, but perfect reductions are difficult both to achieve and to hold.

It would seem at this time that surgical treatment is indicated for younger, athletically active patients, and for those, such as construction workers, whose occupations require walking and standing on uneven ground. It must be stressed that even a recent report[12] from an experienced surgeon demonstrated good results in only about 75% of cases, and, on a subjective basis, surgical and nonsurgical results may be roughly equal. It is thus incumbent on the surgeon to consider every aspect of what Tile[13] has referred to as the "personality of the fracture" before undertaking surgical treatment.

Evolution of Surgical Methods

Essex-Lopresti's[4] method of percutaneous pin manipulation and fixation was the pioneering technique for these fractures. In skilled hands this procedure can produce good results, but it has two serious drawbacks.

There can be no visualization of disrupted joint surfaces, and this method requires casting, which limits early motion. McReynolds,[14] and later Burdeaux,[15,16] proposed a medial surgical approach to the calcaneus, which allows accurate repositioning of the angulated medial wall fracture and reduction of the sustentacular fragment. Elevation of the lateral portion of the posterior articular facet was accomplished without visualization of the joint, and both authors thought that closed compression of the lateral bulge of the calcaneus would be sufficient to restore normal calcaneal width and prevent peroneal tendon impingement. Pennal and Yadav[9] pointed out the advantages of a posterolateral approach, used initially for primary subtalar arthrodesis, but which affords such good visualization of the subtalar joint that they also used it for open reduction and internal fixation. The latter authors also used a simple external-fixation device to provide intraoperative traction and reduction of the fracture. This method was refined recently by Mast and associates[17] using the small-fragment fixator for multiplanar control and reduction of the calcaneus fragments. Using a fixator in this way allows excellent visualization of the subtalar joint, eases reduction by taking full advantage of ligamentotaxis on the fracture fragments, and is simple and quick. Other surgeons using primarily lateral surgical approaches include Fernandez.[18] Stephenson[12] described his combined approach using lateral and medial exposures.

To avoid confusion and unnecessary partisanship, one should again apply the analogy of the acetabular

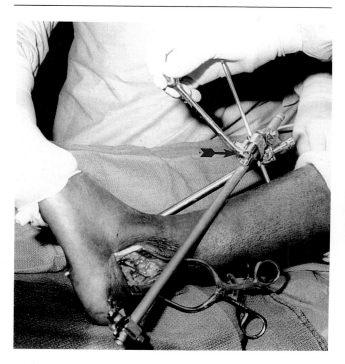

Fig. 2   The AO external fixator used as a distractor is a significant aid to fracture reduction. Clamps are sufficiently rigid to control rotation and angulation with only two pins. The distraction device (arrow) can be used when necessary.

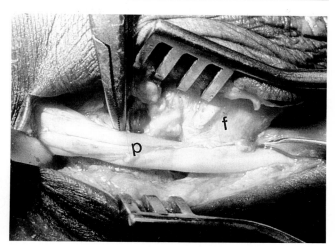

Fig. 3   The peroneal tendons (p) are subluxated from their normal path around the distal fibula (f) by lateral impingement of fracture fragments.

fracture in choosing surgical approaches. Some injuries can be treated by pure medial or pure lateral approaches, and some will require combined surgical approaches from the outset.

Treatment of Specific Fractures

General Principles

Surgical correction of fractures should be undertaken as soon as possible. If delays cannot be avoided, the limb should be cleansed with bacteriostatic soap, wrapped with sheet cotton and a gentle elastic wrap, and elevated on a Bohler-Braun frame or similar support to prevent excessive swelling.

All surgery is done with gentle soft-tissue handling, and full-thickness skin-to-bone flaps should be maintained. Self-retaining retractors should be applied with care, not to the skin but to the deep soft-tissue layers. Skin edges, articular cartilage, and tendons should be kept moist with saline or Ringer's solution, and antibiotics are given in all cases.

Tongue-Type Fractures

Simple tongue-type fractures may be treated by lateral or medial approaches, but nonarticular fractures are easily treated by medial visualization. External-fixation aids are optional.

The patient's position may be supine or prone. Prone positioning facilitates exposure somewhat, but makes the use of regional anesthesia nearly impossible. Under tourniquet control, an incision is made equidistant between the tuberosity of the calcaneus and the medial malleolus, sharply dividing the flexor retinaculum and retracting the neurovascular bundle anteriorly. Burdeaux[16] does not believe that the bundle needs to be dissected out, but those with less experience than he has may be more comfortable doing so. If fibers of the abductor hallucis obscure the medial face of the calcaneus, they can be retracted plantarward. By blunt dissection and use of a small, sharp-edged periosteal elevator, the fracture fragments can be readily identified, reduced, and held, either with bone screws appropriate in size to the fragment or with smooth Steinmann pins. The 2-mm end-threaded pins are ideal for this purpose, if screws are not chosen.

Simple Joint-Depression Fractures (First- and Second-Degree Thalamic Injuries)

Here, the primary problem is visualization of the posterior facet of the subtalar joint and reduction of the posterior facet of the calcaneus. I recommend a posterolateral approach using external fixation.

If supine, the patient should have a sandbag or roll under the ipsilateral hip. A single, 4.5-mm, external-fixator half pin is inserted into the tibia starting anteriorly approximately two fifths from its distal end. A large transfixing pin is then drilled through the posterior portion of the calcaneus. Because the usual fracture deformity is a varus and lateral angulation, the pin should be inserted from the medial side in an anterior-to-posterior direction. Righting the axis of the pin to make it perpendicular to the long axis of the tibia and

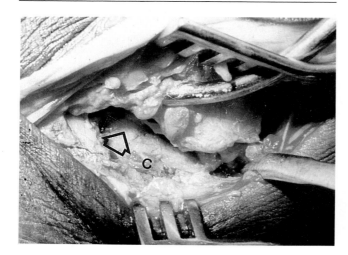

Fig. 4 Limited view of the subtalar joint (arrow) above the calcaneus (c) without distraction.

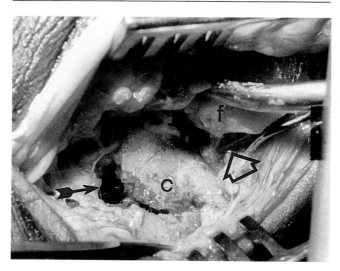

Fig. 6 The calcaneal articular fragment (c) has been elevated, leaving a bony defect (small arrow). The normal space for the peroneal tendons (large arrow) deep to the fibula (f) has been restored.

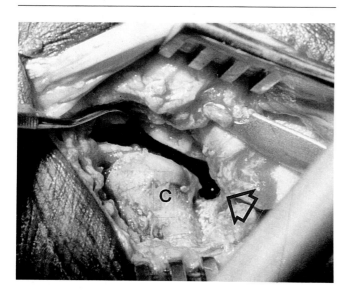

Fig. 5 With distraction applied, the subtalar joint space (arrow) is clearly visualized, and a depressed calcaneal fragment (c) is seen.

foot will help reduce this deformity. A simple triangular frame is then constructed, which can be combined with the external-fixator distraction device, if needed, for traction (Fig. 2).

The lateral surgical approach is made through an incision that starts posterior to the lateral malleolus between the Achilles tendon and the peroneal tendons, and continues with a gentle curve towards the calcaneocuboid joint. The sural nerve should be retracted posteriorly and plantarward. In light-skinned patients, a small branch of the lesser saphenous vein may serve as a cutaneous marker for this nerve. The peroneal

tendons are retracted dorsally in their sheath. If distal exposure is needed, the peroneus longus sheath may be opened distally to approach the calcaneocuboid joint. The fibulocalcaneal ligament complex is divided from the calcaneus and retracted dorsally. More detailed descriptions of the lateral approach to the os calcis are available.[19]

The surgeon may find that the normal space for the passage of the peroneal tendons has been obliterated by lateral displacement of calcaneal fragments (Fig. 3). With dorsal retraction of the peroneal tendons, the subtalar joint may be seen, but not clearly enough to allow accurate fracture reduction (Fig. 4). Distraction with the external fixator opens up the subtalar joint, and the depressed lateral portion of the facet may be seen (Fig. 5). The facet fragment can then be elevated to restore articular alignment. The resulting defect in the calcaneus caused by impaction of cancellous bone will now be apparent (Fig. 6).

Fixation of the joint-depression fracture can be obtained with small cancellous-bone screws, smooth Steinmann pins, or staples. The cancellous-bone defect, if large, should be filled with bone graft. Fernandez[18] obtains this from the distal tibia through his lateral dissection, but I prefer using an iliac crest cancellous graft.

Complex Joint-Depression Fractures (Third-Degree Thalamic Injuries)

These fractures should be viewed as combinations of joint-depression injuries and associated shear injuries through the thalamus that cause the tuber and the sustentaculum to be widely separated and comminuted. Although Burdeaux[16] advocated a medial approach for these injuries, a combined approach is best for this type of complex calcaneal fracture. For these injuries, external fixation also aids reduction and visualization of fracture anatomy. The medial exposure repositions the sustentaculum and corrects medial collapse. These complex fractures frequently involve the calcaneocuboid joint, and if this aspect of the injury is not addressed, persistent pain and disability may result. The combined approach is favored by Stephenson,[12] and I think that most surgeons will find that adding the external fixator will also improve their results.

Fixation techniques must be tailored to the fracture at hand, but the choices are pins, screws, plates, and staples. Longitudinal pin fixation is favored by Fernandez[18] for the larger tuber fragments to realign and fix these to the distal calcaneus, along with screw fixation of the posterior facet fracture. The use of H plates or four-pronged staples may be required to provide fixation of smaller fragments in complex fractures.

The ultimate goal of any fixation must be to allow early subtalar joint motion. If this is not possible and a cast is applied, subtalar joint stiffness is likely, and an inferior result little different from closed treatment, or perhaps worse, will be obtained.

Trickey's[3] allusion to the lateral tibial plateau fracture may be used as a suitable summation to this discussion:

> We have learnt that it is possible to reconstruct [a depressed lateral tibial condyle] in such a way that mobilisation is not delayed, and an excellent result may be obtained, but this is an art that must be mastered: Many attempts to reconstruct the joint surface are done so inadequately that the results are bad. There is nothing wrong with the idea; it is the execution which is at fault.

References

1. Hamilton JJ, Ziemer LK: Functional anatomy of the human ankle and foot, in Kiene RH, Johnson KA (eds): American Academy of Orthopaedic Surgeons *Symposium on the Foot and Ankle*. St. Louis, CV Mosby, 1983, pp 1–2.

2. Paley D, Hall H, McMurtry R, et al: Operative treatment of calcaneal fractures: A long term follow-up; calcaneal protocol score; and factors that affect outcome. *Orthop Trans* 1987;11:484.

3. Trickey EL: Treatment of fractures of the calcaneus, editorial. *J Bone Joint Surg* 1975;57B:411.

4. Essex-Lopresti P: The mechanism, reduction technique, and results in fractures of the os calcis. *Br J Surg* 1952;39:395–419.

5. Soeur R, Remy R: Fractures of the calcaneus with displacement of the thalamic portion. *J Bone Joint Surg* 1975;57B:413–421.

6. Romash MM: Calcaneal fractures: Three-dimensional treatment. *Foot Ankle* 1988;8:180–197.

7. Ostapowicz G, Sateri F, Wessel G: Ergebnisse der Calcaneus-frakturen [Results after fracture of the os calcis]. *Arch Orthop Trauma Surg* 1978;91:11–18.

8. Aaron DA, Howat TW: Intra-articular fractures of the calcaneum. *Injury* 1976;7:205–211.

9. Pennal GF, Yadav MP: Operative treatment of comminuted fractures of the os calcis. *Orthop Clin North Am* 1973;4:197–211.

10. Omoto H, Sakurada K, Sugi M, et al: A new method of manual reduction for intra-articular fracture of the calcaneus. *Clin Orthop* 1983;177:104–111.

11. Järvholm U, Körner L, Thorén O, et al: Fractures of the calcaneus: A comparison of open and closed treatment. *Acta Orthop Scand* 1984;55:652–656.

12. Stephenson JR: Treatment of displaced intra-articular fractures of the calcaneus using medial and lateral approaches, internal fixation, and early motion. *J Bone Joint Surg* 1987;69A:115–130.

13. Tile M: *Fractures of the Pelvis and Acetabulum*. Baltimore, Williams & Wilkins, 1984, p 177.

14. McReynolds IS: The case for operative treatment of fractures of the os calcis, in Leach RE, Hoaglund FT, Riseborough EJ (eds): *Controversies in Orthopaedic Surgery*. Philadelphia, WB Saunders, 1982, pp 232–254.

15. Burdeaux BD: Reduction of calcaneal fractures by the McReynolds medial approach technique and its experimental basis. *Clin Orthop* 1983;177:87–103.

16. Burdeaux BD Jr: Fractures of the calcaneus, in Chapman MW, Madison M (eds): *Operative Orthopaedics*. Philadelphia, JB Lippincott, 1988, vol 3, pp 1723–1736.

17. Mast J, Jakob R, Ganz R: *Planning and Reduction in Fracture Surgery*. Berlin, Springer-Verlag, 1989, pp 185–192.

18. Fernandez DL: Transarticular fracture of the calcaneus: A technical note. *Arch Orthop Trauma Surg* 1984;103:195–200.

19. Gould N: Lateral approach to the os calcis. *Foot Ankle* 1984;4:218–220.

Tibial Pilon Fractures

Michael J. Brennan, MD

Introduction

Tibial pilon fractures, caused by a combination of compression and shear forces, present challenging reconstructive problems. Fractures resulting from compression forces are characterized by marked articular comminution. Shear forces tend to cause fibular, metaphyseal, and soft-tissue disruption. The degree of bony injury reflected by cortical comminution and cancellous crush to a large extent determines the prognosis and serves as the basis for the AO classification of these injuries (Fig. 1). Osteoporosis and comminution may diminish the usefulness of internal fixation.

In both open and closed injuries, the condition of the soft tissue can determine both the timing and type of intervention. I usually treat all tibial pilon fractures as if they were open, and initiate surgery early. If this is not possible, I delay open reduction and internal fixation (ORIF) until I believe the soft tissue can tolerate further trauma. Although surgical incisions are determined by the fracture pattern and the soft-tissue injury, the principles of the surgical approach are fairly constant. It is essential that the surgeon reduce the fibula to restore length, anatomically align the articular surface, anticipate a metaphyseal defect and be prepared to use autogenous bone graft, and plan both provisional and final fixation. It is also important to maintain options for wound closure, because the condition of the soft tissue may change during the course of surgery.

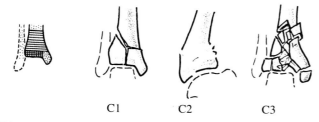

C1 ..., articular simple, metaphyseal simple
C2 ..., articular simple, metaphyseal multifragmentary
C3 ..., multifragmentary

Fig. 1 AO classification of tibial pilon fractures. Reproduced with permission from Müller ME, Nazarion S, Koch P: The AO Classification of Fractures. Springer-Verlag, Berlin, 1988.

Procedure

Incision placement, often determined by the soft-tissue injury, is generally just lateral to the tibial crest, extending along the medial border of the tibialis anterior. To maximize the anterior skin bridge, the second incision is made posterior to the fibula. Surgical intervention always increases soft-tissue trauma, but this can be minimized by operating through soft-tissue defects and between fracture fragments, avoiding excessive periosteal stripping. The use of a calcaneal traction pin and an image intensifier will help assess the effects of traction, and the restored length facilitates reduction of the fracture fragments.[1] Frequently, I accomplish this with the AO femoral retractor, connecting the threaded rod to half-pins in the tibia and calcaneus. If ORIF is selected, first fix the fibula, provisionally fix

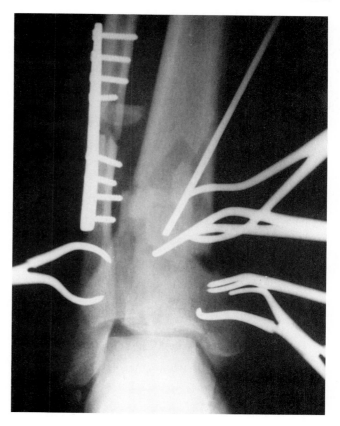

Fig. 2 Restoration of fibular length and provisional fixation of tibia.

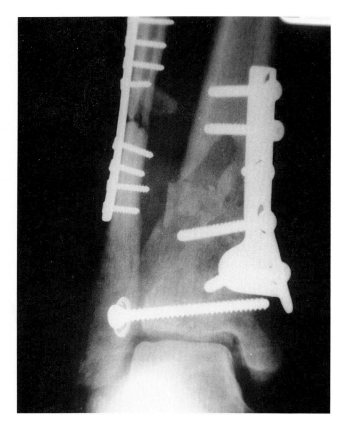

Fig. 3   Definitive fixation of tibia including the lateral tibial plafond.

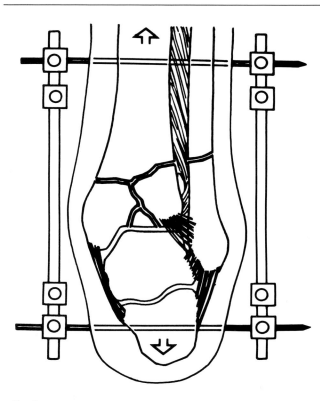

Fig. 4   Ligamentotaxis by distraction. (Reproduced with permission from Schatzker J, Tile M: *The Rationale of Operative Fracture Care.* Berlin, Springer-Verlag, 1987, p 359.)

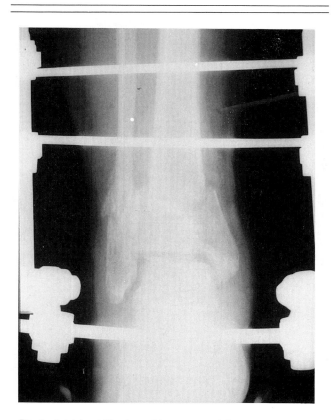

Fig. 5   Initial stabilization with an external fixator.

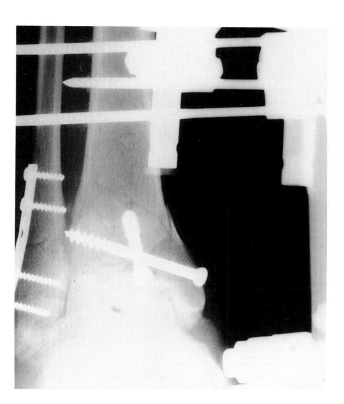

Fig. 6   Limited internal fixation of joint surface used with an external fixator.

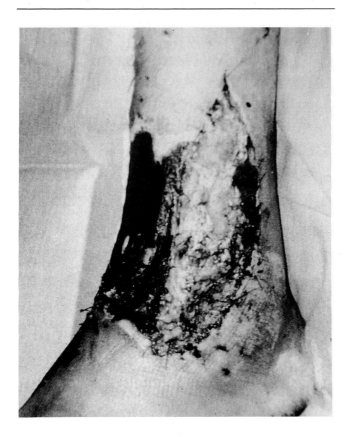

Fig. 7 Necrosis of a rotational flap.

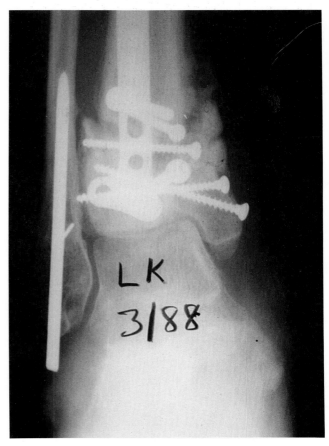

Fig. 8 Nonunion with varus angulation.

the tibia (Fig. 2), and then obtain three standard radiographs of the ankle. If alignment is satisfactory, proceed with definitive fixation and bone grafting. Realignment of the lateral plafond is important, because it restores both the articular surface and the syndesmosis (Fig. 3). Bone grafting of the metaphyseal defect is strongly recommended.

The fracture configuration determines the type of fixation used. When a pilon fracture is associated with a transverse fracture of the fibula, a Rush rod, which maintains length with little soft-tissue dissection, can be used. However, a Rush rod does not provide rigid rotational control, and an anteromedial plate is used to fix the tibia. In a C1-type fracture with the fibula intact, interfragmentary compression-screw fixation of the tibia may suffice. Screws may also be used with long, spiral fractures that extend into the joint, where a plate is impractical.

Distraction methods can be used to maintain length and facilitate the treatment of the soft-tissue injury (Fig. 4). An external fixator (Fig. 5) will stabilize or neutralize the fracture, allowing delayed, limited ORIF of the joint (Fig. 6).

Coverage is vital to the success of the operation. Even in closed injuries, closure can be difficult. I frequently close the medial tibial wound over a drain and leave the wound posterior to the fibula open with peroneal musculature exposed. I return five to seven days later for a delayed primary closure or split-thickness skin graft if tension is still a problem. Local rotation flaps should be avoided because the skin is traumatized and is highly susceptible to necrosis after rotation (Fig. 7). A small problem can become a large one. If a large soft-tissue defect exists, conservative management calls for free-tissue transfer.

Complications

These injuries are fraught with complications. The neurovascular status of the limb must be assessed carefully before surgery. A 40-year-old man sustained a shear, grade IIIC injury with devascularization of the foot. After vein-graft revascularization, he underwent ORIF. Despite initial success, the graft clotted twice during the next two weeks, and the patient ultimately chose to have a below-the-knee amputation rather than undergo another reconstructive attempt.

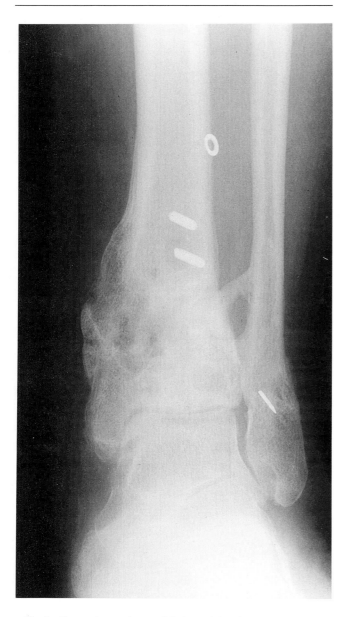

Fig. 9   Correction and consolidation achieved.

Less severe complications also occur. To facilitate detection of infection and compartment syndrome, I use a splint rather than a circumferential cast. Nonunion and malunion, which can be problems, are usually managed with bone grafting and osteotomy. The Ilizarov technique may also have a role. A 30-year-old woman, who eight months earlier had ORIF and bone grafting of a pilon fracture, was admitted with a painful nonunion, loss of fixation, and a varus malalignment (Fig. 8). The hardware was removed, and an Ilizarov frame was applied without supplemental bone graft. The frame was gradually distracted medially until correction was achieved. Once consolidation occurred (Fig. 9), the frame was removed.

All patients with pilon fracture are at risk for posttraumatic ankle arthritis. Eventually some cases will require ankle arthrodesis, and in these cases the prior ORIF should facilitate the alignment of the fusion. Primary ankle arthrodesis at the time of injury is technically demanding and has little or no advantage over late ankle arthrodesis.

Summary

The character of soft-tissue and bony injury in tibial pilon fractures varies widely, and no one treatment method is right for all. Surgery is undertaken to reduce the fibula, to restore length, to align the articular surface, to stabilize the fracture, and to obtain coverage without tension. If bone grafting is required, it should be done as early as possible. Complications, which occur frequently, must be aggressively managed.

Reference

1. Mast JW, Spiegel PG, Pappas JN: Fractures of the tibial pilon. *Clin Orthop* 1988;230:68–82.

External Fixation

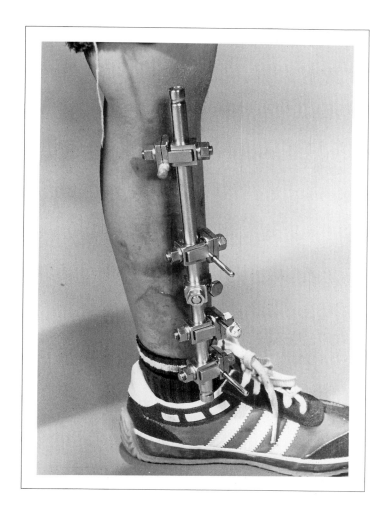

External Fixation:
Special Indications and Techniques

Fred Behrens, MD

Introduction

Since external fixation was last reviewed in *Instructional Course Lectures, XXXIII*, in 1984, our understanding of the method has increased and become more refined. The contributions in this volume examine some of these refinements, present newer indications, and explore biologic processes and devices that only recently have been introduced to surgeons in North America.

Open tibial fractures remain the principal indication for the use of external fixators. With the recognition and application of general principles for safe frame application, the complication rate for this injury has continuously decreased. Yet, as only a few orthopaedic surgeons have become truly comfortable using these devices, there is growing enthusiasm to replace unilateral fixators with intramedullary nails in grade II and possibly grade IIIA open tibial fractures. The risks and advantages of this approach are, at this time, not clear. Although external fixation of the femur has always carried a high complication rate, it remains the method of choice for grade IIIB and grade IIIC open fractures, for some infected lesions, and in the emergency management of pelvic injuries associated with ruptured internal organs or hypovolemia. Other indications are anterior and lateral compression injuries of the pelvis.

External fixation has become an increasingly valuable tool in the management of complex upper-extremity injuries, particularly for the multiply injured patient. As in the femur, fixators in the arm are often used in a staged process. They are used to provide initial stabilization and, once the general circumstances of the patient or the local soft-tissue conditions have sufficiently improved, are replaced by definitive internal fixation. Empirically, it appears that if pin tracts remain clean, a direct switch to internal fixation is possible within two to three weeks after fixator application.

After initial hesitation, orthopaedic surgeons have found that external fixators are well tolerated by children for indications other than limb-lengthening. In addition to their use in severe open fractures, external fixators have proven valuable when treating children with head injuries, unstable diaphyseal fractures, floating knees and elbows, and joint injuries with multiple ligamentous lesions.

During the past three decades, advances in fracture care that were developed in Western countries have relied heavily on metallurgically and mechanically improved implants. In eastern Europe and the Soviet Union, Ilizarov and other surgeons have achieved similar results by perfecting complex and adaptable ring fixators that allow precise manipulation of bony fragments and soft tissues through K-wires placed under tension. Ilizarov and his co-workers also have developed the concept of distraction osteogenesis, which has revolutionized the management of limb-length discrepancies, malalignments, and infected nonunions. Since hearing of these advances, many surgeons in the West have worked to learn how these devices are applied and to understand the biologic basis for distraction osteogenesis. In this volume, these efforts are well described by the contributions of Aronson and Harp and of Paley. In another chapter, Green describes some complications of ring fixators and shows us how these complications can be avoided.

More than any other method of skeletal fixation, external fixation is constantly changing as to fixator design and shape, indications, and acceptability. External-fixation devices appear to be most helpful when other methods of stabilization fail or are too risky. To apply a fixation device safely and effectively demands both an understanding of the basic clinical and mechanical principles and a creative appreciation of the device's potential.

Factors Influencing the Choice of External Fixation for Distraction Osteogenesis

James Aronson, MD

John H. Harp, Jr., BSCE

Distraction osteogenesis is a dynamic process of bone formation that is clinically controlled by an external fixator.[1,2] The resurgence of interest in fracture healing with dynamic external fixation[3-7] and the development of more versatile devices have catalyzed the acceptance of this approach to handling difficult problems of bone deficiency.

Clinically, distraction osteogenesis has expanded the indications for and improved the results of traditional bone-lengthening techniques.[8,9] Distraction osteogenesis has improved results in complicated problems of nonunion, pseudarthrosis, and chronic osteomyelitis.[10] Perhaps most notably, distraction osteogenesis permits bone transportation[11] as a new method to restore major intercalary defects in bone without requiring bone grafts. Distraction osteogenesis also provides an excellent experimental model for the study of mineralization[12-15] and neogenesis of soft tissues, such as nerves and muscles.[16] Drawing from our clinical experience (16 limb lengthenings) and experimental studies (30 dogs), we have outlined some of the factors involved in the process of distraction osteogenesis.

Biology of Distraction Osteogenesis

Our work[1,13,15] closely parallels the findings of Ilizarov and associates,[2,8,10,14,16-18] that distraction osteogenesis proceeds by direct intramembranous ossification. Histologically, the process is similar to that seen beneath the periosteum attached to the ring of Lacroix[19] at a rapidly growing physis (J. Aronson, unpublished data). In both cases, a fibrovascular lattice uniformly spans two bone ends undergoing distraction.[1] In bone growth, the process is controlled by the growth rates of the physes at each end of the bone while, in distraction osteogenesis, the rate of lengthening is controlled mechanically by the external fixator.

The ideal rate of distraction is 1 mm per day, preferably divided into at least four equal increments.[1,2,8,11,13,14,16,17] Depending on such factors as the age of the patient, the location within the bone (metaphysis vs diaphysis) and the local vascularity, the distraction rate ranges from 0.5 to 2.0 mm per day.[1,2,11] Intrinsic biologic distraction rates, estimated from the work of Anderson and associates[20] on femoral and tibial growth, are in the range of 0.05 to 0.2 mm per day.

Because bone is intrinsically stable during load-bearing, the surrounding periosteal intramembranous os-sification is most likely shielded from shearing forces by a dampening effect. At the same time, it is subjected to a gradually increasing tension force exerted by the expanding physis. An external fixator plays a similar role, providing stability for the bone ends while simultaneously exerting controlled strain at the site of osteogenesis.

Before exploring the role of external fixation in distraction osteogenesis, it is important to understand the technique and biologic implications of corticotomy, the special method of bone separation used to enhance local osteogenesis. Ilizarov and associates[2,14,17] strongly emphasized avoiding damage to local vessels and bone tissue during the operation. Through a longitudinal, 1-cm incision, a slightly smaller osteotome is pushed through periosteum to bone and rotated 90 degrees. When the osteotome is carefully directed, only the cortex is cut and the periosteal and endosteal vessels are preserved. Slow twisting of the osteotome and the bone ends fractures the remaining cortex on the contralateral surface with minimal displacement of the bone and surrounding tissues. The goal of this low-energy corticotomy is to minimize damage to local vessels and osteocytes and to keep the periosteal sleeve and internal medullary spongiosa intact. In practice, more than just cortex is cut or fractured, but, with the minimal trauma, tissue integrity can be restored quickly by maintaining the bone surfaces in proximity (less than 1 mm of distraction) with an external fixator for a few days. As normal fracture healing ensues, a fibrovascular network of soft tissue soon bridges the ends. This period of latency may vary from one to ten days depending on local damage, the age of the patient, and the location within the bone. Under normal conditions the recommended period of latency before initiating distraction is four days.[2,8]

The biomechanical implications of a biologically active interface, referred to as the fibrous interzone,[1] between the cut surfaces of bone are significant. Actual distraction of the bone ends must overcome the ultimate tensile strength of the interface unless biologic growth alone can add the necessary length. The force required to lengthen a tibia has been measured in the range of 10 to 15 kg.[21] Along with the biologic interface, skin, muscles, nerves, and vasculature must also contribute resistance to distraction. Understanding the relative contribution of each becomes a complex problem. The combined effect, however, is to place various strains on the external fixator. Load transfer from the

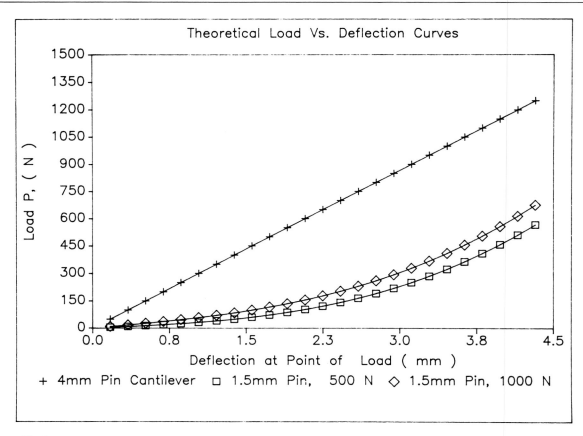

Fig. 1 Theoretical load vs deflection curves.

external fixator to the site of osteogenesis determines the success of distraction osteogenesis, but failure to withstand strains contributed by these other forces may lead to failure of the device itself.

Biomechanical Factors

There are two major variables in external fixator-bone constructs: the pins and the frame itself. Self-tensioning wires (small-diameter full pins used in the Ilizarov device) deserve special attention because they behave differently from the commonly used cantilever pins (large-diameter half pins used in the Wagner and Orthofix devices).

The characteristic rigidity of most frames has already been established under conditions of axial loading, bending, and torsion of an externally fixed test member with and without a gap.[22-28] Most test results were derived by either compression or tension loading of the limb, but no testing had been done using resistance material to bridge the gap (simulating the biologic interface or fibrous interzone). We have employed finite-element analysis to explain some of the failures that were observed experimentally in these frames under

the constant strain of distraction across a fibrous interzone.

The load-deflection behavior of a cantilever pin and a tensioned wire can be modeled with simple mathematical equations. For a tension wire, the slope of the load deflection curve is constantly increasing as the load and deflection increase, while for a cantilever pin the slope is constant. As shown in Figure 1, load deflection for a pin 4 mm in diameter loaded in cantilever is linear from 0 to 4.5 mm of deflection, for loads up to 1,200 N. The smaller-diameter pins (1.5-mm Kirschner wires) loaded at the midpoint between rigidly fixed ends demonstrate nonlinear behavior. Pretensioning the wire between 500 N and 1,000 N shows little variation for 4 mm of deflection and up to a load of 600 N. Because the slope of these two curves is constantly rising, the tensioned wires are considered nonlinear, self-stiffening pins. At approximately 4 mm of deflection, the actual rigidity, or the slope of the curve, for tensioned wires actually exceeds that of the cantilever pin. Deflection at the free end of the cantilever pin is calculated by

$$\frac{PL^3}{3EI}$$

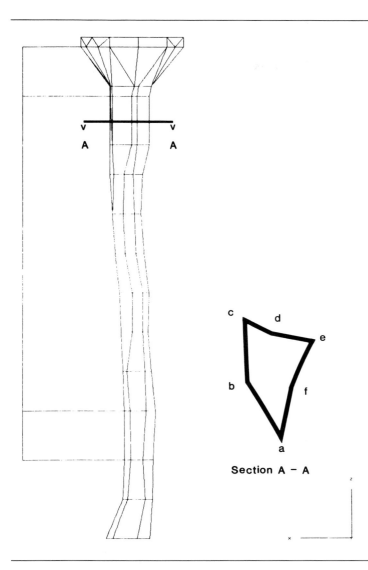

Section A – A

Fig. 2 Finite-element model of externally fixed tibia. The cross section A-A is taken from the proximal metaphyseal-diaphyseal junction, corresponding to the experimental level of corticotomy for distraction osteogenesis. Loads (a to f) are graphically represented in Figure 3. The medial side of the tibia is represented by b, the lateral side by f, and the posterior side by d, while a represents the anterior tibial tuberosity.

where P = applied load at the free end, L = cantilever length, E = modulus of elasticity, and I = moment of inertia.[29] The load on the tensioned wire is equal to:

$$2AE\left[\frac{2Z}{L}\right]\left[\frac{L}{S_o} - \frac{1}{\sqrt{1+(2Z/L)^2}}\right]$$

In this equation, A = the cross-sectional area of the wire, E = the modulus of elasticity, Z = the deflection at the midpoint, L = the distance between supports, and S_o = the unstressed wire length.[30]

The gradually increasing rigidity of self-stiffening wires may enhance osteogenesis by providing a higher level of compatibility with the viscoelastic properties[21] of the fibrous interzone. Experimental evidence indicates that osteogenesis is inhibited by sudden, extreme distractions and is optimized under gradually increasing distraction.[1,12,13,31]

A finite-element analysis was performed to demonstrate the mechanical behavior of a typical unilateral external fixator (Wagner device with 4-mm Schanz pins) during distraction osteogenesis. The finite-element analysis computer program and the processors were used to generate the finite-element models and to analyze the results. The geometric configurations of the bone were obtained from a series of computed tomographic scans of a canine tibia (Fig. 2). The material values used for this analysis were taken from previously published finite-element analyses.[32] The Young's modulus and Poisson's ratio used were 207,000 and 0.30 respectively for the 4-mm steel pin, 18,500 and 0.30 for the 2-mm-thick cortical bone, and 6 and 0.47 for the 4-mm-thick callus. Soft tissue, such as muscle, was not modeled. The load condition used was 1 mm of distraction along the axis of the fixator. The two most proximal pins were located in the coronal plane of the proximal metaphysis. The rigid, telescoping body was fixed to the pins 25 mm from the medial cortex. The fixator was then inclined in the parasagittal plane

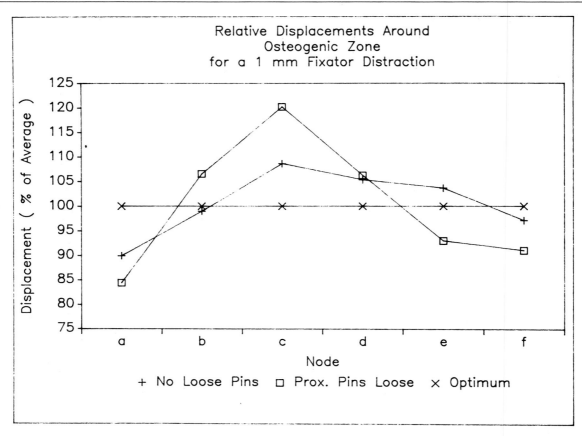

Fig. 3 Relative axial displacement at the osteogenic zone for 1-mm fixator distraction. The optimum condition (1), shown by a horizontal line at 100%, indicates that for 1 mm of fixator distraction, the osteogenic zone will displace 1 mm. In condition 2 with no loose pins (all rigidly fixed), loads c, d, and e exceed the optimum, while a and f are less than optimum. This pattern is exaggerated with loosening of the proximal pins (condition 3). This finite-element analysis indicates that distraction would be asymmetric, tending to valgus and extension deformity.

l.5 degrees posteriorly. This allowed the two most distal pins to be placed in the midcoronal plane of the distal diaphysis.

In the primary analysis with all pins rigidly fixed (no loose pins), the average displacement across the osteogenic zone during a 1-mm distraction of the external fixator was 0.79 mm. This model also indicated stress concentrations at the bone-pin interfaces of the proximal set of pins, which correlated to the location of pin loosening observed during some of the canine experiments. Therefore, a second finite-element analysis was performed modeling proximal pin loosening. With the two proximal pins loose, the average displacement across the osteogenic zone for 1 mm of distraction of the external fixator was 0.62 mm.

Relative displacement of different points within the osteogenic zone (transverse, cross section AA, Fig. 2) is graphically compared for three conditions (Fig. 3). Optimum strain (condition 1) would be a uniform displacement across the entire osteogenic zone, as represented by the horizontal line at the 100% level (Fig.

3). Within the coronal plane, medial displacements (b,c) exceed lateral displacements (e,f), creating the valgus deformity observed experimentally (Fig. 4). This asymmetric strain is attributed to bending moments about rigidly fixed cantilever pins (condition 2) and is accentuated by loosening of the proximal pins (condition 3). In the sagittal plane, the modeled bone rotated into extension with posterior displacements exceeding anterior ones. Our experimental experience has demonstrated the opposite tendency, into a flexion deformity. We speculate that the soft-tissue forces (primarily muscle) play an important role in loading the tibia during distraction. In this case, the strong posterior calf muscles exploit the delicate flexion-extension balance, causing the flexion deformity.

This finite-element analysis indicated that the actual displacement at the osteogenic zone can vary from the distraction applied by the external fixator. Rotations in both the coronal (varus-valgus) and sagittal (flexion-extension) planes resulted in uneven distribution of strain in the osteogenic tissue.[33] Pin loosening accentuates the

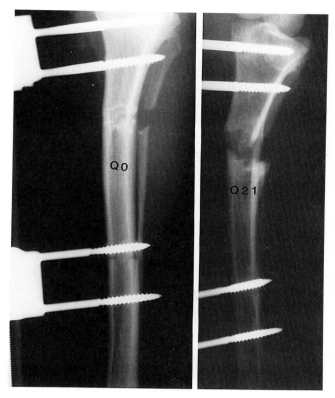

Fig. 4 Experimental distraction osteogenesis with cantilever pins. The left side of the figure demonstrates the position of 4-mm Schanz pins, Wagner external fixator, and the adult canine tibia immediately after a proximal metaphyseal corticotomy. On the right, the same bone after 14 mm of distraction (day 21 of the experiment), demonstrating angulation into valgus. In this case the pin clamps rotated under the forces induced by distraction osteogenesis.

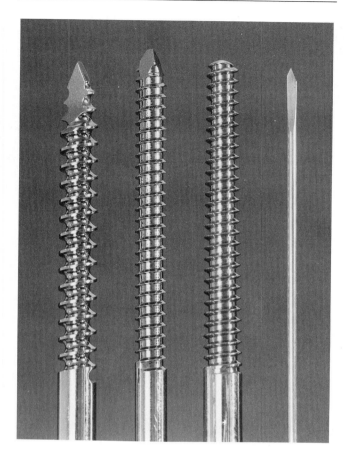

Fig. 5 Four types of pins. **Left to right,** The Schanz pin is used with the standard Wagner external fixator with a sharp trochar tip and thick threads, the AO pin with blunted tip is used with either AO or Wagner external fixators, the conical pin with rounded tip and cortical taper from 8 to 5 mm is used with the Orthofix device, and the smaller K-wire 1.5 mm in diameter with a bayonet tip is used with the Ilizarov device.

asymmetric strain profile resulting from half-pin fixation during distraction osteogenesis. Our experiments indicate that excessive strain and local instability may inhibit osteogenesis (J. Aronson, unpublished data).

Clinical Factors

The two major considerations in using external fixation systems are adaptability and user-friendliness for both the physician and patient. Adaptability implies that the frame can be universally and fully applied to any deformity for the desired correction. Pins must be easy to place; must avoid nerves, vasculature, growth plates, and joints; and should be well-tolerated by the patient. User-friendliness implies that the pins and frame can easily be applied within a reasonable time by the surgeon, and that the patient will have little difficulty performing such functions as pin care, distraction, exercises, and daily activities.

Most of these considerations are highly subjective, and we will use anecdotal experience to describe prac-

tical differences between the systems. First, we would like to divide the systems into half-pin and full-pin types.

Pin Types

Both the Wagner and Orthofix systems types use half pins (Fig. 5). Half pins are adaptable and easy to use. Insertion points into the bone can be found easily and safely because the soft tissues are penetrated on only one side. These pins are usually predrilled and then placed with hand chucks, requiring two maneuvers. Generally, because half-pin systems use fewer pins, there are fewer sites to clean, fewer sites to become infected, and fewer sites to impinge on soft tissues.

The Orthofix system has special drill guides that guide pin placement, providing an extra measure of safety against twirling a nerve or vessel into the threads. The Orthofix pins are blunted at the tip to avoid cutting structures on the opposite side of the bone. They are

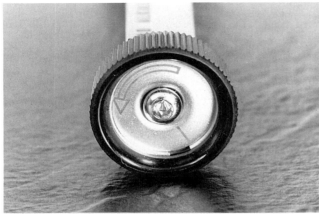

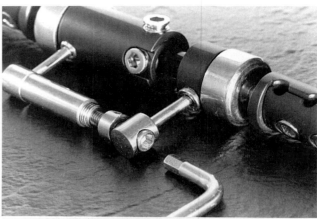

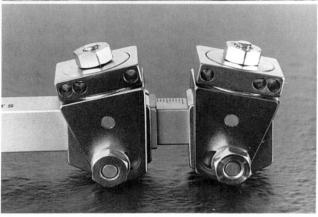

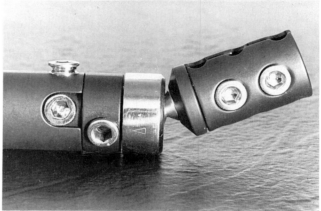

Fig. 6 Wagner external fixator. **Top,** The large plastic handle at the end of the device is quite handy for ease of turning with the direction clearly marked. **Bottom,** The pin clamps are maximally rotated within slotted hinges. The telescoping portion has clearly marked calibrations. Two potential pin spreads are available in each clamp, held by friction fit nuts and washers. The head of the pin clamp also can rotate circumferentially within grooved lock washers held by the nut over the pins. The pin clamp on the left can slide up and down the telescoping shaft for initial length adjustments, while the pin clamp at the end is rigidly fixed.

Fig. 7 Orthofix external fixator. **Top,** The fixator shows the outboard distraction-compression device that must be inserted into the fixator and the hexagonal Allen wrench used for turning. The telescoping body is driven by this outboard device. Set screws in the telescoping body allow for axial dynamization. The pin clamps, which provide three to five pin slots depending on the size of fixator used, are held in the clamp by friction from two hexagonal bolts. **Bottom,** The pin clamp can rotate 360 degrees by virtue of a ball joint but can only angulate approximately 25 degrees on the axis of the telescoping body.

designed with a special tapered thread to allow retightening if the pin becomes loose within the bone. This feature, which is helpful in cases of fracture healing, becomes risky during distraction osteogenesis because it requires loosening the pin clamp to advance an individual pin. All pins in that clamp then become loose, and the tension across the fibrous interzone is lost, resulting in loss of bony alignment. The taper also necessitates a longer thread length, which is more susceptible to plastic deformation under cantilever loads.

The full pins used by Ilizarov are actually K-wires. Because these wires must be attached to the fixator ring on both sides to achieve enough internal tension to become relatively rigid,[29] each wire must enter and exit the soft tissues on either side of a bone. Therefore, fewer portals of entry, as compared with half pins, are available to the surgeon because vascular and neuro-

logic anatomy must be considered on both sides of the bone. Drilling of these wires is a bit more difficult and time-consuming, even though predrilling and drill guides are not necessary. Special techniques for insertion are suggested by Ilizarov to avoid soft-tissue impingement. The wires are pushed or hammered through soft tissues and are drilled only across the bone, using a low RPM setting. To minimize pain during the lengthening, the skin must be positioned with no tension. The muscles, too, must be stretched appropriately as the wire passes through each side of the bone in order to allow for full excursion of adjacent joints. A single wire may require several passes to find its ideal position.

Compared with the half-pin devices, many more wires are required to stabilize a given bone by full-pin techniques, thereby theoretically increasing the potential

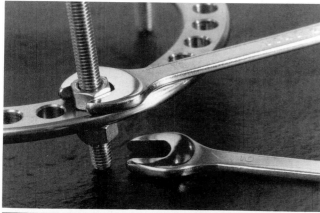

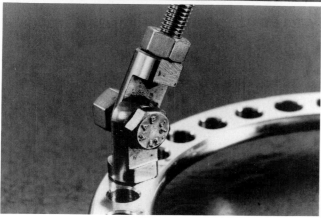

Fig. 8 Ilizarov external fixator. **Top**, Two open-end 10-mm wrenches are necessary to distract or compress the threaded rods. The lock nut is first loosened and then the driving nut is advanced. The nuts must be marked to keep track of direction and degree of rotation. One full rotation is equal to 1 mm of axial change. **Bottom**, Hinges are constructed and connected to threaded rods. Hinge rotation of more than 90 degrees is possible, but may be limited by local anatomy. Two hinges can be placed in series to create a universal joint. The base of the hinge may be rotated 360 degrees. Hinges may be located at any position circumferentially in the ring around the limb.

for soft-tissue impingement and infection. However, the smaller-diameter (1.5 to 1.8 mm) wire is much better tolerated by the patient than a larger-diameter (4 to 6 mm) half pin. If properly placed, the wires seem to allow fuller joint motion and certainly result in fewer skin problems than do the half pins.

It is postulated that smaller-diameter, smooth wires can pass through soft tissues more safely than can the larger-diameter trocars, drill guides, and threaded pins. We have found that the wires are also safer and easier to place near joints and physes (through the epiphyses, if necessary), and that they are much better tolerated by the patient than the larger-diameter half pins. Pin care of the wires seems easier even though more sites must be cleaned. The scars from the wires are much less noticeable.

To summarize the comparison between pin types, the learning curve for proper placement of Ilizarov wires is steeper, but adaptability for the surgeon, user-friendliness for the patient, and the system's usefulness in dealing with certain difficult problems make the technique worth learning.

Frames

The frames fall into two basic categories: the preassembled, rigid-body type, and the modular ring type. Both the Wagner and Orthofix devices are factory-made and have rigid, telescoping bodies for unilateral placement with large-diameter half pins. The Ilizarov device, a totally modular system of partial and complete rings, must be designed and assembled by the surgeon. There is no question that the former type is initially easier for the surgeon to use, but that the latter is more adaptable.

The Wagner device has a long tradition of reliability.[30] Its large plastic handle and large-diameter worm gear allow the patient to turn the distractor more easily in this fixator than in any other (Fig. 6). No wrench is needed, the handle is part of the device and is readily accessible, and the calibrations are clearly marked. When all parts are rigidly applied, the mechanical axis of distraction is parallel to the telescopic portion. The device also strictly limits pin spread and angulation. As discussed above, however, any slippage in the pin connections will lead to bending moments across the distraction site, introducing uncontrolled strains. Angular corrections must be performed manually and necessitate loosening the pin clamps. Even with the patient under general anesthesia, the tension forces in the distraction zone make such a change a formidable task. This device is most appropriate for simple diaphyseal lengthenings of modest proportion without major angular or rotational corrections.

The Orthofix device resembles the Wagner in that pin spread is limited to the channels in each head. Potential angulation between pin clamps is increased by virtue of ball joints that connect the pin clamp to the main body (Fig. 7). Some rotational correction is possible but, because the rotational axis is about the frame itself rather than the bone, some displacement of the bone ends will occur with this maneuver. Distraction is a bit more difficult because two extra parts, the outboard distractor and the large Allen wrench, are required. The threads of the distractor are smaller in diameter than the Wagner worm gear, making turning more difficult even when using the longer lever arm of the Allen wrench. The calibrations are scored into the telescoping member but are difficult to read. Even with the friction-fit cams torqued to factory recommendations, the ball joints have been known to slip under the high cantilever loads of distraction osteogenesis.[23] A special Orthofix device that has no ball joints and more closely resembles the Wagner device is therefore rec-

Table 1
Postoperative control of distraction osteogenesis

Correction Mode	External Fixator		
	Wagner*	Orthofix*	Ilizarov*
Distraction or compression	Mechanical, 0 to 15 cm (screw)	Mechanical, 0 to 8 cm (screw or friction telescope)	Mechanical, unlimited (screw or friction telescope)
Varus or valgus* or flexion or extension*	Manual, 0 to 45 degrees (grooved lock washers, sliding hinge)	Manual, 0 to 45 degrees (universal ball joint)	Mechanical, 0 to 90 degrees (universal hinge joint)
Rotation	None (initial pin placement)	Manual, 0 to 20 degrees, eccentric (depends on pin length and bone diameter)	Mechanical, 360 degrees, concentric

*Pins are assumed to be in coronal plane.

ommended for lengthening. Special transverse heads are available to allow pin placement into the epiphysis for physeal and metaphyseal lengthenings. Unfortunately, the large-diameter pins are not well tolerated near joints. In our experience, persistent synovial fluid leaks, with reduced motion, have occurred near the knee. The standard device, which lengthens up to 4 cm, must be exchanged for the long body during a lengthening to allow up to an additional 8 cm of extension. A femur that displaced into varus and extension during one such exchange procedure proved very difficult to correct, even with the patient under general anesthesia. The angular and rotational modularity of this system is all manual. There is no potential for gradual angular correction during a lengthening.

Once the techniques of application, which include using a template, pin and drill guides, and different head types, are mastered, the Orthofix device has many advantages over its more rigid predecessor, the Wagner device. Pin spread within the standard pin clamp is greater because the clamp has five potential slots rather than the three available on the Wagner device. The ball joints allow some initial rotational correction, as well as angular mobility in multiple planes, an advantage over the two perpendicular planes allowed by the Wagner. Following a lengthening, the Orthofix system can easily be transformed into a dynamic load-sharing device (semicontrolled) by removing the outboard distractor and loosening one set screw. The Wagner has very little load-sharing capability. Finally, the cone-shaped threads on the Orthofix pins are easy to remove, and doing so requires no anesthesia. The Wagner and the Orthofix devices, however, both lack any mechanism for correcting angulation or rotation during lengthening. With these devices, angular and rotational corrections must be made manually with much difficulty and at high risk of losing control under the great tension forces exerted by distraction osteogenesis.

The Ilizarov device is clearly the most modular and universal of external fixators. Circumferential rings, which can be constructed as full or partial circles, allow for circumferential and multiplanar pin placement. Pin spread is unlimited, as either posts or additional rings can be added. The rings can be connected by relatively rigid threaded rods or by threaded rods within telescoping units that increase rigidity and allow for axial dynamization. Rings can also be connected by threaded rods that are hinged in one or more planes (Fig. 8). By appropriate placement of these hinges with a fulcrum effect, angulatory changes can be induced mechanically during distraction osteogenesis.

By special modifications of different diameter rings and threaded rods, mechanical rotational changes can also be induced during distraction osteogenesis. Additional support rods can be added during distraction osteogenesis, which means that longer threaded rods can be individually replaced as needed, allowing indefinite lengthening without loss of stability.

The Ilizarov device must be assembled by the surgeon, and adapting the frame for each situation takes significant time and planning. The frame is also bulky and has wire tips that may catch on clothing. Depending on how extensive a frame is required, the overall weight may exceed that of the half-pin devices. Also, the appearance of the Ilizarov device is not as appealing as the more sleek half-pin designs.

Despite any drawbacks, the Ilizarov device is, without question, the most adaptable of all the external fixation systems. It is not initially easy to use by the surgeon, who must plan and construct an individualized external fixator. During distraction osteogenesis, however, it is the easiest device to use, in that any three-dimensional change, including translation, can be accomplished mechanically, gradually, and with minimal pain to the patient (Table 1).

References

1. Aronson J, Harrison BH, Stewart CL, et al: The histology of distraction osteogenesis using different external fixators. *Clin Orthop* 1989;241:106–116.
2. Ilizarov GA: The significance of the combination of optimum mechanical and biological factors in the regenerative process of transosseous osteosynthesis, in Bianchi-Maiocchi A (ed): *Abstracts of the First International Symposium on Experimental, Theoretical and Clinical Aspects of Transosseous Osteosynthesis in the Method Developed in Kurgan Scientific Research Institute.* Milan, Medi Surgical Video, 1984, p 1.
3. De Bastiani G, Aldegheri R, Renzi Brivio L: The treatment of fractures with a dynamic axial fixator. *J Bone Joint Surg* 1984; 66B:538–545.
4. Goodship AE, Kenwright J: The influence of induced micro-movement upon the healing of experimental tibial fractures. *J Bone Joint Surg* 1985;67B:650–655.
5. Goodship A, Walker P, James S, et al: Modulation of fracture healing by applied mechanical stimulation, abstract. *J Bone Joint Surg* 1988;70B:849.
6. Rubin CT, Lanyon LE: Regulation of bone formation by applied dynamic loads. *J Bone Joint Surg* 1984;66A:397–402.
7. Wu JJ, Shyr HS, Chao EY, et al: Comparison of osteotomy healing under external fixation devices with different stiffness characteristics. *J Bone Joint Surg* 1984;66A:1258–1264.
8. Ilizarov GA, Deviatov AA: Operativnoe udlinenie goleni [Surgical elongation of the leg]. *Ortop Travmatol Protez* 1971;32:20–25.
9. Paley D: Current techniques of limb lengthening. *J Pediatr Orthop* 1988;8:73–92.
10. Ilizarov GA: Basic principles of transosseous compression and distraction osteosynthesis [English abstract]. *Ortop Travmatol Protez* 1975;10:7–15.
11. Aronson J, Johnson E, Harp JH: Local bone transportation for treatment of intercalary defects by the Ilizarov technique: Biomechanical and clinical considerations. *Clin Orthop* 1989;243:71–79.
12. Aronson J, Harrison B: Mechanical induction of osteogenesis by distraction of a metaphyseal osteotomy in long bones. *Trans Orthop Res Soc* 1987;12:180.
13. Aronson J, Harrison B, Boyd CM, et al: Mechanical induction of osteogenesis: Preliminary studies. *Ann Clin Lab Sci* 1988;18:195–203.
14. Ilizarov GA, Lediaev VI, Shitin VP: Techenie reparativnoĭ regeneratsii kompaktnoĭ kosti pri distraktsionnom osteosinteze v razlichnykh usloviiakh fiksatsii kostnykh otlomkov (éksperimental'noe noe issledovanie). *Eksp Khir Anest* 1969;14:3–12.
15. Aronson J, Good B, Stewart C, et al: Preliminary studies of mineralization during distraction osteogenesis. *Clin Orthop*, in press.
16. Sidorenkov OK, Lebedintsev YA: Comparative evaluation of clinical, radiological, vasographic, morphological and biochemical findings in the process of moderate and accelerated experimental bone fragment distraction of the tibia using the Ilizarov apparatus, in Bianchi-Maiocchi A (ed): *Abstracts of the First International Symposium on Experimental, Theoretical and Clinical Aspects of Transosseous Osteosynthesis in the Method Developed in Kurgan Scientific Research Institute.* Milan, Medi Surgical Video, 1984, p 9.
17. Ilizarov GA, Schreinen AA, Imerlishvili IA, et al: On the problem of improving osteogenesis conditions in limb lengthening, in Bianchi-Maiocchi A (ed): *Abstracts of the First International Symposium on Experimental, Theoretical and Clinical Aspects of Transosseous Osteosynthesis in the Method Developed in Kurgan Scientific Research Institute.* Milan, Medi Surgical Video, 1984, p 4.
18. Villa A: Le rigenerazioni dei tessuti secondo GA Ilizarov, in Bianchi-Maiocchi A (ed): *Introduzione alla conoscenza delle metodichi di Ilizarov in ortopedia e traumatologia.* Milan, Medi Surgical Video, 1983, p 217.
19. Lacroix P: *The Organization of Bones.* Philadelphia, Blakiston Co, 1951, p 61.
20. Anderson M, Green WT, Messner MB: Growth and predictions of growth in the lower extremities. *J Bone Joint Surg* 1963;45A:1–14.
21. Leong JC, Ma RY, Clark JA, et al: Viscoelastic behavior of tissue in leg lengthening by distraction. *Clin Orthop* 1979;139:102–109.
22. Behrens F, Johnson WD, Koch TW, et al: Bending stiffness of unilateral and bilateral fixator frames. *Clin Orthop* 1978;178:103–110.
23. Chao EY, Hein TJ: Mechanical performance of the standard Orthofix external fixator. *Orthopedics* 1988;11:1057–1069.
24. Chao EY, Kasman RA, An KN: Rigidity and stress analyses of external fracture fixation devices: A theoretical approach. *J Biomech* 1982;15:971–983.
25. Gasser B, Wyder D, Schneider E: Comparative investigation on the biomechanical properties of the circular and other three-dimensional external fixators, in Bergmann G, Kölbel R, Rohlmann A (eds): *Biomechanics: Basic and Applied Research. Selected Proceedings of the Fifth Meeting of the European Society of Biomechanics, September 8–10, 1986, Berlin, FRG.* Dordrecht, The Netherlands, Martinus Nijhoff, 1987, pp 429–434.
26. Karaharju EO, Aalto K: The deformation of external fixation devices during loading. *Int Orthop* 1983;7:179–183.
27. McCoy MT, Chao EY, Kasman RA: Comparison of mechanical performance in four types of external fixators. *Clin Orthop* 1983;180:23–33.
28. Paley D, Fleming B, Pope M, et al: A comparative study of fracture gap motion and shear in external fixation. Presented at the Meeting on Advances in External Fixation, Riva del Garda, Italy, Sept 28–30, 1986.
29. Wagner H: Operative lengthening of the femur. *Clin Orthop* 1978;136:125–142.
30. Higdon A, Ohlsen EH, Stiles WB, et al: *Mechanics of Materials.* New York, John Wiley & Sons, 1967, p 570.
31. Aronson J, Harrison B, Boyd CM, et al: Mechanical induction of osteogenesis: The importance of pin rigidity. *J Pediatr Orthop* 1988;8:396–401.
32. Leonard JW: *Tension Structures.* New York, McGraw Hill, 1988, p 20.
33. Carter DR, Blenman PR, Beaupré GS: Correlations between mechanical stress history and tissue differentiation in initial fracture healing. *J Orthop Res* 1988;6:736–748.

Treatment of Tibial Nonunion and Bone Loss With the Ilizarov Technique

Dror Paley, MD

The Ilizarov apparatus for the fixation of fractures[1] was developed by Gavriil Abramovich Ilizarov in Kurgan, Western Siberia, USSR, in 1951. Using the modular-construction capability of this innovative device, Ilizarov was able to develop new orthopaedic methods to deal with a number of different skeletal problems.[2] His greatest contribution, however, was pioneering the science of bone and soft-tissue regeneration under tensile forces. He calls this the "theory of tension stress."[3-5] The methods he uses to treat nonunions and bone defects are based on these biologic principles.

The Apparatus

The Ilizarov apparatus, shown in Figure 1, is a circular external fixator that uses 1.5- or 1.8-mm smooth Kirschner wires for fixation to bone. The wires pierce the bone in multiple directions and multiple planes and cross within the bone.[6] The ends of the wires are attached to the metal rings of the apparatus with special bolts. The wires are placed under 80 to 130 kg of tension, which stiffens them, giving the construct its stability. Some special wires, called olive wires or stopper wires, have a bead on them. These beaded wires can be used to lock in bone fragments, thereby increasing fixation stability (static olive), or they can be used to displace and reduce a bone fragment (dynamic olive).

The Ilizarov apparatus is modular and has numerous parts. These include special hinges for deformity correction, posts used to suspend wires that are not fastened to the rings, threaded rods used for distraction or compression, compression plates, threaded sockets, bushings, bolts, and nuts. Once fixation to bone is achieved with the appropriate construct, three-dimensional corrections can be performed, including manipulations of length, rotation, angulation, and translation.

Although the wires used in the Ilizarov apparatus pass through skin, muscle, and bone, they are generally free of the problems experienced with the transfixion pins of the quadrilateral Hoffmann frame.[7] This is probably because they are smaller in diameter and do not cluster in one plane. In addition, the technique of inserting the pin while the muscle is placed in a stretched position avoids restricting the passive range of joint motion.

Biology of Distraction Histogenesis

Reports on limb lengtheners since 1905[8] have stated that bone can regenerate between two bone ends that are distracted apart (Fig. 2). Bone regeneration was thought to be an unreliable phenomena that occurred only in young children. Even today, many surgeons rely on the method of Wagner, which uses bone grafting and plating of the distraction gap to resolve bone-gap problems.[9]

Ilizarov showed that distraction osteogenesis can be reliably produced and consists of membranous bone formation without having an enchondral intermediary.[4,5] The fibrous-like interzone that forms in the distraction gap between longitudinally oriented new trabeculae is seen radiographically as a lucent line with longitudinal trabeculae radiating from it towards the opposite cortices.[10] Histologic examination reveals that the interzone is a region of undifferentiated mesenchymal spindle-shaped cells, which under appropriate conditions differentiate into osteoblasts and form parallel columns of trabeculae.[4,5] In this way the interzone acts as a pseudo growth plate. To optimize this new bone formation while lengthening the limb, the following conditions should be satisfied[4,5,11-13]: (1) stable fixation; (2) osteotomy by corticotomy (a percutaneous subperiosteal cutting of the bony cortex while sparing the periosteal and endosteal tissues); (3) metaphyseal rather than diaphyseal level for the corticotomy; (4) no initial diastasis between bone ends; (5) a seven- to 14-day latency period after corticotomy before initiating distraction; and (6) a controlled rate and rhythm of distraction, usually 0.25 mm four times each day, giving a distraction rate total of 1 mm per day.

Treatment Considerations in Nonunions

The word nonunion is misleading because it conjures up an image of a bone whose only problem is a lack of union. Common associated problems include deformity, shortening, bone defects, and infection. It is also important to consider the type of nonunion. The two basic types are hypertrophic and atrophic.[14] These are further divided into infected and noninfected. Another useful consideration is whether the nonunion is stiff or lax. In stiff, or stable, nonunions the gap contains fibrocartilage or dense fibrous tissue, which has the ability to ossify. Lax, or unstable, nonunions have either

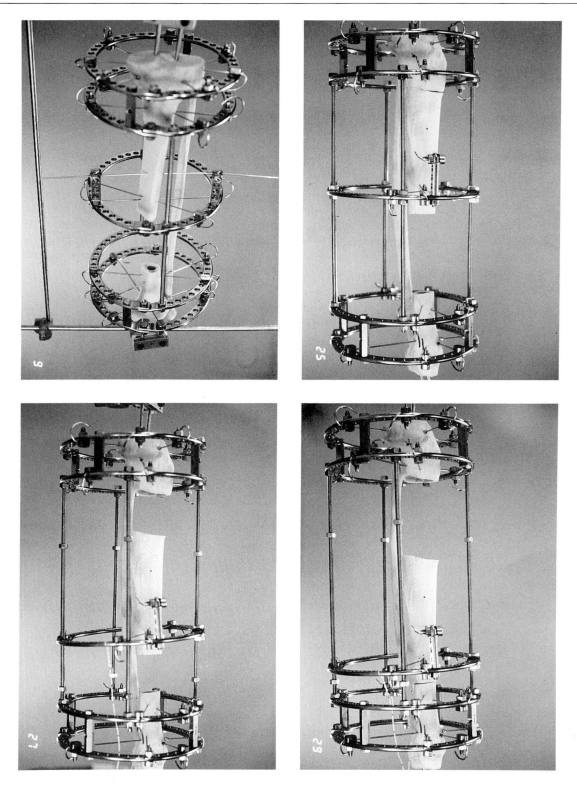

Fig. 1 **Top left**, Ilizarov apparatus for bone transport applied to tibial bone defect model (anteroposterior view). **Top right**, Lateral view of bone transport immediately after corticotomy of proximal tibia. **Bottom left**, Transport of the segment halfway across the bone defect, as seen. **Bottom right**, Bone transport across the bone defect is complete and compression is applied to the distal nonunion.

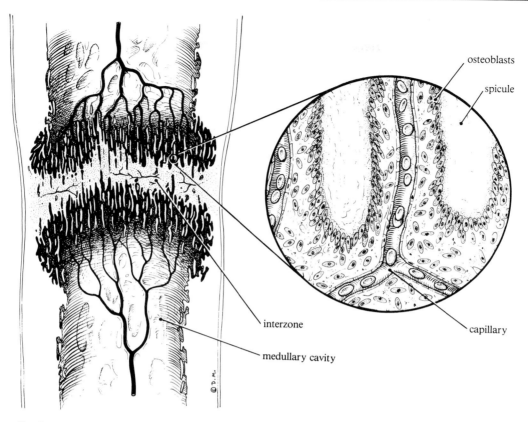

Fig. 2 During distraction the interzone is the site of longitudinal growth of the trabeculae. In comparison to the richly hypervascular trabeculated regions on either side, the interzone is relatively hypovascular and, thus, sensitive to changes in distraction rate. Between each pair of bony trabeculae is found a vascular channel. The appearance is that of cascades of bone and vessels. The osteoblasts seen around the tips of the trabeculae seem to be generated from the cells of the interzone. There is no cartilaginous intermediary between the interzonal cells and these osteoblasts. This process is, therefore, considered to be intramembranous bone formation rather than enchondral.

less dense fibrous tissue or a true synovial space connecting the bone ends. This tissue will rarely ossify.[15-17]

Other factors must also be evaluated in each individual case, for example, whether the medullary cavity is open or closed; whether osteoporosis, sclerosis, or osteonecrosis is present; and whether the fibula is intact. The relative displacement of the bone ends, the status of the surrounding soft tissues, the presence of current or preexisting infection, the circulatory and neurologic status of the limb, the shape of the bone ends, the location in the bone, the specific bone involved, and the presence of shortening must also be considered. An analysis of these and other factors, together with such specific factors as the patient's general health, age, ability to comply, and other socioeconomic factors, allows the surgeon to plan an individual treatment for each case.

The following discussion therefore presents only general guidelines for treatment methods available using the Ilizarov technique (Figs. 3 to 8). These guidelines,

based on general principles, will have to be modified by the surgeon, taking into account the parameters outlined above.

Ilizarov Modalities of Treatment

Compression Osteosynthesis

Nonunions without bone loss, with or without deformity, can be treated by applying the Ilizarov apparatus with two levels of fixation, above and below the nonunion site (Fig. 9).[18] Deformity is corrected acutely at the initial surgery if the nonunion is lax, or gradually if it is stiff. Gradual compression is then applied. Compression is added, at the rate of 0.5 mm per day, for approximately two to four weeks. This will cause bowing of the wires on either side of the nonunion and will stimulate most hypertrophic, stiff nonunions to heal. This method is commonly unsuccessful in treating atrophic, lax nonunions or nonunions where there is interposed dead bone.

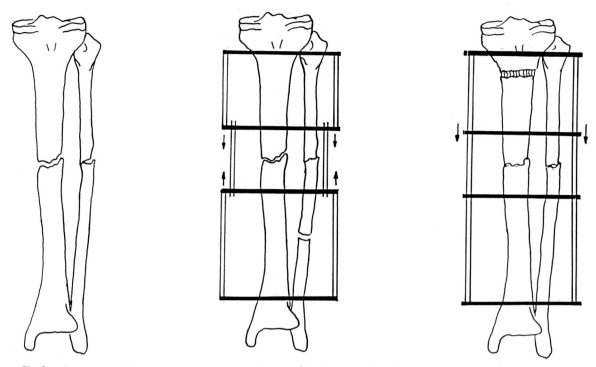

Fig. 3 Lax nonunions without bone loss with and without deformity can be treated by acute correction of the deformity and then compression osteosynthesis and fibulectomy. Alternatively, the compression in the more atrophic types can be achieved by a distraction compression osteosynthesis with bone transport.

Distraction Osteosynthesis

Distraction of the nonunion (Figs. 10 and 11) may be used with stiff hypertrophic nonunion and requires

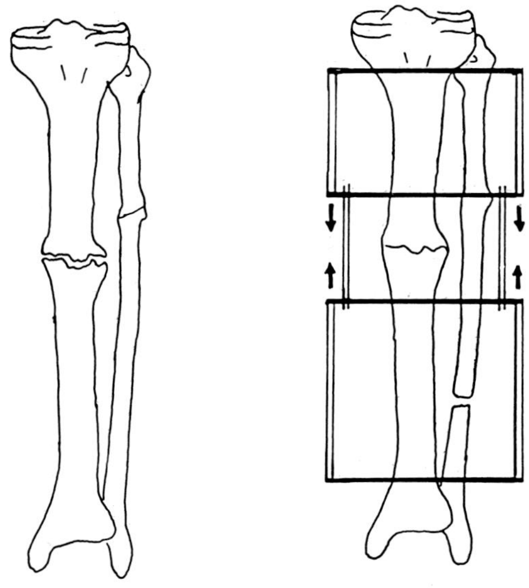

Fig. 4 Stiff nonunions without bone loss or deformity can be treated by compression osteosynthesis and fibulectomy.

correction of the deformity at the level of the nonunion and/or lengthening of the limb. This method succeeds only with very stiff hypertrophic nonunions. The dense fibrous tissue between the bone ends acts as the interzone for distraction osteogenesis.

Monofocal Compression-Distraction Lengthening Osteosynthesis

Osteogenesis involves initial compression of the nonunion site followed by gradual distraction of the same site (Fig. 9). It can be used to lengthen and to correct deformity as needed. This method is applicable to hypertrophic and normotrophic stiff nonunions that have limited motion at the nonunion site. It is often unreliable in atrophic, infected, and lax nonunions.[19]

Sequential Monofocal Distraction-Compression Osteosynthesis

This method is used to stimulate healing at the nonunion site. The apparatus is used to distract the pseudoarthrosis, followed by compression at the same site until the bone ends come into contact. This method can be used with atrophic and hypertrophic nonunions that show significant instability. Distraction disrupts the tissue at the nonunion site, frequently leading to some poor bone regeneration. This poor bone regeneration is stimulated to consolidate when the two bone ends are brought back together again. Although the new bone formation is inadequate for limb lengthening, the

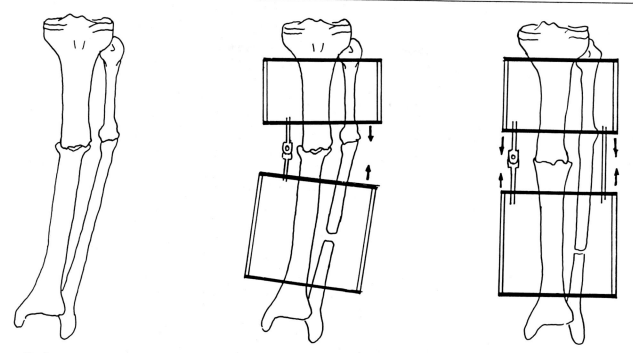

Fig. 5 Stiff nonunions without bone loss but with fixed deformity can be treated by fibulectomy and gradual correction of deformity followed by compression osteosynthesis.

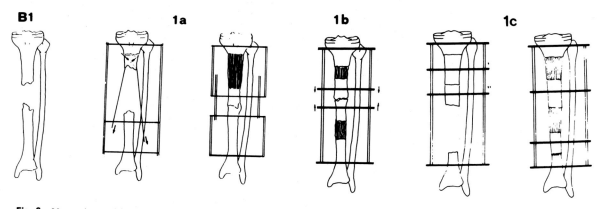

Fig. 6 Nonunions with bone defects but no shortening can be treated by bifocal distraction-compression transport osteosynthesis—unilateral (1a), contralateral (1b), and ipsilateral (1c). This can be performed using longitudinally oriented transport wires or transversely oriented transport wires.

compression augments the callus by causing it to bulge around the nonunion site, and, therefore, the atrophic nonunion will heal.

Bifocal Compression-Distraction Lengthening Osteosynthesis (Bone Lengthening)

In this method, the nonunion site is compressed, and the length discrepancy is corrected through an adjacent corticotomy (Fig. 12). The corticotomy lengthening serves as an osteogenic stimulus to the healing of an adjacent nonunion.[7] This method is used to correct atrophic nonunions with shortening.

Bifocal Distraction-Compression Transport Osteosynthesis (Bone Transport)

This method allows the healing of large bone defects without the use of bone grafting. A corticotomy is performed on one or both sides of a bone defect and the bone segment produced by the corticotomy is transported across the bone defect at a gradual rate. When

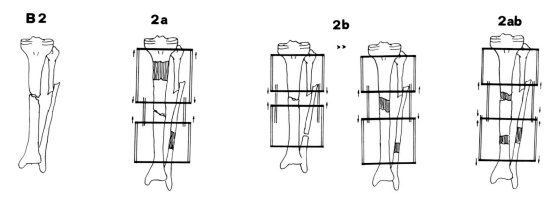

Fig. 7 Nonunions with shortening but no bone defect can be treated by: bifocal compression distraction lengthening osteosynthesis (2a): monofocal distraction osteosynthesis or monofocal compression distraction lengthening osteosynthesis (2b); or by the combination of 2a and 2b at two different sites. In all of these varieties a fibular osteotomy is necessary if there is no fibular nonunion.

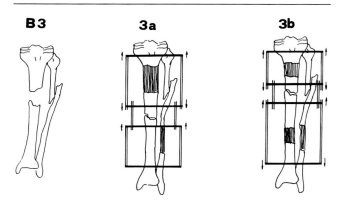

Fig. 8 Nonunions with bone defects and shortening can be treated by bifocal distraction transport type and then of the lengthening type. This may be unilateral (3a), contralateral (3b), or ipsilateral as shown in Figure 6, type 1c.

the transported bone segment arrives at the other end, it is compressed across the nonunion site and allowed to consolidate with the bone column behind it.

Soft-Tissue Defects

As the bone segment is transported, it brings with it its surrounding soft tissues. Where there is no soft-tissue defect, this causes temporary edema and bunching of soft tissues. For bone transport, it is a good idea to use rings a size larger than usual to allow room for edema. Soft-tissue transport can be minimized, by using longitudinal distraction wires for the bone transport, or maximized, by using horizontal wires supported on a transport ring. In any event, the bunching of the soft tissue resolves with cessation of transport.

Many soft-tissue defects associated with bone gaps can be closed by means of soft-tissue transport, thus avoiding complicated operations to obtain coverage.

This technique is especially useful after resection for osteomyelitis, when soft tissues are routinely left open to drain.

Nonunions With Bone Loss

Classification

As shown in Figures 3 through 8, there are three basic types of bone loss: bone defect, called type 1; shortening, called type 2; or a combination of a defect and shortening, called type 3.[7] This classification helps one plan the simultaneous resolution of other problems. In general, bone defects are treated by bone transport; shortening is treated by relengthening. Correction of deformity, compression of the nonunion, and fibular osteotomy are components of all of these forms of treatment. If distraction of a corticotomy is used to regenerate the bone lost, the essential difference between bone transport and limb lengthening is that lengthening involves changing the total length of the limb, which increases soft-tissue tension. In bone transport, limb length remains the same; only the length of the transport segment increases. Limb lengthening involves external lengthening, while bone transport lengthens internally. The other means of regenerating length is monofocal compression-distraction, in which both compression and distraction occur at the nonunion site.

To shorten treatment time, lengthening may be performed at two sites within the bone, either through two separate corticotomies or by using one corticotomy and the nonunion site. Bone transport may also be performed at two sites, one proximal and another distal to the bone defect (Fig. 13). Alternatively, when a short segment remains on one side of the defect and a long segment on the other, the longer segment can be cut

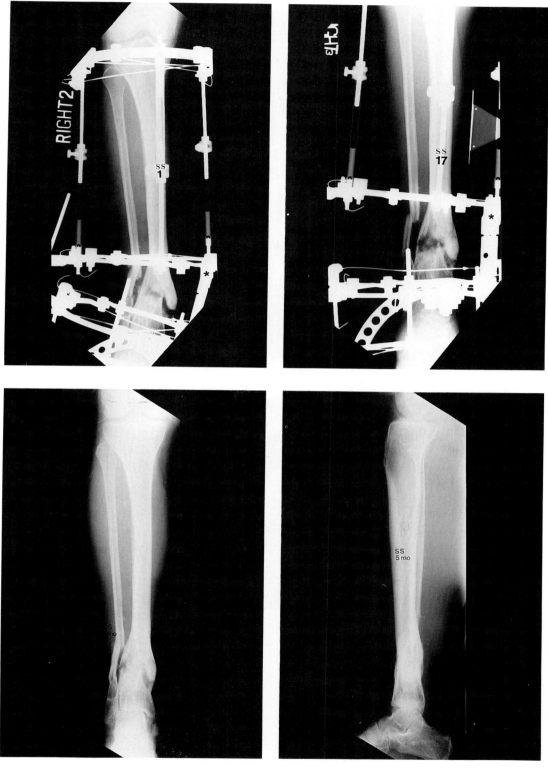

Fig. 9 **Top left,** Stiff nonunion of distal tibia with valgus, lateral translation, and recurvatum deformities. The Ilizarov apparatus has been applied with two levels of fixation in the proximal tibia and two levels in the distal tibia and foot. A distraction translation type of hinge articulates between them (*). **Top right,** With distraction of the convex lateral aspect, the deformity is corrected and the rings are parallel. The hinge (*) is now straight. Notice the medial translation of the distal fragment. **Bottom left** and **bottom right,** The apparatus was removed after six months. The alignment on the anteroposterior and lateral views is almost anatomic with some mild residual lateral translation deformity.

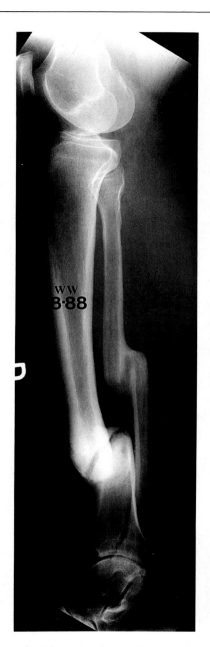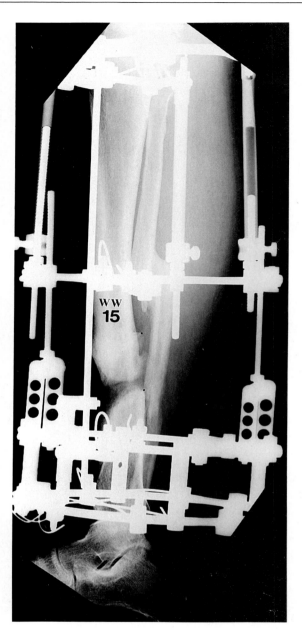

Fig. 10 **Left**, A very stiff hypertrophic nonunion with shortening of 3 cm of the distal tibia (Fig. 7, type B2). **Right**, Treatment by fibular osteotomy and distraction osteosynthesis to reestablish length. Notice the distraction osteogenesis new bone formation from the nonunion site. The lengthening achieved is indicated by the two black dots.

in two places to achieve the same result in less time. Finally, to correct shortening and a bone defect, transport and lengthening can be performed at a single corticotomy site, or transport can be done at one site and lengthening at another.

Bone transport may also be used to treat partial-thickness bone defects. This method involves transporting a segment of bone created by a corticotomy of the partial circumference of the adjacent bone, rather like closing a window from above or from the side.

Problems and Obstacles During Treatment

Problems may arise during treatment that can block treatment or prolong treatment time.

Soft-Tissue Obstruction to Bone Transport Transporting bone across a previously scarred region may become difficult. If the scarring is limited, a second corticotomy may solve the problem. For example, performing a second corticotomy in the coronal plane will liberate the portion of bone that lies in the posterior unscarred region

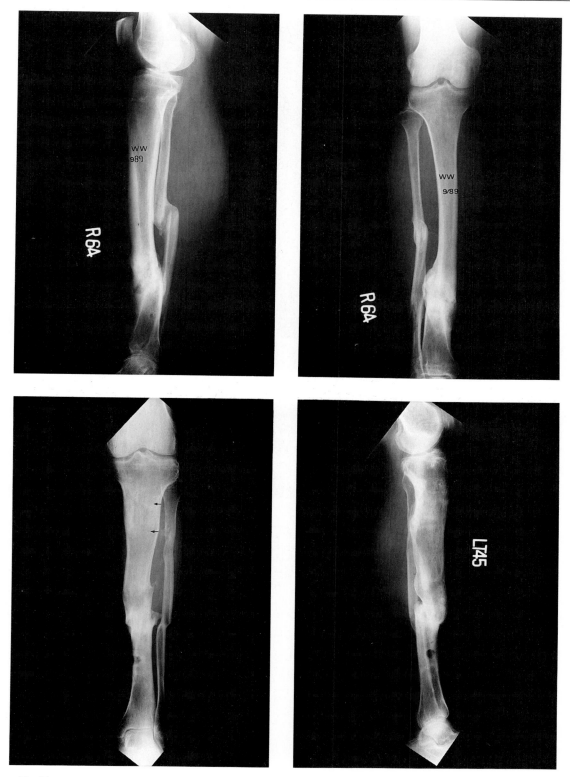

Fig. 11   The final result, with correction of the lateral and posterior translation deformities.

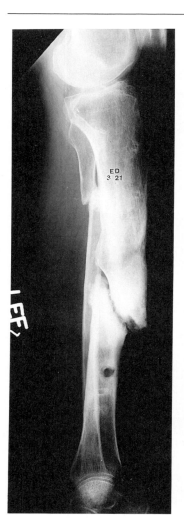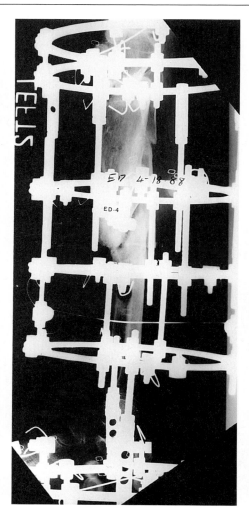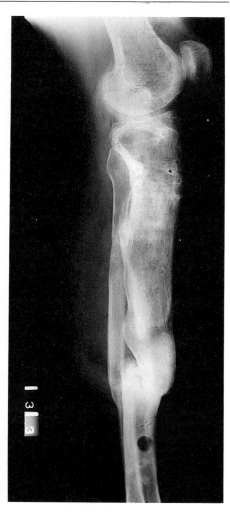

Fig. 12   Left, Lax nonunion with 5 cm of shortening (type B2). This nonunion was extremely unstable and proved to be a synovial pseudoarthrosis at surgery. **Center**, Bifocal compression-distraction lengthening osteosynthesis was performed. The nonunion was opened through a limited exposure, the bone ends reshaped to establish internal stability for end-to-end compression, and the medullary cavity opened on either side. **Right**, Union and 5 cm of lengthening were achieved in ten months of treatment.

and allow it to pass unimpeded through the soft tissues. In some situations, a negative soft-tissue defect may block passage of a transported segment. In such cases, the negative defect can be elevated by passing multiple wires under the skin of the negative defect and slowly elevating the soft tissues. Once the negative defect is elevated, the bone can continue its movement.

Delayed Bone Regeneration Poor osteogenesis may develop in the distraction gap. Treatment for this problem is to go in reverse and compress the new bone. Once osteogenesis begins, distraction can proceed again. In extreme cases, it may even be necessary to bone graft the distraction gap.

Delayed Consolidation of the Nonunion Site Despite excellent bone formation in the distraction gap, consolidation of the nonunion site may be delayed, especially in

atrophic nonunions.[19] Treatment for this problem may involve opening the nonunion site and reshaping the bone ends so that the medullary cavity is open on both sides and the configuration of contact is stable and broad. One may also bone graft the site of a delayed consolidation, but this is rarely necessary. Premature consolidation of the fibula may delay union and necessitate a fibular ostectomy. Bone grafting the nonunion site is also a modality of treatment that may shorten the treatment time.

Osteonecrosis of the transport segment may contribute to the delay in bony consolidation. In one case, in which I retrieved a pathologic specimen from a patient undergoing bone transport, the transported segment was avascular. It is not known whether this was caused by the original trauma; the debilitated, elderly, malnourished state of the patient; or vascular decompen-

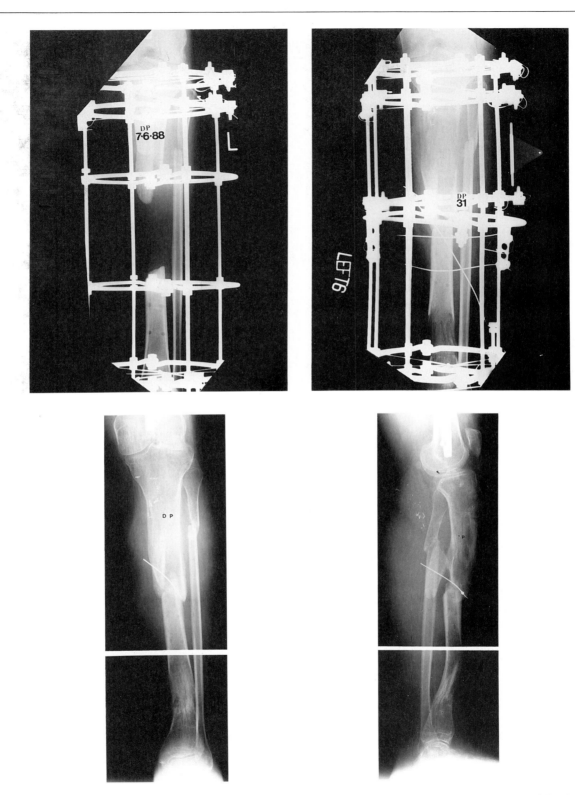

Fig. 13 Top left, A 16-cm bone defect of the tibia has been stabilized with the Ilizarov apparatus. **Top right**, A two-level bone transport was performed moving one bone segment from proximal to distal and one from distal to proximal. Note the new bone regeneration in the two distraction gaps. The ends of the two transport segments have made contact and are placed under compression. **Bottom left** and **bottom right**, At 12 months solid union had been achieved and the apparatus was removed.

sation of the bone due resulting from bone transport. Frame instability after bone transport contributed to refracture at the nonunion site in another patient.

Results of Ilizarov Method of Treatment

Aronovich and associates from Kurgan, USSR, described the results of 170 tibial bone defects treated by these techniques.[20] The nonunions had been present from five to ten years, and 39% had osteomyelitis. Of the 170, 68.9% had excellent results, with union, no length discrepancy, no infection, and no deformity. The results were rated only fair in 28.7%, despite the presence of union, no infection, and no deformity, because a residual limb-length discrepancy of more than 3 cm remained. In 2.4% the results were considered poor because of the recurrence of osteomyelitis. Seventy-five percent of the patients returned to work.

Kuftiryev and Meshkov[21] reported another study from Ilizarov's center that included 154 femoral defects ranging from 1 to 23 cm. In 45 of the 154, osteomyelitis was present. Union was achieved in all 154 cases, with elimination of infection, deformity, and limb-length discrepancy in 147. Residual fistulous drainage remained in four. Other Russian authors have reported similar results.[22-24]

In a review of 25 patients 19 to 62 years old treated for tibial nonunions with bone loss at the Hospital of Lecco and Bergamo in Italy,[7] there were 22 atrophic and three hypertrophic nonunions. Bone loss ranged from 1 to 23 cm with a mean of 6.2 cm. Thirteen had chronic osteomyelitis, 19 had a limb-length discrepancy (2 to 11 cm), 12 had a bone defect (1 to 16 cm), and 13 had a deformity. Six had a bone defect with no shortening, 13 had shortening with no defect, and six had both a bone defect and shortening. In ten cases with shortening, monofocal compression-distraction was applied. This was successful in all three of the hypertrophic nonunions, but failed in the seven atrophic and/or infected nonunions treated in this way. Noninfected atrophic nonunions were treated by bifocal compression-distraction, and infected nonunions were treated by resection of the infected necrotic bone and bone transport. Union was achieved in all cases. The mean time to union was 13.6 months.

Using conventional methods, hypertrophic nonunions are treated by stability alone, and atrophic nonunions by stability and osteogenic stimulus, usually in the form of a bone graft. The Ilizarov analog of the bone graft is the corticotomy, which, it is believed, stimulates osteogenesis in the adjacent nonunion. Thus, while the methods are different, the principles of treatment underlying conventional and Ilizarov methods are the same. Hypertrophic nonunions are treated by stabilization, using the Ilizarov apparatus. Atrophic unstable nonunions are treated by stabilization, a corticotomy for bone regeneration, and sometimes local

decortication of the bone ends. Infected nonunions are treated by resection and bone transport.

In this study from Italy, union was ultimately achieved in all cases, infection was eliminated in all but three cases, deformity in all but four, and limb shortening in all but one. On the basis of these criteria, the results were rated as excellent in 18, good in five, and fair in two.

Functional results, based on return to work and activities of daily living, were excellent in 16, good in seven, fair in one, and poor in one. Defects included a significant limp in four patients, dystrophy in four patients, pain in four patients, and residual untreated equinus deformity in five patients. Preexisting neurologic damage was the usual cause of the dysfunction. For example, one patient who achieved an excellent bony result later requested a voluntary amputation to relieve persistent, unrelenting neurogenic pain. This case illustrates the limits of this technique. This method broadens the capabilities of orthopaedic treatment, but its use must be tempered by common sense. For example, the man with the elective amputation had, in fact, an insensate painful clawfoot with poor skin and a decubitus on his heel. Although his bone was restored to normal in an acceptable period of time, his soft-tissue injury was such that he was a poor candidate for reconstructive treatment.[25] An elective amputation for pain relief was carried out two years later.

Conclusions

The Ilizarov technique offers many advantages over conventional methods of treatment for nonunions with and without bone loss. The technique is less invasive, allows immediate weightbearing, and has few failures and few complications. It leaves the pathologic focus of the bone alone and operates on the healthy bone. The technique is a comprehensive one in that it treats not only the nonunion but also the length discrepancy, the deformity, the infection, and the bone defect.

References

1. Ilizarov GA: The principles of the Ilizarov method. *Bull Hosp Joint Dis Orthop Inst* 1988;48:1–11.
2. Special Communication: Kurgan Revolution in Orthopedics. *J Am Podiatr Med Assoc* 1973;63:667–668.
3. Paley D: Current techniques of limb lengthening. *J Pediatr Orthop* 1988;8:73–92.
4. Ilizarov GA: The tension-stress effect on the genesis and growth of tissues: Part I. The influence of stability of fixation and soft-tissue preservation. *Clin Orthop* 1989;238:249–281.
5. Ilizarov GA: The tension-stress effect on the genesis and growth of tissues: Part II. The influence of the rate and frequency of distraction. *Clin Orthop* 1989;239:263–285.
6. Fleming B, Paley D, Kristiansen T, et al: A biomechanical analysis of the Ilizarov external fixator. *Clin Orthop* 1989;241:95–105.

7. Paley D, Catagni MA, Argnani F, et al: Ilizarov treatment of tibial nonunions with bone loss. *Clin Orthop* 1989;241:146–165.

8. Codivilla A: On the means of lengthening, in the lower limbs, the muscles and tissues which are shortened through deformity. *Am J Orthop Surg* 1905;2:353–369.

9. Wagner H: Operative lengthening of the femur. *Clin Orthop* 1978;136:125–142.

10. Ilizarov GA, Berko VG: Rentgenologicht eskai sinamika razvitiia kostnogo regenerata pri udlinenii bedra v eksperimente [Roentgenographic dynamics of the bone regenerate development in elongation of the hip in experiment]. *Ortop Travmatol Protez* 1976;12:25–31.

11. Ilizarov GA, Berko VG: Morfologicheskaia kharakteristika regenerata, obrazuiushchegosia pri udlinenii bedra v eksperimente [Morphologic characteristic of the regenerate formed in elongation of the hip in experiment]. *Ortop Travmatol Protez* 1980;7: 54–59.

12. Ledeyev, Ilizarov G: Regeneration of the bone tissue of the diaphysis under different conditions of osteosynthetic traction under experimental conditions. *Exp Chir* 1975;2:

13. Shtin VP, Nikitenko ET: O tempe distraktsii pri udlinenii dlinnykh trubchatykh kostei [The rate of the distraction in elongation of the long tibular bones]. *Ortop Travmatol Protez* 1975;10:40–44.

14. Weber BG, Cech O: *Pseudoarthrosis.* Bern, Hans Huber, 1976.

15. Gyulnazarova SV, Shtin VP: Reparative bone tissue regeneration in treatment of pseudoarthroses with simultaneous elongation in the pathologic focus region (experimental study). *Ortop Travmatol Protez* 1983;4:10.

16. Kravchuk VI: Kliniko-rentgenolgicheskaia dinamika reparativnoi regeneratsii v usloviiakh distracktsii pri psevdoartrozakh trubchatykh kostei nizhnykh knoechnostei [Clinico-roentgenographic dynamics of the reparative regeneration in conditions of distraction in pseudoarthroses of tubular bones of the lower extremities]. *Ortop Travmatol Protez* 1977;2:28–32.

17. Sveshnikov AA, Desiatnik EG, Smotrova LA: Obmennye protsessy v kostnoi tkani pri lechenii psevdoartroyov goleni po Ilizarovu [Metabolic processes in the bone tissue in the therapy of pseudarthoses of the tibia according to Ilizarov]. *Ortop Travmatol Protez* 1982;2:48–52.

18. Ilizarov GA: Basic principles of transosseous compression and distraction osteosynthesis. *Ortop Travmatol Protez* 1975;10:7–15.

19. Gyulnazarova SV, Nadirshina IK: Variants of osteogenesis in the treatment of flail pseudoarthroses by the compression/distraction method. *Ortop Travmatol Protez* 1985;5:20–23.

20. Aronovich AM, Shlyachov VI, Payevski SA, et al: Rehabilitation by Ilizarov technique of patients with bony defects of the tibia complicated by chronic osteomyelitis. Presented at the Second International Conference on Experimental Theoretical and Clinical Aspects of Transosseous Osteosynthesis Developed at the KNIIEKOT, Kurgan, USSR, Sept 3–5, 1986.

21. Kuftiryev LM, Meshkov AN: The treatment of bony defects of the femur by the Ilizarov method. Presented at the Second International Conference on Experimental Theoretical and Clinical Aspects of Transosseous Osteosynthesis Developed at the KNIIEKOT, Kurgan, USSR, Sept 3–5, 1986.

22. Lebyedev AA, Kisyelev VY, Chizhenkov GA, et al: The treatment of nonunions with bony defects of the tibia complicated by osteomyelitis. Presented at the Second International Conference on Experimental Theoretical and Clinical Aspects of Transosseous Osteosynthesis Developed at the KNIIEKOT, Kurgan, USSR, Sept 3–5, 1986.

23. Voronovic IP, Volchkevich PL: The treatment of bony defects of the tibia by the Ilizarov method. Presented at the Second International Conference on Experimental Theoretical and Clinical Aspects of Transosseous Osteosynthesis Developed at the KNIIEKOT, Kurgan, USSR, Sept 3–5, 1986.

24. Zhadenov II, Reshetnikov NP, Philipov VV, et al: The treatment of long tubular bone defects with the transosseous osteosynthesis apparatus of Ilizarov. Presented at the Second International Conference on Experimental Theoretical and Clinical Aspects of Transosseous Osteosynthesis Developed at the KNIIEKOT, Kurgan, USSR, Sept 3–5, 1986.

25. Hansen ST Jr: The type-IIIC tibial fracture: Salvage or amputation, editorial. *J Bone Joint Surg* 1987;69A:799–800.

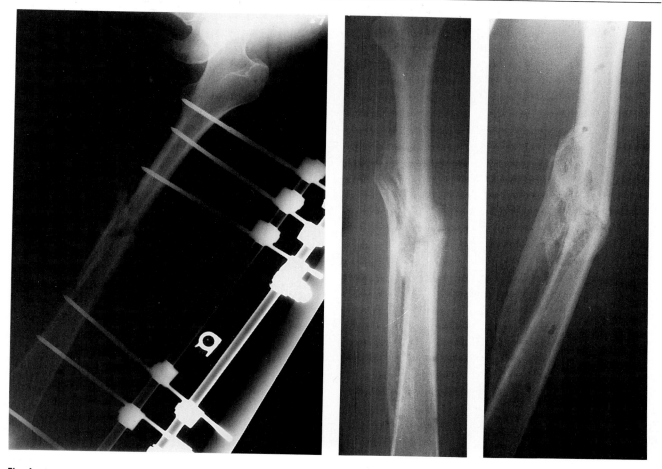

Fig. 4 Same case shown in Figure 3. **Left,** To avoid the use of general anesthesia, a femoral fixator was applied under regional block. **Center,** Anteroposterior view of the healed fracture after a successful delivery. **Right,** Lateral view of the healed fracture.

lateral to medial. Anterior pins can be used, but they restrict knee motion more than do pins from the lateral position.

Safe Corridor

By reviewing the cross section of the thigh (Fig. 5), and visualizing the safe zone of half-pin insertion, an adequate frame can be applied without injury to nerves or vascular structures. In the most proximal part of the femur the safe zone encompasses an arc of 200 degrees. In the midshaft the safe arc of half-pin insertion is only 180 degrees. In the distal femur this arc expands to 250 degrees, and it is only in this distal third of the femur that transfixion pins may be used. They are used mainly in knee arthrodesis.

Frame Application

In order to construct an appropriate frame, the mechanical properties of each fixation must be understood because adjustments can be difficult once the pins have been inserted.[14]

Simple-Pin Fixators In this type of fixator, each pin is connected to the bar separately. This provides a mechanical advantage because the pins can be separated from each other, which adds rigidity to the frame. Three pins are placed in each fragment, separated as widely as possible, and each of the two middle pins are placed at least 2 cm from the fracture site.

With simple-pin fixators, the pins are inserted in the following order (Fig. 6). (1) The most proximal and most distal pins are inserted first. Do not use the power drill when inserting the pins because to do so can cause bone necrosis. Some pins can be predrilled before insertion. (2) One or two bars of the appropriate length are applied, with a minimum of three clamps on each side of the fracture. The fracture is reduced and the clamps retightened. (3) The inner pins are inserted. They should be at least 2 cm from the fracture site. (4) The rest of the pins are inserted, the fixator is adjusted, and the pins are prestressed. Finally, the fixator is secured and retightened.

Cluster-Pin Fixators/Transfixion With Fixators With this type

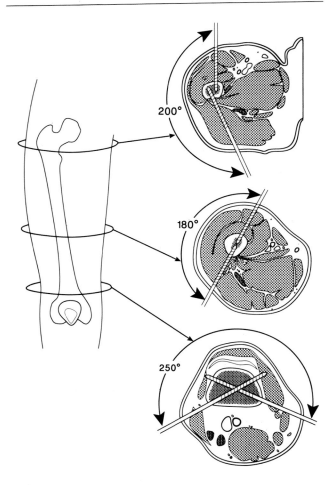

Fig. 5   The "safe corridor"

of fixator, the surgeon can apply the fixator first and then reduce the fracture. There are two or three pins per clamp, and each clamp is connected to the bar. These pins are closer together, which decreases the stability of the frame.

This type of device should be inserted in the following order (Fig. 7). (1) The most proximal and most distal pins are inserted first. (2) The third pin is inserted using a guide or template to keep the pins in each fragment parallel to one another. (3) The fourth pin is inserted in the other fragment, placed at least 2 cm from the fracture site. (4) The fracture is reduced and all of the joints are tightened.

Postoperative Management

Postoperative management includes elevation of the extremity, pin care, and frame care. The pins are cleaned daily with a cotton applicator and hydrogen peroxide. Any loose pins should be removed and reapplied.

The external fixation device can be used for temporary treatment while the soft tissues heal, after which the definitive treatment may be by intramedullary nailing, plating, and/or casting.

Once the soft tissues have healed and bony union has begun, some frames can be dynamized, which encourages fracture healing. De Bastiani and associates[11] reported a healing rate of 98% in closed and 89% in open femoral fractures using this procedure. Other frames can be made less rigid by sequential disassembly.

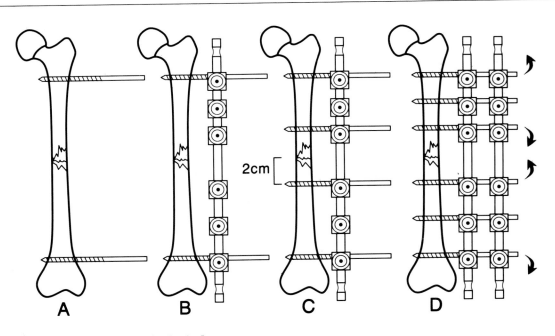

Fig. 6   Application of the simple-pin fixator.

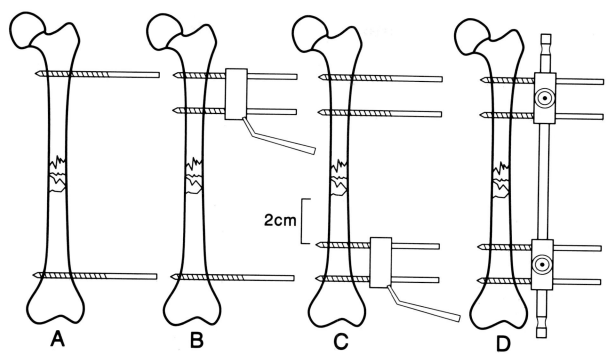

Fig. 7   Application of the cluster-pin fixator.

Case Study

A retrospective review of 24 femoral fractures treated between 1983 and 1986 delineated the indications and limitations of external fixation in treated femoral fractures.[4] The review included 13 open fractures, of which eight were grade II and five were grade III. There were six comminuted fractures, and five cases involved unstable medical patients requiring immediate surgical management.

Temporary Treatment In 14 patients, the fixator was used for initial fixation, after which the definitive method of fixation was achieved in six patients by intramedullary nailing, in four patients by plating, and in four patients by long leg casting.

In this group, a complication was encountered in the group treated by intramedullary nailing, when one patient developed osteomyelitis. Among the patients treated by plating or casting after temporary stabilization by external fixation, there were no complications.

Definitive Treatment In ten patients, the fixator was used for both initial and definitive treatment. Five of the ten patients were children, none of whom required any external support after removal of the fixator. The other five patients were adults with complex fractures and complex frames. In three patients, the frame was disassembled, making these fractures less stable. In two patients the frames were dynamized and bony union ensued. In this group the average time the fixator was in place was four months, with a range of three to 28 months.

The only complication in this group was shortening— 2.1 cm in one patient and 3.2 cm in a second patient with a comminuted fracture.

Solid union was achieved in 21 patients. Two patients had delayed union. One patient developed a septic nonunion after exchanging a fixator for an interlocking nail.

Diminished knee motion was seen in 11 patients from both groups. The average loss in range of motion was 56 degrees.

Summary

External fixation of the femur remains a viable option in the acute treatment of fractures or in reconstructive procedures. As in any method of fixation, the surgeon must be familiar with the device used, the mechanical properties of the device, the application technique of such devices, and, most importantly, the postoperative management of the patient.

References

1. Lhowe DW, Hansen ST: Immediate nailing of open fractures of the femoral shaft. *J Bone Joint Surg* 1988;70A:812–820.
2. Chapman MW: The role of intramedullary fixation in open fractures. *Clin Orthop* 1986;212:26–34.
3. Alonso JE, Horowitz M: Use of the AO/ASIF external fixator in children. *J Pediatr Orthop* 1987;7:594–600.
4. Baird RA, Kreitenberg A, Eltorai I: External fixation of femoral shaft fractures in spinal cord injury patients. *Paraplegia* 1986;24:183–190.
5. Behrens F, Jones RE III, Mears DC, et al: External skeletal Fixation, in Murray DG (ed): American Academy of Orthopaedic Surgeons *Instructional Course Lectures, XXX.* St. Louis, CV Mosby, 1981, pp 112–182.
6. Klemm KW: Use of the external fixator in thigh fractures, in Uhthoff HK (ed): *Current Concepts of External Fixation of Fractures.* Berlin, Springer-Verlag, 1982, pp 207–214.
7. Seligson D, Kristiansen TK: Use of the Wagner apparatus in complicated fractures of the distal femur. *J Trauma* 1978;18:795-799.
8. Stein H, Makin M: Use of the Wagner apparatus in fractures of lower limb. *Orthop Review* 1980;9:96–99.
9. Rüedi TP, Lüscher JN: Results after internal fixation of comminuted fractures of the femoral shaft with DC plates. *Clin Orthop* 1979;138:74–76.
10. Alonso J, Geissler W, Hughes JL: External fixation of femoral fractures: Indications and limitations. *Clin Orthop* 1989;241:83–88.
11. De Bastini G, Aldegheri R, Renzi Brivio L: The treatment of fractures with a dynamic axial fixator. *J Bone Joint Surg* 1984;66B:538–545.
12. Behrens A: External fixation: General principles and application in the lower leg, in Chapman MW (ed): *Operative Orthopaedics.* Philadelphia, JB Lippincott, 1988, vol 1, pp 161–171.
13. Giachino A: Anatomic considerations in the placement of percutaneous pins, in Uhthoff HK (ed): *Current Concepts of External Fixation of Fractures.* Berlin, Springer-Verlag, 1982, pp 203–206.
14. Hughes JL, Sauer BW: Wagner apparatus: A portable traction device, in Seligson D, Pope M (eds): *Concepts in External Fixation.* New York, Grune & Stratton, 1982, pp 203–217.

External Fixation in Children: Lower Extremity

Fred Behrens, MD

During the past two decades, external fixation has gained widespread acceptance for the management of adult extremity injuries and deformities. However, most surgeons are reluctant to use these devices in children, except to correct limb-length discrepancies and malalignments. This attitude is based largely on fears of a high complication rate and concerns that children find these devices too cumbersome or otherwise unacceptable. The introduction of more rational concepts,[1] simpler designs, and tissue-protecting instrumentation has made serious complications a rare event. Furthermore, the accumulated experience from different pediatric centers suggests that children tolerate fixators well.[2-7]

Equipment

Fixators

The same components and frame configurations appropriate for adults are generally used in the management of musculoskeletal injuries in teenagers. In the absence of specifically designed devices, external fixation in smaller children generally relies on modified adult equipment, in particular on devices originally developed for the management of upper extremity injuries. Hybrids, which combine small pin sizes with standard clamps and connecting rods, are another option.

For children less than 12 years old, pin diameters ranging from 2.5 to 4 mm should be used, with the provision that the pin diameter is not to exceed one third of the bony diameter. Because many clamps cannot be adjusted to hold pins of smaller diameters, tight fits between clamp and pin must be achieved with the help of shims. I have found small segments of K-wires, which are readily available in different diameters, most useful. If properly fitted, such shims will provide a tight clamp fit for several months.

Frames

The use of large components and the smaller forces generated by children make many of the methods used to build stiffer frames unnecessary. Therefore, universal joints, which have a limited pin spread, and simple, one-plane unilateral frames are routinely used.[7] These frames provide sufficient strength for full early weightbearing as long as there is no segmental bone loss. In teenagers, the severity of the injuries and the mechanical needs set higher demands. Thus, more complex frame designs, such as double-bar one-plane unilateral frames or two-plane unilateral frames,[6] and a more judicious schedule for weightbearing may be appropriate. However, transfixion pins and bilateral frame configurations are even less justified than in adults.[8]

Fixator Application and Care

In order to be acceptable, an external fixation frame should be safe and nonobstructive, should accommodate a wide variety of injuries, should be of sufficient stiffness to maintain alignment, and should allow full weightbearing. It should also have a low rate of serious complications. These goals can be achieved by adhering to three basic principles. In order of decreasing importance, frames should not damage vital anatomic structures, should provide sufficient wound access for debridement and secondary procedures, and, finally, should fulfill the mechanical demands of patient and injury.[6]

Principles

In children, as in adults, external fixators are best suited for limb segments in which the principal bone lies eccentrically and all pins can be inserted through a safe corridor, one free of major neurovascular and myotendinous structures. Fixators so applied do not limit the function of myotendinous units and generally have a low rate of pin-tract infections. Limb segments in which the principal bone is centrally located (for instance in the femur) are less ideal. Here muscle transfixion cannot be avoided, and at least temporary limitation of motion in the distal joint is inevitable. This can lead to permanent restrictions of motion in adults, but most children will regain full motion once the fixator is removed.

When pins are placed periarticularly, the location of the physis must be carefully considered.[8] Although the thickness of the physis rarely exceeds 5 to 8 mm, its undulating shape creates an unsafe zone that is 1 to 2 cm wide. Pin injuries to the physis can lead to serious growth disturbances and should be avoided at all costs. Outside the physeal zone, and within the safe corridor, pins can be freely inserted into the epiphysis and the metaphysis (Fig. 1). Epiphyseal pins demand particular care, as an infected pin tract will not only jeopardize the physis but also the adjacent joint.

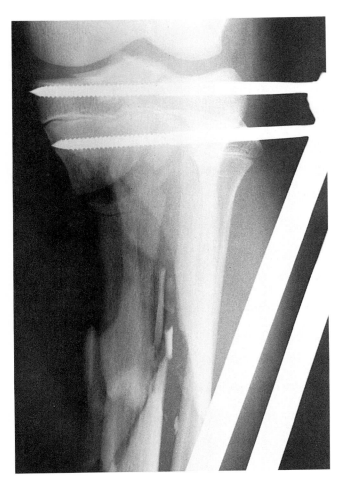

Fig. 1 Stabilization with an external fixator of an open comminuted fracture of the proximal tibia in a 12-year-old boy. Pins are placed into the epiphysis and proximal metaphysis without injury to the epiphyseal plate.

Application

As in adults, the fixator should be applied under sterile conditions, using general or regional anesthesia. To prevent malalignments, the limbs should be draped so that the two joints adjacent to the lesion under treatment lie within the operating field. An image intensifier is of great advantage during pin insertion and for the assessment of overall alignment and is mandatory for pin placement in the vicinity of the physis. The pin holes should be predrilled with a sharp drill bit. Insert the pins with the help of one of the newer triple trochar systems to ensure soft-tissue protection and accurate alignment of the pins.[8] As universal articulations are used for most pediatric frames, fracture alignment or its correction is generally no problem. The final position of the bony fragments should be checked in two planes, on long films that include the two adjacent joints.

Frame Care

In children with head injuries, it may be necessary to cover the protruding fixator parts with cotton wool held in place by a bandage. Most children quickly grow accustomed to the external fixator and often treat it as a curious, attention-getting part of their anatomy rather than an unpleasant obstacle. Pin and frame care can be carried out independently by teenagers, but parents must be responsible for younger children.

Indications

The principal indications for external fixation in children are (1) open fractures, particularly grade III lesions (Figs. 2 and 3) and fractures with segmental bone loss[1,4,6,8]; (2) closed fractures that are unstable, associated with burns or dermatologic conditions, or treated after fasciotomy; (3) fractures associated with neurovascular lesions; (4) unstable periarticular fractures, which present difficulties that may require a combination of internal and external fixation; (5) severe joint injuries with multiple ligamentous disruptions or an open joint; (6) fractures in the presence of a closed head injury or spasticity[3,4]; (7) multiple fractures such as floating knees or bilateral extremity lesions[9]; (8) polytrauma, in which it facilitates mobilization and patient care; (9) certain unstable pelvic fractures[8]; (10) fixation of osteotomies; and (11) limb-length discrepancies and malalignments.

External Fixation in the Lower Extremity

External fixators are more often used on the tibia than on any other extremity segment. As a broad subcutaneous surface of bone is available for pin insertion, frame application rarely causes problems. Unless prevented by segmental bone loss or injuries elsewhere, most patients are able to walk with full weightbearing within three weeks. Depending on the age of the patient, bone grafting is necessary only if there is substantial bone loss or if no significant callus is seen within ten to 12 weeks. For comminuted fractures with large diaphyseal or metaphyseal fragments, a combination of internal and external fixation is often the best way to achieve bony continuity. Nonunions, which often occur when this approach is used in adults, are not seen in children.

For femoral fractures, it is preferable to position the patient on the fracture table, applying the frame only when proper length and alignment have been secured. One-plane unilateral frames applied from a lateral direction are used exclusively, and the pins are inserted somewhat anterior to the frontal plane. In patients who

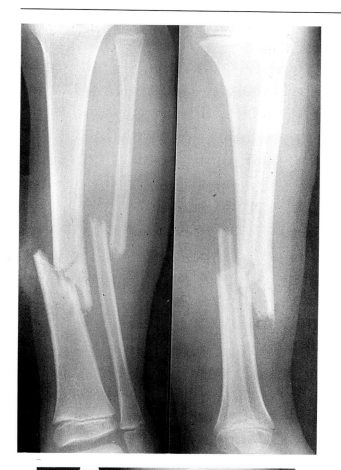

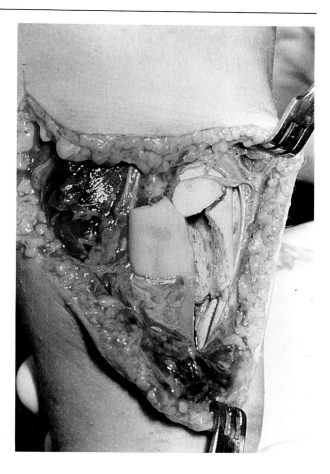

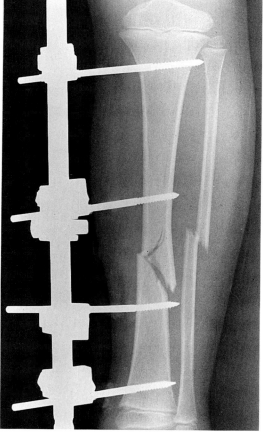

Fig. 2   Top left, Admission radiographs of grade III tibial fracture. **Top right,** Appearance of leg after initial debridement. **Bottom,** Alignment after application of external fixator.

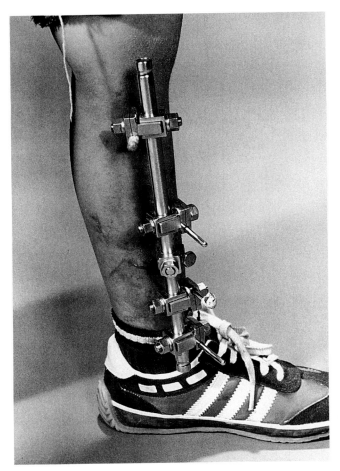 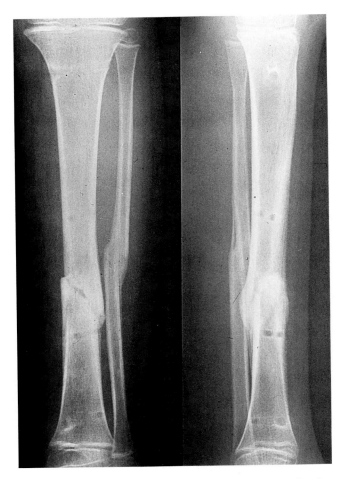

Fig. 3 Left, Four weeks after the injury shown in Figure 2, the soft-tissue wounds are healed and the patient walks full weightbearing without support. **Right,** After ten weeks the fractures have healed and the fixator is removed.

are bedridden, this frame location avoids entanglement with the bed sheets. Although femoral fixators limit knee motion, they generally do not prevent the patients from walking. While the fixator is in place, vigorous physical therapy is contraindicated as it only increases pain, pin drainage, and the risk of a serious pin-tract infection. However, as soon as the fixator is removed, the patient should be encouraged to move the knee actively. Full range of motion is frequently reestablished within two to three weeks.

In the knee, the multiligamentous injury, particularly when it is open, is an excellent indication for an external fixator. Because some pins penetrate the distal femur, the situation is managed as if a full femoral frame were in place. When used for the stabilization of extensive ligamentous reconstructions, the fixator should not be applied for longer than two to four weeks.

References

1. Behrens F, Searls K: External fixation of the tibia: Basic concepts and prospective evaluation. *J Bone Joint Surg* 1986;68B:246–254.
2. Engert J: Indikation und Anwendung des Fixateur externe im Kindesalter. *Z Kinderchir* 1982;36:133–137.
3. Porat S, Milgrom C, Nyska M, et al: Femoral fracture treatment in head-injured children: Use of external fixation. *J Trauma* 1986;26:81–84.
4. Quintin J, Evrard H, Gouat P, et al: External fixation in child traumatology. *Orthopedics* 1984;7:463–467.
5. Reff RB: The use of external fixation devices in the management of severe lower-extremity trauma and pelvic injuries in children. *Clin Orthop* 1984;188:21–33.
6. Schwartz N: Der fixateur externe als Behandlungs method beim Oberschenkeibruch des Kindes. *Unfallheilkunde* 1983;86:359–365.
7. Tolo VT: External skeletal fixation in children's fractures. *J Pediatr Orthop* 1983;3:435–442.
8. Alonso JE, Horowitz M: Use of the AO/ASIF external fixator in children. *J Pediatr Orthop* 1987;7:594–600.
9. Letts M, Vincent N, Gouw G: The 'floating knee' in children. *J Bone Joint Surg* 1986;68B:442–446.

External Fixation in the Upper Extremity

Jesse B. Jupiter, MD

Introduction

External fixation has been used less frequently to correct traumatic and reconstructive problems in the upper limb than in the lower extremity. Several factors account for this discrepancy. In the first place, the number of severely traumatized upper limbs is lower. Secondly, shortening is better tolerated in the upper limb, permitting the zone of trauma to be resected and the skeleton stabilized with internal fixation. Finally, mobility is fundamental to upper-extremity function, and therefore prolonged transarticular fixation or arthrodesis is avoided whenever possible.

At the same time, a number of clinical situations lend themselves to external fixation of the upper-extremity skeleton. In addition to complex skeletal injuries that have severe soft-tissue damage, external fixation has seen increasing application in the management of complex distal radius fractures, fracture-dislocations of the carpus, distraction arthroplasty of the elbow, digital lengthening, and fixation of complex injuries involving the smaller tubular skeleton of the hand.

The History of External Fixation in the Upper Limb

From the outset, the developers of external fixation extended its application to problems of the upper limb. Lambotte, who coined the term "fixateur externe" (external fixator), designed a unilateral frame at the turn of this century. He applied it to a wide variety of upper-extremity problems,[1] including open clavicular fractures, floating elbows, and metacarpal and phalangeal fractures. His fixator, which consisted of half pins connected by a metal frame, required fracture alignment prior to attachment of the frame to the pins.

In the 1930s, in North America, Haynes[2] developed a fixation frame using multiple half pins and a rigid external support that incorporated telescopic bars and sleeve adjustments. He demonstrated its effectiveness in fractures of the forearm. Later, Stader[3] and Anderson and O'Neil[4] also developed external fixation frames applicable to upper-extremity problems.

Hoffmann[5] of Geneva, who reported on his external fixation device in 1938, similarly extended its application to the upper extremity skeleton. A type of frame still used today bears his name and is similar to his original designs.

Finally, Jakob in Switzerland and Jaquet in France

developed smaller, more versatile frames that allow external skeletal fixation to be used on the metacarpals and phalanges.[6,7] These scaled-down devices are increasingly used to handle articular fractures, soft-tissue injuries, and reconstructive problems previously considered too complex for stable skeletal fixation.

Upper-Extremity External Fixation: General Applications

Trauma

The indications for external fixation of traumatic problems in the upper extremity parallel those for the lower limb. These include complex skeletal and soft-tissue wounds, thermal or electrical injuries associated with fractures, gunshot wounds, and certain complex articular fractures. It is often used for unstable fractures of the distal radius.

Reconstruction

External fixation is used in conjunction with soft-tissue reconstructions, as well as for injuries with infection, infected nonunion, distraction arthroplasty of the elbow, lengthening, and arthrodesis of smaller joints.

Shoulder Girdle

The role of external fixation for traumatic and reconstructive problems of the shoulder is limited and deserves only brief mention. It is noteworthy, however, that in 1905 Lambotte effectively used a unilateral external frame to stabilize an open clavicle fracture. More recently, Schuind and associates[8] reported 20 such cases with no vascular, neurologic, or pulmonary complications from the pins. They extended the indications to include nonunions, clavicle fractures that threaten to penetrate the skin, and fractures associated with polytrauma. They stated that the cortical middle third of the clavicle affords excellent pin anchorage for predrilled, 3-mm, blunt-tipped, model C Hoffmann pins.

External skeletal fixation is also useful in managing such complex injuries of the shoulder as gunshot wounds, high-energy trauma with neurovascular compromise (Fig. 1), or thermal or electrical burns with associated fractures.[9] External fixation for arthrodesis of the shoulder associated with a complex soft-tissue injury has also been described.[10]

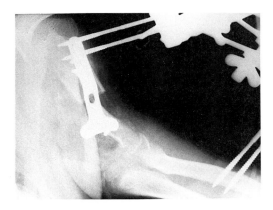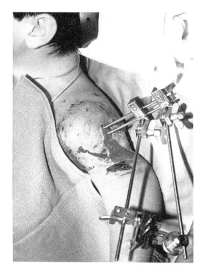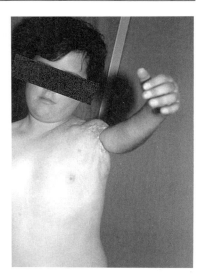

Fig. 1 A 10-year-old boy sustained a severe injury to his left arm during a train accident. In addition to the comminuted humeral fracture, a nearly circumferential zone of trauma extended from the shoulder girdle to the elbow. Although stripped from their surrounding soft tissue for several centimeters, the median and radial nerves were intact. Revascularization was necessary. **Left** and **center,** A unilateral half frame in conjunction with a T-plate stabilized the limb, permitting full access to the soft tissue. **Right,** A sensate limb resulted with some recovery of digital motion.

Humeral Shaft

The vast majority of diaphyseal humeral fractures can be treated effectively either by closed means or surgically with plate or intramedullary rod fixation. For this reason, the indications for external skeletal fixation have traditionally been limited to special situations, including fractures with complex soft-tissue injuries,[11-13] segmental fractures with bone loss,[14] heavily contaminated fractures,[15] gunshot injuries, and fractures associated with thermal or electrical burns.[12,16]

On the other hand, two recent studies employing less rigid unilateral fixation frames for uncomplicated humeral shaft fractures have observed excellent results. Burney and associates[17] treated 100 patients using a unilateral Hoffmann frame with two to three threaded half pins proximal and distal to the fracture. They reported a 95% union rate within four months after injury and a low incidence of pin-related problems. De Bastiani and associates[18] in 1984, in 40 closed humeral-shaft fractures, noted a 98% union rate within an average of 3.4 months, a low incidence of pin-tract problems, and only one case of refracture. They employed a frame that had a connecting rod with telescoping features that allowed its conversion from rigid to dynamic fixation. The Wagner external fixation device, which has the advantage of using the large half-threaded Schanz pins,[19] has also proven effective as a unilateral assembly for the humeral shaft.

In reconstructive situations, the infected nonunion is perhaps the major indication for external fixation of the humerus.[13,15] Humeral lengthening, although less common than lengthening of bones in the lower limb, has had some applications after physeal arrests or post-traumatic loss.[20]

Elbow

Because mobility is fundamental to elbow function, the basic treatment for most articular fractures and dislocations of the elbow involves internal fixation and early mobilization. In some circumstances, however, where there is extensive soft-tissue trauma,[11] infection, or posttraumatic contractures, such goals are not easily achieved. In these situations, external fixation has a place.[21]

In cases involving acute trauma, most elbows can be sufficiently stabilized with a unilateral frame incorporating half pins in the distal third of the humeral shaft and in the proximal third of either the radius or ulna. As with all external fixation applied in the upper extremity, these pins are best placed through limited incisions made at normal intervals. After the bone is exposed by blunt dissection between muscle planes, drill sleeves are used for predrilling and for placement of the half-threaded, blunt-tipped pins. On rare occasions, as with extensive soft-tissue loss and extreme instability, a triangular frame can be constructed in which transfixion pins placed through the distal humerus are connected laterally to half pins in the ulna. As a rule, external fixation of the elbow should be of brief duration, remaining in place only until soft tissues heal sufficiently to tolerate mobility.

A unique application of external fixation is found in the treatment, by distraction arthroplasty, of posttraumatic joint dysfunction.[21] Volkov and Oganesian[22] in 1975 helped introduce a hinged distractor that featured transosseous pins, external hinge joints, and an external fixation frame. Problems were noted, however, with accurate centering of flexible transosseous pins and with pin-track drainage.

In 1983 Deland and associates[23] reported a simpler elbow hinge distractor developed at the biomechanics laboratory of the Brigham and Women's Hospital. Each of these units is custom-made, using radiographs taken before surgery to ensure accurate positioning of the transosseous pins in the center of rotation of the distal humerus. A lock screw separates the humeral and ulnar components, and distraction can be achieved separately on the ulnar and radial side. This device can be also used with excisional arthroplasties of the elbow.

Forearm

The vast majority of displaced fractures of the forearm are suitably treated by internal fixation.[24] Even open fractures, including most grade I and grade II soft-tissue wounds, can safely be treated with plate fixation. In fact, in some cases of grade III injuries, plate fixation has been successful if suitable forearm musculature remains to cover the plate and underlying skeleton. For certain injuries, however, extensive internal fixation on the day of injury may not be advisable. Included in this category are heavily contaminated farm-related injuries, thermal burns, gunshots, or fractures associated with significant skeletal loss.

In some cases we have placed external fixation on the day of injury and defined the extent and depth of the wound. If at a second look, 24 to 48 hours later, the wound was clean and acceptable for secondary flap coverage, the external fixation was replaced by plate fixation.

In contrast to fractures of the humeral shaft, the goals with forearm fractures include the maintenance of length, angular and rotational alignment, and interosseous space. In many respects, such fractures resemble articular injuries in that the forearm joint is responsible for pronation and supination. Thus, when external skeletal fixation is considered for forearm fractures, care must be taken to use individual half-frames for each bone and to check for forearm rotation.

Because the neurovascular structures and gliding tendons are closely aligned to the forearm skeleton, placement of forearm pins requires direct exposure of the bone. Generally, two or three pins proximal and a like number distal to the fractures will suffice. In distal-third fractures, it is often best to place the distal pins

into the metacarpals (Fig. 2). Predrilled, blunt-tipped 4-mm half pins are recommended for most forearm fractures. Smaller pins should be considered for the metacarpals.

The placement of pins may also be dictated by the requirements, if any, for soft-tissue coverage. If an axial-pattern groin flap is needed, this must be taken into consideration in placing the pins. If the patient is agitated, it is sometimes advisable to place pins in the ipsilateral iliac crest and attach the forearm frame to the pelvis for a limited period of time. For reconstruction after posttraumatic infection or skeletal loss, external fixation may be used in the forearm to maintain skeletal length and alignment during the reconstructive procedures.

Fractures of the Distal Radius

In a patient with an unstable fracture pattern in whom anatomic restoration is deemed advantageous, external skeletal fixation is more likely than plaster to maintain the anatomy. External fixation also allows freer motion of the digits, forearm rotation, and elbow motion, which, among other advantages, helps reduce soft-tissue swelling.

It has been suggested that external fixation could cause wrist stiffness, but results of a number of studies fail to support this concern. In the landmark study at the Mayo Clinic by Cooney and associates,[25] only five of 60 patients lost more than 50% of wrist motion after treatment with external fixation. The average wrist dorsiflexion in healed wrists was 58 degrees compared with 62 degrees in uninjured wrists. Wrist palmar flexion figures were 52 degrees vs 62 degrees. Fixation devices with hinges are available,[26] but they are difficult to apply and do not give significantly better results.

External fixation in the upper extremity is most frequently used to treat complex distal radius fractures. Pin stabilization was popularized by Böhler[27] in 1929, and a number of surgeons have advocated the use of pins incorporated in plaster.[28] These methods led to a number of complications, however,[29,30] and the use of more rigid metal external fixators has been advocated by many authors.[25,26,31–40]

Despite the popularity of external fixation for fractures of the distal radius, basic questions still remain regarding its indications and applications. These included questions about the indications, the optimal frame configuration, the length of time the fixator is to be left in place, the use of a hinged distractor to provide early motion, possible complications and their prevention, and the role of combined external and internal fixation.

Indications Studies of distal radius fractures reveal some consensus regarding the indications of external fixations.[40,41] These include (1) such unstable fractures as those with metaphyseal comminution extending vo-

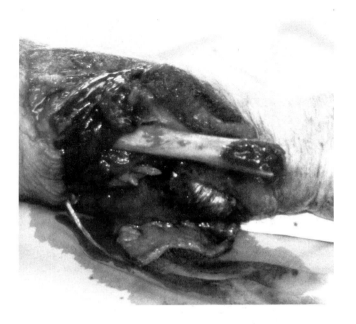

Fig. 2 A 48-year-old man sustained a grade III open fracture of his distal radius and ulna. **Top,** Extensive stripping and devascularization of the distal third of the radius is shown in this clinical photograph. **Bottom left,** An anteroposterior radiograph shows the fracture reduction with plating of the ulna and an external fixator to stabilize the radius. **Bottom right,** Six weeks later, a corticocancellous graft was placed in the defect of the distal radius.

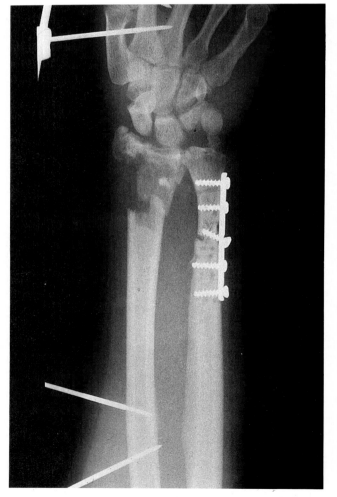

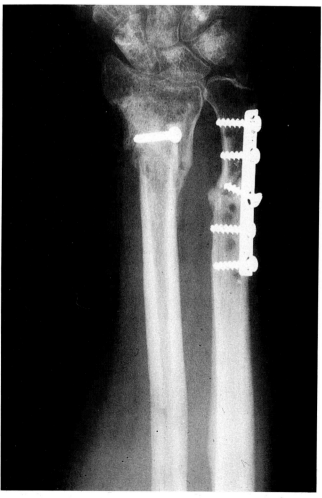

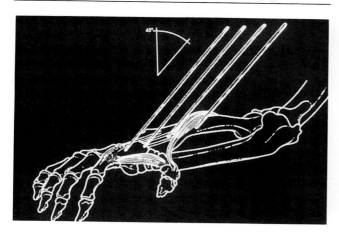

Fig. 3 The placement of the pins in the distal radius and metacarpal should be at least 45 degrees off the horizontal plane. (Reproduced with permission from Jakob RP: *The Small External Fixator.* Berne, Switzerland, AO Publications, 1983.)

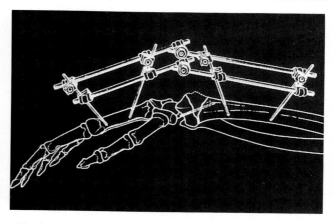

Fig. 4 A pin-bar external fixation frame should be versatile to permit correction in three planes. (Reproduced with permission from Jakob RP: *The Small External Fixator.* Berne, Switzerland, AO Publications, 1983.)

lar to the midaxial plane, fractures with severe displacement, intra-articular Frykman III to VIII fractures, and those with impacted articular fragments; (2) fractures that have redisplaced despite a closed reduction and appropriate plaster immobilization; (3) bilateral fractures; and (4) open fractures or fractures associated with major soft-tissue trauma.

Techniques The procedure is readily accomplished with regional Bier block anesthesia, axillary anesthesia, or general anesthesia.

There is some difference of opinion as to whether or not the fracture should be reduced and held in traction before the external fixator is applied. In general, unless a surgical approach to the fracture is anticipated, we find it easier to place the pins with the patient's arm resting on a hand table. Then, using image control, vertical traction is applied to reduce the fracture. The frame is then assembled and the pins connected.

Pin type and placement depend on the type of external frame available to the surgeon. In general, pin sites should be predrilled with a smaller core diameter drill bit, and the pins placed into the bone using a high-torque, low-speed power drill. This procedure minimizes bone necrosis and resultant pin loosening.

Our experience has been with frames supporting pins inserted along the dorsoradial side of the forearm and hand. We place two pins into the second metacarpal and two into the distal third of the radius.[42,43] As shown in Figures 3 and 4, the pins should be placed (1) 45 degrees off the horizontal plane to permit full extension of the thumb and (2) through small incisions with drill guides to prevent injury to nerves or tendons.

The two pins in the radius should parallel each other, as do the pins in the metacarpals. The position of the pins should be confirmed by radiograph before proceeding with fracture reduction and/or frame assembly.

It is most important to ensure that fracture reduction corrects not only radial length and volar tilt of the articular surface, but also rotational alignment. This latter consideration influenced our choice of a unilateral frame design that permits three-dimensional corrections during frame assembly. If possible, a 0.62-inch Kirschner wire should be inserted obliquely through the radial styloid into the opposite cortex to function as an internal splint. This pin is cut off just below the skin. Finally, attention is directed to the distal radioulnar joint. Instability there may be corrected by pinning the distal ulna to the radius. A larger ulnar styloid fracture can be stabilized by internally fixing the styloid, either with Kirschner wires or with a small screw.

Skin tension around the pins should be relieved, if necessary, before leaving the operating room. We generally place a compression gauze dressing around each pin and leave it in place for four to five days after surgery before beginning pin care. Additionally, we have found a short arm splint placed on the volar and ulnar surface to be helpful during the first week.

Patients are encouraged to begin shoulder, elbow, forearm, and digital motion as soon as they can do so comfortably. Follow-up with a therapist provides a useful means of monitoring a patient's progress. Follow-up radiographs are obtained 24 to 48 hours, one week, two weeks, and four weeks after surgery. After the fourth or fifth day, patients are encouraged to clean their pin sites two to three times a day with hydrogen peroxide (Figs. 5 to 7).

How long the external fixator must remain in place depends on a number of factors. Addition of a percutaneous styloid pin will permit frame removal for most fracture patterns after six to eight weeks. Ex-

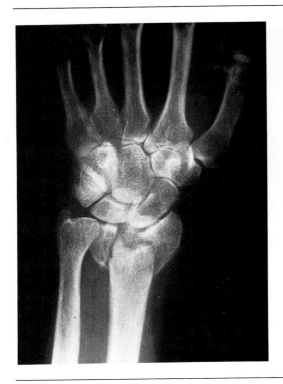

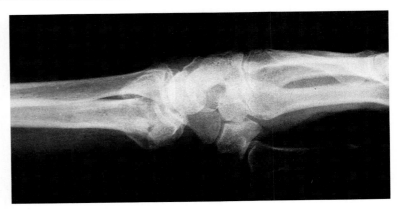

Fig. 5 A 62-year-old active woman sustained a comminuted unstable intra-articular fracture of the distal radius. Treatment consisted of closed reduction with longitudinal traction and manipulation, external fixation, and a percutaneous K-wire through the radial styloid. Anteroposterior **(left)** and lateral **(right)** radiographs reveal metaphyseal comminution and articular involvement.

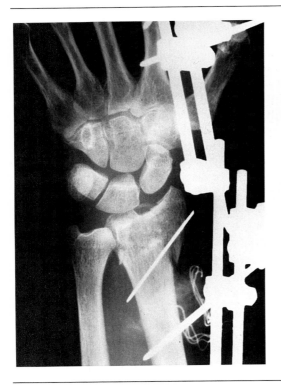

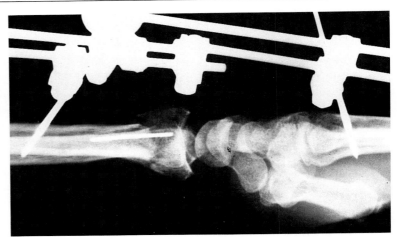

Fig. 6 Anteroposterior **(left)** and lateral **(right)** radiographs of the patient shown in Figure 5 made after reduction and application of the fixator and percutaneous K-wire.

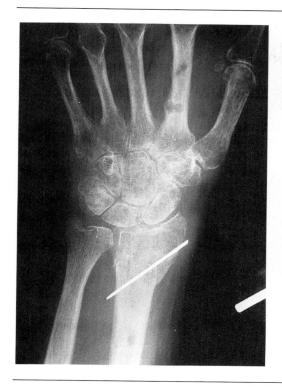

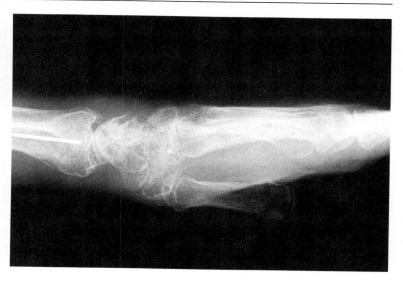

Fig. 7   Anteroposterior (**left**) and lateral (**right**) radiographs of the patient shown in Figures 5 and 6 at the time of frame removal, six weeks after the injury.

tremely comminuted, high-energy, metaphyseal-diaphyseal fractures in younger patients may require eight to ten weeks of immobilization. After frame removal, the patient should wear a volar splint for seven to 14 days and should begin wrist exercise during that time.

The most frequently reported complications of external fixation of distal radius fracture are infection, nerve injury, pin loosening or breakage, and loss of reduction.[30] Attention to detail, proper patient selection, careful follow-up, and willingness to change a pin or remove the frame will help minimize the risk of complications.

Fracture-Dislocation of the Carpus

Carpal fracture-dislocations usually respond to traction, closed or open reduction, internal fixation, and a two- to three-month period of cast immobilization.[44] The use of external fixation for carpal immobilization has several advantages. Reduction and internal fixation of the fractures is easier, carpal reduction is maintained, and the adjacent joints remain mobile.[45] External fixation is particularly useful in dealing with combined injuries of the same limb.[46]

Placement of the frame with two pins in the second metacarpal and two into the radial shaft, followed by manual reduction, facilitates the repositioning of ligaments.[45] After reduction, the frame and clamps are tightened, and surgical procedures can proceed with no assistance needed to maintain longitudinal traction.

The external fixator may be left in place until fracture union or ligamentous healing has taken place. The rigidity of the frame, in contrast to a cast, decreases the tendency of the capitate to migrate proximally and helps protect internal skeletal and ligamentous repairs. Such procedures as skin or bone grafting are easily accomplished with the frame in place.

The Hand

Many traumatic and reconstructive problems involving the tubular skeleton of the hand lend themselves to external fixation using scaled-down fixators and pins. Early methods of fixation included pins anchored in acrylic frames. These could not be adjusted after application and on occasion proved unstable.[47-50] The small Roger Anderson fixator, adjustable in only one plane, was also not very stable.[51,52]

Jaquet designed an improved minifixator in 1970 that has greatly expanded the applications of external fixation for hand problems.[7,53-60] His system is readily adjustable in three planes both during and after surgery. It can be applied before reducing the fracture and can be adjusted to either compress or distract the fracture site.

Few parts are required for a stable mounting with the Jaquet frame: a simple swiveling clamp, straight or offset pin holders, partially threaded self-tapping, blunt-tipped pins, and connecting bars. With 90 de-

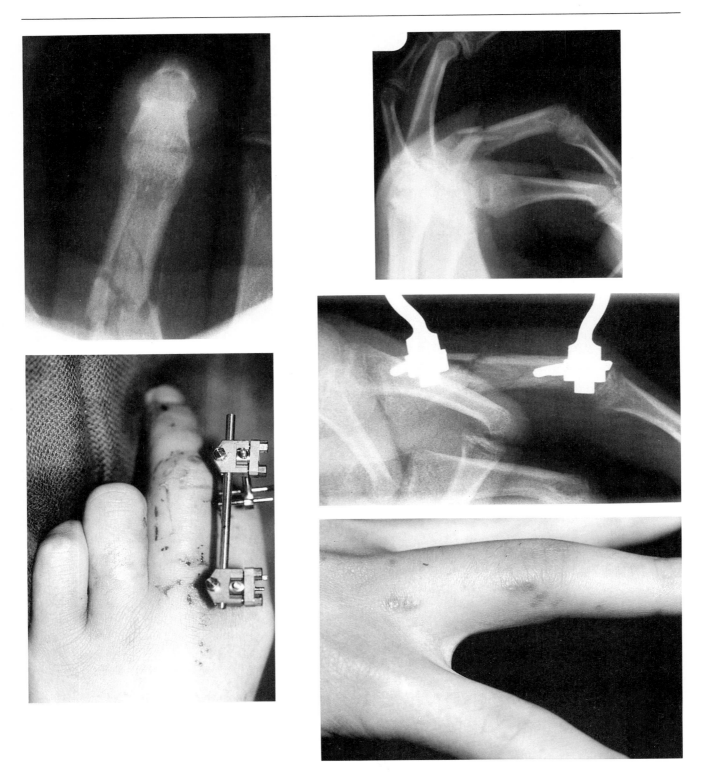

Fig. 8   A 14-year-old boy was admitted 2.5 weeks after injury with malposition of a comminuted proximal phalangeal fracture of his dominant long finger. The joints were stiff and digit malrotated and angulated. Anteroposterior and lateral radiographs (**top left** and **top right**) show the comminuted proximal phalangeal fracture with deformity. Early periosteal callus is visible. **Bottom left** and **center right**, A unilateral Jaquet frame was applied, the fracture manipulated, and the frame secured. **Bottom right**, Full motion and alignment and excellent fracture healing resulted.

grees of motion in the swiveling clamp and unlimited rotation of the pin holders, the frame can be adjusted to nearly any position.

Indications for external fixation of traumatic injuries in the hand include gunshot injuries, severely comminuted diaphyseal fractures (Fig. 8), comminuted articular fractures and fracture-dislocations, and fractures with loss of bone stock.

Digital lengthening, infected nonunions, and soft-tissue reconstructions are good candidates for external fixation for hand reconstruction.

Technique (Jaquet)

Several frame configurations are available for the phalanges and metacarpals. The unilateral frame is the most applicable. Pins should be inserted obliquely to the mid-axial line to avoid tethering of the extensor tendons and to reduce contact with neighboring digits. Drill holes are made through small incisions with 1.5-mm drill bits, and 2-mm blunt-tipped pins are inserted with a hand chuck. Because insertion of the pins is not limited by the technical restrictions of the frame, their placement can be adjusted to the anatomic and pathologic conditions of the involved skeletal unit. Two pins are inserted proximal and two are inserted distal to the fracture.

The pins are connected to straight or offset pinholders. Offset holders are used where there is limited distance between the pins. The pinholders are connected to swivel clamps, which are joined to a connecting rod of desired length. Once the entire frame is assembled, the surgeon reduces the bone manually, and the screws and swiveling clamps are tightened by an assistant. In some cases, particularly when crossing a joint or into the distal phalanx, 2-mm, central-threaded transfixion pins are used, held in place by triangular frames.

References

1. Lambotte A: *Chirurgie operatoire des fractures.* Paris, Masson, 1913.
2. Haynes HH: Treating fractures by skeletal fixation of the individual bone. *South Med J* 1939;32:720–724.
3. Stader O: A preliminary announcement of new method of treating fractures. *North Am Vet* 1937;18:37.
4. Anderson R, O'Neil G: Comminuted fractures of the distal end of the radius. *Surg Gynecol Obstet* 1944;78:434–440.
5. Hoffmann R: *Rotules à os pour la réduction dirigee non sanglante des fractures.* Paris, Congrès Français de Chirurgie, 1938, pp 601–610.
6. Jakob RP: Die Distraktion instabiler distaler Radiustrummerfrakturen mit einem Fixateur externe—ein neuer Behandlungsweg. *Z Unfallmed Berufskr* 1980;73:115–120.
7. Asche G, Haas HG, Klemm K: First experiences with the external mini fixator of Jaquet. *Aktuel Traumatol* 1979;9:261–268.
8. Schuind F, Pay-Pay E, Andrianne Y, et al: External fixation of the clavicle for fracture or non-union in adults. *J Bone Joint Surg* 1988;70A:692–695.
9. Brooker AF Jr: The use of external fixation in the treatment of burn patients with fractures, in Brooker AF Jr, Edwards CC (eds): *External Fixation: The Current State of the Art. Proceedings of the 6th International Conference on Hoffmann External Fixation.* Baltimore, Williams & Wilkins, 1979, pp 225–237.
10. Mears DC: The use of external fixation in arthrodesis, in Brooker AF Jr, Edwards CC (eds): *External Fixation: The Current State of the Art. Proceedings of the 6th International Conference on Hoffmann External Fixation.* Baltimore, Williams & Wilkins, 1979, pp 241–275.
11. Wild JJ Jr, Hanson GW, Bennett JB, et al: External fixation use in the management of massive upper extremity trauma. *Clin Orthop* 1982;164:172–176.
12. Santavirta S, Karaharju E, Korkala O: The use of osteotaxis as limb salvage procedure in severe compound injuries of the upper extremity. *Orthopedics* 1984;7:642–648.
13. Hierholzer G, Kleining R, Hörster G, et al: External fixation: Classification and indications. *Arch Orthop Trauma Surg* 1978;92:175–182.
14. Kamlin M, Michaelson M, Waisbrad H: The use of external fixation in the treatment of fractures of the humeral shaft. *Injury* 1988;19:245–248.
15. Hierholzer G, Hax P-M: External fixation of the upper extremity with the ASIF tubular set and Wagner apparatus, in Uhthoff HK (ed): *Current Concepts of External Fixation of Fractures.* Berlin, Springer-Verlag, 1982, pp 303–306.
16. Hinsenkamp M, Burny F: External fixation of the fracture of the humerus. *Orthopedics* 1984;7:1309–1314.
17. Burney F, Hinsenkamp, Donkerwolcke M: External fixation of the fractures of the humerus: Analysis of 100 cases, in Vidal J (ed): *Hoffmann External Fixator.* Montpellier, 1979, pp 191–202.
18. De Bastiani G, Aldegheri R, Renzi Brivio L: The treatment of fractures with a dynamic axial fixator. *J Bone Joint Surg* 1984;66B:538–545.
19. Wagner H: Tecnik un indikation der operativen verkurzing and verladerung von ober- und unterschenkel. *Orthopaedic* 1972;1:59.
20. Olerud S, Henriksson TG, Engkvist O: A free vascularized fibular graft in lengthening of the humerus with the Wagner apparatus: Report of a case in a twenty-year-old man. *J Bone Joint Surg* 1983;65A:111–114.
21. Cooney WP III: Contractures and burns, in Morrey BF (ed): *The Elbow and Its Disorders.* Philadelphia, WB Saunders, 1985, pp 433–451.
22. Volkov MV, Oganesian OV: Restoration of function in the knee and elbow with a hinge-distractor apparatus. *J Bone Joint Surg* 1975;57A:591–600.
23. Deland JJ, Walker PS, Sledge CB, et al: Treatment of posttraumatic elbows with a new hinge-distractor. *Orthopedics* 1983;6:732.
24. Moed BR, Kellam JF, Foster RJ, et al: Immediate internal fixation of open fractures of the diaphysis of the forearm. *J Bone Joint Surg* 1986;68A:1008–1017.
25. Cooney WP III, Linscheid RL, Dobyns JH: External pin fixation for unstable Colles' fractures. *J Bone Joint Surg* 1979;61A:840–845.
26. Clyburn TA: Dynamic external fixation for comminuted intra-articular fractures of the distal end of the radius. *J Bone Joint Surg* 1987;69A:248–254.
27. Böhler L: *The Treatment of Fractures,* ed 4. Baltimore, William Wood, 1935.
28. Green DP: Pins and plaster treatment of comminuted fractures of the distal end of the radius. *J Bone Joint Surg* 1975;57A:304–310.
29. Chapman DR, Bennett JB, Bryan WJ, et al: Complications of distal radial fractures: Pins and plaster treatment. *J Hand Surg* 1982;7:509–512.
30. Weber SC, Szabo RM: Severely comminuted distal radial fracture as an unsolved problem: Complications associated with external

fixation and pins and plaster techniques. *J Hand Surg* 1986;11A: 157–165.

31. Cooney WP III: External fixation of fractures of the distal radius, in Brooker AF Jr, Cooney WP III, Chao EY: *Principles of External Fixation.* Baltimore, Williams & Wilkins, 1983, pp 103–121.

32. Cooney WP: External fixation of distal radial fractures. *Clin Orthop* 1983;180:44–49.

33. Foster DE, Kopta JA: Update on external fixators in the treatment of wrist fractures. *Clin Orthop* 1986;204:177–183.

34. Grana WA, Kopta JA: The Roger Anderson device in the treatment of fractures of the distal end of the radius. *J Bone Joint Surg* 1979;61A:1234–1238.

35. Jenkins NH, Jones DG, Johnson SR, et al: External fixation of Colles' fractures: An anatomical study. *J Bone Joint Surg* 1987; 69B:207–211.

36. Kongsholm J, Olerud C: Comminuted Colles' fractures treated with external fixation. *Arch Orthop Trauma Surg* 1987;106:220–225.

37. Nakata RY, Chand Y, Matiko JD, et al: External fixators for wrist fractures: A biomechanical and clinical study. *J Hand Surg* 1985; 10A:845–851.

38. Ricciardi L, Diquigiovanni W: The external fixation treatment of distal articular fractures of the radius. *Orthopedics* 1984;7:637–641.

39. Vaughan PA, Lui SM, Harrington IJ, et al: Treatment of unstable fractures of the distal radius by external fixation. *J Bone Joint Surg* 1985;67B:385–389.

40. Vidal J, Buscayret CH, Paran M, et al: Ligamentotaxis, in Mears DC (ed): *External Skeletal Fixation.* Baltimore, Williams & Wilkins, 1983, pp 493–496.

41. Knirk JL, Jupiter JB: Intra-articular fractures of the distal end of the radius in young adults. *J Bone Joint Surg* 1986;68A:647–659.

42. Jakob RP: The small external fixator. *AO Bull*, 1983, pp 3–52.

43. Fernandez DL, Jakob RP, Büchler U: External fixation of the wrist: Current indications and technique. *Ann Chir Gynaecol* 1983;72:298–302.

44. Green DP, O'Brien ET: Open reduction of carpal dislocations: Indications and operative techniques. *J Hand Surg* 1978;3:250–265.

45. Fernandez DL, Ghillani R: External fixation of complex carpal dislocations: A preliminary report. *J Hand Surg* 1987;12A:335–347.

46. Jupiter JB: The management of multiple fractures in one upper extremity: A case report. *J Hand Surg* 1986;11A:279–282.

47. Aron JD: Brief Note: Using methylmethacrylate to make external fixation splints. *J Bone Joint Surg* 1976;58A:151.

48. Crockett DJ: Rigid fixation of bones of the hand using K wires bonded with acrylic resin. *Hand* 1974;6:106–107.

49. Dickson RA: Rigid fixation of unstable metacarpal fractures using transverse K-wires bonded with acrylic resin. *Hand* 1975;7: 284–286.

50. Pritsch M, Engel J, Farin I: Manipulation and external fixation of metacarpal fractures. *J Bone Joint Surg* 1981;63A:1289–1291.

51. Bilos ZJ, Eskestrand T: External fixator use in comminuted gunshot fractures of the proximal phalanx. *J Hand Surg* 1979;4:357–359.

52. Morton HS: Fractures of the wrist and hand. *Can Med Assoc J* 1944;51:430–434.

53. Freeland AE, Sparks DR: Hand injury: Repair and reconstruction with an external mini-fixator. *Hosp Physician* 1985;21:19.

54. Freeland AE: External fixation for skeletal stabilization of severe open fractures of the hand. *Clin Orthop* 1987;214:93–100.

55. Riggs SA Jr, Cooney WP III: External fixation of complex hand and wrist fractures. *J Trauma* 1983;23:332–336.

56. Seitz WH Jr, Gomez W, Putnam MD, et al: Management of severe hand trauma with a mini external fixateur. *Orthopedics* 1987;10: 601–610.

57. Asche G: Operative Versorgung von Verletzungen und Erkrankungen der Hand mit dem Minifixateur externe [Operative treatment of injuries and diseases of the hand with external mini fixateur]. *Beitr Orthop Traumatol* 1980;27:711–717.

58. Asche G: Stabilisierungsmöglichkeit einer intraartikulären Trummerfraktur des ersten Mittelhandknochens mit dem Minifexateur externe [Possibilities for stabilization of an intra-articular comminuted fracture of the first metacarpal: Use of the external mini fixator]. *Handchirurgie* 1981;13:247–249.

59. Richard JC, Latouche X, Lemerle JP, et al: La place du fixateur externe dans le traitement en urgence des traumatismes graves ouverts de la main: Présentation d'une technique originale [External fixation in emergency treatment of severe open traumatisms of the hand: An original technique]. *Ann Chir* 1980;34: 699–701.

60. Nonnenmacher J: Osteosynthesis of fractures of the base of the first metacarpal by an external fixator. *Ann Chir Main* 1983;2: 250–257.

Complications of Pin and Wire External Fixation

Stuart A. Green, MD

Introduction

Recent interest in circular transfixion-wire external fixation has been stimulated by reports from Professor Gavriil A. Ilizarov, MD, of Kurgan, USSR. These reports describe dramatic clinical results achieved when the Ilizarov circular fixator, designed in 1951, is used in conjunction with a system of orthopaedic procedures he developed between 1955 and 1965.

At first, Ilizarov did not mention the complications associated with his method, but a review of reports from his Institute in Kurgan, and from other hospitals in the Soviet Union and Italy, indicates that the complication rates associated with transfixion-wire external fixation are about the same as those noted by orthopaedic surgeons elsewhere who were using threaded pins for external skeletal fixation. The trend in threaded-pin external fixation techniques during the past decade has been away from half-pin and toward transfixion-wire applications, with the pins inserted into subcutaneous bone wherever possible. Biomechanical studies[1] have shown that a circular transfixion-wire external fixator resists shear motion better than half-pin and full-pin frames. At the same time, they are more dynamic in axial loading, a feature, according to proponents of circular fixation, that stimulates osseous healing.

Various kinds of difficulties can arise with the use of a fixator. The least severe of these may be resolved by modifying the frame or changing patient management. Certain other difficulties are more serious and can only be alleviated either by a return trip to the operating room while the fixator is in place or by physical therapy or some other intensive management program once the fixator is removed.

The most serious difficulties are those that adversely affect the final outcome. Such problems, which may or may not be relieved by additional surgical procedures, include permanent numbness, shortening, residual angulation, permanent limitation of motion, and so forth. For purposes of comparing pin and wire external fixation, it is simplest to consider all these levels of difficulties as complications.

In this chapter, I will consider complications that are common to pin and wire fixators, as well as complications unique to one or the other of these two fixation systems. I will also discuss the preventive measures common to both types of fixators as well as those unique to each category of fixator.

Pin- or Wire-Tract Infections

In 1983, I reviewed the English-language literature published between 1944 and 1980 dealing with external fixation pin sepsis.[2] Tabulating the total number of major pin-tract infections, such as purulent discharge, osteolysis, and pin-hole osteomyelitis, I calculated an 8.4% overall major pin infection rate when pin fixators were employed. At about the same time, researchers at Ilizarov's institute summarized the complications associated with 3,669 fixator applications during the period from 1970 through 1975.[3] Analyzing wire-tract infections, they found an 8.3% rate of purulent soft-tissue sepsis and a 0.2% rate of wire-hole osteomyelitis, for a total infection rate of 8.5%. This similarity in implant sepsis rates between pin and wire fixators should not be a surprise. After all, limb transfixion, whether by smooth wire or threaded pin, violates the body's principal barrier to bacterial invasion—the intact skin.

Threaded pins offer enhanced osseous fixation in exchange for a larger foreign body and perhaps greater tissue damage at insertion. Smooth wires cause less tissue damage but attach less securely to bone than do threaded pins; hence, the propensity for bone-fixator instability is greater. For this reason, smooth-wire external fixators must employ two or more tensioned wires at each ring level to prevent the bone from shuttling back and forth. Ideally, these wires should be at a 90-degree angle to each other, but anatomic constraints limit such mountings to a few regions of the body. For this reason, it is often necessary to insert more than two wires at acute angles to each other, and this increases the total number of wire-skin interfaces.

Although the principles that have evolved to prevent either pin or wire infections are the same for both types of implants, the techniques employed are different. The first principle is to avoid necrosis of tissues at the time of pin or wire insertion. Necrosis of the soft tissues can be caused by winding of tissues around the implant, by excessive tension, or by thermal injury from heat generated during drilling.

A threaded pin—especially a modern one with self-cutting flutes at the tip—can wind soft tissues into the thread's grooves. For this reason, one should always use a trochar and sleeve to insert threaded pins into bone. With transfixion wires, the bayonet point used for cortical bone transfixion might also ensnare soft tissues; therefore, push transfixion wires straight

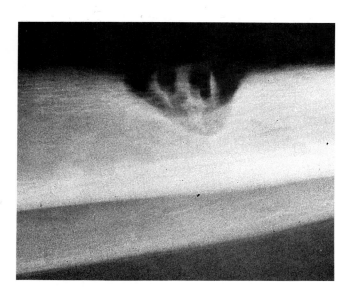

Fig. 1 A double ring sequestrum probably caused by a thermal injury related to intracortical (rather than transmedullary) pin insertion. (Reproduced with permission from Green SA: *Complications of External Skeletal Fixation.* Springfield, Ilinois, Charles C Thomas, 1981.)

through the tissue to bone before turning on the drill. If the wire misses the bone, do not redirect it within the limb's tissues. Instead, reinsert it only after withdrawing it completely. As soon as a transfixion wire penetrates the bone's far cortex, stop the drill to keep tissues on the limb's opposite side from winding around

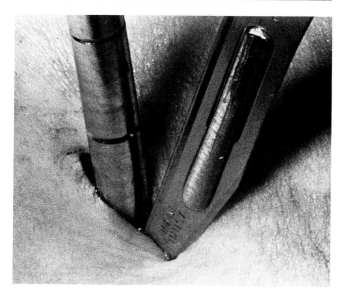

Fig. 2 Releasing tension adjacent to a transosseous pin: insert a No. 11 blade into the ridge of skin adjacent to the pin to enlarge the hole.

the wire-tip. To drive the wire through these tissues, grasp the wire with pliers and hit the pliers with a mallet.

Do not use a power drill to insert a threaded pin directly into bone. Heat buildup at the pin's point could cause a thermal injury to bone. Instead, predrill the bone hole with a sharp fluted drill bit and a drill sleeve and insert the pin with a hand drill.

When drilling with a drill bit, a self-drilling threaded pin, or a transfixion wire, stop the drill every few seconds to allow the cutting tip to cool down. The heat generated by drilling not only damages the bone, but also work-hardens the osseous tissue, causing it to resist further advancement. A worthwhile practice is to irrigate the exposed portion of the drill bit or wire to cool it and conduct heat away from the tip.

If much resistance is encountered during drilling, when finished, grasp the drill-bit tip or emerging transfixion-wire tip between your fingers to check its temperature. If the tip cannot be comfortably held for 15 or 20 seconds, do not leave the implant in the bonehole. To do so would risk chronic osteomyelitis by placing necrotic, thermally injured bone in communication with the pinhole's bacteriologic environment. Instead, remove the implant, allow the point to cool off, and reinsert it elsewhere.

In a report published in 1984, Ripley and I[4] observed that most cases of sequestrum-associated chronic pintract osteomyelitis were associated with intracortical, rather than transmedullary, pin insertion (Fig. 1). We advised that pins be inserted through a wide portion of a bone, advice that seems appropriate for smooth transfixion wires as well. Two distinct cortices will be felt if a pin crosses the medullary canal. Moreover, whenever osseous resistance to pin or wire progress is encountered, a slow stop-and-start insertion technique is essential to prevent burning of bone.

Once the pin or wire is in place, soft-tissue tension around the implant can produce necrosis and lead to local sepsis. With pins, tension is released by pushing a No. 11 blade into the ridge of skin on the tensioned side of the pin hole, thereby enlarging the hole in the opposite direction (Fig. 2). With transfixion wires, a different tension-release strategy is employed. Do not incise the redundant skin ridge adjacent to the wire; instead, slowly withdraw the wire (with pliers and a mallet) until its tip drops below the skin's surface. Allow the skin to shift to a more neutral location and advance the wire again until it pokes through the skin in an improved position (Fig. 3). If the soft-tissue tension occurs on the insertion side of a limb, cut off the wire's blunt end obliquely to create a point, advance the wire to just below the skin's surface as described above, and tap the wire back through the skin after adjusting the skin's position.

When an olive wire (a wire, thicker at one point, that is used to move or stabilize bone segments) causes ten-

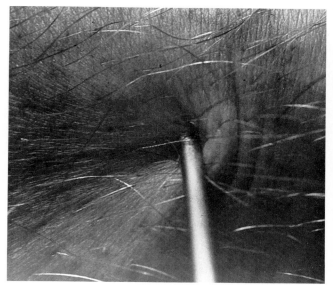

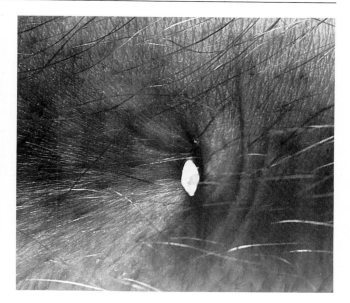

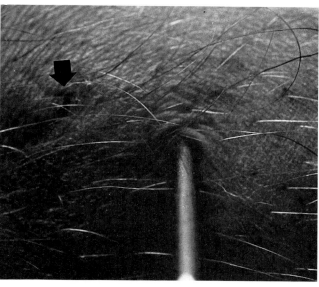

Fig. 3 Top left, Tension adjacent to a transcutaneous wire appears as a ridge of skin on the compression side of the wire. **Top right,** To release tension, back the wire out until the point drops below the skin surface. **Bottom,** Push the point forward after readjusting the skin position. (The arrow points to the original wire-hole.)

sion on the side of the limb adjacent to the olive, merely enlarge the hole initially made to pass the olive through the skin. If the tension occurs on the limb's side opposite the olive, back the olive wire out with the pliers-mallet technique, and readjust the skin position.

With transfixion wires, it is necessary to check the range of motion to make sure that no undue tension occurs within the range that will be required while the fixator is on the limb. If necessary, a wire should be reinserted if movement of an adjacent joint causes undue skin tension around a wire.

Occasionally, a full- or half-pin must be bent slightly to fit into its pin-gripping clamp. Similarly, the Swiss AO group recommends bending pins slightly within each cluster to help stiffen the bone-fixator configu-

ration. In either situation, slight bending of a pin will be tolerated by the soft tissues, as the tissue pressure is distributed across the pin's broad surface. However, when transfixion wires are used, bending the wire for ring attachment may cause excessive soft-tissue damage, because the narrow wire concentrates pressure over a smaller area. For this reason, transfixion-wire fixator systems use special strategies to avoid bending a wire during frame attachment. The original Ilizarov equipment employs washers, posts, and other hardware to achieve this goal (Fig. 4). Other circular fixators use other techniques. In any case, not bending a wire when attaching it to a frame is critical to successful smooth-wire external fixation.

Preventing tissue motion at the implant is another

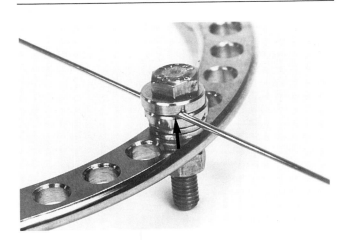

Fig. 4   With the Ilizarov system, washers and other hardware are used to build up from a ring to a wire to avoid bending the wire when attaching it to the ring.

principle in avoiding pin or wire sepsis. A bulky wrap of gauze filling the space between the skin and the fixator (Fig. 5) should be used in the first month or so after the frame is applied. Special slotted sponges have been developed that accomplish the same purpose with transfixion wire fixators. In the Soviet Union and Italy, medicine-bottle stoppers are placed over each transfixion wire to hold gauze sponges against the skin, thereby achieving skin-wire interface stability. Smooth wires do not hold the bone securely (leading to possible sliding of bone and soft tissues along the wire), and so more than one wire must be employed at each level of fixation

to secure the bone within the ring, and this, too, helps to prevent soft-tissue sepsis along the implant.

Various pin- and wire-care protocols have been suggested over the years, but no technique seems to be best. I prefer to cover pin or wire sites with a bulky wrap, and to leave them untouched while the frame is on the patient, unless a problem develops at the site. The patient can shower with the frame on, but should rewrap the pin-sites afterwards with the bulky wrap.

At the first sign of soft-tissue inflammation, oral antistaphylococcal antibiotics should be started, and the patient's activities should be curtailed. If these measures do not relieve the problem within a 48- to 72-hour period, the patient should be admitted to the hospital for parenteral antibiotic therapy. If necessary, an implant may have to be removed and another inserted elsewhere to control sepsis. When removing an infected pin or wire, be sure to curette the bone hole if there is radiographic evidence of osteolysis or sequestrum formation. Chronic pin-site or wire-site osteomyelitis should be treated with a parenteral course of antibiotics, curettage, and perhaps bone grafting or some other technique used to deal with chronic osteomyelitis.

Nerve and Vessel Injury

In 1981[5] I estimated the incidence of nerve and vessel injury associated with pin external fixation (based on a review of the English-language literature) to be about 0.5%. The rate of wire-associated neurovascular injuries in the Kurgan series[3] was 0.41%.

Smooth transfixion wires measuring 1.5 or 1.8 mm

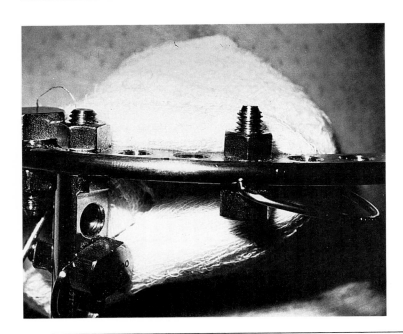

Fig. 5   A bulky gauze wrap should fill the space between the skin and the frame.

are about the same diameter as 18- and 16-gauge needles, respectively. Therefore, a transfixion wire may pass straight through a nerve—especially a large one—without causing much harm. If the wire's bayonet tip is rotating as the nerve is penetrated, greater damage might occur. This possibility supports the recommendation that wires be pushed directly through soft tissues to bone before the drill is turned on. A wire can also traverse a major vein or artery without causing much harm, because the hole in the vessel is about the same size as one created by an intravenous catheter. When a vessel is penetrated, bleeding may be encountered at either the wire's insertion or its exit hole. When this happens, use the pliers-mallet technique to withdraw the wire without spinning it, and insert the wire elsewhere. Slight pressure on the hole will usually stop the bleeding within a few minutes.

Delayed bleeding may occur about a month after the fixator is applied. The problem, which is not common, is cause by delayed erosion of the vessel resting against a pin or wire. Obviously, the implant should be removed when such bleeding is encountered. If the bleeding does not stop, arteriography may identify the problem. In some cases, vessel-wall erosion and bleeding may become apparent only when the implant is removed.

Limb elongation can also produce nerve or vessel problems. If tingling, numbness, or other trophic disturbances occur during limb lengthening, the distraction should be stopped or even reversed for several days until neuromotor function returns to normal.

Pin or Wire Placement

In 1981, I wrote a monograph[5] that featured a zone system for pin placement. The method was developed to lessen the possibility of neurovascular injuries. With the use of threaded half-pin external fixation, insertion into subcutaneous bone greatly reduces the likelihood of damage to a nerve, vessel, or tendon. With the introduction of transfixion-wire external fixation into Western countries, the zone system, which makes use of the cross-sectional anatomy of the leg, is helpful for application of a circular external fixator.

Certain danger areas should generally be avoided at the time a fixator is applied. In the lower portion of the leg, at the junction of the third and fourth quarters of the tibia, the anterior tibial artery and deep peroneal nerve cross the lateral surface of the tibia. This region is unsafe for transfixion-wire insertion unless the location of this neurovascular bundle is known.

In the thigh, the profundus femoris artery crosses the medial femoral cortex in the proximal part of the second quarter. Half-pins in the proximal femur should not penetrate beyond the far cortex of the bone, lest the profundus femoris artery be damaged. The super-

ficial femoral artery passes the coronal plane of the femur at midshaft; pins inserted into the mid-femur may transfix this vessel if care is not taken to avoid the coronal plane at the time of insertion.

In the upper limb, the radial nerve surrounds the humeral shaft's lateral cortex throughout the second and third quarters of the bone's length. I recommend open pin insertion in this area when threaded half-pins are used and careful palpation to determine the location and extent of the nerve before transfixion wire insertion.

In the forearm, transfixion-wire insertion is dangerous in many regions. For this reason, I suspect most surgeons trained in Western countries will prefer to use half-pins, even when a circular external fixator is applied to correct a complex musculoskeletal problem.

Broken Components

The manufacturers of external fixator components provide no warranty for the parts if used for more than one patient application. Nevertheless, the components can be used over and over again without concern for breakage, provided the parts are inspected before attachment to a patient. The head of a threaded bolt used for transfixion wire attachment or in a pin-gripping clamp may break off during tightening. If this occurs, merely replace the broken bolt.

Long threaded rods used in either pin or wire systems can become damaged when grasped by pliers. The surgical team will encounter difficulty moving nuts along such damaged hardware. Bent or damaged threaded components should be discarded.

Pin breakage can occur, especially if the pin is subjected to substantial stresses when the patient walks. Pins usually break at the junction of the threaded and smooth portions. Such breakage may occur at the bone's surface, leaving the threaded portion of the pin within the bone. To minimize this problem, do not prestress threaded half-pins by bending them during fixator attachment.

Smooth transfixion wires occasionally break while a frame is on a patient. When this happens, I suspect that the wire was damaged at the time of insertion, possibly by an overtight wire chuck or when the wire was grasped with pliers during insertion. If enough wires have been incorporated into the configuration, it may not be necessary to replace the broken wire; merely remove it. If the frame becomes unstable when a wire breaks, remove the broken wire and insert another at a nearby location.

Fixator Problems

The fixator itself may impinge on the soft tissues if inadequate room has been allowed for postoperative

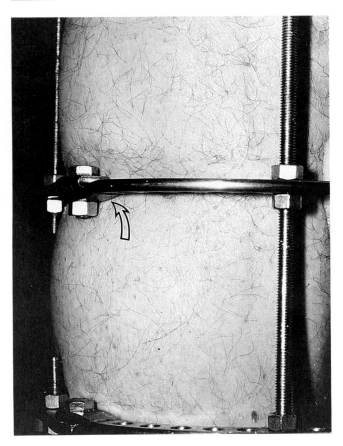

Fig. 6 Be sure to allow enough room for limb swelling when applying an external fixator. A half-pin fixator can usually be slid away from the skin along the pins, but a circular fixator cannot. (Arrow points to compressed skin and calf muscle.)

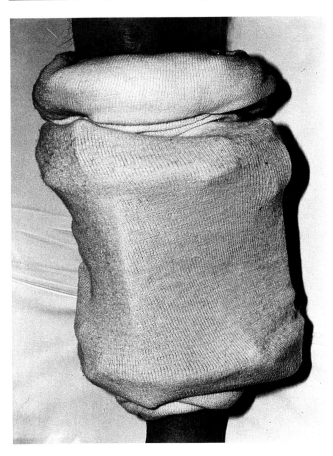

Fig. 7 A double-thickness 6-inch stockinette can be used for psychological and hygienic reasons to cover an external fixator.

swelling (Fig. 6). Similarly, when a fixator is used to correct a deformity, some element of the frame may impede movement of the limb segments. In either situation, an adjustment may be necessary. Be sure to stabilize the fixator with a temporary strut before moving any important structural elements of a frame.

The tips of pins or wires can catch on clothing and bedding, even when they are properly covered or curled into the frame. For this reason, I now routinely enclothe every external fixator with a double-thickness stockinette (Fig. 7).

As a patient with a circular external fixator in place lies in bed, it is possible for the limb to displace within the frame. To avoid this possibility, position olive wires in positions to prevent such shifting. Usually, the olive must be resting against the bone's posterior surface to prevent the frame from displacing anteriorly. Where neurovascular and tendinous structures lie along a bone's posterior surface, use of this technique may not be possible. It is also helps to modify the patient's bed so that the fixator-stabilized limb can rest in a comfortable position at the same plane as the rest of the

body. This modification can be accomplished by placing such supports as mats or folded blankets so that they raise the rest of the patient's body to the level of the stabilized limb.

Tardy Union

The subject of delayed bone healing in external fixation has been considered in prior instructional course lectures. The fixator's rigidity may inhibit callus formation yet not be stiff enough to allow primary bone healing.[6] Whether the fixator uses pins or wires, certain principles are helpful in preventing tardy bone healing. These are (1) accurate anatomic reduction with restoration of the limb's mechanical axis; (2) functional use of the limb stabilized in an external fixator; (3) interfragmentary compression where possible; (4) early autogenous cancellous bone grafting; (5) dynamization of the fixator during the course of fracture or nonunion healing.

The importance of anatomic reduction cannot be overemphasized. One of the principal advantages of a modular fixation system incorporating threaded rods, posts, and other hardware is the ability to reduce mal-aligned and malrotated bone segments gradually, thereby restoring a limb's mechanical axis (Fig. 8). Often, correction of the axis seems to promote rapid osseous healing.

During the final stages of healing, a fixator—whether pin or wire—must be dynamized to encourage final maturation and corticalization of the new osseous tissue. With pin fixators, dynamization can be achieved by removing pins, by increasing the pin-clamp distance from the limb, or by reducing the number of connecting rods between pin-clamps. In one recently developed fixation system, it is possible to exchange the connecting rods for less rigid ones. Other fixators dynamize when locking nuts are released along telescopic connecting rods. With transfixion-wire frames, the fixator, which is already quite axially dynamic, can be further dynamized by loosening nuts that secure the rings to connecting rods, or by eliminating redundant wires from the configuration.

If there is any doubt about the quality of osseous union, a patient should be placed in an orthotic support when either a pin or wire fixator is removed.

Contractures

Limb lengthening with any external fixator may produce joint contractures, subluxations, or dislocations, because myofascial tissue resists stretching.[7] The problem is most noticeable with muscles that cross two joints, because the patient may flex either joint to relieve discomfort in the elongating muscle. Thus, lengthening a tibia can produce either knee flexion or ankle equinus because of tension on the gastrocnemius muscle. In principle, such problems associated with limb lengthening can be avoided or managed by one of the following methods: (1) proper placement of pins or wires near joints to avoid interfering with joint function; (2) intensive physiotherapy to maintain joint motion; (3) frequent roentgenographic assessment of joints likely to dislocate or subluxate; or (4) joint distraction with external fixation if needed to overcome a fixed contracture.

Angulation

During limb lengthening, a bone segment may angulate, rotate, or translate at the level of the distraction gap (Fig. 9). As with joint contractures, the deformity is related to resistance of myofascial tissues to elongation; hence, the direction of the deformity can usually be predicted by the location of a limb's main muscle bulk. In the lower leg, for example, the tibia tends to angulate anteriorly because of the gastrocnemius-soleus muscles. It moves into valgus proximally because of the anterior compartment muscles, and into varus distally because of the deep posterior compartment muscles. The femur angulates anteriorly because of the hamstrings, moving into varus proximally, pulled by the adductor muscles, and usually into valgus distally because of the iliotibial band. The humerus will angulate into varus proximally and recurvatum distally.

Appropriate preventive measures include placement of olive wires in strategic locations when wire fixators are used, frame modifications to anticipate such deformities, or use of a stiff half-pin frame capable of resisting deformity. Once a deformity occurs, the fixator frame must be modified to achieve correction.[8] This time-consuming procedure can usually be accomplished in an outpatient setting, unless supplementary wires or pins are needed to secure bone fragments.

Problems With Regenerating Bone

Ilizarov's method often includes the creation of a distraction gap where new bone regenerates during elongation or angulation of the osteotomized segments.[9,10] The regenerating bone in a distraction gap may ossify too rapidly, limiting distraction, or, more commonly, may mature too slowly, prolonging the fixator application for the patient.[11]

Ordinarily, the distraction gap will show small hazy patches of calcification, often within the first two weeks following cortical osteotomy of a long bone. This two-week period consists of five days of predistraction fixation, followed by nine days of distraction at a rate of 1 mm/day. If no calcification appears within the distraction gap by the end of the second week, do not be concerned. Merely adjust the rate of distraction to a slower rate for the next two weeks. By the fourth week after surgery, some calcification should be visible within the distraction gap. If it is not, reverse the distraction, and compress the gap over a period of two to three days. Then, after a brief rest of three or four days, commence distraction once again. Usually, bone will form during the second distraction interval.

If at any point during elongation the quality of neo-osteogenesis within the distraction gap causes concern, the distraction can be stopped or reversed briefly in what has been called an "accordion" procedure. Ideally, the regenerate bone should appear on roentgenograms as longitudinal striations attached to both cortical fragments and a clear radiolucent growth zone will remain in the center.

Once elongation or correction has been completed, leave the fixator in place for at least as long as the time spent during elongation or deformity correction. Note that this period of neutral fixation following correction is often difficult for the patient to tolerate, so the surgeon should emphasize the importance of this step.

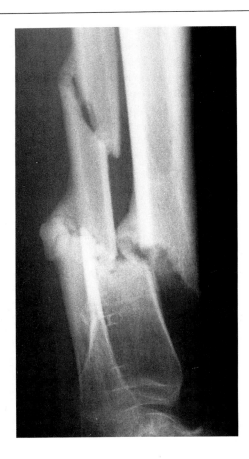

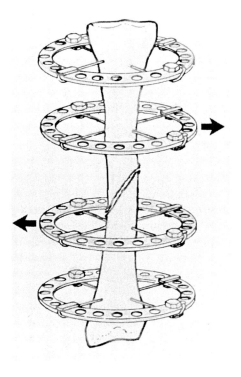

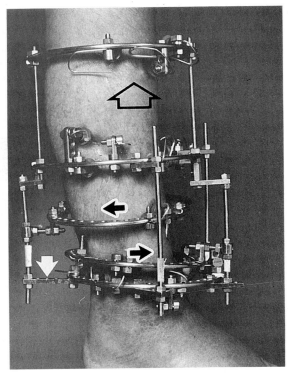

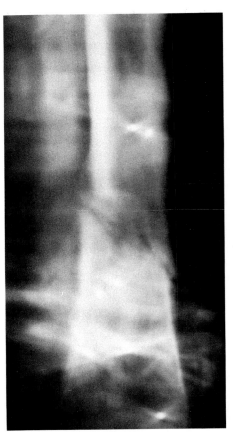

Fig. 8   Top left, A fully displaced overlapping tibial nonunion at eight months. Anteroposterior interfragmentary compression in this position will not result in union. Instead, the fracture site must be distracted prior to interfragmentary compression. **Top right,** The scheme of interfragmentary compression using countertension on rings adjacent to the fracture site. **Bottom left,** The apparatus used to realign the fracture can simultaneously lengthen the limb and apply interfragmentary compression with rings adjacent to the fracture site. **Bottom right,** An anatomic reduction (seen on a tomogram) obtained with the apparatus. The fracture healed ten weeks after reduction was accomplished.

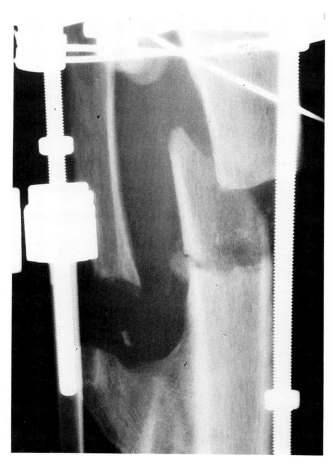

Fig. 9 Valgus angulation occurring during limb elongation for posttraumatic shortening. Appropriately placed olive wires and prophylactic ring positioning would have prevented this problem.

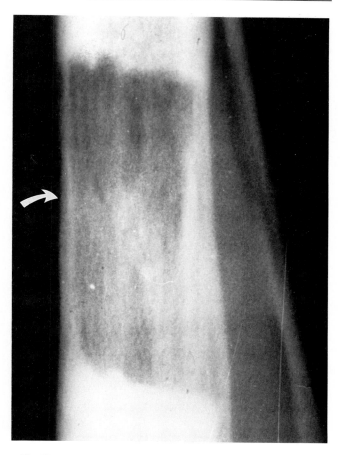

Fig. 10 Maturation of the distraction-gap regenerate bone. Prior to fixator removal, the bone in the distraction gap should be fully corticalized (arrow) without scalloping along the edge and should have relatively uniform density without large radiolucencies ("cysts") within its substance.

Towards the end of the neutral-fixation period, Ilizarov recommends compressing the frame about 0.25 mm twice a week. This maneuver is used for both the regenerate bone in a distraction gap and for any areas of tardy bone healing at a fracture or nonunion site.

The fixator can be removed when the regenerate is mature (Fig. 10) and demonstrates (1) no defects or scalloping along the regenerated bone edge farthest from the periosteal blood supply (for example, along the anterior tibial edge), (2) complete ossification of the radiolucent central growth zone of the regenerated bone, and (3) uniform radiographic density of the regenerated bone in both projections. At this time the regenerated bone should have a radiographic density that is midway between that seen in the adjacent cortical bone and that seen in its marrow canal.

Prior to removal of either a pin or a wire fixator, loosen the frame and allow it to "float" on the limb to test osseous stability. If the threaded connecting rods are loosened, the rings above and below the distraction region may not be secure enough for patient comfort.

Also, if the frame must be restabilized because the limb is not ready for fixator removal, the wires will be loose. For these reasons, it is often necessary to renew the tension on the wires if ring positions are altered at the end of the neutral fixation period.

A cast or brace is rarely needed after removal of a dynamized external fixator. A stiff fixator that does not permit dynamization, however, should be followed by some sort of external support for at least one to two months following fixator removal. Otherwise, the poorly ossified, newly formed bone will deform with weightbearing.

Conclusion

It is obvious from the foregoing discussion that both transfixion-wire and threaded-pin external fixators are associated with a multitude of problems. Moreover, the expanded indications for external fixation now coming to us from the Soviet Union will present a new constellation of difficulties as surgeons perform limb lengthening and deformity correction to correct an expanding array of problems. With attention to detail, many complications of external fixation can be avoided. Prompt recognition and action can avert other impending problems. Further studies will clarify the best use for pin fixators, wire fixators, and combinations of these types of transosseous stabilization.

References

1. Fleming B, Paley D, Kristensen T, et al: A biomechanical analysis of the Ilizarov external fixator. *Clin Orthop* 1989;241:95–105.
2. Green SA: Complications of external skeletal fixation. *Clin Orthop* 1983;180:109–116.
3. Deviatov A, Kaplunov A: Complications with the use of the Ilizarov apparatus: Applications of compression distraction osteosynthesis, in *Traumatology and Orthopaedics*. Kurgan, 1978.
4. Green SA, Ripley MJ: Chronic osteomyelitis in pin tracks. *J Bone Joint Surg* 1984;66A:1092–1098.
5. Green SA: *Complications of External Skeletal Fixation: Causes, Prevention, and Treatment*. Springfield, Illinois, Charles C Thomas, 1981.
6. Green SA: Complications of external fixation, in Murray JA (ed): American Academy of Orthopaedic Surgeons *Instructional Course Lectures, XXXIII*. St. Louis, CV Mosby, 1984, pp 138–143.
7. Paley D: Current techniques of limb lengthening. *J Pediatr Orthop* 1988;8:73–92.
8. Ilizarov GA: Angular deformities with shortening, in Coombs R, Green SA, Sarmiento A (eds): *External Fixation and Functional Bracing*. London, Orthotext, 1989.
9. Ilizarov GA: The tension-stress effect on the genesis and growth of tissues: Part I. The influence of stability of fixation and soft-tissue preservation. *Clin Orthop* 1989;238:249–281.
10. Ilizarov GA: The tension-stress effect on the genesis and growth of tissues: Part II. The influence of the rate and frequency of distraction. *Clin Orthop* 1989;239:263–285.
11. Green SA: Ilizarov external fixation: Technical and anatomic considerations. *Bull Hosp Dis Orthop Inst* 1988;48:28–35.

External Fixation in the Multiply Injured Patient

Andrew R. Burgess, MD

Introduction

In many cases, the patient who has suffered multiple injuries as a result of blunt trauma goes into shock, usually from hypovolemia caused by bleeding. The team treating such a patient must reverse the shock state as quickly as possible, directing immediate efforts toward airway control, breathing, and circulation.[1]

Hemorrhagic shock results from external or internal bleeding. External bleeding can be seen, and the assessment and examination that accompany the first resuscitation efforts will quickly determine its extent and significance. Internal bleeding can occur only in the chest, the peritoneal cavity, the retroperitoneal space, or at the site of a major extremity fracture. The initial physical examination plus radiographic studies will aid in locating any internal bleeding.

Clinical Intervention

External fixation in the multiply injured patient is indicated when there is a need (1) to treat major hemorrhage, related to bleeding from the pelvic ring or closed long-bone fractures; (2) to stabilize skeletal injuries to aid in the treatment of combined musculoskeletal and vascular injuries severe enough to threaten limb loss or death; and (3) to temporize severe extremity injuries while addressing other life-threatening injuries. Although the preferred treatment of certain musculoskeletal injuries, especially intra-articular injuries, may involve open reduction and internal fixation[2] by complex intramedullary rodding or plating procedures, these procedures may have to be delayed while such injuries or conditions as hypothermia and coagulopathy are addressed. Under such circumstances, external fixation stabilizes long-bone fractures and allows access to open wounds, while minimizing surgical intervention and further loss of blood. This combination of virtues makes external fixation a logical choice for temporary stabilization.

Later, the external fixation may be converted to a more definitive external or internal fixation, or additional periarticular or articular reconstruction may be undertaken.[3] If the patient's overall status precludes such treatment, the external fixation already in place can be adjusted to provide increased stabilization. This versatility—the fact that it stabilizes long-bone and intra-articular fractures, decreases additional hemorrhage, and provides wound access—makes external fixation particularly useful in multitrauma treatment.

Pelvis

Although bleeding associated with pelvic-ring disruption is sometimes related to the bony fracture itself, it more frequently results from rupture of retroperitoneal vessels. The way the pelvic ring is disrupted is important because the amount of force required for pelvic-ring disruption and the direction in which that force is applied[4] determine the amount of vascular damage. Vessels at risk in pelvic-ring fractures include the internal iliac artery; its branches, which are the lateral sacral, iliolumbar, and superior gluteal, obturator, and pudendal arteries; and the veins that accompany these vessels. The vasculature associated with the viscera contained within the true pelvis is also at risk.

A lateral compression fracture of the pelvis can cause significant skeletal disruption, but is not usually associated with major vascular disruption. Frequently, however, there is significant intraperitoneal hemorrhage secondary to viscus organ injury and/or thoracic injury, usually on the injured side. Anteroposterior compression injuries to the pelvis often create a complete diastasis anteriorly through the pubic symphysis and partial or complete diastasis posteriorly, through one of the sacroiliac joints. In this type of injury, tensile and shear forces to the adjacent vasculature usually cause more bleeding than is seen in a lateral compression injury. A high-energy, vertical shear injury may also disrupt the pelvic vasculature.

The function of external fixation in such a milieu is to reestablish the boundaries of the potential retroperitoneal space enclosed within the true pelvis (Fig. 1). By controlling the radius of the true pelvis, the external fixator limits the volume of the retroperitoneum and the volume of the hemorrhage. Nonstabilized anteroposterior compression or vertical shear injuries of the pelvis allow expansion of the retroperitoneal hematoma through bleeding that would be checked by the pelvic ring if it were not damaged. Resuscitative efforts based on fluid replacement and restoration of pressure diminish the patient's coagulation profile and may make the bleeding more severe.

During resuscitative and assessment procedures, the patient with blunt trauma is often moved about the emergency room or admitting area for further diag-

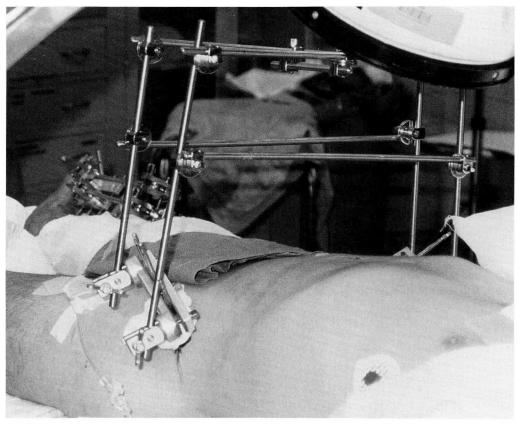

Fig. 1 A typical "double frame" pelvic fixator used for a multiply injured patient with a severe pelvic fracture. Although biomechanically suboptimal, these tall frames may be rotated caudad over the thighs and/ or cephalad over the thorax to permit access for laparotomy or other procedures while maintaining the environment of a stabilized pelvic ring.

nostic tests. The nonstabilized pelvic ring, surrounding an expanding retroperitoneal hematoma, tolerates such repeated stress poorly, especially if a transfusion coagulopathy is developing. Newly formed, tenuous clots, especially those located just anterior to the sacroiliac joint, may break loose. External fixation, by stabilizing the area during transport and transfer, promotes clot retention and diminishes additional hemorrhage.

A third benefit of using external fixation for a pelvic fracture in a multiply injured patient is early mobilization. With external fixation of the pelvic ring, the patient can sit up or may be rolled from side to side in bed, reducing the danger of pneumonia and making nursing care easier.

Stabilization: Combined Musculoskeletal and Vascular Injuries

For patients with multiple injuries or severe musculoskeletal and associated vascular injuries, the timing of treatment is crucial. Although treatment of a limb

at risk from vascular interruption is best done within the first one to three hours, conditions often preclude such ideal therapy. For example, a patient may be referred after diagnosis from a facility incapable of treating such severe injuries, or difficulties associated with patient extrication may delay therapeutic intervention. In the multiply injured patient, it often happens that life-threatening injuries, specifically those of the central nervous system and cardiovascular system, must be addressed first, delaying the treatment of extremity injuries.[5] Ideally, using a multiple-team approach, such injuries would be addressed simultaneously. For the patient with a completely ischemic limb and associated skeletal injuries, we have developed a dual, preplanned approach. The first treatment, if possible, is to use a shunt to provide temporary inflow to the ischemic limb. The vascular surgical team decides whether to place a shunt.

Next, I recommend simultaneous treatment by an orthopaedic surgeon and a vascular surgeon. The vascular surgeon gains proximal vascular control, while the orthopaedic surgeon performs distal fasciotomies.

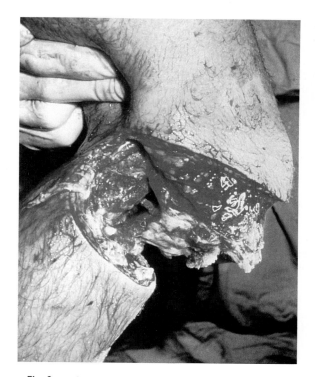
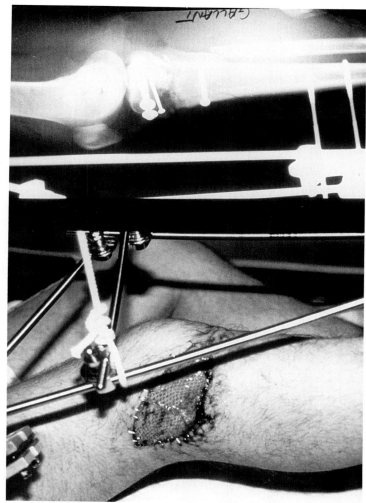

Fig. 2 **Left,** Preoperative clinical photograph of a contaminated, open, incomplete amputation through the proximal tibia in a multiply injured patient. **Right,** Seven days postoperatively, clinical photograph and radiograph show a "salvage" fixator crossing the knee joint, minimal internal fixation, and a split-thickness skin graft. A buttress plate was applied at a later date and the fixator was removed to allow knee motion.

This combined surgical intervention saves time and allows both surgeons to make incisions that can be used for subsequent reconstructive procedures. For example, with regard to the upper extremity, a reverse Henry incision used by the orthopaedic surgeon for forearm fasciotomies would connect well with a medial incision used by the vascular surgeon for brachial artery repair. Similarly, fasciotomy and vascular incisions of the lower extremity could be positioned to permit later open reduction and internal fixation of either proximal tibial or distal femoral fractures.

After fasciotomy and proximal vascular control, the orthopaedic surgeon applies external fixation to provide temporary fracture stabilization, while the vascular surgeon performs a vein harvest on a noninjured extremity, usually a contralateral lower extremity.

The orthopaedic surgeon now either leaves the field

or assists the vascular surgeon in performing the definitive vascular repair. After vascular repair, an angiogram is used to assess both vascular integrity and fracture position, after which the external fixation is revised to optimize pin placement and correct fracture reduction.

Staging and Temporizing

Salvage external frames are constructed for the severely injured extremity in the patient who has life-threatening injuries. These frames permit access for wound care while maintaining skeletal length and protecting associated vascular repairs. Salvage frames are usually applied after debridement of open wounds (Fig. 2).

If fracture patterns and surgical judgment indicate that later detailed open reduction and internal fixation is likely, the external fixator used in the salvage frame should avoid these areas. In this way, open pin tracts will not later coexist next to freshly placed plates and screws. Periarticular areas are to be avoided, especially those that require future complex reconstructive efforts. If there are large, free-floating articular fragments, and if time permits, minimal internal fixation may be added to the external fixation.[6]

Sometimes, to provide soft-tissue or vascular stability, a joint must be crossed by the external fixator. Obviously, crossing the articular surface using external fixation may compromise eventual joint mobility; but, in this situation, external fixation is a temporary or short-term treatment device, the primary goals being survival of the patient and gross stabilization of soft tissues near any skeletal injury. Conversion to a more definitive type of fracture treatment can be undertaken after fracture management has achieved the goal of a clean, healed, noninfected soft-tissue envelope.[7]

Conclusions

External fixation in the multiply injured patient should be thought of in terms of treating the overall patient, not in terms of treating individual injuries. Its use is of particular benefit in the management of pelvic hemorrhage, the management of associated orthopaedic and vascular injuries, and the temporary management of complex extremity injuries in a patient with other severe life-threatening problems.

References

1. Cowley RA, Dunham CM (eds): *Shock Trauma/Critical Care Manual: Initial Assessment and Management.* Baltimore, University Park Press, 1982.
2. Goris RJ, Gimbrère JS, van Niekerk JL, et al: Early osteosynthesis and prophylactic mechanical ventilation in the multitrauma patient. *J Trauma* 1982;22:895–903.
3. Burgess AR, Poka A: Principles of external fixation, in Browner BD, Jupiter JB, Levine AM, et al (eds): *Skeletal Trauma.* Philadelphia, WB Saunders, in press.
4. Young JWR, Burgess AR: *Radiologic Management of Pelvic Ring Fractures: Systematic Radiographic Diagnosis.* Baltimore, Urban & Schwarzenberg, 1987.
5. Committee on Trauma, American College of Surgeons: *Advanced Trauma Life Support Manual.* Chicago, American College of Surgeons, 1981.
6. Burgess AR: Fracture fixation, in Yaremchuk MJ, Burgess AR, Brumback RJ (eds): *Lower Extremity Salvage and Reconstruction: Orthopaedic and Plastic Surgical Management.* New York, Elsevier, in press.
7. Burgess AR, Poka A, Brumback RJ, et al: Management of open grade III tibial fractures. *Orthop Clin North Am* 1987;18:85–93.

Management Decisions in Complex Upper-Extremity Fractures

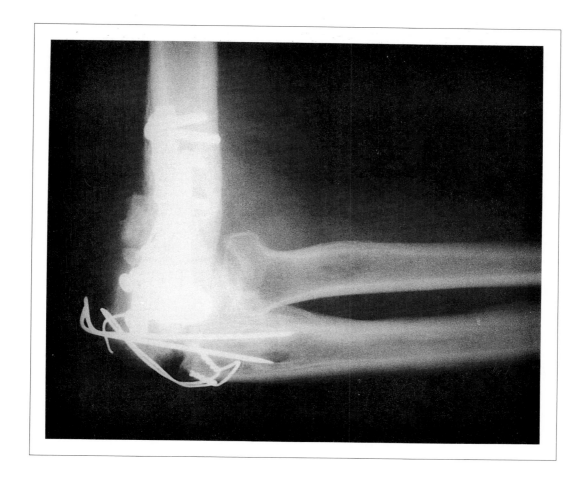

Choosing Upper-Limb Fracture Fixation

Loren L. Latta, PhD

Rationale

The goal of fracture fixation is to control the skeletal parts sufficiently to allow an acceptable level of function while healing takes place. Healing occurs best in an environment controlled by symptoms rather than hardware. However, in many cases, although fixation involves surgical intervention and placement of devices that can delay healing, these things provide mechanical advantages that allow for earlier joint motion and muscle activity. In general, the benefits often outweigh the disadvantages. Thus, bone healing is not the only priority in allowing the patient to return to a preinjury function level as soon as possible.[1]

The ideal fixation system adds no rigidity to the bone after it has healed.[2-4] All of the stresses of normal functional activity should then pass through the bone in the normal manner.[1,5] In reality, however, current treatment techniques and devices accomplish this to varying degrees depending how much strength and rigidity was required at the time of early treatment.[2,6-11] Fixation must be strong enough to hold the parts in position during normal functional activities. Rigidity or stiffness of fixation affects the speed and type of healing that take place,[12,13] but the strength and rigidity of fixation may or may not be related to the actual rigidity and strength of the device used for fixation. As an example, if a screw is used to fix two bone fragments together, the metal screw is stiffer than bone, but the stiffness of the fixation is related to the area of bone held in contact by the screw and to the ability of the screw to compress the surfaces of the fracture together so that the stresses from functional activity pass more through the bone than through the screw.[14] Also, although the screw is stronger than the surrounding bone, the strength of the fixation depends on how well the screw transfers stress to the bone and maintains the rigidity of fixation. If the screw loosens before the fracture has healed, the fixation will lose its rigidity and will be less strong, but the rigidity and strength of the screw will not change. This underlines the important distinction between the strength of the device and the strength of its fixation as well as the rigidity of the device and the rigidity of its fixation.

Increasing the rigidity of the fixation does not always increase the strength of fixation, although generally this relationship is true for a given type of fixation. For instance, if the rigidity of fixation with a single screw increases, there is more stress through the bone and less stress in the screw as well as more rapid increase in strength of healing of bone fragments. Thus, the increase in rigidity of fixation increases the strength of fixation. However, other forms of fixation that are less rigid may be as strong as or stronger than single-screw fixation. For instance, intramedullary rod fixation is generally stronger than single-screw fixation, but its rigidity is likely to be much less.

The strength of fixation of any device is the stability the device provides. Malposition and malunion occur in a fracture after initial reduction only if the strength of fixation is lost and progressive deformity accompanies early functional activity. Thus, while strength of fixation is synonymous with stability, rigidity of fixation is related to healing, but not necessarily to stability. Stability implies a permanent change in position or a plastic deformation of the construction and progressive deformity with continued loading.

Rigidity of Fixation and Healing

Rigidity of fixation influences the type and rate of healing of bone fragments and may also influence the healing of soft tissues surrounding the fracture. In general, plate-and-screw fixation provides the most rigid fixation of bone fragments, allowing only a few microns of motion between the fragments.[6] Because of the limited motion and the close approximation of the fragments, the healing involves primary bone formation, with minimal or no formation of fibrous tissue and cartilage.[7,12,13] Therefore, little or no callus is seen on radiographs taken during the healing. Plate fixation for the large diaphyseal bones with dynamic or outboard compression plates provides maximum strength and rigidity because the plates are able to compress the bony fragments. When good bone contact is accomplished, this type of fixation provides minimal callus formation and maximum primary bone healing. However, the plates used to fix small bones of the hand are relatively small, making it more difficult to accomplish direct bone apposition and compression. Here the rigidity of fixation is significantly less. Although the tension-band effect of these plates is quite good, there is more callus and secondary bone formation associated with the use of these devices in the metacarpals or phalanges.

COMPARATIVE STIFFNESS
TYPES OF FRACTURE FIXATION

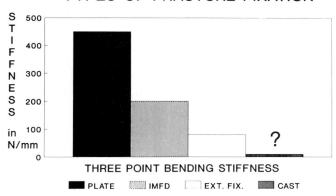

Fig. 1 Measurement of fixation stiffness for a model bone without any soft tissues provides the most typical form of comparison between internal and external means of fixation. In this case the bone was modeled with a tube of acrylic 1 inch in diameter with a ⅛-inch wall, the plate was a 3.5-mm DCP, the intramedullary device (IMFD) was an 18-mm GK, and the external fixator was a single half-pin Hoffmann with four 5-mm pins.

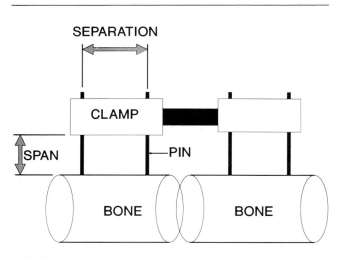

Fig. 2 Pin span is the distance between the pin-bone interface and the pin-clamp interface for each pin. Pin separation is the distance between adjacent pins at the pin-bone interface.

Internal fixation with intramedullary fixation devices allows a wide range of fixation stiffnesses and degrees of motion at the fracture site.[5] Relative motion of the fragments at the fracture site may vary from a fraction of a millimeter to several millimeters, depending on the rigidity of fixation and the configuration and location of the fracture. In general, intramedullary fixation is less rigid than plate-and-screw fixation for the same type of fracture (Fig. 1). Because this degree of motion is significantly greater than that allowed by plate-and-screw fixation, and because the bony parts need not be

EFFECT OF PIN SPAN
5 mm Hoffman

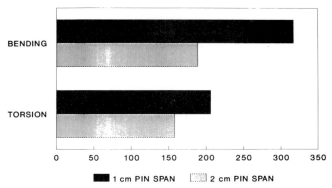

EFFECT OF PIN SEPARATION
ON BENDING STIFFNESS

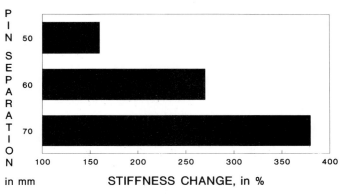

EFFECT OF PIN DIAMETER
ON STIFFNESS

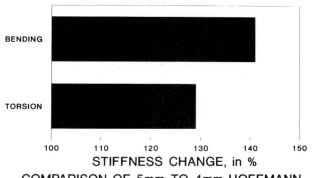

Fig. 3 **Top**, The rigidity of external fixation is significantly affected by the pin span in both bending and torsion. Pin separation (**center**) and pin diameter (**bottom**) have less of an effect on torsional rigidity than on bending.

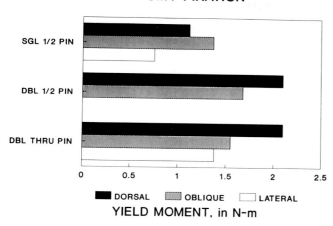

Fig. 4 Isolated metacarpal bones with midshaft, transverse osteotomies were tested in three-point apex dorsal bending to compare the stiffness of available forms of internal and external fixation systems. Plate fixation, as it is with most long bones, was much more rigid than wire, intramedullary (IMFD), and double half-pin external fixation (with the mini-Hoffmann). But double half-pin fixation with the very rigid vice clamp provided about as much rigidity as the plate.

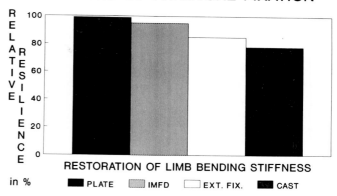

Fig. 5 Tests on above-knee amputation specimens with all soft tissues intact except for the damage caused by the creation of a closed, diaphyseal fracture and the surgical insult associated with plate-and-screw fixation allowed for comparison of fracture-site motion in a controlled laboratory environment for plate, single half-pin external fixator, reamed IMFD, and a fracture brace in bending, rotation, and axial compression. Relative resilience measures the change in motion at the fracture site for each loading condition by comparing motion before and after each type of fixation was applied.

compressed rigidly together to obtain good intramedullary fixation, the healing is usually of a secondary nature marked by peripheral callus formation and a significant degree of bone formation secondary to cartilage and fibrous tissue formation.[5,7] The degree to which this peripheral callus forms is related to the degree of biologic insult to the medullary canal during application of the device, to the amount of gap between fragments of the bone, and to the rigidity of fixation provided by the particular device. A wide variety of device stiffnesses are available for reamed or nonreamed intramedullary fixation of upper limb fractures. Nonreamed applications for diaphyseal fractures commonly include the use of Ender pins, Rush rods, or simple Steinmann pins, usually applied by closed blind technique. These provide a very elastic or nonrigid fixation of the bone fragments and are associated with abundant peripheral callus formation when function is introduced early. Reamed diaphysis devices are available with optional proximal and/or distal locking.

External fixation devices allow anywhere from fractions of a millimeter to several millimeters of motion at the fracture site, depending on the configuration and rigidity of the particular frame applied and the bone to which it has been applied.[15,16] Many factors affect the relative rigidity of external fixation systems in the upper limb. Pin separation, pin diameter, and pin span are three important factors that determine the strength and stiffness of fixation by an external fixator (Figs. 2 and 3), but the apposition of the bone fragments is even more important. Very rigid constructions can be

assembled using rigid pin-clamp assemblies, multiple pins, and multiple planes of application. On the other hand, the easiest system and most popular system to use, single half-pin fixation, provides significantly less rigidity.[15,17] In general, external fixation systems provide significantly less rigidity than does plate fixation (Fig. 1). However, the single exception to this seems to be in the application to metacarpal or phalangeal fractures, where a rigid pin-clamp assembly and dual half-pin fixation is comparable in rigidity to single-plate fixation in selected loading conditions (Fig. 4).[17] In most applications, external fixation provides significantly less rigidity than plate fixation does and is most often associated with secondary bone formation and significant peripheral callus. One advantage in using external fixation is the ability to reduce the fixation's stiffness as the bone heals, thus eliminating the effects of long-term rigidity of fixation.[18-20] Because closed treatment with fracture braces, splints, or casts allows several millimeters of motion at the fracture site in most applications with early functional activity (Fig. 5), these types of treatment are consistently associated with abundant peripheral callus formation and secondary bone healing.[13,21,22] With closed treatment techniques, soft tissues play a major role in both fixation stiffness and its strength.[22] Thus, the condition of the soft tissues must be considered when choosing this method of fixation. Soft tissues are also important when choosing a method of mechanical testing for any fixation system that is more compliant than plate-and-screw fixation (Fig. 6).[23]

METACARPAL FRACTURE FIXATION
The Role of Soft Tissues

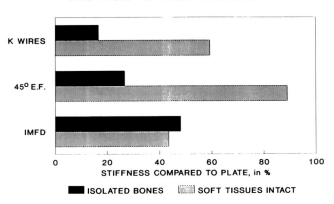

Fig. 6 For the more compliant forms of fixation, the soft tissues can provide a mechanically significant tension band, particularly in the hand, where large tendons and minimal muscle surround the bone. Here a comparison is shown for apex dorsal bending stiffness measurements in the metacarpal fracture model described in Figure 4, and the same fixation applied through a surgical wound and tested in metacarpals in intact hands compared to plate fixation under the same conditions.

Strength of Fixation and Stability

With rigid screw and/or plate fixation, the strength of fixation is related to the rigidity of fixation. With good bone apposition, plate-and-screw fixation is strong enough to allow early functional activity and to protect injured and repaired soft tissues until they heal. If good bone apposition cannot be accomplished with plate-and-screw fixation, the strength of fixation is severely compromised (Fig. 7), because the stresses will pass through the device, significantly increasing the stresses at the fixation points in the bone.[17,24] Fixation is weakest at those fixation points because the threading of the bone where the screws are attached causes significant stress concentration, weakening the bone by at least 50% (Fig. 8).[25–27]

Intramedullary fixation devices, at the time of application, are usually as strong as plate fixation, if there is good bone apposition. This is because most of the stress placed on the bone during activity passes through the bone rather than through the fixation device. If there is a gap, the intramedullary device has to transfer the load from one bone fragment to the other, as in plate fixation, in which case the strength of the device relates directly to the strength of fixation.[28] Because of the lack of rigid fixation of the intramedullary device to the bone itself, as healing progresses more of the stress goes through the bone until the stress through the device decreases to nearly zero. Thus, the long-term effect of the device is minimal once the bone has healed.[5]

The strength of fixation of an intramedullary device

ISOLATED METACARPALS
OSTEOTOMY FIXATION

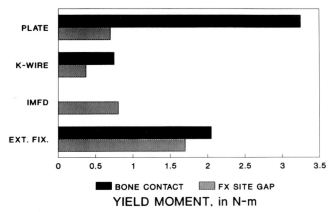

Fig. 7 Coaption and compression are important factors in providing rigidity to the more rigid forms of fixation, because bone contact is essential for the transmission of load through bone. For more compliant forms of fixation, a gap at the fracture site reduced the strength of fixation to less than that measured for plate fixation in this model of isolated metacarpals (as described in Figure 4).

PLATED FRACTURE HEALING
BENDING REFRACTURE STRENGTH

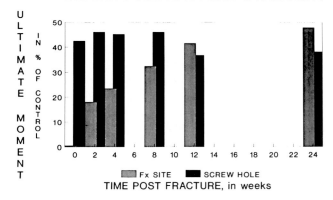

Fig. 8 In the plated fracture of the dog's radius, measurement of refracture strength in three-point bending (after plate removal) as long as six months after fracture was compared with the strength of the unfractured control radius. There was a significant reduction in refracture moment no matter whether the failure occurred at the screw holes or at the original fracture site. But the fracture site tended to become stronger with time, whereas the screw holes did not appear to gain strength.

depends on its frictional fit within the medullary canal and its points of contact along the medullary canal. These resist bending and torsion. The leverage of the device in resisting bending is directly related to the length of its contact points. Important factors in resisting torsion are the configuration of the fracture site and the degree of bone apposition. Most torsional loads

METACARPAL FRACTURE STABILITY
The Role of Soft Tissues

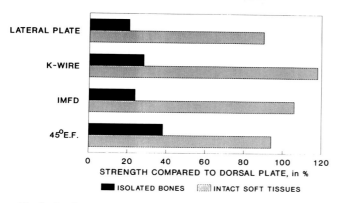

Fig. 9 In the metacarpal model, the soft-tissue tension band increased the strength of fixation significantly in apex dorsal bending with all forms of fixation except for the dorsal plate. The most likely reason that the less rigid fixation systems could approach the strength of the dorsal plate fixation is that perfect coaptation was not possible with any of the devices with the hand intact. Plate fixation is the most sensitive to changes in coaptation (see Figure 7).

ISOLATED METACARPALS
OSTEOTOMY FIXATION

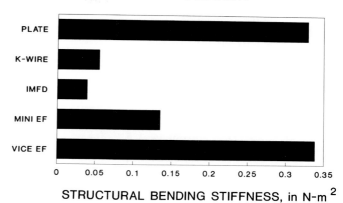

Fig. 10 In the isolated metacarpal fracture model described in Figure 4, variations in external fixation frame configurations and pin cluster planes provided a wide variety of fixation stiffnesses in apex dorsal bending.

are transferred directly at the fracture site if the site is adequately interdigitated. If there is a gap or poor fracture interdigitation, much of the torsional load is transferred to the device, and its strength of fixation in resisting torsion is reduced. Thus, in cases in which the strength of the fixation depends on the device, proximal or distal locking strategies may be necessary. Such devices are now available for the humerus, distal radius, radial or ulnar diaphyseal fractures, and metacarpal and proximal phalangeal fractures. A soft-tissue tension band can also aid in obtaining coaptation and load transfer through the bone if no gap is present (Fig. 9).

In the case of external fixation, a wide variety of strengths of fixation are available, depending on the configuration of the devices applied. Failure of an external fixator is usually caused when a pin loosens, slides in the bone, or bends, and these must be minimized to provide strong fixation. Pins applied only in one plane have good strength in that plane, but poor strength of fixation in bending or torsion outside that plane. Thus, the use of multiple planes is important in providing strong fixation (Fig. 10).[15,17] Because the bending strength of the pins is directly related to pin diameter, pin diameter is another important factor in providing strength of fixation. If small pins must be used, this lack of strength can be avoided by using more pins, by spacing them as far apart as possible, and by minimizing pin span to reduce the leverage of the external frame on the pin as the bone fragments attempt to move beneath the skin.

With soft tissue compressed in a brace or cast, strength of fixation is related to the intrinsic strength

SOFT TISSUE STABILITY
Intrinsic vs. Hydraulic Support

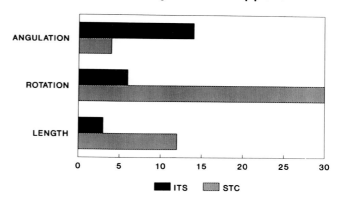

Fig. 11 Localized soft-tissue tension banding at the fracture site provides good resistance to shortening and rotation but is not so effective at angulation. Soft-tissue compression of the surrounding musculature provides good angulatory control but is less resistant to shortening and rotation. Calculations were made from a simple theoretical model of a soft callus vs surrounding soft tissue in a size and shape similar to a humerus and arm. An arbitrary soft-tissue resistance was set at a mechanical strain of 10% in the soft tissues for relative comparison.

of soft tissues left intact in the area of the fracture and the degree of soft-tissue healing and soft callus to provide added intrinsic strength. Within this envelope of motion allowed at the fracture site, the incompressible fluid nature of the surrounding soft tissues provides strength during loading conditions.[29] Thus, two mech-

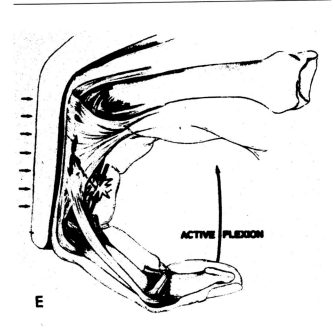

E

Fig. 12 In the hand and about distal joints where no bulky muscular tissues cross the joints, joint positioning can be used to place a preload tension on the local soft tissues to supply the tension band. (Reproduced with permission from Reyes FA, Latta LL: Conservative management of difficult phalangeal fractures. *Clin Orthop* 1987;214: 23–30.)

anisms from the soft tissues provide support—the incompressible fluid contained within the brace or cast and the intrinsic strength of tissues near the fracture site that are intact or have healed. The relative importance of these two varies depending on the loading condition and location of the fracture. The intrinsic strength of soft tissues resists overriding, which changes the length of the bone, and torsion (Fig. 11). The surrounding soft tissues resist angulation of the bone fragments. Although soft-tissue compression in a brace provides an incompressible fluid effect in the soft tissues, it does not provide intrinsic strength at the fracture site. Intrinsic strength near the fracture site depends on minimal soft-tissue injury, as in closed injuries, or early soft-tissue healing in order for fracture braces to provide adequate stability.[29,30]

Mechanical Principles

Adequate strength and rigidity of fixation depends on three mechanical principles—buttress, tension band, and neutralization.[14] The best means of applying a buttress is good coaptation of the bone fragments and direct apposition of bone on bone. The buttress portion of the configuration of fractured bone, soft tissue, and fixation device is the area where compression stresses are transferred from one portion of the limb to the

other. Because bones are best able to translate compression, they should be used as the buttress whenever possible. When a gap exists and length must be maintained, a bone buttress may be provided by bone grafting or by bone healing over an extended period of time. In internal and external fixation, stresses on the device are significantly increased if a bone buttress is not available.[24,28] In effect, a race takes place between the bone's ability to supply a buttress and the mechanical failure of the fixation of the device. In general, fixation devices are not designed to be prostheses and cannot take the stresses that are normally taken by the bone.

Once a buttress is accomplished, a tension band is applied to maintain that buttress by compressing it during loading. The tension band can be a plate with screw fixation, direct wire fixation of the bone, an intramedullary device that withstands the tension stresses and transfers compression to the bone, or an external fixation system that holds the bones in apposition. Soft tissues can also passively or actively apply tension band and maintain compression on the bone.[23,31] Because of the rigidity of plate-and-screw fixation, a plate provides the most rigid tension band.[14] Because intramedullary fixation depends on the frictional fit of the device in the medullary canal and the rigidity of the device, its tension band effect is less than that of a plate.[5] The frame of the external fixator can provide a tension band. Because soft tissues are more compliant than a plate is, their tension banding effect is quite compliant compared with plate-and-screw fixation.[15] The soft tissues around the fracture are often strong enough to make the tension-band strength quite adequate. For instance, tendons and adjacent ligamentous structures provide a good tension band for fractures near a joint and in the hand.[23,30] In the case of intra-articular fractures or fractures near joints, joint positioning by splinting and combination fracture-bracing techniques can provide a passive soft-tissue tension band by ligamentaxis[30] or tensioning of a tendon on the tension side of the fracture by passive lengthening of the musculotendinous unit (Fig. 12).[29]

Neutralization, which provides strength to the fixation and reduces its vulnerability to mechanical failure, must provide resistance to load within the strain tolerance of the method of fixation. This means that neutralization must resist any displacement of the major fixation method that would lead to mechanical failure. In the case of screw fixation, rigid neutralization is necessary because a small amount of motion at the screw-bone interface can cause mechanical failure. Therefore, plate neutralization is necessary for most screw fixations.[14]

Wire fixation and pin fixation, on the other hand, are more compliant than screw fixation and will allow more displacement before mechanical failure takes place. External fixation or, in some instances, a cast or

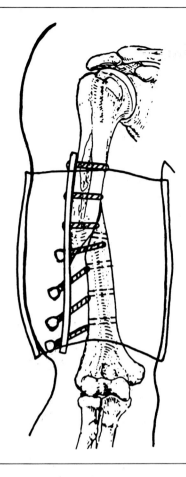

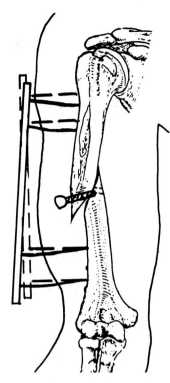

Fig. 13 Screw fixation cannot be adequately supplemented by an external fixator or brace for the tension band, because the degree of fracture site motion allowed by these devices in order to provide resistance to load is beyond the motion causing failure of the screw fixation. These devices are mechanically incompatible.

brace is used to provide neutralization for wire or pin fixation. In the case of intramedullary fixation, neutralization is generally adequately supplied by the device itself, if there is good bone apposition and the device fits the canal tightly in the area of the fracture. However, if either good bone apposition or fit near the fracture site is lacking, neutralization may be provided by an external cast or brace[32-34] or by proximal or distal locking of the device[35] to resist rotation and axial translation. With fracture brace application to diaphyseal fractures in the arm and forearm, soft-tissue compression and molding of the soft tissues provides neutralization for the fracture site.[29]

Combining Fixation Techniques

As described above, more than one type of fixation can be used at once to accomplish the neutralization and tension banding needed to maintain the bony buttress of a given fracture. The most important factor related to this combined application is the mechanical compatibility of the techniques. One must recognize that the strength of fixation of any particular technique is related to its ability to limit the amount of movement of the parts below the point at which fixation would be lost or compromised. If one kind of neutralization or tension band is combined with another kind of coaptation and/or compression, the resistance from these tension bands or neutralization must be sufficient to limit displacement to the range tolerated by the coaptation-compression fixation technique. Otherwise, fixation may fail before adequate tension band or neutralization resistance is accomplished. These relative differences become obvious when one thinks about the rigidity of fixation associated with a particular strength of fixation for a given technique. With plate-and-screw fixation or isolated screw fixation, the motion of the fragments is relatively small, within an order of microns. With other techniques, the motion allowed for given functional activities is significantly greater than that allowed by rigid plate-and-screw fixation. This is why rigid plate-and-screw fixation is consistently associated with primary bone healing, and other techniques are associated with secondary types of bone formation. The only exception to this is with extremely rigid external fixation, particularly of the small bones of the hand, which may provide rigidity and strength com-

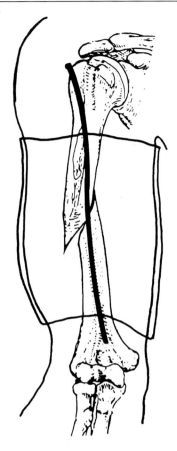

Fig. 14 Intramedullary devices (particularly of the elastic type) and pin fixation are mechanically compatible with casts or fracture braces. Thus bracing can be expected to provide supplemental support to properly selected cases of intramedullary devices or pin fixation.

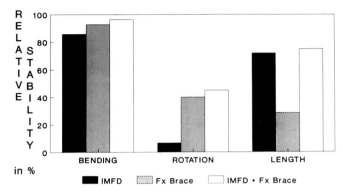

COMBINED FIXATION
Elastic IMFD + Fx Brace

Fig. 15 This example provides relative information on the supplemental effect of bracing on diaphyseal fracture fixation. The measurements were made in an above-knee amputation specimen with a tibial fracture, but the same relative values should apply generally to forearm or humeral diaphyseal fractures.

parable to that achieved by a plate and/or screws.[17] Thus, in combining techniques, there must be mechanical compatibility. In general, a brace, cast, external fixator, or intramedullary device cannot be expected to adequately neutralize a single-screw fixation of a diaphyseal fracture (Fig. 13).[36,37] Only a plate provides the rigidity required to neutralize lag-screw fixation. A cast or brace can be used to neutralize a flexible intramedullary device or external fixation in bending, but it will not substantially support rotation or length stability (Figs. 14 and 15).[32,34,38]

However, sequential use of techniques does not require mechanical compatibility. For instance, external fixation or internal fixation may be used while soft tissues heal and soft callus forms at the fracture site. These techniques can then be followed by functional bracing or cast immobilization to accomplish bone healing.[32] In another instance, one may choose to use traction, cast, or splint immobilization to accomplish wound management and soft-tissue healing, followed by delayed internal fixation to accomplish early joint motion and soft-tissue function during bone healing.

In these instances, the techniques do not require mechanical compatibility in order to maintain stability for all phases of the rehabilitation process. Each technique provides its own stability during its use, and biologic compatibility is a more important factor. For instance, intramedullary fixation after removal of external fixation is associated with a high incidence of infection even though mechanically these techniques may be compatible.[39] On the other hand, rigid internal fixation of an infected, open fracture will protect soft tissues from further damage and will localize the infection until the bone can heal, even though the surgeon recognizes that the infection will not resolve with metal in the wound, which must be left open. After the limb is stable, the fixation is removed and the wound and infection managed with the limb in a splint, a cast, or a simple dressing.[40]

References

1. Sarmiento A, Latta LL, Tarr RR: Principles of fracture healing: Part II: The effect of function on fracture healing and stability, in Murray JA (ed): American Academy of Orthopaedic Surgeons *Instructional Course Lectures, XXXIII*. St. Louis, CV Mosby, 1984, pp 83–106.
2. Uhthoff HK, Dubuc FL: Bone structure changes in the dog under rigid internal fixation. *Clin Orthop* 1971;81:165–170.
3. Carter DR, Vasu R, Harris WH: The plated femur: Relationships between the changes in bone stresses and bone loss. *Acta Orthop Scand* 1981;52:241–248.
4. Akeson WH, Woo SL, Rutherford L, et al: The effects of rigidity of internal fixation plates on long bone remodeling: A biomechanical and quantitative histological study. *Acta Orthop Scand* 1976;47:241–249.
5. Tarr RR, Wiss DA: The mechanics and biology of intramedullary fracture fixation. *Clin Orthop* 1986;212:10–17.

6. Perren SM, Rahn BA: Biomechanics of fracture healing: Historical review and mechanical aspects of internal fixation. *Orthop Surv* 1978;2:108.

7. Yamagishi M, Yoshimura Y: The biomechanics of fracture healing. *J Bone Joint Surg* 1955;37A:1035–1068.

8. Terjesen T, Johnson E: Effects of fixation stiffness on fracture healing: External fixation of tibial osteotomy in the rabbit. *Acta Orthop Scand* 1986;57:146–148.

9. Woo SL-Y, Lothringer KS, Akeson WH, et al: Less rigid internal fixation plates: Historical perspectives and new concepts. *J Orthop Res* 1984;1:431–449.

10. Goodship AE, Kenwright J: The influence of induced micromovement upon the healing of experimental tibial fractures. *J Bone Joint Surg* 1985;67B:650–655.

11. Møster AO, Gjerdet NR, Langeland N, et al: Controlled bending instability in the healing of diaphyseal osteotomies in the rat femur. *J Orthop Res* 1987;5:29–35.

12. Rahn BA, Gallinaro P, Baltensperger A, et al: Primary bone healing: An experimental study in the rabbit. *J Bone Joint Surg* 1971; 53A:783–786.

13. Lindholm RV, Lindholm TS, Toikkanen S, et al: Effect of forced interfragmental movements on the healing of tibial fractures in rats. *Acta Orthop Scand* 1969;40:721–728.

14. Muller ME, Allgower M, Schneider R, et al: *Manual of Internal Fixation: Techniques Recommended by the AO Group*, ed 2. Berlin, Springer-Verlag, 1979.

15. McCoy MT, Chao EYS, Kasman RA: Comparison of mechanical performance in four types of external fixators. *Clin Orthop* 1983; 180:23–33.

16. Ritter G, Weigand H, Ahlers J: Necessary stability and biomechanics of fracture healing in external fixation osteosyntheses. *Unfallchirurgie* 1983;9:92–97.

17. Kato S, Latta L, Burkhalter WE: Mechanical evaluation of external and internal fixation for metacarpal fractures. *Trans Orthop Res Soc* 1986;11:316.

18. Egger EL, Lewallen DG, Norrdin RW, et al: Effects of destabilizing rigid external fixation on healing of unstable canine osteotomies. Presented at the 13th International Conference on Hoffmann External Fixation, 1989.

19. Kenwright J, Richardson JB, Goodship AE, et al: Effect of controlled axial micromovement on healing of tibial fractures. *Lancet* 1986;2:1185–1187.

20. Wolf JW Jr, White AA III, Panjabi MM, et al: The superiority of cyclic loading over constant compression in the treatment of long bone fractures: A quantitative biomechanical study in rabbits. *Trans Orthop Res Soc* 1980;5:174.

21. Lippert FG III, Hirsch C: The three dimensional measurement of tibia fracture motion by photogrammetry. *Clin Orthop* 1974; 105:130–143.

22. Latta LL, Sarmiento A, Tarr RR: The rationale of functional bracing of fractures. *Clin Orthop* 1980;146:28–36.

23. Ouillette EA, Dennis J, Milne EL, et al: The tension band effect of soft tissues in the bending behavior of external and internal metacarpal fixation. Presented at the 13th International Conference on Hoffmann External Fixation, 1989.

24. Pawluk RJ, Tzitzikalakis GI, Larrison W, et al: Effects of bone gaps on internal fixation stability. *Trans Orthop Res Soc* 1982;7: 325.

25. Kato S, Malinin T, Wagner J, et al: The weakest link in the bone-plate-fracture system: Changes with time. *Trans Orthop Res Soc* 1986;11:474.

26. Malone CB, Heiple KG, Burstein AH: Bone strength: Before and after removal of unthreaded and threaded pins and screws. *Clin Orthop* 1977;123:259–260.

27. Hidaka S, Gustilo RB: Refracture of bones of the forearm after plate removal. *J Bone Joint Surg* 1984;66A:1241–1243.

28. Kyle RF: Biomechanics of intramedullary fracture fixation. *Orthopedics* 1985;8:1356–1359.

29. Zagorski JB, Zych GA, Latta LL, et al: Modern concepts in functional fracture bracing: The upper limb, in Griffin PP (ed): American Academy of Orthopaedic Surgeons *Instructional Course Lectures, XXXVI.* Park Ridge, Illinois, American Academy of Orthopaedic Surgeons, 1987, pp 377–401.

30. White AA III, Panjabi MM, Southwick WO: The four biomechanical stages of fracture repair. *J Bone Joint Surg* 1977;59A: 188–192.

31. Reyes FA, Latta LL: Conservative management of difficult phalangeal fractures. *Clin Orthop* 1987;214:23–30.

32. Zych GA, Zagorski JB, Latta LL, et al: Modern concepts in functional fracture bracing: The lower limb, in Griffin PP (ed): American Academy of Orthopaedic Surgeons *Instructional Course Lectures, XXXVI.* Park Ridge, Illinois, American Academy of Orthopaedic Surgeons, 1987, pp 403–425.

33. Wiss DA, Segal D, Gumbs VL, et al: Flexible medullary nailing of tibial shaft fractures. *J Trauma* 1986;26:1106–1112.

34. Brumback RJ, Bosse MJ, Poka A, et al: Intramedullary stabilization of humeral shaft fractures in patients with multiple trauma. *J Bone Joint Surg* 1986;68A:960–970.

35. Seidel H: Humeral locking nail: A preliminary report. *Orthopedics* 1989;12:219.

36. Green S: Combined internal and external fixation, in Coombs R, Green S, Sarmiento A (eds): *External Fixation and Functional Bracing.* London, Orthotext, 1989, p 233.

37. Krettek C, Haas N, Wippermann B, et al: One hundred thirty-two open tibial fractures treated with external fixation: Advantages with additional lag screws? Presented at the 13th International Conference on Hoffmann External Fixation, 1989.

38. Rinaldi E, Marenghi P, Corradi M: The treatment of tibial fractures by elastic nailing and functional plaster cast. *Ital J Orthop Trauma* 1987;13:173.

39. Bone LB, Johnson KD: Treatment of tibial fractures by reaming and intramedullary nailing. *J Bone Joint Surg* 1986;68A:877–887.

40. Calkins MS, Burkhalter W, Reyes F: Traumatic segmental bone defects in the upper extremity: Treatment with exposed grafts of corticocancellous bone. *J Bone Joint Surg* 1987;69A:19–27.

Open Fractures and Wound Management

William E. Burkhalter, MD

Introduction

In dealing with wound management and its relation to fracture management, Rank and Wakefield's[1] concept of tidy and untidy wounds does not always apply. The amount of injury required to create an open fracture in an adult long bone is almost certain to result in an untidy wound. An untidy injury is a diffuse injury located at a distance from the actual fracture site and complicated by contamination with viable organisms and perhaps foreign bodies.

Debridement is the removal of all material detrimental to wound healing, basically, devitalized and nonessential tissue that cannot contribute to the overall usefulness of the extremity. These tissues include the fascia, as well as pieces of skin, fat, and contused muscle. Tendons, nerves, and blood vessels are not excised, and these should be exposed and protected during the surgical procedure of debridement. To debride an open fracture, an elective incision is made to the fracture site. In this way, wide exposure can be obtained and vessels and nerves protected. Even if it were possible, it would be dangerous to attempt to debride an open fracture through an approach limited to the compound wound laceration. As the energy inflicted on the extremity increases to explosive and crush proportions, the exposure likewise must increase in size and extent. Exposure should be handled segmentally, especially with high-energy injuries to the upper limb. The segment from the wrist to the elbow and that from the elbow to the shoulder are addressed separately when exposing this type of injury. Only by exploration, exposure, and fasciotomy is it possible to debride an open upper-extremity fracture (Figs. 1 to 4).

In the open fracture, once debridement has been completed, the next concern is skeletal stability. Multiple metacarpal fractures in the hand or multiple fractures in the radius require skeletal stability to allow rehabilitation of the extremity. The upper extremity is

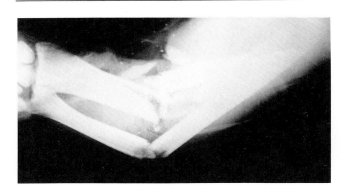

Fig. 1 The exit wound of a 30-caliber gunshot injury to the forearm of a 25-year-old man.

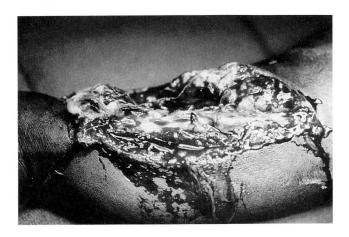

Fig. 2 Radiograph showing the highly comminuted fracture of the midshaft of the radius.

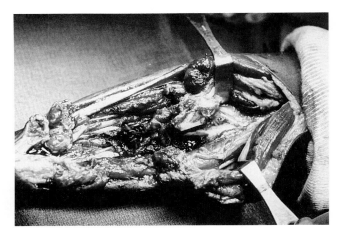

Fig. 3 With such severe destruction to bone and soft tissue, segmental exposure is necessary in order to debride adequately, do adequate fasciotomies, and protect undamaged structures.

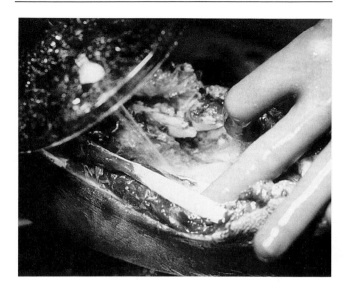

Fig. 4   Following fasciotomies, wound debridement, and exploration, irrigation further reduces bacterial contamination.

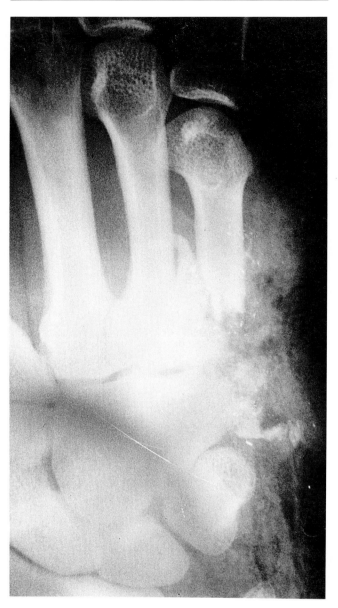

Fig. 6   Radiograph showing extensive loss of bone, with involvement of the basilar joint of the fifth metacarpal and its articulation with the hamate.

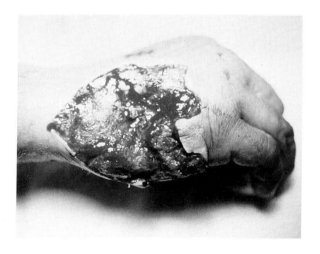

Fig. 5   A gunshot wound to the ulnar border of the hand with loss of skin, intrinsic muscles, and extensor tendon to the ring and small fingers in a 50-year-old man.

essentially a system of motion, not a system of support, and without early mobility of the entire upper extremity, motion will be lost. Because prevention is less spectacular but more effective than treatment, an effort should be made to avoid the stiffness that can occur with upper-extremity fractures.[2]

If an open fracture involves injury to major blood vessels, they must be stabilized and repaired by direct suture or graft. Necrotic tissue and tissue that lacks a blood supply are debrided at the initial surgery, and,

in the same way, improving tissue perfusion to tissues with diminished circulation will aid in preventing infection and achieving prompt wound healing. This cannot be accomplished without a stable skeleton. Once the wound has been debrided, the skeleton should be stabilized and then the vessels should be repaired. Wound closure is still not a matter of urgency. Blood-vessel repairs, especially grafts, must be covered, but it is not necessary to close the wound. If no vessels require repair, rehabilitation can begin within a few days. If small vessels, such as digital vessels, have been sutured, it is likely that early mobility will compromise the overall

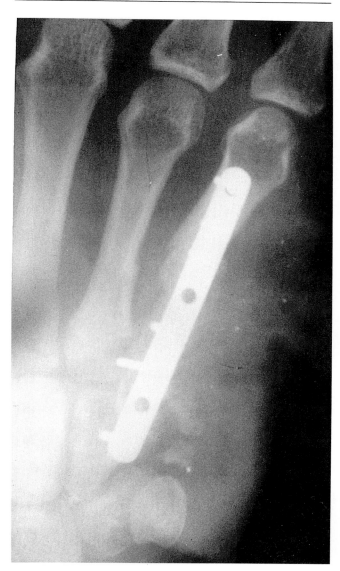

Fig. 7 Four days after initial wound surgery, the patient returned to the operating room for internal fixation with intercalary bone graft and arthrodesis of the carpometacarpal joint of the fifth metacarpal.

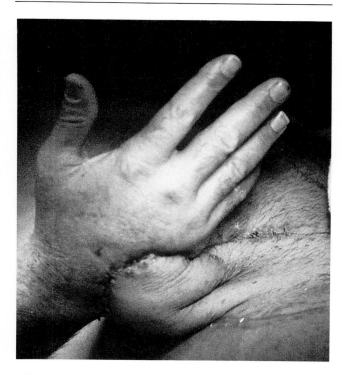

Fig. 8 Three days later, a groin flap was applied to the defect on the ulnar border of the hand. Rehabilitation during the period of immobilization was possible because of the fact that the hand could be placed in supination during the rehabilitation period.

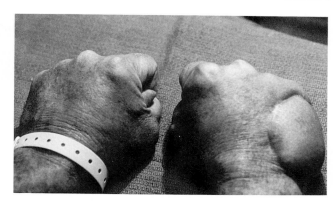

Fig. 9 At six months the patient demonstrates full digital flexion with no loss of length of the metacarpal.

result. In larger vessels, however, mobility probably does not carry this risk, and rehabilitation of the upper extremity can be started.

In bone-loss injuries of the upper extremity, delayed primary bone grafting can provide ultimate stability with tissue that has a potential for healing (Figs. 5 to 10). I have had good results with this method and have avoided the use of the external fixator except for extensively comminuted fractures in which small-vessel vascular repair is required. In my opinion, the external fixator delays rehabilitation of the upper extremity. I believe that applying an autogenous bone graft and rigid internal fixation in a surgically clean wound provides optimum circumstances for rapid union and, at the same time, avoids the problem of reexploring the fracture area once wound healing and tissue equilibrium have been achieved.[3] Weeks or months after injury, the dense scar tissue makes the exposure difficult. Secondary operations also have an extremely high breakdown rate. Skeletal stability allows early or even immediate rehabilitation of the extremity.

If there is any question about whether closure of a

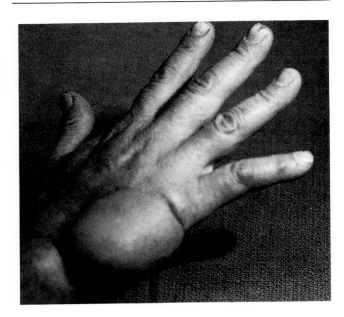

Fig. 10 Shows full extension of the small finger at six months in spite of the fact that there was no real extensor tendon in the area. Simple protective motion and dynamic splinting in extension with the patient working into active flexion frequently will make an "extensor tendon" on the dorsum of the hand.

wound will be successful, it should not be closed. Military and civilian experience and laboratory tests have shown that delayed closure is more effective for contaminated wounds than primary closure.[4-6] It is better to err on the side of leaving the wound open than to close it and have it break down secondary to sepsis. This may not be gross sepsis with purulence. A wound of the hand that is red, swollen, and reactive for a number of days poses a problem. It is difficult to get the extensor mechanism, the collateral ligaments, and the flexor tendon system to work in this kind of an environment. The increased edema and tenderness associated with this inflammatory process can limit tendon gliding and invite stiffness.

Wound closure can be accomplished by delayed primary closure or by a secondary closure. Delayed primary closure means wound closure three to five days after the initial injury. Secondary closure is accomplished after the wound has already begun to granulate—usually after five days or longer. Secondary wound closure is a traumatic operation that requires undermining. Because of the additional surgical trauma, it has a higher wound breakdown rate than does delayed primary closure. Split-thickness skin grafting can also provide wound closure. Other techniques, such as random flaps or axial pattern flaps, initially have better blood supply than split graft, but once they are separated from their donor site they become dependent on the vasculature of the limb to which they have been transferred. Also, these types of flaps may require positions that are awkward and limit rehabilitation. I avoid using this type of coverage in upper-extremity injuries, preferring some type of free-tissue transfer. It is then possible to maintain mobility of the proximal joints, maintain elevation of the hand, maintain a range of motion of the extremity, and avoid the problem of stiffness. The proper approach for an untidy wound of the upper extremity is initial wound exploration to achieve a surgically clean wound, followed by skeletal stabilization, rehabilitation of the extremity, and, finally, wound cover or closure. The use of grafts and internal fixation does not mean that wound closure must be accomplished at once. An exposed plate that stabilizes a deep bone graft will have to be removed following union, because a wound will not granulate over an exposed plate. Once union has been obtained through deep, well-vascularized tissue, the plate can be removed as an elective procedure.[7]

References

1. Rank BK, Wakefield: *Surgery of Repair as Applied to Hand Injuries,* ed 2. Edinburgh, Livingstone, 1970.
2. Peimer CA, Smith RJ, Leffert RD: Distraction-fixation in the primary treatment of metacarpal bone loss. *J Hand Surg* 1981;6:111–124.
3. Freeland AE, Jabaley ME, Burkhalter WE, et al: Delayed primary bone grafting in the hand and wrist after traumatic bone loss. *J Hand Surg* 1984;9A:22–28.
4. Brown PW: The prevention of infection in open wounds. *Clin Orthop* 1973;96:42–50.
5. Jabaley ME, Peterson HD: Early treatment of war wounds of the hand and forearm in Vietnam. *Ann Surg* 1973;177:167–173.
6. Burkhalter WE, Butler B, Metz W, et al: Experiences with delayed primary closure of war wounds of the hand in Viet Nam. *J Bone Joint Surg* 1968;50A:945–954.
7. Calkins MS, Burkhalter WE, Reyes F: Exposed corticocancellous bone grafts in open injuries of the upper extremity. Presented at the 52nd Annual Meeting of the American Academy of Orthopaedic Surgeons, Las Vegas, Jan 24–29, 1985.

Hand Fractures

William E. Burkhalter, MD

Introduction

I believe that most fractures of the diaphysis of the metacarpal and phalanges can be treated by closed means. Individuals interested in internal fixation tend to compare bad closed treatment of fractures with good open treatment of fractures, a patently unfair comparison.[1] Absolute anatomic restoration is not necessary for an excellent functional result.[2] Many patients with terrible bony anatomy nonetheless have excellent function, and have had for a number of years.

Most metacarpal and phalangeal fractures can be reduced satisfactorily by putting the hand in the James safe position, accomplished by applying a plaster cast while the wrist is in 30 to 45 degrees of dorsiflexion maintaining the transverse arch of the hand. At the same time, a dorsal hood is applied to bring 70 degrees or more of metacarpophalangeal (MP) joint flexion. In this way, with the proximal interphalangeal (PIP) joints free, interphalangeal joint motion can be instituted on the day of the fracture and continued during rehabilitation. The MP joint stiff in extension is not seen.[3]

Metacarpal Fractures

The mere presence or absence of shortening in the metacarpal is not an indication for internal fixation except in bone-loss injuries and perhaps in multiple displaced and irreducible metacarpal fractures. The hand tolerates shortening of the metacarpal of the small finger least. Internal metacarpals shorten only in a controlled fashion. The index metacarpal, in point of fact, does not seem to shorten a great deal unless multiple fractures are overriding because ligamentous restraint has been lost. Shortening of the small finger, on the other hand, seems to pull the other fingers into ulnar drift, which can be very destructive of hand function. Metacarpals are often shortened as much as 0.5 cm without loss of function as long as the hand is not al-

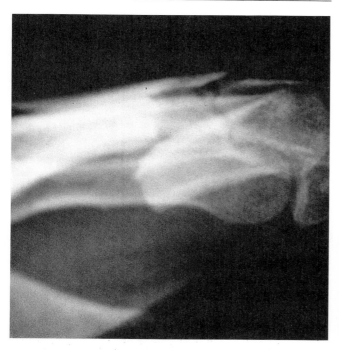

Fig. 1 A radiograph demonstrating a fracture of the index metacarpal with displacement and overriding. Angulatory deformity is minimal. Treatment consisted of applying a short arm cast with the MP joints flexed to approximately 60 degrees and with the PIP joints free to move.

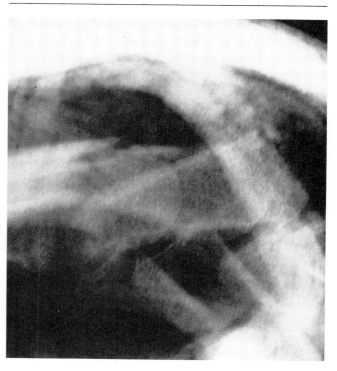

Fig. 2 Radiographs through the cast showing persisting deformity, but flexed MP joints.

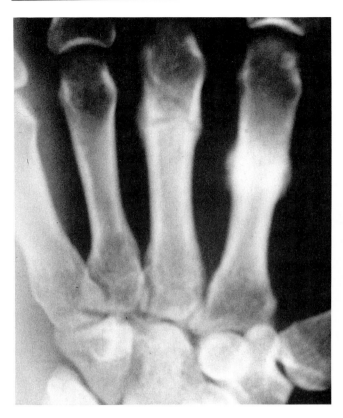

Fig. 3 At five weeks union was secure.

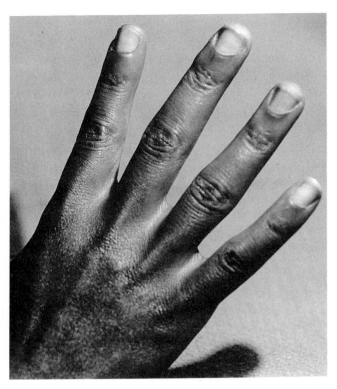

Fig. 4 Shows full extension of the index MP joint with no great discrepancy in digital length.

lowed to stiffen during the time of the shortening. If the hand is actively moved, beginning from the functional or the James position, no loss of function will occur (Figs. 1 to 5).

Another problem is rotational alignment. An oblique or spiral fracture of a metacarpal is more susceptible to rotational deformity because that configuration tends to rotate into malposition as the bone shortens. The best way to correct rotational malalignment is to flex the MP joints of all of the fingers simultaneously. Placing the hand in this position takes care of the rotational abnormalities and virtually eliminates the problem of MP joint stiffness. Shortening without bone loss rarely affects hand function in these fractures.

A patient must maintain this position for about four weeks to gain union. Although fracture lines may still be visible, in most metacarpal fractures in which the patient is actively moving, osseous callus will also be visible at this time and will provide the needed stability. When the cast is removed, at three to four weeks, the patient will have a significant extensor lag through the MP joint. This is not a matter of great concern. Once the patient starts to move the wrist and starts to move the MP joint into extension, the extensor lag will disappear. Any adherence of the extensor mechanism should be relieved by closing the fingers into a tight

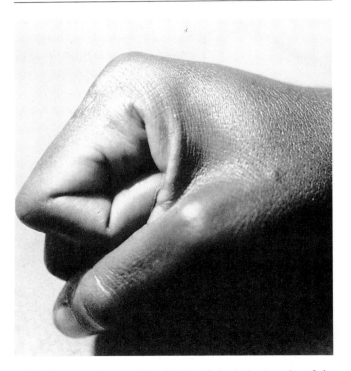

Fig. 5 Shows full MP joint flexion of the index in spite of the overriding and shortened metacarpal. Although there is deformity with union, there is no secondary joint stiffness following the fracture treatment.

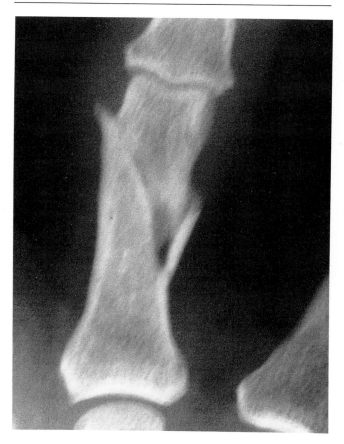

Fig. 6 Anteroposterior radiograph of a slightly comminuted oblique fracture of the proximal phalanx of the ring finger of a 60-year-old woman. This patient was treated in a similar cast with MP joint flexion and the PIP joints free to move in full flexion and extension.

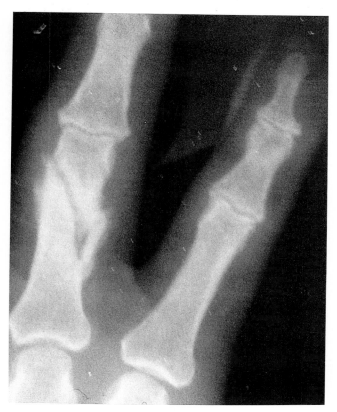

Fig. 7 Union of the fracture at six weeks with no rotational abnormality but with slight ulnar translation of the distal in relation to the proximal fragment.

fist and flexing the wrist maximally to give the greatest possible excursion of the extensor. Increasing the tendon's excursion frees it from its adhesions, precluding concern about loss of extension. Increased excursion will lead to complete MP joint extension.

Proximal phalanx fractures can be treated in like fashion. The proximal phalanx is unusual in that 90% of it is covered by tendon. Only distally, at the area of the PIP joint, can the bone be easily exposed surgically. Plate fixation of transverse fractures of the proximal phalanx is difficult because there is not adequate room beneath the extensor mechanism for plate and screws. Screw fixation, as opposed to plate fixation, avoids this problem and is preferable if internal fixation is required. I believe, however, that the tendon system that surrounds most of this bone can be used for diaphyseal fracture management. The Swiss AO group have demonstrated the value of the tension band in internal fixation. This principle also applies in closed reduction.[4,5] As the fingers close into a tight fist, the extensor is brought close against the dorsal cortex of the proximal

phalanx. A fracture hematoma and edema beneath the extensor create a tension band dorsally (F. Reyes, unpublished data). Reduction of the distal fragment to the proximal is a standard orthopaedic maneuver. The same method can be used to manage proximal phalanx fractures. The fingers are put in flexion through the MP joints and simultaneous PIP joint flexion is allowed. Also, as in metacarpal fracture, rotation can be controlled. The adjacent fingers control angulation and the dorsal extension of the cast puts slight pressure in the area of the PIP joint, gently reducing the distal to the proximal fragment.[6] Most patients with proximal phalanx fractures have a problem with extension of the PIP joint because of swelling and hematoma beneath the extensor mechanism. Patients must be taught how to extend the PIP joint passively and then actively flex the joint from the James safe position. By using anatomy's help, it is possible to avoid the open reduction and resultant adhesion formation associated with internal fixation (Figs. 6 to 9).

With fractures closer to the ends of the phalanges or metacarpals, joint subluxation and dislocation, in addition to the fracture, become an important part of the injury. A common intra-articular fracture in the

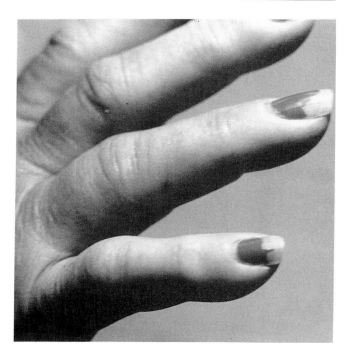

Fig. 8   The patient demonstrates nearly full extension of the PIP joint at seven weeks.

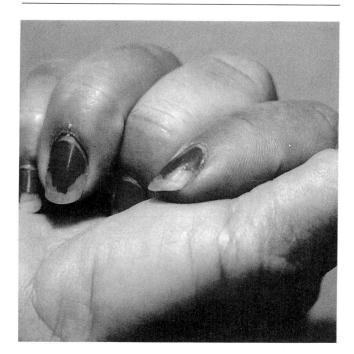

Fig. 9   She has nearly full digital flexion. This type of result in older patients is difficult to achieve by any treatment mode, but prevention of stiffness should be the hallmark of any treatment, certainly in older patients.

hand is the fracture of the base of the thumb, the Bennett's or Rolando's fracture. On the opposite side of the hand, the fracture of the base of the fifth metacarpal is similar, in that a small piece toward the center of the hand holds the ligament support system of the carpometacarpal joint and a large muscle-tendon unit works to displace the fragments and subluxate the joint. Other intra-articular fractures of relative importance in the hand are fracture-dislocations or subluxations, either volar or dorsal, of the PIP joint and the intra-articular fracture through the distal phalanx with the extensor digitorum communis tendon attached to one piece and the flexor digitorum profundus attached to the volar piece.

These fractures are inherently unstable because of muscle forces that pull them apart, resulting in displacement, intra-articular incongruity, or gross dislocation. Because of this, some type of internal fixation will probably be required to achieve reduction and maintain it until union occurs. Clearly, in metaphyseal fractures with intra-articular components, there is a place for internal fixation.

In addition to fractures with gross dislocation and those in which muscle forces act to displace the fractures, there are chip fractures in which a portion of the articular surface is dislocated by the external violence that caused the fracture. Condylar fractures of the distal portion of the proximal phalanx at the PIP joint create special surgical problems. The collateral ligament remains attached to this condylar fracture. Sometimes, maintaining a varus or valgus force on the digit and applying a plaster finger cast to the finger will obtain reduction. Often, however, fractures of this type are difficult to reduce and even more difficult to maintain. For this reason, metaphyseal intra-articular fractures are more apt to require internal fixation than are those in the more diaphyseal portions of the bone, most of which can be treated by closed means.

Basilar thumb fractures, both intra- and extra-articular, may be overlooked for one reason or another. Often, these fractures heal with some deformity, but with little functional impairment.[7] Arthroplasties or fusions at the base of the thumb are rare in men with malunited or Bennett's or Rolando's fractures. Arthroplasty of the basilar joint of the thumb is more likely to be performed for osteoarthritis that is not related to previous joint fracture. There are many persons whose basilar joints of the thumb are deformed, but who remain asymptomatic.

References

1. Burkhalter WE: Closed treatment of hand fractures. *J Hand Surg* 1989;14A:390–393.
2. Burkhalter WE, Reyes FA: Closed treatment of fractures of the hand. *Bull Hosp Joint Dis Orthop Inst* 1984;44:145–162.

3. Coonrad RW, Pohlman MH: Impacted fractures in the proximal portion of the proximal phalanx of the finger. *J Bone Joint Surg* 1969;51A:1291–1296.

4. Freeland AE, Jabaley ME, Hughes JL: *Stable Fixation of the Hand and Wrist*. New York, Springer-Verlag, 1986.

5. Segmüller G: *Surgical Stabilization of the Skeleton of the Hand*. Baltimore, Williams & Wilkins, 1977.

6. Jahss SA: Fractures of the proximal phalanges: Alignment and immobilization. *J Bone Joint Surg* 1936;18:726–731.

7. Cannon SR, Dowd GSE, Williams DH, et al: A long term study following Bennett's fracture. *J Hand Surg* 1986;11B:426.

Comminuted Fractures of the Distal Radius

Joseph B. Zagorski, MD

Introduction

Fractures of the distal radius, among the most common of all fractures, are unfortunately also among the most commonly mismanaged. The goals of treatment are restoration of anatomy, restoration of function, and prevention of arthrosis. However, realization of these goals depends on a number of patient variables, including age, sex, occupation, associated injuries, and comminution of the fracture. Obviously, the selection of treatment and method of management will depend on the interplay of these variables. It is the author's purpose to assist the reader in formulating a plan of management based on fracture mechanics and personal experience.

Although there are numerous classification schemes for distal radius fractures,[1-6] other than for anatomic significance they are generally cumbersome and of little use in planning treatment. Therefore, I prefer using two determinants to assess and classify injuries. First, is the injury a high- or a low-energy fracture? Second, is the fracture stable or unstable?

Low-energy injuries are usually the result of a fall or direct blow and are generally stable. The majority of these fractures can be managed by nonsurgical means.

High-energy injuries, usually the result of a motor-vehicle accident or a fall from a height, are often unstable and require surgical treatment. In addition to instability, other indications for surgical treatment include irreducibility, progressive median neuropathy requiring carpal tunnel release, severe open fractures, and fractures with an associated ipsilateral injury requiring fixation.

Closed Treatment

Reduction after closed manipulation can be maintained in these fractures by understanding the mechanical, anatomic, and physiologic factors that determine stability. The normal forces across the radiocarpal joint are volarly oriented. That is, the axial joint line, as designated by a line bisecting the lateral arc of the radiolunate joint, will fall volar to the midaxial line of the radius (Fig. 1).

If radiographs taken after reduction do not show restoration of the volar position of the axial joint line, then the probability of collapse of a distal radius fracture is significant.[7,8] This is essentially consistent with dorsal translation of the distal fragment, and, in the

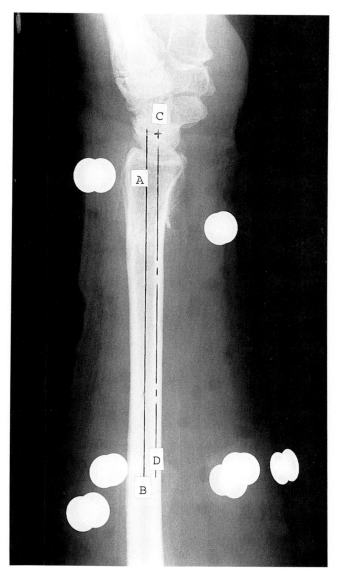

Fig. 1 Lateral radiograph demonstrating axial joint line (line CD).

presence of a dorsally comminuted fracture, collapse is imminent.

Anatomic Factors

The reduction should attempt to restore volar cortical abutment (not over-reduction) of the fracture fragments in order to maintain stability. However, if volar

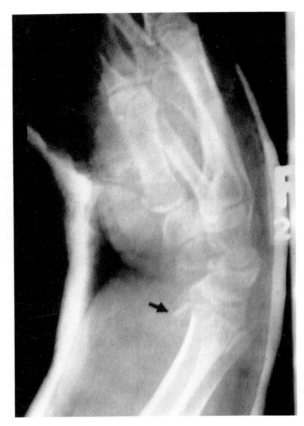

Fig. 2 Lateral radiograph demonstrating volar comminution.

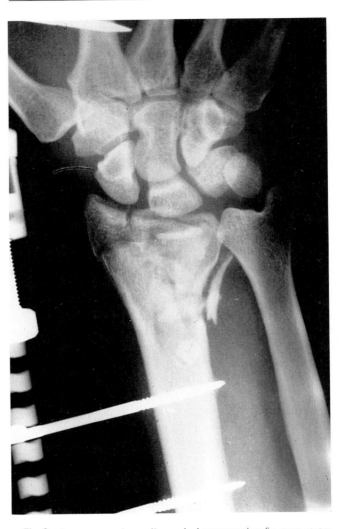

Fig. 3 Anteroposterior radiograph demonstrating fracture status after external fixator application with residual articular incongruity.

cortical comminution is present (Fig. 2) on either the distal or the proximal fragment, then stability is jeopardized and collapse of the fracture often occurs.[8] Therefore, even low-energy fractures that are volarly comminuted are at risk for further deformity and may require internal or external fixation.

Physiologic Factors

The muscle forces of the dorsal forearm, including the extensor carpi radialis brevis, the extensor carpi radialis longus, the extensor digitorum longus, and the brachioradialis, tend to deform distal radius fractures dorsally. In previous studies,[8-11] it has been shown that positioning the forearm in supination minimizes the deforming muscular forces. This is particularly important in closed treatment in which orthopaedists have historically tended to position the forearm in pronation.

Surgical Treatment

The current trend has been to use external fixation for the vast majority of comminuted displaced distal radius fractures.[12-14] This trend results in part from the current vogue for external fixation and the availability of improved fixators and in part from the difficulty of

open reduction and internal fixation if the injury is comminuted. Additionally, the use of plates and screws in the distal radius often proves to be more difficult than anticipated, leading, in many cases, to frustration and suboptimal fixation.

External fixation can provide satisfactory treatment, but this technique is also associated with complications. Pin-tract infections, tendon injuries, nerve injuries, prolonged stiffness, nonunion, reflex sympathetic dystrophy, and disuse osteoporosis can occur with this treatment.[15-18] Weber and Szabo[16] recently reported complication rates as high as 62% with external fixation. On the basis of my experience, I use external fixation only when absolutely necessary to maintain reduction, and generally leave it in place for no longer than six weeks.

One problem frequently associated with external fixation is failure to achieve joint restoration despite

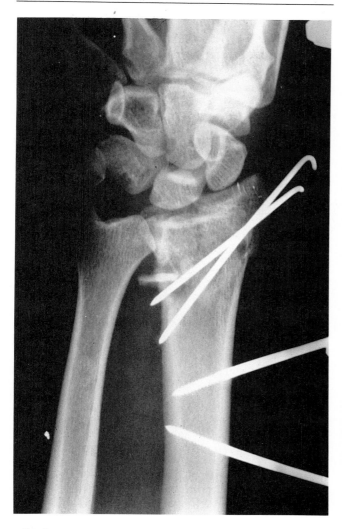

Fig. 4 Anteroposterior radiograph demonstrating intra-articular fracture with external fixator and K-wire supplementation for articular fracture.

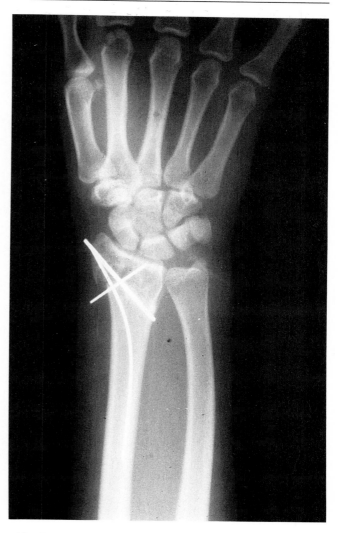

Fig. 5 Anteroposterior radiograph after percutaneous pin fixation.

length and angular restoration (Fig. 3). Unless the distal radial articular surface is reapproximated, the use of an external fixator (or any other fixation device) will not give a predictably satisfactory end result. Therefore, when the articular surface is incongruous and cannot be restored by external fixation alone, it is imperative to use additional Kirschner wires (Fig. 4), screws, or some other means to realign the joint surface and to give the best possible end result.

Discussion

My preference for most unstable distal radius fractures is to use percutaneous K-wire fixation whenever possible. I insert at least two wires from the radial styloid proximally and ulnarward to maintain length, stability, and position. Additional K-wires may be used as

necessary to hold the position of the articular fragments. Accurate positioning is crucial. The procedure should be performed using image intensification. The use of 0.62-mm and 0.45-mm wire for major fragment stability effectively maintains length. The 0.45-mm K-wire frequently does not penetrate the ulnar cortex of the radius, but stays in the intramedullary canal, where it causes a bending or "spring" effect that helps maintain radial length (Figs. 5 and 6).

At our institution, my colleagues and I have tried nearly all of the available external fixators for distal radius fractures and have found none that has an apparent advantage over the others. I recommend using the fixator that is most familiar and that can be applied most easily and quickly. The most common error in applying an external fixator is failure to achieve an accurate reduction. Using a fixator to hold an inaccurate reduction will only lead to malunion, nonunion,

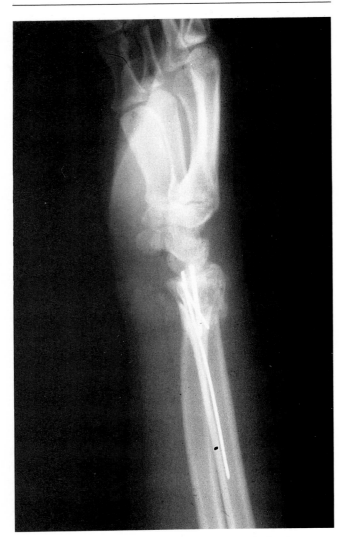

Fig. 6 Lateral radiograph after percutaneous pin fixation.

or late collapse of the fracture upon removal of the fixator. This frequently necessitates arthrodesis or some other salvage-type procedure leading to an unsatisfactory result. Similarly, the same principle applies when pins[6,19] or other types of internal fixation are used. To minimize the number of poor results, every effort must be made to achieve an anatomic reduction. The best way to accomplish this is to use intraoperative image intensification, to pay attention to detail, and to strive for perfection.

Whatever method is used to treat these fractures, the patient must be initiated into an early hand therapy program, preferably within the first 24 to 48 hours after surgery. Anatomic alignment alone cannot guarantee an excellent functional result. Early range of motion and early function are essential if the outcome is to be satisfactory.

References

1. Frykman G: Fracture of the distal radius including sequelae: Shoulder-hand-finger syndrome, disturbance in the distal radio-ulnar joint and impairment of nerve function. *Acta Orthop Scand* 1967;108(suppl):1–153.
2. Lidstrom A: Fractures of the distal end of the radius: A clinical and statistical study of end results. *Acta Orthop Scand* 1959;41(suppl):1–118.
3. Gartland JJ Jr, Werley CW: Evaluation of healed Colles' fractures. *J Bone Joint Surg* 1951;33A:895–907.
4. Sarmiento A, Pratt GW, Berry NC, et al: Colles' fractures: Functional bracing in supination. *J Bone Joint Surg* 1975;57A:311–317.
5. De Oliveira JC: Barton's fractures. *J Bone Joint Surg* 1973;55A:586–594.
6. Melone CP, Jr: Articular fractures of the distal radius. *Orthop Clin North Am* 1984;15:217–236.
7. Charnley J: *The Closed Treatment of Common Fractures.* London, E & S Livingston, 1972, p 128.
8. Zagorski JB, Zych GA, Latta LL, et al: Modern concepts in functional fracture bracing: The upper limb, in Griffin PP (ed): American Academy of Orthopaedic Surgeons *Instructional Course Lectures, XXXVI.* Park Ridge, Illinois, American Academy of Orthopaedic Surgeons, 1987, pp 377–401.
9. Sarmiento A: The brachioradialis as a deforming force in Colles' fractures. *Clin Orthop* 1965;38:86–92.
10. Zagorski JB: Functional bracing of Colles' fractures: A prospective study of immobilization in supination vs pronation. *Orthop Trans* 1979;3:62.
11. Sarmiento A, Zagorski JB, Sinclair WF: Functional bracing of Colles' fractures: A prospective study of immobilization in supination vs pronation. *Clin Orthop* 1980;146:175–183.
12. Cooney WP III, Linscheid RL, Dobyns JH: External pin fixation for unstable Colles' fractures. *J Bone Joint Surg* 1979;61A:840–845.
13. Clyburn TA: Dynamic external fixation for comminuted intra-articular fractures of the distal end of the radius. *J Bone Joint Surg* 1987;69A:248–254.
14. Knirk JL, Jupiter JB: Intra-articular fractures of the distal end of the radius in young adults. *J Bone Joint Surg* 1986;68A:647–659.
15. Cooney WP III, Dobyns JH, Linscheid RL: Complications of Colles' fractures. *J Bone Joint Surg* 1980;62A:613–619.
16. Weber SC, Szabo RM: Severely comminuted distal radial fracture as an unsolved problem: Complications associated with external fixation and pins and plaster techniques. *J Hand Surg* 1986;11A:157–165.
17. Chapman DR, Bennett JB, Bryan WJ, et al: Complications of distal radial fractures: Pins and plaster treatment. *J Hand Surg* 1982;7:509–512.
18. Green DP: Pins and plaster treatment of comminuted fractures of the distal end of the radius. *J Bone Joint Surg* 1975;57A:304–310.
19. Melone CP Jr: Open treatment for displaced articular fractures of the distal radius. *Clin Orthop* 1986;202:103–111.

Complex Upper-Extremity Fractures

Gregory A. Zych, DO

Complex Forearm Fractures

Segmental Fractures

Segmental fractures of the radius and ulna are usually the result of high-energy motor-vehicle accidents, which produce greater soft-tissue damage than trauma producing single-level fractures. There is often a crush component and more instability. Although it is generally agreed that stable internal fixation is required, few surgical techniques have been specifically developed to handle this clinical situation.[1-3]

Two types of segmental fractures are seen. The most common is characterized by diaphyseal fractures at two or more levels, with no joint involvement. These levels may be separated by several centimeters, often with a short proximal or distal segment. The radius, the ulna, or both may be involved. The other type is characterized by an intra-articular fracture level, frequently at the humeroulnar joint.

There are several considerations in choosing internal fixation for these fractures. Short segments may prevent adequate screw purchase if one plate is applied. A second smaller plate, placed perpendicular to the first, will improve fixation within the same segment. The 3.5-mm compression plates permit a greater number of screws per length of bone and should be used in this situation when possible. Fractures of the ulna will often have one level minimally displaced and can be stabilized with minimal soft-tissue dissection[3,4] by an intramedullary device such as a Rush rod. Angulation of the ulna toward the radius, especially in the proximal third, will produce loss of rotation or synostosis. Therefore, if angulation occurs, this method is contraindicated.

Surgical approaches are standard but tend to be extensile owing to multiple fracture levels. The longest exposure is required for plate fixation of displaced fractures. Preservation of the osseous blood supply assumes prime importance. Plate contouring may be difficult, and twisting it around the long axis is often necessary. Single long plates can apply dynamic compression across only one fracture level at best; therefore, fracture compression is achieved by lag screw intrafragmentary compression, with the plate used in the neutralization mode. To avoid a significant stress riser, plates should not be placed end to end.

Fracture lines with intra-articular extension into the humeroulnar joint and associated distal fracture levels can be stabilized using combined techniques. Conventional tension-band wiring will fix the proximal fracture, with the antirotation Kirschner wires of the tension band being used for intramedullary fixation of the distal fracture (Fig. 1). Plates and tension-band wiring are used to fix highly comminuted fractures.

References

1. Anderson LD, Sisk TD, Tooms RE, et al: Compression-plate fixation in acute diaphyseal fractures of the radius and ulna. *J Bone Joint Surg* 1975;57A:287–297.
2. Mast J, Jakob R, Ganz R: *Planning and Reduction Technique in Fracture Surgery.* Springer-Verlag, 1989, pp 85–90.
3. Sage FP: Medullary fixation of fractures of the forearm: A study of the medullary canal of the radius and a report of fifty fractures of the radius treated with a prebent triangular nail. *J Bone Joint Surg* 1959;41A:1489–1516.
4. Rush L: *Atlas of Rush Pin Technics.* Bervion Co, 1965.

Complex Proximal Humeral Fractures

Introduction

Although complex three- and four-part fractures and proximal humeral fractures have a relatively low incidence, they present formidable diagnostic and therapeutic challenges. Neer[1] has created an excellent classification system that allows the orthopaedist to understand the injury and arrive at a reasonably accurate prognosis for most proximal humeral fractures. The basis of this system is recognition of the importance of the blood supply to the humeral head and displacement of the four major fracture fragments. However, discerning or diagnosing the exact nature of the injury before undertaking surgery may be difficult, because the spherical shape of the humeral head and overlapping bones make these injuries difficult to evaluate radiographically. Therefore, the surgeon must be prepared mentally and technically to handle all possibilities. This, in addition to the frequent comminution, marked osteopenia, and the need for expert rehabilitation, makes these fractures a therapeutic challenge.

Three-Part Fracture or Fracture-Dislocation

The most common pattern is a surgical neck fracture with a displaced greater or lesser tuberosity. Because

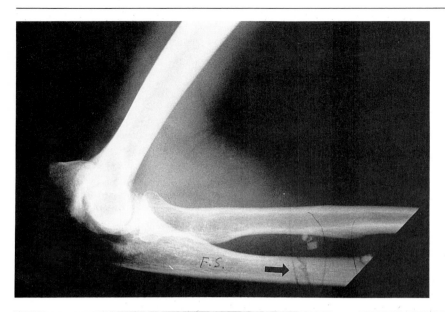

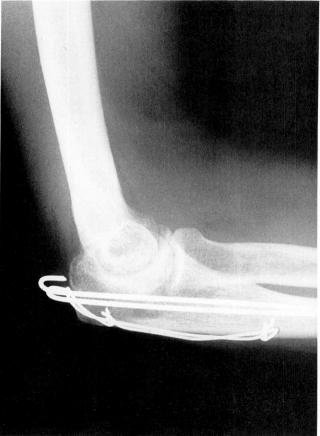

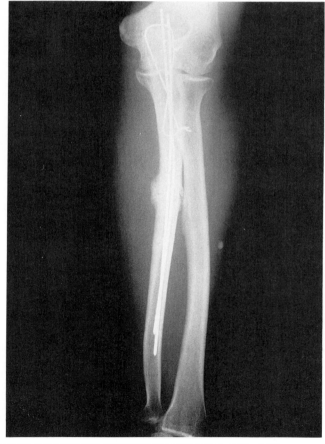

Fig. 1 Top, Radiograph showing displaced fracture of olecranon and ipsilateral midshaft ulnar fracture (solid arrow). **Bottom left**, Five months postoperatively the olecranon fracture has healed with the tension-band wiring. **Bottom right**, Extension of the K-wires across the midshaft ulnar fracture with excellent healing and alignment.

the majority of the circulating blood arrives through the greater tuberosity, these fractures have a poorer prognosis than fractures of the lesser tuberosity. The distal humeral shaft is usually medially displaced and may even be in side-to-side apposition with the proxi-

mal segment. The greater tuberosity is superior and posterior to the normal position. If the lesser tuberosity is intact, the articular segment may be internally rotated as a result of action of the subscapularis. Conversely, the head may be externally rotated if the lesser tuberosity is displaced. Dislocations, if present, commonly occur in the anterior direction.

Major problems secondary to these fractures are malunion and loss of motion. Malunited segments may cause bone or soft-tissue impingement. A displaced greater tuberosity fragment will impinge on the acromion or posterior glenoid. Malposition of the head leads to rotational deformity, although this may be well compensated. Muscle power of the rotator cuff could be decreased from loss of effective length. Less frequently, osteonecrosis is seen, generally associated with greater tuberosity fracture and head dislocation.

Treatment should be directed, therefore, to obtaining an anatomic reduction and instituting early motion. Unlike two-part surgical neck fractures,[2] when the three-part fractures are treated by closed reduction and some form of immobilization,[1,2] most reports in the literature state that unsatisfactory results are common. Malunion is the detrimental factor in most of these cases.

The most appropriate form of treatment is open reduction and internal fixation.[3-5] The goal should be stable fixation of the tuberosity to the proximal and distal humeral segments. Methods include cerclage wiring or suturing, with or without intramedullary rods, and buttress plating. Cerclage technique uses heavy wire or sutures passed through drill holes to secure the fragments. An intramedullary device may be passed antegrade from the proximal to the distal segments to improve axial stability, but it should not be used as the sole form of fixation because rotational control is poor. I believe this form of fixation is unpredictable, and its applications are limited.

Buttress plating uses several types of plates affixed to the proximal and distal humeral segments with a combination of cortical and cancellous screws. These plates are "T-plates," "L-plates," cloverleaf, and modified semitubular, according to the AO/ASIF terminology. The advantages of this type of fixation are multiple points of purchase on the humeral head or proximal segment and the ability to encompass or hold together the tuberosity and head segment by the contouring of the proximal plate. These advantages become clear when the bone is osteopenic and comminuted.

The preferred surgical approach is a straight anterior deltopectoral incision extending from the clavicle to the medial edge of the deltoid humeral insertion. It should not be necessary to detach either end of the deltoid muscle, as abduction of the arm will provide wide exposure. After incision of the clavipectoral fascia, the long head of the biceps tendon is identified and traced proximally to the bicipital groove. This groove defines the border between the greater and lesser tuberosities, one of which will be displaced. The greater tuberosity will frequently be found posterior and perhaps superior to the humeral head because of pull of the posterior rotator cuff. The humeral head is often rotated into flexion, with the fracture surface facing anteriorly. Initial reduction proceeds after the surgeon identifies and curettes all fracture edges. A heavy mattress suture is placed in the insertion of the rotator cuff to assist in derotating and reducing the greater tuberosity fragment. Care must be taken to ensure that all of the greater tuberosity is reduced, as comminuted pieces with rotator cuff muscle attachments are commonly seen. If not comminuted, alignment of the lateral cortex will provide a good assessment of how well length and rotation have been restored. It is quite difficult to judge reduction on the medial cortical border, because of the capsular attachments, which should not be violated. Provisional fixation of the greater tuberosity can be accomplished with pointed fracture reduction clamps or temporary suturing. Except in comminuted cases, a good reduction will be quite stable to gentle passive motion.

Once the reduction is accomplished, the buttress plate must be selected. I believe that all plates should be placed posterior to the bicipital groove, where maximal contact is achieved between the plate and tuberosity. The "L-plate," with the "L" extension directed posteriorly, facilitates screw insertion, because the long axis of the plate is actually anterior to the long axis of the shaft. To minimize impingement, the surgeon should place the upper border of the plate no higher than one half the vertical distance of the greater tuberosity. It is desirable to have a minimum of three screws with six-cortex fixation in the distal humeral segment, so plate length is important. The three most proximal plate holes will accept 6.5-mm cancellous screws, which should be placed in a divergent fashion in the head segment. Fully threaded cancellous screws are recommended for maximal purchase (Fig. 2). Great care must be taken to prevent penetration of the articular surface or head with either the drills or screws. Intraoperative radiographs are mandatory.

The cloverleaf plate is especially suited for use in osteopenic bone. As many as seven 3.5-mm or 4-mm cancellous screws can be placed through the proximal portion of the plate into the humeral head (Fig. 3). The anterior "leaf" may be removed to allow for more anterior placement of the plate so as not to disturb the biceps tendon. I preserve the biceps tendon whenever possible.

A different technique advocated recently[6] uses a modified semitubular plate described originally by Weber. In essence, a "blade plate" is created by bending the proximal plate 90 degrees. Limited clinical experience has been reported with this implant, but it does appear promising for some fractures.

Four-Part Fracture or Fracture-Dislocation

In this injury, vascularity of the humeral head is thought to be completely interrupted, because the tub-

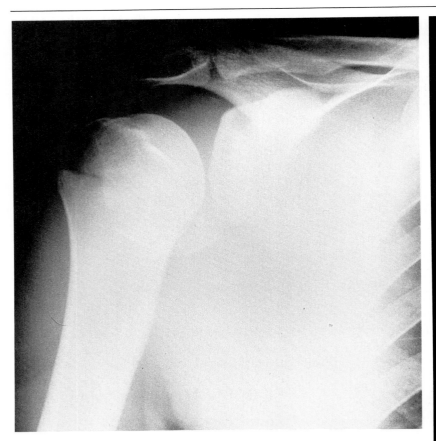
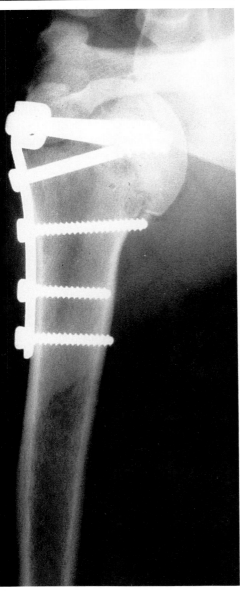

Fig. 2   **Left**, Three-part fracture of the proximal humerus. **Right**, Open reduction and internal fixation with an "L-plate."

erosities are dissociated totally from the articular segment. In my experience, dislocation occurs almost equally in both anterior and posterior directions.

Neer's original studies of this fracture reported a 38% rate of osteonecrosis of the humeral head.[1] Subsequent series have all documented the occurrence of this complication but with an average incidence of only 20%.[2,4,5] Furthermore, many patients with radiographic evidence of osteonecrosis have not developed humeral head collapse or symptomatic arthrosis.[7] If internal fixation is technically feasible, it may be considered the treatment of choice in selected patients; however, good bone quality, minimal comminution between the major fragments, and patient compliance are prerequisites

that are seldom found in one patient. If any of these three is absent, prosthetic replacement is recommended. Extensive comminution of the proximal humeral shaft is an indication for implantation of an intercalary allograft cortical segment to provide reliable bone support for the humeral prosthesis.

The surgical approach is the same as previously described for three-part fractures. In fracture-dislocation, the humeral head segment may be found outside the capsule, and in one of my cases it was in the axilla. It must be carefully replaced within the glenoid cavity if internal fixation is performed. The next challenge is to decide whether the surgical findings indicate either internal fixation or prosthetic replacement. Loss of me-

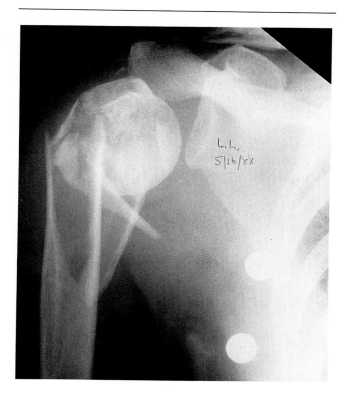

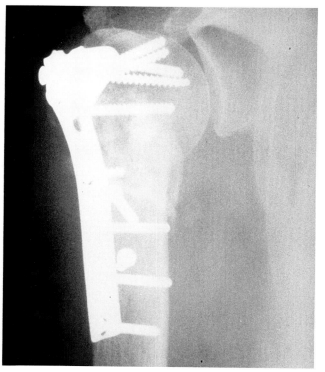

Fig. 3 Top, Comminuted proximal humerus with extension into the diaphysis. **Bottom,** Open reduction and internal fixation with a cloverleaf plate. The proximal plate extension has been removed.

dial bone makes it difficult to reposition the head on the shaft and fix it securely while maintaining proper length. At times, there may be only 2 to 3 cm of cancellous bone left in the head for screw purchase, mandating accurate screw placement. Cancellous screws 4 mm in diameter are favored, because more screws can be placed than with the 6.5-mm variety. Fixation of the tuberosities to the head is usually not possible, because the head segment is composed of or covered entirely with articular cartilage. Stabilization to the humeral shaft will allow healing to occur between the head and tuberosities. The lesser tuberosity is sutured to the greater tuberosity as well as to the shaft. The most suitable buttress plate for this purpose is the cloverleaf.

The humeral prosthetic replacement technique has been well described in the literature and will not be discussed here.

Rehabilitation

Among the most important aspects of treatment are a well planned rehabilitation program and a cooperative patient.[1,8] In severe fractures, only stable internal fixation will permit the early humeral motion so necessary to prevent shoulder adhesions and to minimize pain. Likewise, with prosthetic replacement, early motion will yield the best functional results.

Passive motion, using sling support between exercise periods, in the sagittal (flexion) and coronal (external rotation) planes is begun within the first postoperative week. Emphasis is placed on regaining range of motion first, with muscle strengthening as a later objective. Active motion should be avoided for the first six weeks or until the tuberosities are healed. Patients with buttress-plate fixation will often require removal of the plate within four to six months postoperatively to achieve maximal range of motion. If the fixation is removed early, the final motion will not be compromised.

Summary

Complex proximal humeral fractures are a challenge to the orthopaedic surgeon. Achieving fracture healing while avoiding loss of function is best accomplished by early rigid fixation or prosthetic replacement, depending on the fracture type and characteristics.

References

1. Neer CS II: Displaced proximal humeral fractures: Part I. Classification and evaluation. Part II. Treatment of three-part and four-part displacement. *J Bone Joint Surg* 1970:52A:1077–1103.
2. Young TB, Wallace WA: Conservative treatment of fractures and fracture-dislocations of the upper end of the humerus. *J Bone Joint Surg* 1985;67B:373–377.

3. Paavolainen P, Björkenheim JM, Slätis P, et al: Operative treatment of severe proximal humeral fractures. *Acta Orthop Scand* 1983;54:374–379.
4. Siebler G, Kuner EH: Spätergebnisse nach operativer Behandlung proximaler Humerusfrakturen bei Erwachsenen [Late results following the surgical treatment of proximal humerus fractures in adults]. *Unfallchirurgie* 1985;11:119–127.
5. Kristiansen B, Christensen SW: Plate fixation of proximal humeral fractures. *Acta Orthop Scand* 1986;57:320–323.
6. Sehr JR, Szabo RM: Semitubular blade plate for fixation in the proximal humerus. *J Orthop Trauma* 1988;4:327–332.
7. Lee CK, Hansen HR: Post-traumatic avascular necrosis of the humeral head in displaced proximal humeral fractures. *J Trauma* 1981;21:788–791.
8. Stableforth PG: Four-part fractures of the neck of the humerus. *J Bone Joint Surg* 1984;66B:104–108.

Complex Fractures About the Elbow

Joseph B. Zagorski, MD

Introduction

In the past decade, advances in internal fixation have offered additional treatment modalities for intra-articular fractures of the distal humerus and radial head. This chapter describes the management of these two injuries.

Intra-articular Comminuted Fractures of the Humeral Condyles

Historically, controversy regarding the management of displaced intra-articular comminuted fractures of the distal humerus has caused a great deal of confusion for the practicing orthopaedist. There have been strong advocates of both nonsurgical[1-7] and surgical[8-19] treatment for these fractures. Recently,[14-19] however, surgical treatment has become increasingly popular, probably because of the availability of better instrumentation and implants. Without exception, in the recent decade all of the proponents of surgical treatment have strongly advocated rigid internal fixation. My own experience[17] has confirmed that open reduction and rigid internal fixation provides the most predictably satisfactory results in the management of

intracondylar humeral fractures. Certain principles, however, must be emphasized if consistently satisfactory results are to be achieved.

Surgical Principles

Even under ideal circumstances, surgery about the elbow is difficult because of the anatomic structures and complex anatomy of the elbow joint. In severely displaced fractures the morbid anatomy makes surgery even more difficult.

Achieving an extensile exposure to the elbow is among the most important principles in surgical management. The skin incision may be made in an inverted posterior U-shape as described by MacAusland and Wyman[14] or it may be longitudinal with the underlying tissues exposed in a posterior U-shape. The latter has been my preference over the last several years because it allows essentially the same exposure and is cosmetically superior to the other.

It is essential to identify the ulnar nerve, to retract it carefully, and to be aware of its location throughout the surgical procedure. An osteotomy of the olecranon is necessary and may be performed either in an intra-articular or extra-articular manner. Most fractures can

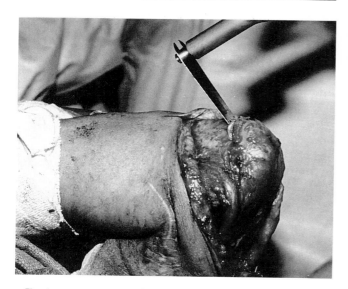

Fig. 1 Extra-articular osteotomy using oscillating saw.

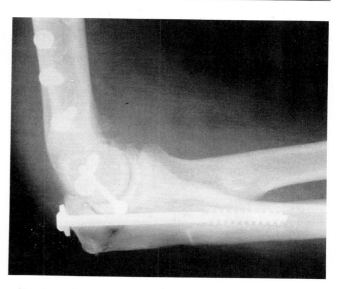

Fig. 2 Lateral radiograph demonstrating ''V'' intra-articular osteotomy.

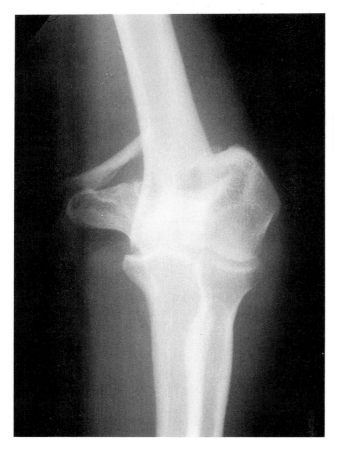

Fig. 3   Anteroposterior radiograph demonstrating intracondylar fracture.

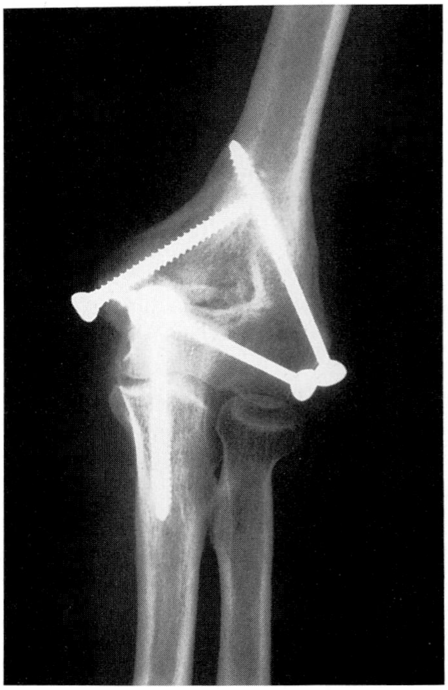

Fig. 4   Anteroposterior radiograph after open reduction and internal fixation demonstrating triangular pattern of screw fixation.

be approached using the extra-articular osteotomy.[17] This has the advantage of avoiding further joint damage and also prevents the subsequent nonunions of the olecranon that can occur when an intra-articular osteotomy is used. Before the osteotomy of the olecranon is done, the proximal ulna should be predrilled with a 3.2-mm drill. The osteotomy is then performed with a micro saw blade held at a 45-degree angle to the long axis of the ulna (Fig. 1). I prefer to perform an extra-articular osteotomy for most fractures except for anteriorly displaced condylar fractures. When the condyles or articular fragments are displaced proximally and anterior to the joint, an intra-articular osteotomy is better. Recently, when an intra-articular osteotomy is indicated, I have used a chevron olecranon osteotomy, which, although technically more difficult, gives increased stability and greater cancellous bone contact, minimizing the possibility of olecranon nonunion (Fig. 2).

A pulsatile jet lavage system is useful for cleansing the fracture fragments of obscuring clots. The intra-articular fragments should be reapproximated first, with special attention directed toward preserving all

bone stock. Once this is accomplished, the condyles and reconstructed distal fragments are rigidly fixed to the proximal fragment using AO technique. I prefer to use screw fixation rather than plate fixation whenever possible. When using screws, careful planning of the screw placement is essential. Usually the first attempt at screw placement provides the best fixation, because multiple attempts often lead to further comminution and destruction of bone. When using screws, a triangular configuration is optimal (Figs. 3 and 4). Kirschner wires are used only for temporary or supplemental fixation and should never be used as a primary implant because they do not provide rigid fixation. Frequently, however, screw fixation alone is not sufficient, and the use of either a one-third tubular or reconstruction plate is necessary. Careful planning is required to achieve satisfactory screw and plate position and to prevent impingement of joint motion from poor implant placement. Before closure, stability and range of motion are evaluated. The osteotomy is fixed with a 6.5-mm cancellous bone screw and a washer. A closed drainage system is used, and closure is performed in the routine fashion.

Table 1
Radial head fractures

Clinical Data	Excision	No Surgery	Open Reduction/ Internal Fixation
Isolated Fractures			
No. of cases	9	9	2
Mean range of motion			
Extension	21°	14°	18°
Flexion	110°	123°	125°
Pronation	62°	78°	50°
Supination	72°	90°	53°
Fracture-Dislocations			
No. of cases	8	1	3
Mean range of motion			
Extension	25°	12°	15°
Flexion	122°	130°	125°
Pronation	60°	80°	60°
Supination	73°	85°	75°

Rehabilitation after surgery is nearly as important as the surgical technique. Therapy is initiated by the second or third day after surgery. Active and active assisted range of motion is emphasized for the first four to six weeks. Cast fixation or supplementation is contraindicated in these fractures. Prolonged immobilization will almost guarantee permanent stiffness, arthrofibrosis, and loss of motion. Recently, my colleagues and I reported on a large series of patients treated surgically and nonsurgically and concluded that all patients who were immobilized had poor results, whereas 76% of patients who had surgical intervention with early motion demonstrated good to excellent results.[17]

The goals of management therefore are threefold: (1) anatomic reduction, (2) rigid fixation, and (3) early joint motion. Failure to achieve any one of these goals will yield predictably unsatisfactory results.

Displaced Fractures of the Radial Head

Although many recommendations for management of radial head fractures have been proposed,[20-31] none has been universally accepted. It is therefore important to approach these injuries with a rational, goal-oriented protocol. This chapter seeks to clarify the indications for various methods of treatment using information gleaned through personal and collective experience.

Because the radial head has a role as a significant stabilizer of the elbow,[23,25,27,30,32] it seems unusual that one of the most common methods of treatment for a radial head fracture is its excision. Excision may be acceptable for the severely comminuted, isolated radial head injury, but in the presence of an associated dislocation, it is far from optimal treatment.

Materials and Methods

I recently evaluated 32 comminuted fractures of the radial head. Of 12 with associated elbow dislocations, eight had surgical excision of the fragments, three had an open reduction and internal fixation of the radial head, and one patient had closed treatment with early motion. Of the 20 isolated displaced fractures, nine had excisions of the radial head, nine had no surgical treatment, and two patients had open reduction and internal fixation. All patients were evaluated as to their elbow stability and range of motion. The average follow-up was one year.

Results

Of the eight patients with fracture-dislocations who had radial head excisions, five (62%) had recurrence of the dislocation. These patients were immobilized for two to three weeks in a long arm splint or cast and then placed in a fracture brace that limited extension (30 to 45 degrees) for three weeks. Three elbows redislocated in the brace and two redislocated after brace removal. All five patients continued to complain of pain in their elbows at one-year follow-up. Of the three patients who had an open reduction and internal fixation, none suffered redislocation. One of the three ORIF patients continued to have occasional discomfort but was not in constant pain. The single patient who was treated by closed means (seven days) and early motion remained stable.

Analysis of the entire series revealed that the average range of motion in the nonsurgical group (Table 1) was slightly better than that of the group treated by excision or open reduction and internal fixation. One must take into account however, that several of the excisions were performed because range of motion was impeded.

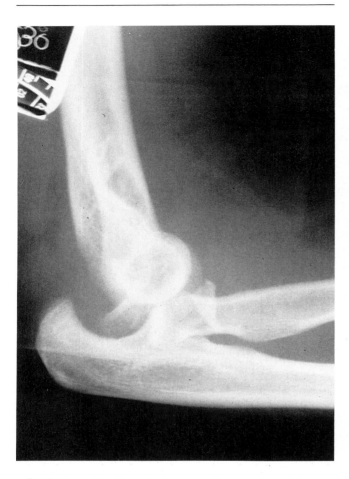

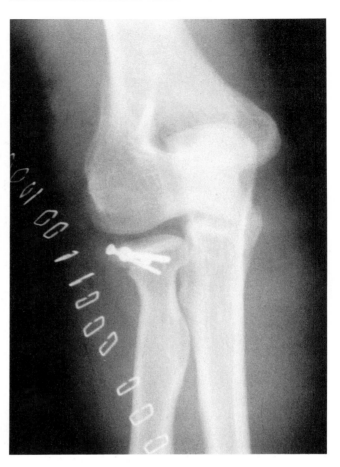

Fig. 5 Lateral radiograph demonstrating comminuted fracture dislocation.

Fig. 6 Anteroposterior radiograph demonstrating open reduction and internal fixation after fracture-dislocation.

These preliminary findings, as well as the experience of others,[22,24,26] suggest that preservation of the radial head may be a better alternative with an associated dislocation of the elbow. Additionally, even if the radial head cannot be internally fixed, it appears that as long as there are no fragments impeding motion, early excision has no advantage over early motion treatment without surgery.[20,21,28,29]

Protocol

My preferred treatment, therefore, is immediate aspiration of the elbow, injection of 1% lidocaine, and evaluation of the range of motion of the elbow with respect to flexion-extension and pronation-supination. If there is impingement, then surgical excision is indicated. If there is no impingement, I recommend five to seven days of immobilization, followed by active range-of-motion exercises. If an associated dislocation accompanies the fracture, stability should be assessed,

and open reduction and internal fixation should be considered if the elbow is unstable.

Technical Points

When open reduction is selected, one should attempt to achieve rigid fixation.[22,24,26,33] Therefore, the use of screws is preferable to pins. I find AO mini-screws particularly suitable for fixation in these fractures. The screw heads may be buried by countersinking them into the articular surface (Figs. 5 to 7).

On certain occasions a mini-plate may be needed to fix the radial head to the shaft. When this is necessary, care should be taken to place the plate on the lateral side of the radial head and neck. (Ideal placement is at the level of the 3- or 4-o'clock position when the forearm is in full supination.) This will prevent metal impingement at the proximal radioulnar joint. The fixation must be checked prior to closure and stability and range of motion must be evaluated carefully. If an el-

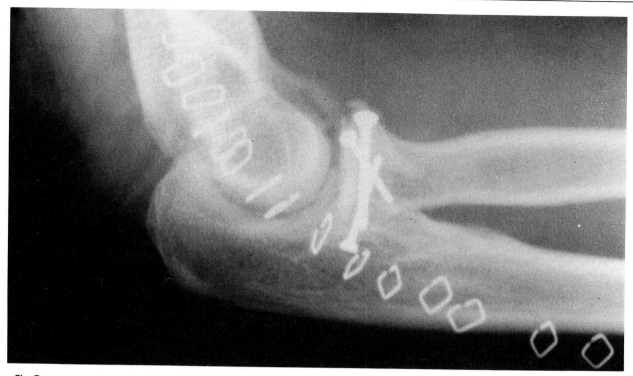

Fig. 7 Lateral radiograph after open reduction and internal fixation of the radial head.

bow dislocation was present, any instability in extension should be noted so that the physical therapy program can be modified appropriately. Early motion is instituted on the first or second day after surgery. Motion is limited to within a range of stability for three weeks, then gradually increased until the sixth week, at which time full range of motion is allowed.

Discussion

Recent reports may have made open reduction[22,24,26,33] for isolated radial head fractures seem attractive, but there have been no conclusive results to indicate that surgical repair is superior to excision or even nonsurgical treatment. My experience, while encouraging, is too preliminary to recommend open reduction and internal fixation routinely. Despite some advocates for silicone radial head replacement,[30,34] recent reports of inconclusive results, silicone synovitis, and implant failure[23,27,35] make this a questionable management alternative at best.

Whatever method of treatment is selected, prolonged immobilization should be avoided. Casts are never used and early range of motion and functional activity should be initiated. With an early exercise program stressing active control and motion of the elbow, satisfactory results may be achieved in the majority of patients.

References

1. Eastwood WJ: The T-shaped fracture of the lower end of the humerus. *J Bone Joint Surg* 1937;19:364–369.
2. Van Gorder GW: Surgical approach in supracondylar "T" fractures of the humerus requiring open reduction. *J Bone Joint Surg* 1940;22:278–292.
3. Watson-Jones R: *Fractures and Joint Injuries*, ed 4. Baltimore, Williams & Wilkins, 1952, vol 2, p 534.
4. Conn J Jr, Wade PA: Injuries of the elbow: A ten year review. *J Trauma* 1961;1:248–268.
5. Riseborough EJ, Radin EL: Intercondylar T fractures of the humerus in the adult: A comparison of operative and non-operative treatment in twenty-nine cases. *J Bone Joint Surg* 1969; 51A:130–141.
6. Brown RF, Morgan RG: Intercondylar T-shaped fractures of the humerus: Results in ten cases treated by early mobilisation. *J Bone Joint Surg* 1971;53B:425–428.
7. Horne G: Supracondylar fractures of the humerus in adults. *J Trauma* 1980;20:71–74.
8. Speed JS: Fractures: Number 1. Surgical treatment of condylar fractures of the humerus, in Pease CN (ed): American Academy of Orthopaedic Surgeons *Instructional Course Lectures, VII.* Ann Arbor, JW Edwards, 1950, pp 187–194.
9. Cassebaum WH: Operative treatment of T and Y fractures of the lower end of the humerus. *Am J Surg* 1952;83:265–270.
10. Evans EM: Supracondylar-Y fractures of the humerus. *J Bone Joint Surg* 1953;35B:381–385.
11. Knight RA: The management of fractures about the elbow in adults, in Raney RB (ed): American Academy of Orthopaedic Surgeons *Instructional Course Lectures, XIV.* Ann Arbor, JW Edwards, 1957, pp 123–141.

12. Bickel WE, Perry RE: Comminuted fractures of the distal humerus. *JAMA* 1963;184:553–557.

13. Wickstrom J, Meyer PR Jr: Fractures of the distal humerus in adults. *Clin Orthop* 1967;50:43–51.

14. MacAusland WR Jr, Wyman ET Jr: Fractures of the adult elbow in American Academy of Orthopaedic Surgeons *Instructional Course Lectures, XXIV*. St. Louis, CV Mosby 1975, pp 169–181.

15. Bryan RS: Fractures about the elbow in adults, in Murray DG (ed): American Academy of Orthopaedic Surgeons *Instructional Course Lectures, XXX*. St. Louis, CV Mosby, 1981, pp 200–223.

16. Jupiter JB, Neff U, Holzach P, et al: Intercondylar fractures of the humerus: An operative approach. *J Bone Joint Surg* 1985; 67A:226–239.

17. Zagorski JB, Jennings JJ, Burkhalter WE, et al: Comminuted intraarticular fractures of the distal humeral condyles: Surgical vs. nonsurgical treatment. *Clin Orthop* 1986;202:197–204.

18. Gabel GT, Hanson G, Bennett JB, et al: Intraarticular fractures of the distal humerus in the adult. *Clin Orthop* 1987;216:99–108.

19. Henley MB: Intra-articular distal humeral fractures in adults. *Orthop Clin North Am* 1987;18:11–23.

20. Radin EL, Riseborough EJ: Fractures of the radial head: A review of eighty-eight cases and analysis of the indications for excision of the radial head and non-operative treatment. *J Bone Joint Surg* 1966;48A:1055–1064.

21. Miller GK, Drennan DB, Maylahn DJ: Treatment of displaced segmental radial-head fractures: Long-term follow-up. *J Bone Joint Surg* 1981;63A:712–717.

22. Odenheimer K, Harvey JP Jr: Internal fixation of fracture of the head of the radius: Two case reports. *J Bone Joint Surg* 1979; 61A:785–787.

23. Morrey BF, Askew L, Chao EY: Silastic prosthetic replacement for the radial head. *J Bone Joint Surg* 1981;63A:454–458.

24. Shmueli G, Herold HZ: Compression screwing of displaced fractures of the head of the radius. *J Bone Joint Surg* 1981;63B:535–538.

25. Broberg MA, Morrey BF: Results of treatment of fracture-dislocations of the elbow. *Clin Orthop* 1987;216:109–119.

26. Sanders RA, French HG: Open reduction and internal fixation of comminuted radial head fractures. *Am J Sports Med* 1986;14:130–135.

27. Carn RM, Medige J, Curtain D, et al: Silicone rubber replacement of the severely fractured radial head. *Clin Orthop* 1986;209:259–269.

28. Broberg MA, Morrey BF: Results of delayed excision of the radial head after fracture. *J Bone Joint Surg* 1986;68A:669–674.

29. Goldberg I, Peylan J, Yosipovitch Z: Late results of excision of the radial head for an isolated closed fracture. *J Bone Joint Surg* 1986;68A:675–679.

30. Swanson AB, Jaeger SH, La Rochelle D: Comminuted fractures of the radial head: The role of silicone-implant replacement arthroplasty. *J Bone Joint Surg* 1981;63A:1039–1049.

31. Coleman DA, Blair WF, Shurr D: Resection of the radial head for fracture of the radial head: Long-term follow-up of seventeen cases. *J Bone Joint Surg* 1987;69A:385–392.

32. Morrey BF, Chao EY, Hui FC: Biomechanical study of the elbow following excision of the radial head. *J Bone Joint Surg* 1979; 61A:63–68.

33. McArthur RA: Herbert screw fixation of fracture of the head of the radius. *Clin Orthop* 1987;224:79–87.

34. Mackay I, Fitzgerald B, Miller JH: Silastic replacement of the head of the radius in trauma. *J Bone Joint Surg* 1979;61B:494–497.

35. Mayhall WS, Tiley FT, Paluska DL: Fracture of silastic radial-head prosthesis: Case report. *J Bone Joint Surg* 1981;63A:459–460.

Wrist and Forearm Reconstructive Procedures After Complex Upper-Extremity Trauma

William E. Burkhalter, MD

Introduction

After complex upper-extremity trauma to the wrist and forearm, degenerative arthritis and/or instability may severely impair function. Wrist arthrodesis, creation of an ulnar nonunion (three-bone forearm), and stabilization of the extremity by making a one-bone forearm are procedures that may greatly improve function. This chapter discusses the indications for and techniques of these procedures.

The use of these procedures for rheumatoid arthritis or other nontraumatic conditions will also be described.

P A R T A

Arthrodesis

In recent years, numerous reports on prosthetic replacements, limited carpal fusions, and tendon transfer to the ligament to increase stability have obscured the

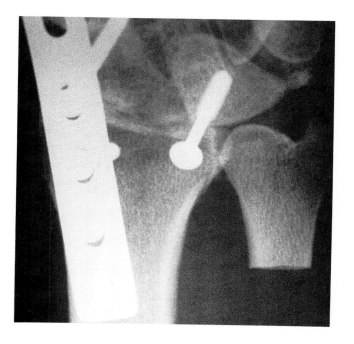

Fig. 2 A partial ostectomy of the ulna was carried out.

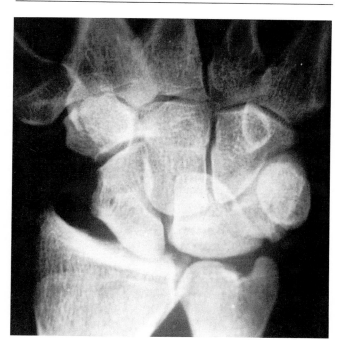

Fig. 1 This 30-year-old-man was injured in a motor-vehicle accident and sustained injuries to all four extremities. This intercarpal and radiocarpal dislocation was treated by immediate arthrodesis as a primary treatment.

use of total wrist arthrodesis as an alternative in patient rehabilitation. Ryu[1] and Palmer and associates,[2] after studies using the electric goniometer, reported that between 30 and 40 degrees of volar flexion and dorsiflexion are used in the normal activities of daily living. Although this suggests that the wrist and therefore the hand require this much dorsiflexion and volar flexion to function normally, this is actually not the case. Compensatory finger and elbow rotation will permit performance of most activities without difficulty.

No known surgical procedure involving intercarpal fusion or ligament augmentation can increase the range of motion of the wrist. Rather, all procedures performed on the wrist, except for capsular releases, result in loss of motion, and if a procedure does not succeed in relieving pain, it has accomplished very little. On the other hand, if losing motion makes it possible to get completely away from pain, is it not better to think in terms of using a wrist arthrodesis as a primary procedure, rather than as an alternative only to be considered after other procedures have failed? Although wrist ar-

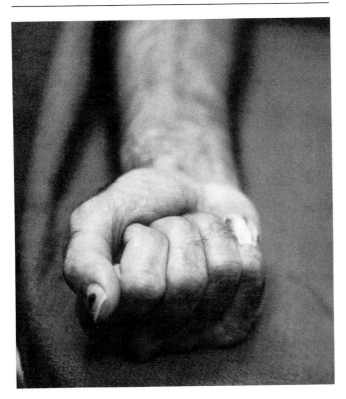

Fig. 3   Shows full digital flexion and full supination five weeks after the accident.

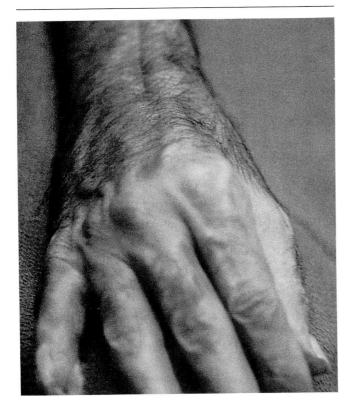

Fig. 4   Full forearm pronation is possible.

throdesis is rarely done if there is some chance of saving wrist motion, it is undeniably frustrating to perform an intercarpal fusion, with its subsequent loss of motion, rehabilitate the patient, and then find that there is incomplete relief from pain. Performing a wrist arthrodesis at this point means that a year of the patient's life will have passed while this problem was being corrected. In such a case, total arthrodesis, the alternative used after failure of an intercarpal fusion or prosthetic replacement, should probably have been considered as a primary treatment (Figs. 1 to 4). Furthermore, intercarpal fusions have not been used long enough to establish with any degree of certainty that they will last the life of the patient. The wrist arthrodesis definitely will last that long. Wide and associates[3] have found that, for their arthrodesis patients, perianal care is the sole functional problem. Because wrist flexion makes this task easier, however, even patients with bilateral wrist fusion can function normally as long as the arthrodesis is done in neutral position rather than dorsiflexion. Using a compression plate, with or without iliac bone graft, and reducing the intercarpal bones to living cancellous bone grafts has improved our fusion rate considerably and has also diminished the risks involved in this surgery.[4]

References

1. Ryu J: Fracture evaluation of the wrist: Range of motion and strength. Presented at the 41st Annual Meeting of the American Society for Surgery of the Hand, February 1986.
2. Palmer AK, Werner FW, Murphy D, et al: Functional wrist motion: A biomechanical study. *J Hand Surg* 1985;10A:39–46.
3. Wide G, Quezer D, Strickland J, et al: Arthrodesis for post traumatic arthritis of the wrist: Reliability and function. Presented at the 42nd Annual Meeting of the American Society for Surgery of the Hand, San Antonio, Sept 9–12, 1987.
4. Hajj A, Burkhalter W, Dorin D: Arthrodesis of the wrist using a compression plate. Presented at the 37th Annual Meeting of the American Society for Surgery of the Hand, New Orleans, January 1982.

P   A   R   T   B

Three-Bone Forearm

In the three-bone forearm, nonunion of the ulna has been achieved through a reconstructive procedure. The three-bone forearm, mentioned by Steindler in his book on orthopaedics as an alternative to the Darrach procedure, has various indications[1-5] for treatment of an abnormal distal radioulnar joint. An arthritic distal radioulnar joint, whether the result of trauma or secondary to rheumatoid arthritis, will maintain carpal support but limit forearm pronation and supination. Creating an ulnar nonunion an inch or so proximal to the distal radial joint will allow the patient to have forearm rotation. Most patients with an ulnar ostectomy

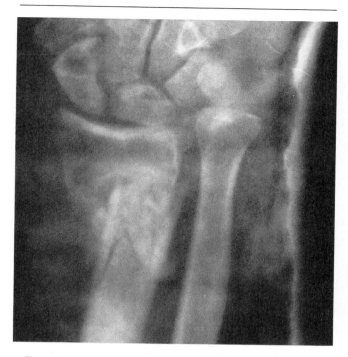

Fig. 1 Radiograph of a 55-year-old man treated for multiple gunshot wounds including this one of the radius. Union occurred with deformity and with considerable pain and limitation of forearm rotation.

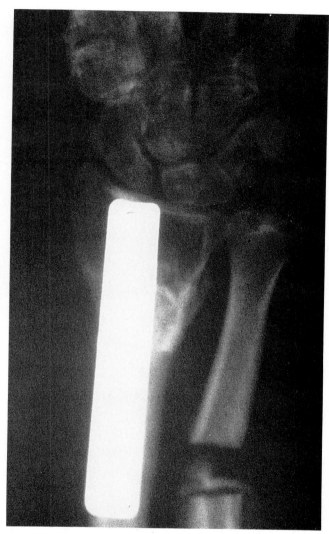

Fig. 2 An osteotomy to realign but not necessarily lengthen the radius was carried out, and a partial ulnar ostectomy was performed to improve forearm rotation.

substitution have a greater-than-normal range of motion of forearm rotation. The three-bone forearm concept, with or without arthrodesis of the distal radial ulnar joint, also has drawbacks. After a partial ulnar ostectomy, the stability of the proximal ulna depends on an intact interosseous membrane. This membrane, which runs from proximal radial to distal ulnar, is not capable of healing like other ligamentous tissues. The central portion of it is the significant part. A Monteggia lesion with an ulnar shaft fracture and dislocation of the radial head proximally is an example. Because of interosseous membrane continuity distal to the ulnar fracture, the radius is only stable once the ulna has been reduced and maintained. Without the interosseous membrane, stabilization of the ulna cannot stabilize the radius. If the interosseous membrane, in this case, is torn from the ulnar fracture to the proximal radial ulnar joint, but not distally, plating the ulna essentially produces an intact interosseous membrane to aid in relocation of the radial head. The Essex-Lopresti fracture is another example of an interosseous membrane tear associated with subluxation of the distal radial ulnar joint and radial head fracture proximally. In this situation, creating a nonunion of the ulna will lead to extensive instability and is contraindicated.[6]

The Darrach operation is used to relieve arthritis of the distal radial ulnar joint. Like the three-bone forearm, it is not applicable when there is instability of the

distal radioulnar joint.[7] That is, treating the instability of the distal radioulnar joint by partial excision of the ulna, either at its most distal extent or more proximally, is only to risk further instability. Compared with the Darrach, the three-bone forearm procedure has the advantage of being easier to perform and easier to rehabilitate, and of having more applications. For example, a partial ulnar ostectomy is valuable to allow controlled shortening of the radius to achieve union in a highly comminuted radial fracture. Likewise, in performing an osteotomy of the distal radius to realign an articular surface, bone grafting is not necessary. Length need not be restored to maintain forearm rotation. A closing wedge osteotomy will correct the deformity without either bone graft or osseous lengthening (Figs. 1 to 4).

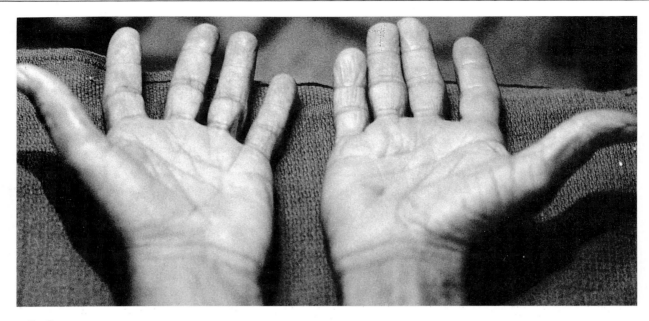

Fig. 3   Shows the supination possibility with this partial ulnar ostectomy.

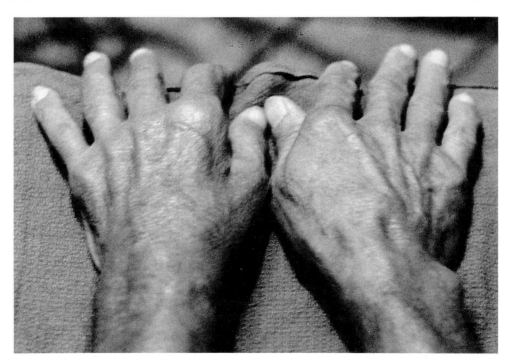

Fig. 4   Shows pronation that is possible with this partial ulnar ostectomy without distal radioulnar joint fusion.

One discouraging aspect of a Darrach procedure done to correct instability is continuing or increased instability of the proximal ulna following excision.[8] Multiple procedures using tendons in various combi-nations from the extensor carpi ulnaris and the flexor carpi ulnaris have been tried to correct this distressing problem, but none of these is 100% effective.[9,10] Ar-throdesis or the creation of a synostosis between the radius and ulna may be necessary to get rid of the instability that limits the patient's use of the forearm. If instability of the radius and ulna limits function and cannot be improved by tendon transfer, it should be treated by creation of a one-bone forearm.

References

1. Sauvé: Constitution d'un ligament annulaire péricubital inférieur (luxation de la tête cubitale lors de al supination). *Bull Mem Soc Nat Chir* 1933;59:628–629.
2. Sauvé: Nouvelle technique de traitement chirurgical des luxations récidivantes isolées de l' extrémité inférieure du cubitus. *J Chir* 1936;47:589–594.
3. Goncalves D: Correction of disorders of the distal radio-ulnar joint by artificial pseudarthrosis of the ulna. *J Bone Joint Surg* 1974;56B:462–464.
4. Sulkosky JM, Ballard A, Burkhalter WE: The three bone forearm: A salvage procedure for treatment of ulnar non-union. Presented at the 44th Annual Meeting of the American of Academy Orthopaedic Surgeons, Las Vegas, Feb 3–8, 1977.
5. Hales W, Burkhalter W: The three-bone forearm procedure in reconstruction of the distal radio-ulnar joint. Presented at the 40th Annual Meeting of the American Society for Surgery of the Hand, Las Vegas, January 1985.
6. Essex-Lopresti P: Fractures of the radial head with distal radio-ulnar dislocation: Report of 2 cases. *J Bone Joint Surg* 1951;33B:244–247.
7. Hui FC, Linscheid RL: Ulnotriquetral augmentation tenodesis: A reconstructive procedure for dorsal subluxation of the distal radioulnar joint. *J Hand Surg* 1982;7:230–236.
8. Dingman PVC: Resection of the distal end of the ulna (Darrach operation): An end-result study of twenty-four cases. *J Bone Joint Surg* 1952;34A:893–900.
9. Goldner JL, Hayes MG: Stabilization of the remaining ulna using one-half of the extensor carpi ulnaris tendon after resection of the distal ulna. *Orthop Trans* 1979;3:330.
10. Tsai TM, Stilwell JH: Repair of chronic subluxation of the distal radioulnar joint (ulnar dorsal) using flexor carpi ulnaris tendon. *J Hand Surg* 1984;9B:289–294.

P A R T C

One-Bone Forearm

Creation of a one-bone forearm for radial ulnar instability with interosseous membrane tear, bone loss, or severe proximal forearm soft-tissue loss may not be easy. If there is good bone stock distally, with ulnar continuity, then arthrodesis of the distal radioulnar joint through the distal cancellous bone and intercalary bone grafting may be all that is required. If, however, a significant portion of the distal ulna has been excised, the problem may be more serious. In this case, the medullary canal of both the radius and ulna must be opened. A corticocancellous bone graft is extended from the medullary canal of the radius into the medullary canal of the ulna. This sheet of bone graft is 3 to 4 cm wide and its length depends on the distance between the radius and ulna. The arthrodesis should be as distal as possible to avoid complications associated

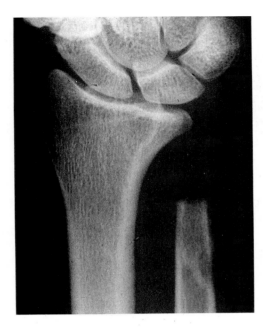

Fig. 1 This is a radiograph of a 40-year-old who had several operations to stabilize an unstable Darrach surgical procedure.

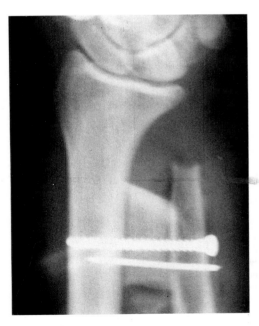

Fig. 2 An attempt was made to stabilize the radius to the ulna by bone graft between radius and ulna.

with surgery in the upper forearm. If iliac bone is used, and I prefer to use it, one side of the graft will be cortical and the other side cancellous. Before fixing the graft into the medullary canals of the radius and ulna,

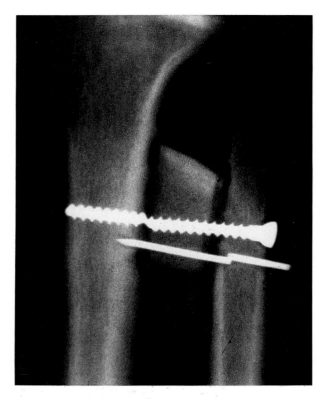

Fig. 3 The procedure failed because the medullary canals of the radius and ulna were not opened.

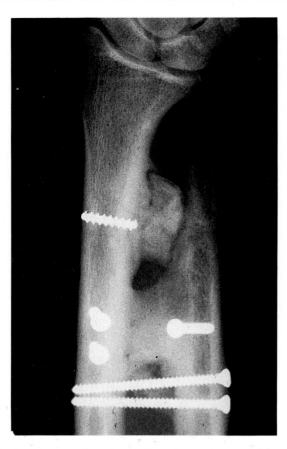

Fig. 4 Subsequently, union of the radius to ulna was achieved by opening the medullary canals and transfixing a unicortical iliac crest bone graft to the radius and ulna with screws. A stable forearm resulted with normal hand, wrist, and elbow function.

transfixing screws are placed between the ulna and radius to compress the bones together. Immobilization, to control forearm rotation, will be required for about 90 days to obtain solid union. If there are problems about the exact position of the forearm, 0.062-cm Kirschner wires can be used temporarily to transfix the radius to the ulna before making the cortical openings into the medullary canals of the radius and ulna. The opposing surfaces of the bone can then be opened to accept the bone graft. I use a straight dorsal incision, working on both sides of the finger extensors, and have found this gives adequate exposure and, if done distally enough, does not interfere with tendon glide because most of the surgery is done under the muscle tissue rather than under the tendons (Figs. 1–4).

If forearm rotation will be lost, what position of the forearm is best regarding pronation and supination? A combination of shoulder abduction and internal rotation can compensate for loss of pronation. Supination has no similar compensatory maneuver. In daily activities, loss of forearm rotation is a more serious problem

than loss of wrist motion. Typing, writing, picking up a telephone, and eating an apple are all movements that require forearm rotation. For patients without nerve injury, I feel that the neutral position is probably best. With median nerve loss, more supination allows the patient to see the palm of the hand and aids manipulation within the grasp. If the radial nerve is destroyed along with muscle loss and severe proximal scarring, more supination may be helpful. With 30 to 40 degrees of supination, wrist flexion will open the hand by tenodesis, and dorsiflexion can be accomplished by gravity. In addition to these variables, hand dominance, occupation, and avocations must be considered in selecting the optimal position. If possible, as in elbow or wrist fusion, it is helpful to use casts or splints to simulate the final position before carrying out surgical fusion.

The Management of Nonunions of the Humerus

Fred G. Corley, MD

Gerald R. Williams, MD

John C. Pearce, MD

Charles A. Rockwood, Jr., MD

Introduction

Fractures of the humerus represent somewhere between 2% and 7% of all fractures.[1-3] In 1985, the Northeastern Ohio Trauma Study predicted there would be 4.6 million emergency room visits for fractures in the United States. Visits for humerus fractures were expected to account for 5% of the total.[1] Early authors reported that humerus fractures, particularly those involving the shaft, resulted in nonunion more frequently than any other long-bone fractures.[3,4] Campbell[3] reported on the management of 226 nonunited long bone fractures, of which 52 involved the humerus.[3] These 52 nonunions represented 17% of the 293 fresh humeral fractures. Improved methods of closed treatment, including the properly applied hanging arm cast, functional bracing, and early isometric exercises, as well as more rigid internal fixation techniques, have helped to lower the nonunion rate for all humerus fractures to less than 13%.[5-9]

Proximal Humerus

Proximal humerus fractures occur most commonly in osteoporotic, elderly women.[10-13] The poor bone stock associated with prolonged nonunion in this population can make surgical reconstruction quite challenging.

The incidence of nonunion of proximal humerus fractures is difficult to determine. Previous reports of proximal humerus nonunion have been scant and were based on small numbers of patients.[13-25] In our experience of 40 patients with proximal humeral nonunion, all fracture patterns described by Neer[11,12,26] were represented, but two-part fractures proceeded to nonunion most commonly.[13,19,27]

Several factors predisposing to nonunion, in addition to the original trauma and displacement, have been identified.[15,17,18,28-33] Neer[12] cited soft-tissue interposition (primarily the deltoid muscle or the long head of the biceps), treatment involving a heavy hanging arm cast or some other element of distraction or overdistraction, inadequate immobilization, alcoholism, and systemic diseases, such as diabetes mellitus. Rooney and Cockshott[18] proposed pre-existing glenohumeral stiffness as a factor. Rockwood and Pearce[34] cited two additional predisposing factors: inadequate primary internal fixation and prolonged immobilization with no isometric deltoid exercises.

Treatment

Nonsurgical treatment is often the most appropriate therapeutic option.[13,16,26,31,35-41] In Rockwood and Pearce's series,[34] 18 of the 40 patients with proximal

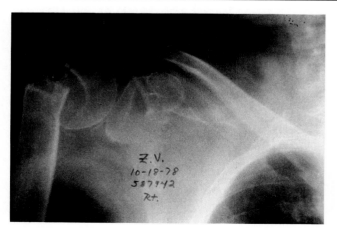
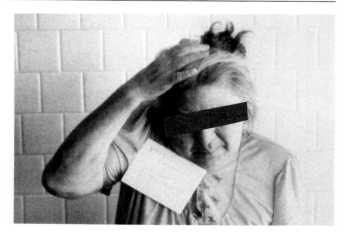

Fig. 1 Despite nonunion of the proximal humerus (**left**), this patient has a functional range of motion and minimal symptoms (**right**). She was treated nonsurgically.

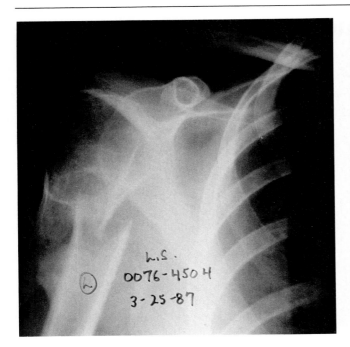
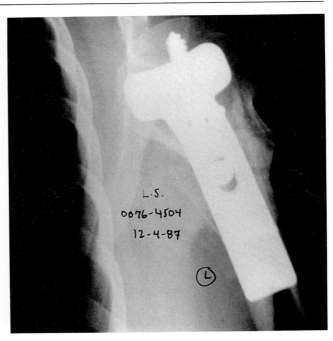

Fig. 2 **Left**, Bone stock is adequate, there has been no infection, the head is vascular, and the joint is congruent and not degenerative. **Right**, Open reduction, rigid internal fixation, and bone grafting are the preferred treatment.

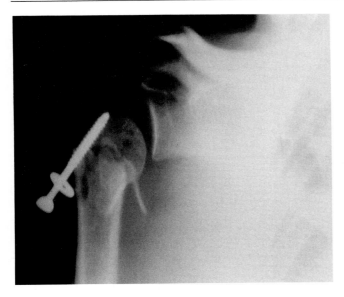
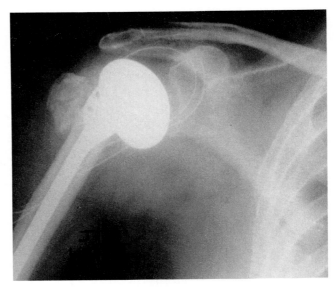

Fig. 3 In this case involving an atrophic proximal fragment (**left**), hemiarthroplasty was performed (**right**).

humerus nonunions were managed nonsurgically. Of these 18, 16 had no or minimal pain and two were poor surgical risks. Six of these patients had no anterior deltoid function and therefore were not good candidates for surgical reconstruction. If the six patients with denervated anterior deltoids are excluded, the patients treated nonsurgically had a functional range of motion of the shoulder and were not particularly limited by their humeral nonunion (Fig. 1).

Many patients with nonunions of the proximal humerus have symptoms that require surgical intervention. The quality and quantity of the remaining bone, the status of the glenohumeral articular surfaces, the vascularity of the head,[41] and the presence or absence

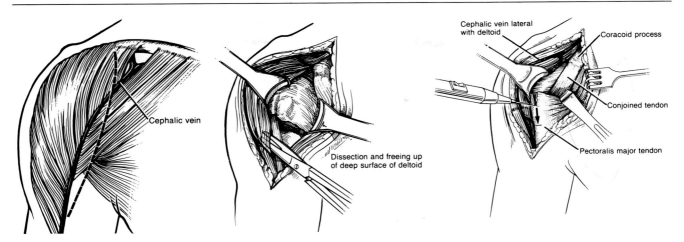

Fig. 4 **Left,** The proximal humerus is approached through a long deltopectoral incision and the cephalic vein is retracted laterally with the deltoid. **Center** and **right,** Exposure is enhanced by freeing the scarred undersurface of the deltoid and by incising the upper portion of the pectoralis major insertion.

of infection are all factors that the surgeon should consider when deciding on a specific surgical procedure. In general, if the bone stock is adequate, the articular surfaces are not incongruent or degenerative, the head is vascular, and there has been no documented infection, open reduction with rigid internal fixation and bone grafting are preferable to prosthetic replacement (Fig. 2).[15,19,26,31,33,42,43] Resectional arthroplasty may be warranted in patients with previous infection or severe bone loss. Hemiarthroplasty and total shoulder arthroplasty are reserved for patients with small, osteopenic proximal fragments, avascular humeral heads, or significant glenohumeral arthritis (Fig. 3).[21,44,45] Because, in many cases, the final decision can only be made at surgery, the surgeon should be prepared for either open reduction and bone grafting or prosthetic replacement.

Technique

The patient is placed on the operating table in the supine position with the hips and knees flexed. A narrow headrest is used to allow full access to the top of the shoulder. The involved shoulder should be positioned at the edge of the table, to allow unobstructed hyperextension down toward the floor and external rotation should it become necessary to dislocate the joint for prosthetic replacement.

The shoulder is approached through a long deltopectoral incision extending from the clavicle to the deltoid insertion. This long incision allows wide exposure. Subcutaneous hemostasis must be meticulous, because previous scarring may increase deep bleeding. The deltopectoral interval is identified and the deltoid is retracted laterally along with the cephalic vein. Care must be taken to mobilize completely the scarred undersurface of the deltoid, which frequently adheres to the

proximal humerus. Exposure can be further improved by releasing the superior half or two thirds of the pectoralis major insertion from the humerus (Fig. 4). After developing the deltopectoral interval, the surgeon must next identify and protect the musculocutaneous and axillary nerves (Fig. 5). The tendon of the long head of the biceps is identified distal to the nonunion site and is traced proximally to the transverse humeral ligament (Fig. 5, *bottom right*). Not infrequently, the tendon will be found trapped within the nonunion site. The proximal humerus and nonunion site are exposed subperiosteally, the fragments are displaced, the nonunion tissue is removed, and the medullary canals of both fragments are opened. The fragments are fashioned into a cup and cone configuration and impacted. Any remaining cortex on the distal fragment is "rose petalled" before impaction. Fixation is obtained with an ASIF T-shaped or cloverleaf plate from the AO small fragment set. Interfragmentary lag screws should be used if possible. Autogenous corticocancellous graft is then added (Fig. 6).

If the proximal fragment is atrophic and inadequate for internal fixation or if the glenohumeral joint is degenerative, prosthetic replacement is undertaken. After the biceps tendon has been traced to the interval between the greater and lesser tuberosities, the tuberosities, along with their musculotendinous attachments to the rotator cuff, are removed from the proximal fragment. The remainder of the proximal fragment is excised and the articular surface of the glenoid is inspected. If it is arthritic, a glenoid component can be cemented into place. A proximal humeral prosthesis is inserted, usually requiring cement for stabilization. The prosthesis should be cemented in a raised position to restore proper tension in the deltoid and the rotator cuff muscles. The tuberosities are then reattached. Can-

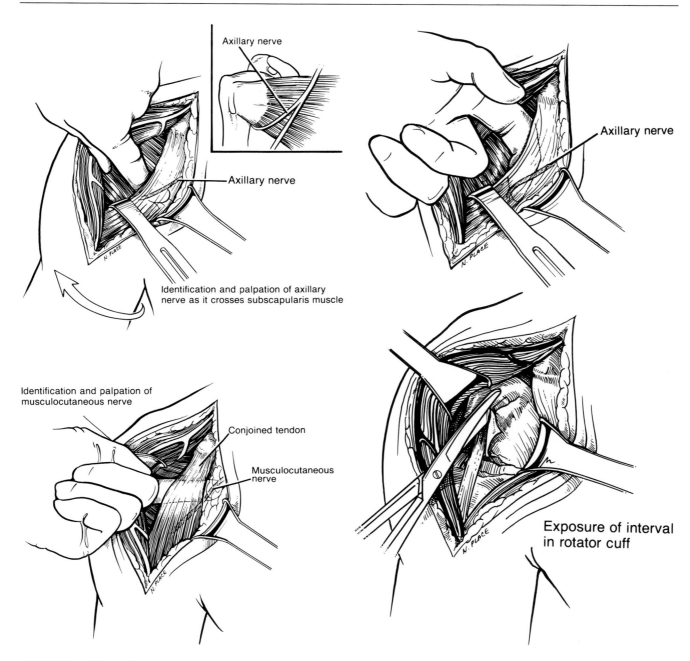

Axillary nerve

Axillary nerve

Identification and palpation of axillary
nerve as it crosses subscapularis muscle

Axillary nerve

Identification and palpation of
musculocutaneous nerve

Conjoined tendon

Musculocutaneous
nerve

Exposure of interval
in rotator cuff

Fig. 5   The axillary and musculocutaneous nerves must be identified and protected before the long head of the biceps and the supraspinatus-infraspinatus interval are identified.

cellous graft from the excised proximal fragment can be used to fill any defects deep to the tuberosities (Fig. 7).

Humeral Shaft

Humeral shaft fractures represent 1% to 1.5% of all fractures.[1,2,10,46] The incidence of nonunion of the shaft of the humerus has changed substantially in the past 50 years. With the introduction by Caldwell[6] of the hanging cast, functional bracing by Sarmiento and associates,[9] and isometric deltoid exercises, the incidence of nonunion has dropped to 13% or less in nonpathologic fractures.[5,8,47-55] Several factors have been implicated in the development of nonunion. These include soft-tissue interposition, location in the middle third, open fracture, inadequate open reduction, comminution, distraction by a heavy hanging arm cast or

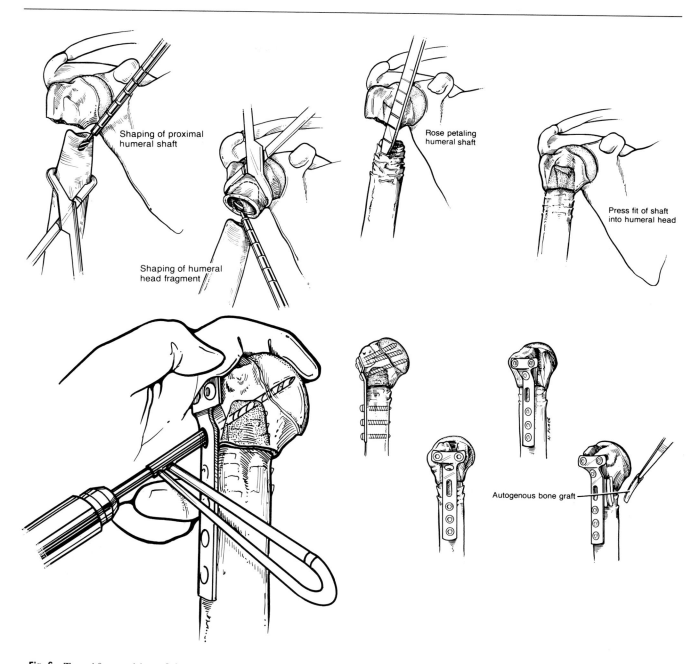

Labels in figure: Shaping of proximal humeral shaft; Shaping of humeral head fragment; Rose petaling humeral shaft; Press fit of shaft into humeral head; Autogenous bone graft

Fig. 6 **Top**, After excision of the nonunion, the medullary canal of each fragment is opened, the fragments are fashioned into a cup and cone configuration and impacted. **Bottom**, An ASIF T-plate and bone graft are then applied.

other cause, pathologic fracture, poor muscle function, alcoholism, and a transverse or short oblique fracture line.[3,8,46,56-58] Our experience confirms the association of several of these factors, especially open fractures, with nonunion.

Treatment

Nonunion of the humeral shaft has been treated using inlay and onlay tibial grafts with bone pegs or bone screws, dual tibial onlay grafts, dual fibular only grafts, cerclage wires, Küntscher nails and other intramedullary devices, compression plates with and without bone grafts, dual compression plates, and electrical stimulation.[3,4,7,8,59-68] The reported union rates using these procedures range from 46% to 96%. Rosen[68] recommended compression plating and adds cancellous bone graft for atrophic nonunions. Healy and associates[8] reported on 26 patients who underwent compression

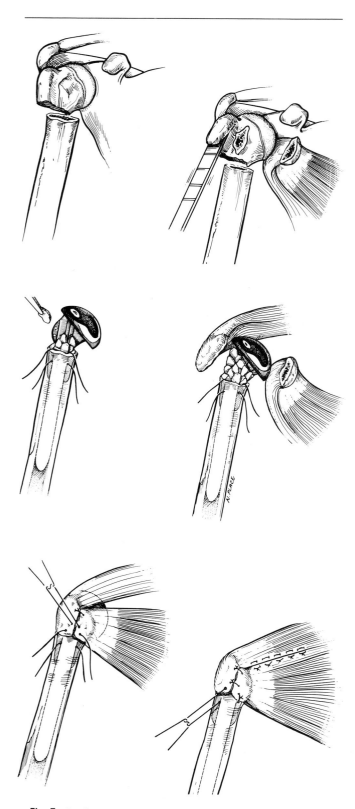

Fig. 7 In the case of hemiarthroplasty, the tuberosities are removed from the proximal fragment for later reattachment to the prosthesis. Any defects deep to the tuberosities can be filled with autogenous graft from the head fragment.

plating for humeral shaft nonunions. Their union rate was 96% with rigid fixation and bone grafting. Factors associated with persistent nonunion were lack of bone graft and failure to obtain rigid internal fixation. Several other reports have confirmed excellent union rates using rigid compression plating and bone grafting.[7,59,61,64,67] Consequently, this is the preferred treatment (Fig. 8).

Technique

With the patient in the supine position, the arm is prepared and draped without a tourniquet to insure complete access to its proximal aspect. A sterile tourniquet should be available.

The humerus is approached anterolaterally between the brachialis and the triceps proximally and the brachioradialis and brachialis distally.[48] The radial nerve is identified distally between the brachioradialis and the brachialis. It is traced proximally to its passage through the lateral intermuscular septum with the radial collateral artery. With the radial nerve protected, the nonunion site is exposed subperiosterally, the nonunion tissue is excised, the intramedullary canal of each fragment is entered, and the sclerotic bone ends are freshened. The bleeding surfaces are approximated and fixed with a 4.5-mm dynamic compression plate. If possible, plates with offset screw holes should be used in order to minimize the stress riser effect of colinear holes in this frequently osteoporotic bone. Healy and associates[8] recommended six cortices on either side of the nonunion site. Rosen,[68] on the other hand, recommended eight cortices. Eight cortices, as well as an interfragmentary compression screw, are preferable, if at all possible. Autogenous cancellous graft is then added (Fig. 9). The operative note should state whether or not the radial nerve crosses the plate and at which hole, because this information is useful if plate removal becomes necessary.

Distal Humerus

In comparison to fractures in other locations, fractures of the distal humerus are uncommon. Wilson[69] reported that fractures or dislocations involving the elbow accounted for only 10% of fractures and dislocations in all locations. Of 4,066 fractures or dislocations seen over a seven-year period and involving all locations, 189 (4.6%) involved the distal humerus. If supracondylar fractures in children are excluded, the incidence drops to 2.6%. The Northeastern Ohio Trauma study[1] reported 11 (1.2%) distal humeral fractures in a series of 886 fractures from all locations. Rose and associates[10] reported 186 distal humeral fractures in the residents of Rochester, Minnesota, over a 10-year period. If fractures in patients under 10 years of age are excluded, there were 79 distal humerus frac-

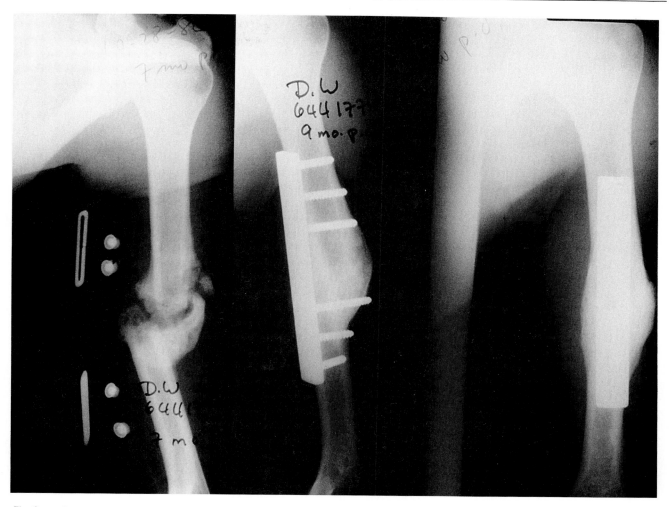

Fig. 8 **Left,** Nonunion of the humeral shaft. **Right,** Treatment is by open reduction, rigid internal fixation, and bone grafting.

tures in 53,000 persons over a ten-year period—an incidence of 1.5 such fractures per 10,000 population per year. Fracture of the distal humerus in adults is clearly uncommon and probably represents approximately 2% of all fractures.[70]

Because fracture of the distal humerus is uncommon, nonunion is rare.[70-77] Consequently, experience with treatment of distal humeral nonunion is limited. Wilson[69] reported a 2% incidence of nonunion in the 50 condylar fractures in his series. Bryan and Bickel[72] identified two (7%) pseudarthroses in 30 T-condylar fractures treated at the Mayo clinic. Knight[76] stated that nonunion of the supracondylar component of a T-condylar fracture occurs more frequently than nonunion of the intercondylar portion. Some predisposing factors to nonunion include inadequate internal fixation, comminution, infection, osteonecrosis, overdistraction, and severe soft-tissue injury, as in open fracture.[70,77,78] Inadequate internal fixation and severe soft-tissue in-

jury appear to be the most common causes of nonunion.

Treatment

Treatment options for condylar nonunions include benign neglect; osteosynthesis using open reduction, internal fixation, and bone grafting; resectional arthroplasty; interpositional arthroplasty; total elbow replacement (B.F. Morrey, unpublished data); distal humeral allograft; vascularized autograft; and arthrodesis.[77,79-88] Anteroposterior and lateral polytomograms taken before surgery are helpful in delineating persistent fracture lines and in evaluating remaining bone stock. Osteosynthesis with open reduction, rigid internal fixation, and bone grafting is the preferred management in most cases (Fig. 10).[74,77] Combining lysis of intra-articular adhesions with osteosynthesis has been recommended in cases in which the arc of joint motion is less than 70 or 80 degrees (B.F.

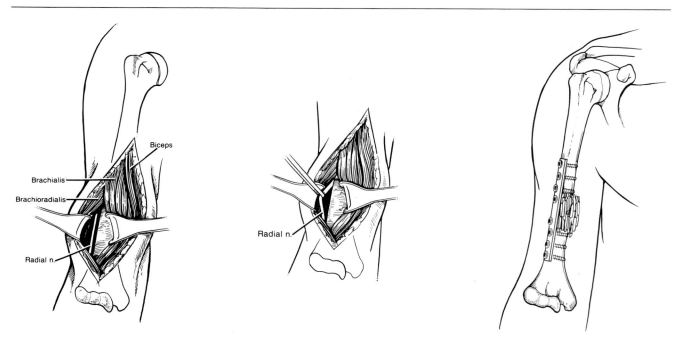

Fig. 9 **Left** and **center**, The humeral shaft is approached anterolaterally and the radial nerve is identified distally between the brachialis and brachioradialis muscles. **Right**, The nonunion is excised, the medullary canal is opened, the shaft is "rose petalled," and the fragments are rigidly fixed and bone grafted.

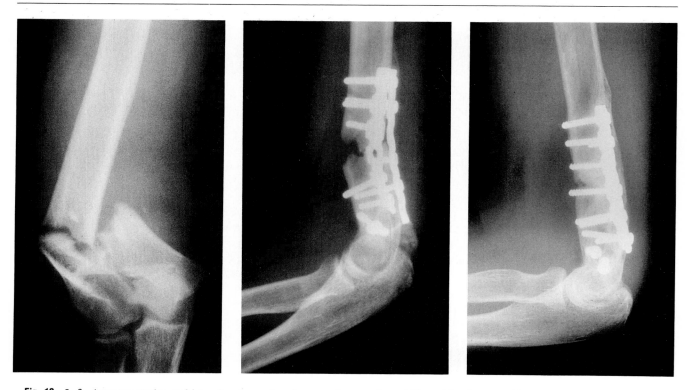

Fig. 10 **Left**, Anteroposterior and lateral radiographs of a severely comminuted T-condylar fracture. **Center**, Treatment with the supracondylar component in hyperextension. **Right**, The nonunion was excised and the fragments were reduced anatomically, rigidly fixed, and bone grafted.

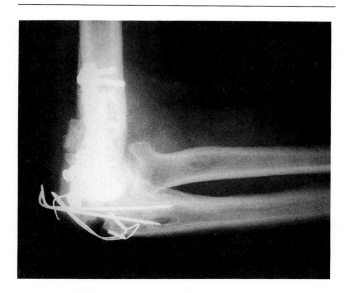

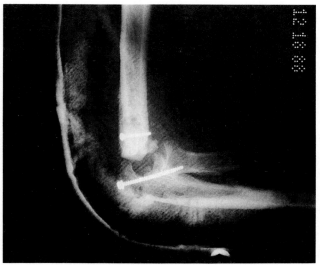

Fig. 11 **Top,** This severely comminuted T-condylar fracture in a 50-year-old man was fixed and went to nonunion. At the time of attempted osteosynthesis, the condylar fragments were found to be avascular and necrotic. **Bottom,** Fascial interpositional arthroplasty was performed.

Morrey; unpublished data). If significant bone loss, marked osteoporosis, or severe arthrosis is present, resectional or interpositional arthroplasty may be indicated (Fig. 11).[80,82,86] Although difficult to obtain, arthrodesis is an excellent alternative in the younger, more active patient.[74] Total elbow replacement is reserved for patients 60 years of age or older.[77,79,84] Early experience with distal humeral allografts is encouraging, but infection, nonunion of the graft, and joint degeneration are significant problems that require further investigation.[87]

Several approaches to the distal humerus and elbow have been described. Combined medial and lateral ap-

proaches are not recommended, because exposure is inadequate. Posterior approaches are subdivided into triceps splitting, triceps reflecting, and transosseous varieties. The triceps splitting approach, as described by Campbell,[88] has limited utility because of inadequate exposure. The triceps can be reflected from proximal to distal to expose the distal humerus,[89,90] but visualization of the anterior and articular surfaces of the distal humerus is limited. The triceps expansion can be reflected off the distal humerus and olecranon in continuity either from lateral to medial, as reported by Kocher,[90] or from medial to lateral, according to Bryan and Morrey.[91] These approaches seem especially well suited for total elbow replacement and resectional arthroplasty. The transolecranon approach can be done either through an extra-articular osteotomy,[92,93] or through an intra-articular osteotomy.[94] The intra-articular osteotomy, because of the excellent exposure of the articular and anterior surfaces of the distal humerus it affords, is preferable. Neither nonunion nor malunion of the olecranon osteotomy has been a problem.

Technique

Open reduction with rigid internal fixation and autogenous cancellous grafting is the preferred treatment. It is performed with the patient in the prone or semiprone position. A sterile tourniquet should be available. The distal humerus is approached through a posterior incision that curves laterally around the olecranon. Full-thickness flaps are raised medially and laterally. The ulnar nerve is mobilized from the cubital tunnel and is retracted, using a moist Penrose drain. The olecranon is exposed and an intra-articular osteotomy is made. The osteotomy is started on the dorsal surface with an oscillating saw, but this technique is discontinued at the subchondral bone. An osteotome is then used to complete the osteotomy by continuing partially through the subchondral plate and then levering the proximal fragment free. This leaves small irregularities at the articular surface of the bone, which interdigitate nicely upon reduction and aid in aligning the fragment anatomically. The olecranon fragment, along with the triceps, is then reflected proximally to expose the distal end of the humerus. The articular surface as well as the anterior aspect of the distal humerus are visualized by dislocating the ulnohumeral joint and reflecting the anterior capsule. The nonunion tissue is identified and excised and the fracture surfaces are freshened. In the case of a T-condylar nonunion, the intercondylar fragments are lagged together with a 4.5-mm ASIF screw. The supracondylar component is then reduced and provisionally fixed with crossed Kirschner wires. Two pelvic reconstruction plates are contoured to fit the distal humerus. One is placed along the posterior aspect of the medial column and the other is placed along the relatively flat lateral surface of the lateral column. This construct offers enhanced rigidity

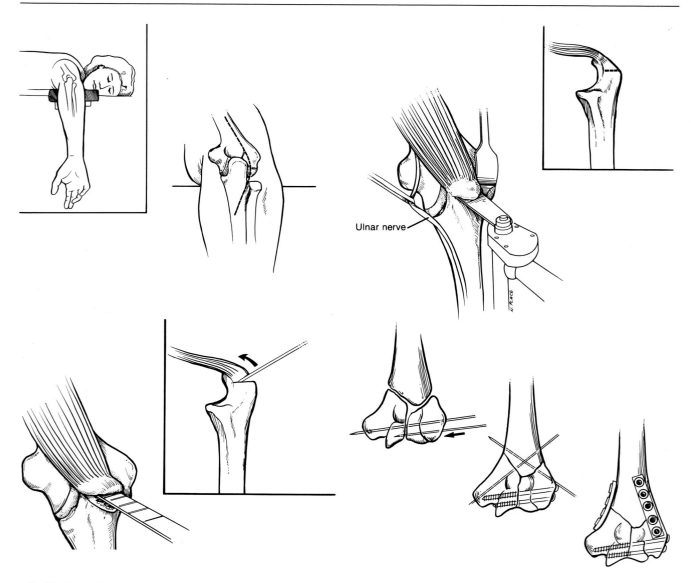

Fig. 12   **Top left,** The distal humerus is approached posteriorly and the ulnar nerve is isolated and retracted medially. **Top right** and **Bottom left,** An intra-articular olecranon osteotomy is performed using a saw and an osteotome. Bottom right, The condylar fragments are lagged together, the supracondylar component is reduced and fixed, and the olecranon is reattached.

because of fixation in two planes at a 90-degree angle to one another. If the fracture pattern permits, an anteroposterior interfragmentary compression screw is placed. The nonunion is then bone grafted with autogenous cancellous graft. The ulnar nerve is not routinely transposed but instead is permitted to seek its own course of least tension. The olecranon is fixed with a tension band wire (B.F. Morrey, unpublished data). The hole in the ulnar metaphysis for passing the tension band wire is drilled far enough anterior in the ulna to prevent the articular surface of the osteotomy from gapping open as the wire is tightened (Fig. 12).

Conclusions

The vast majority of humerus fractures proceed to uneventful union without surgery. In fact, previous open reduction, particularly with inadequate internal fixation, has been associated with the development of nonunion in all three regions of the humerus. When nonunion does occur, successful management can be difficult. Osteosynthesis is the primary objective of surgical management in most patients. However, in some instances this can be difficult, if not impossible. At the proximal and distal ends of the humerus, prosthetic replacement is possible in the elderly patient with poor bone quality or an incongruent or arthritic joint. In the younger patient, arthrodesis, resectional arthroplasty, and interpositional arthroplasty are options. The young patient with substantial loss of the humerus—either segmental or at either end—presents problems that remain to be solved. Preliminary results with allografts are promising but require further investigation. Recent advances in microsurgical techniques have made free, vascularized autografts an attractive alternative.

References

1. Fife D, Barancik JI: Northeastern Ohio Trauma Study: III. Incidence of fractures. *Ann Emerg Med* 1985;14:244–248.
2. Holbrook TL, Grazier K, Kelsey JL, et al: *The Frequency of Occurrence, Impact and Cost of Selected Musculoskeletal Conditions in the United States.* Park Ridge, Illinois, American Academy of Orthopaedic Surgeons, 1984, p 79.
3. Campbell WC: Ununited fractures of the shaft of the humerus. *Ann Surg* 1937;105:135–149.
4. Bennett GE: Fractures of the humerus with particular reference to non-union and its treatment. *Ann Surg* 1936;103:994–1006.
5. Balfour GW, Mooney V, Ashby ME: Diaphyseal fractures of the humerus treated with a ready-made fracture brace. *J Bone Joint Surg* 1982;64A:11–13.
6. Caldwell JA: Treatment of fractures of the shaft of the humerus by hanging cast. *Surg Gynecol Obstet* 1940;70:421–425.
7. Foster RJ, Dixon GL Jr, Bach AW, et al: Internal fixation of fractures and non-unions of the humeral shaft: Indications and results in a multi-center study. *J Bone Joint Surg* 1985;67A:857–864.
8. Healy WL, White GM, Mick CA, et al: Nonunion of the humeral shaft. *Clin Orthop* 1987;219:206–213.
9. Sarmiento A, Kinman PB, Galvin EG, et al: Functional bracing of fractures of the shaft of the humerus. *J Bone Joint Surg* 1977;59:596–601.
10. Rose SH, Melton LJ III, Morrey BF, et al: Epidemiologic features of humeral fractures. *Clin Orthop* 1982;168:24–30.
11. Neer CS II: Displaced proximal humeral fractures: Part I. Classification and evaluation. *J Bone Joint Surg* 1970;52A:1077–1089.
12. Neer CS II: Four-segment classification of displaced proximal humeral fractures, in American Academy of Orthopaedic Surgeons *Instructional Course Lectures, XXIV.* St. Louis, CV Mosby, 1975, pp 160–168.
13. Sorensen KH: Pseudarthrosis of the surgical neck of the humerus: Two cases, one bilateral. *Acta Orthop Scand* 1964;34:132–138.
14. Bosworth, DM: Blade plate fixation: Technic suitable for fractures of the surgical neck of the humerus and similar lesions. Chairman's address. *JAMA* 1949;141:1111–1113.
15. Coventry MB, Laurnen EL: Ununited fractures of the middle and upper humerus: Special problems in treatment. *Clin Orthop* 1970;69:192–198.
16. Leach RE, Premer RF: Nonunion of the surgical neck of the humerus: Method of internal fixation. *Minn Med* 1965;48:318–322.
17. Ray RD, Sankaran B, Fetrow KO: Delayed union and non-union of fractures. *J Bone Joint Surg* 1964;46A:627–643.
18. Rooney PJ, Cockshott WP: Pseudarthrosis following proximal humeral fractures: A possible mechanism. *Skeletal Radiol* 1986;15:21–24.
19. Scheck M: Surgical treatment of nonunions of the surgical neck of the humerus. *Clin Orthop* 1982;167:255–259.
20. Howard NJ, Eloesser L: Treatment of fractures of the upper end of the humerus: An experimental and clinical study. *J Bone Joint Surg* 1934;16:1–29.
21. Lee CK, Hansen HT, Weiss AB: Surgical treatment of the difficult humeral neck fracture: Acromial shortening anterolateral approach. *J Trauma* 1980;20:67–70.
22. Lorenzo FT: Osteosynthesis with Blount's staples in fractures of the proximal end of the humerus: A preliminary report. *J Bone Joint Surg* 1955;37A:45–48.
23. Mills KLG: Severe injuries of the upper end of the humerus. *Injury* 1974;6:13–21.
24. Mouradian WH: Displaced proximal humeral fractures: Seven year's experience with a modified Zickel supracondylar device. *Clin Orthop* 1986;212:209–218.
25. Nicola FG, Eilman H, Eckardt J, et al: Bilateral posterior fracture-dislocation of the shoulder treated with a modification of the McLaughlin procedure: A case report. *J Bone Joint Surg* 1981;63A:1175–1176.
26. Neer CS II: Fractures and dislocations of the shoulder: Part I. Fractures about the shoulder, in Rockwood CA Jr, Green DP (eds): *Fractures in Adults,* ed 2. Philadelphia, JB Lippincott, 1984, vol 1, pp 675–721.
27. Goss TP: Proximal humeral fractures revisited. *Orthop Rev* 1987;16:17–24.
28. Epps CH Jr, Cotler JM: Complications of treatment of fractures of the humeral shaft, in Epps CH Jr (ed): *Complications in Orthopaedic Surgery,* ed 2. Philadelphia, JB Lippincott, 1986, vol 1, pp 277–304.
29. Mayer PJ, Evarts CM: Nonunion, delayed union, malunion, and avascular necrosis, in Epps CH Jr (ed): *Complications in Orthopaedic Surgery,* ed 2. Philadelphia, JB Lippincott, 1986, vol 1, pp 207–230.
30. Muller ME, Thomas RJ: Treatment of non-union in fractures of long bones. *Clin Orthop* 1979;138:141–153.
31. Gristina AG, Bigliani LU, Neviaser RJ, et al: Symposium: Management of displaced fractures of the proximal humerus. *Cont Orthop* 1987;15:61–93.
32. Neviaser JS: Complicated fractures and dislocations about the shoulder joint. *J Bone Joint Surg* 1962;44A:984–998.
33. Paavolainen P, Björkenheim JM, Slätis P, et al: Operative treatment of severe proximal humeral fractures. *Acta Orthop Scand* 1983;54:374–379.
34. Rockwood CA, Pearce J: Nonunions of the proximal humerus: Treatment options. Presented at the meeting of the Southern Medical Association, New Orleans, 1988.
35. DePalma AF, Cautilli RA: Fractures of the upper end of the humerus. *Clin Orthop* 1961;20:73–93.
36. Dingley A, Denham R: Fracture-dislocation of the humeral head: A method of reduction. *J Bone Joint Surg* 1973;55A:1299–1300.
37. Drapanas T, McDonald J, Hale HW Jr: A rational approach to classification and treatment of fractures of the surgical neck of the humerus. *Am J Surg* 1960;99:617–624.
38. Keene JS, Huizengia RE, Engber WD, et al: Proximal humeral fractures: A correlation of residual deformity with long-term function. *Orthopedics* 1983;6:173–178.
39. Perkins G: Rest and movement. *J Bone Joint Surg* 1953;35B:521–539.
40. Young TB, Wallace WA: Conservation treatment of fractures and fracture-dislocations of the upper end of the humerus. *J Bone Joint Surg* 1985;67B:373–377.
41. Laing PG: The arterial supply of the adult humerus. *J Bone Joint Surg* 1956;38A:1105–1116.
42. Thompson AG, Batten RL: The application of rigid internal fixation to the treatment of non-union and delayed union using the AO technique. *Injury* 1977;8:188–198.
43. Svend-Hansen H: Displaced proximal humeral fractures: A review of 49 patients. *Acta Orthop Scand* 1974;45:359–364.

44. Stableforth PG: Four-part fractures of the neck of the humerus. *J Bone Joint Surg* 1984;66B:104–108.

45. Tanner MW, Cofield RH: Prosthetic arthroplasty for fractures and fracture-dislocations of the proximal humerus. *Clin Orthop* 1983;179:116–128.

46. Emmett JE, Breck LW: A review and analysis of 11,000 fractures seen in a private practice of orthopaedic surgery 1937–1956. *J Bone Joint Surg* 1958;40A:1169–1175.

47. D'Aubigne and Solal: Le traitment des pseudarthroses de la diaphyse humerale. *Rev Orthop* 36:373.

48. Hoppenfeld S, deBoer P: *Surgical Exposures in Orthopaedics: The Anatomic Approach.* Philadelphia, JB Lippincott, 1984, p 55.

49. Kennedy JC, Wyatt JK: An evaluation of the management of fractures through the middle third of the humerus. *Can J Surg* 1957;1:26–33.

50. Klenerman L: Fractures of the shaft of the humerus. *J Bone Joint Surg* 1966;48B:105–111.

51. La Ferté AD, Nutter PD: The treatment of fractures of the humerus by means of a hanging plaster case—"hanging cast." *Ann Surg* 1941;114:919–930.

52. Mann RJ, Neal EG: Fractures of the shaft of the humerus in adults. *South Med J* 1942;55:264–268.

53. Pennsylvania Orthopedic Society Scientific Research Committee: Fresh midshaft fractures of the humerus in adults. *Pa Med J* 1959; 62:848–850.

54. Raney RB: The treatment of fractures of the humerus with the hanging cast. *N C Med J* 1945;6:88–92.

55. Stewart MJ, Hundley JM: Fractures of the humerus: A comparative study in methods of treatment. *J Bone Joint Surg* 1955;37A: 681–692.

56. Epps CH Jr: Fractures of the shaft of the humerus, in Rockwood CA Jr, Green DP (eds): *Fractures in Adults,* ed 2. Philadelphia, JB Lippincott, 1984, vol 1, pp 653–674.

57. Fenyö G: On fractures of the shaft of the humerus: A review covering a 12-year period with special consideration of the surgically treated cases. *Acta Chir Scand* 1971;137:221–226.

58. Mnaymneh WA, Smith-Petersen M, Aufranc OE: The treatment of non-union of humeral-shaft fractures, abstract. *J Bone Joint Surg* 1963;45A:1548–1549.

59. Chacha PB: Compression plating without bone grafts for delayed and non-union of humeral shaft fractures. *Injury* 1974;5:283–290.

60. Christensen NO: Küntscher intramedullary reaming and nail fixation for nonunion of the Humerus. *Clin Orthop* 1976;116:222–225.

61. Day L: Humeral nonunions best treated with plating soon after injury. *Orthop Today,* 1984.

62. Durbin RA, Gottesman MJ, Saunders KC: Hackethal stacked nailing of humeral shaft fractures: Experience with 30 patients. *Clin Orthop* 1983;179:168–174.

63. Esterhai JL Jr, Brighton CT, Heppenstall RB, et al: Nonunion of the humerus: Clinical, roentgenographic, scintigraphic, and response characteristics to treatment with constant direct current stimulation of osteogenesis. *Clin Orthop* 1986;211:228–234.

64. Fattah HA, Halawa EE, Shafy TH: Non-union of the humeral shaft: A report on 25 cases. *Injury* 1982;14:255–262.

65. Fischer KA, Leatherman KD, Kotcamp WW: Fibular bone grafting in non-union of the humerus. *J Ky Med Assoc* 1972;70:921–923.

66. Gupta RC, Gaur SC, Tiwari RC, et al: Treatment of un-united fractures of the shaft of the humerus with bent nail. *Injury* 1985; 16:276–280.

67. Loomer R, Kokan P: Non-union in fractures of the humeral shaft. *Injury* 1976;7:274–278.

68. Rosen H: Compression treatment of long bone pseudarthroses. *Clin Orthop* 1979;138:154–166.

69. Wilson PD: Fractures and dislocations in the region of the elbow. *Surg Gynecol Obstet* 1933;56:335–359.

70. Sim FH: Nonunion and delayed union of distal humeral fractures, in Morrey BF (ed): *The Elbow and Its Disorders.* Philadelphia, WB Saunders, 1985, pp 340–354.

71. Bickel WE, Perry RE: Comminuted fractures of the distal humerus. *JAMA* 1963;184:553–557.

72. Bryan RS, Bickel WH: "T" condylar fractures of distal humerus. *J Trauma* 1971;11:830–835.

73. Conn J Jr, Wade PA: Injuries of the elbow: A ten year review. *J Trauma* 1961;1:248–268.

74. Gabel GT, Hanson G, Bennett JB, et al: Intraarticular fractures of the distal humerus in the adult. *Clin Orthop* 1987;216:99–108.

75. Hitzrot JM: Fractures at the lower end of the humerus in adults. *Surg Clin North Am* 1932;12:291–304.

76. Knight RA: The management of fractures about the elbow in adults, in Raney RB (ed): American Academy of Orthopaedic Surgeons *Instructional Course Lectures, XIV.* Ann Arbor, JW Edwards, 1957, pp 123–141.

77. Mitsunaga MM, Bryan RS, Linscheid RL: Condylar nonunions of the elbow. *J Trauma* 1982;22:787–791.

78. Figgie HE III, Inglis AE, Ranawat CS, et al: Results of total elbow arthroplasty as a salvage procedure for failed elbow reconstructive operations. *Clin Orthop* 1987;219:185–193.

79. Anderson LD: Fractures, in Crenshaw AH (ed): *Campbell's Operative Orthopaedics,* ed 5. St. Louis, CV Mosby, 1971, vol 1, pp 477–691.

80. Hurri L, Pulkki T, Vainio K: Arthroplasty of the elbow in rheumatoid arthritis. *Acta Chir Scand* 1964;127:459–465.

81. Koch M, Lipscomb PR: Arthrodesis of the elbow. *Clin Orthop* 1967;50:151–157.

82. MacAusland WR: Arthroplasty of the elbow. *N Engl J Med* 1947; 236:97–99.

83. Moss AL, Waterhouse N, Townsend PL: Free vascularized fibular graft to reconstruct early a traumatic humeral defect. *Injury* 1984;16:41–46.

84. Ross AC, Sneath RS, Scales JT: Endoprosthetic replacement of the humerus and elbow joint. *J Bone Joint Surg* 1987;69B:652–655.

85. Sowa DT, Weiland AJ: Clinical applications of vascularized bone autografts. *Orthop Clin North Am* 1987;18:257–273.

86. Tsuge K, Murakami T, Yasunaga T, et al: Arthroplasty of the elbow: Twenty years' experience of a new approach. *J Bone Joint Surg* 1987;69B:116–120.

87. Urbaniak JR, Aitken M: Clinical use of bone allografts in the elbow. *Orthop Clin North Am* 1987;18:311–321.

88. Campbell WC: Incision for exposure of the elbow joint. *Am J Surg* 1932;15:65–67.

89. Van Gorder GW: Surgical approach in supracondylar "T" fractures of the humerus requiring open reduction. *J Bone Joint Surg* 1940;22:278–292.

90. Kocher T: *Text-Book of Operative Surgery,* ed 3, Stiles HJ, Paul CB (trans). New York, Macmillan, 1911.

91. Bryan RS, Morrey BF: Extensive posterior exposure of the elbow: A triceps-sparing approach. *Clin Orthop* 1982;166:188–192.

92. Cassebaum WH: Operative treatment of T and Y fractures of the lower end of the humerus. *Am J Surg* 1952;83:265–270.

93. Müller ME, Allgöwer M, Willenegger H: *Manual of Internal Fixation: Technique Recommended by the AO-Group.* Berlin, Springer-Verlag, 1970.

94. MacAusland WR: Ankylosis of the elbow: With report of four cases treated by arthroplasty. *JAMA* 1915;64:312–318.

Gait Analysis

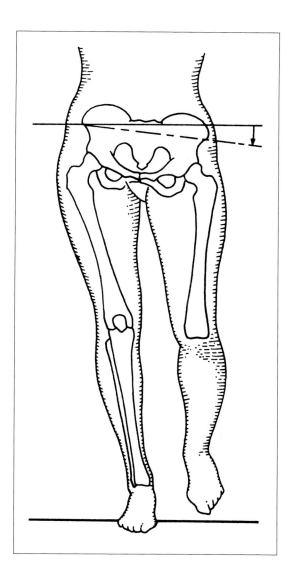

An Overview of Normal Walking

James R. Gage, MD

Introduction

Walking is an activity that appears simple until one takes a closer look at it. Normal gait is an extremely complex activity that is learned spontaneously, and yet all of us walk in a very similar manner. If the kinematics findings in normal subjects are compared, the graphs will be nearly identical. The reasons for this are not fully understood, but it is thought that as we learn to walk we inherently find the most energy-efficient method. Unfortunately, the same is not true for activities such as golf and tennis, in which mediocre performance often persists despite extensive coaching. Although the precise mechanisms by which we learn to walk are not fully understood, normal gait has been studied extensively, and much is known about it.

The Gait Cycle

When describing how a person walks, it is conventional to do so in terms of the gait cycle (Fig. 1). A complete gait cycle or stride begins when one foot strikes the ground and ends when it strikes the ground again. The cycle is divided into two major phases, stance and swing. Stance phase begins with initial contact of the heel with the ground, and ends at toe-off when swing phase begins.

Events in the gait cycle are defined sequentially as occurring at specific percentages of the cycle. Initial contact occurs at 0% and 100% of gait cycle. During normal walking, toe-off occurs at approximately 60% of the cycle. Therefore, stance represents approximately 60% of the gait cycle and swing 40%. Opposite toe-off and opposite heelstrike occur at 10% and 50% of the cycle, respectively. Double support periods occur twice during the gait cycle, and each phase of double support lasts about 10% of the cycle. During these periods of double support, the body's center of mass is at its lowest. The first period of double support, which begins when the foot touches the ground at initial contact, is called loading response. Loading response is a period of deceleration when the shock of impact is absorbed. This is followed by a period of single stance occupying about 40% of the cycle, during which the opposite limb is going through its swing phase. Thus, single support on the stance side must be equal to the period of swing of the opposite limb. In late stance there is a second period of double support called preswing, which begins at approximately 50% of the gait cycle and lasts until toe-off on the stance side. Therefore, loading response is equivalent in time and is, in fact, the same event as preswing on the opposite side. Since normal gait is symmetric, it is important to remember these relationships in order to form a mental picture of where the opposite limb is in the cycle.

The period of single stance can be divided into midstance and terminal stance. During midstance, the body's center of mass is decelerating as it climbs to its zenith and passes over the base of support. In terminal stance, the center of mass has passed in front of the base of support and is accelerating as it falls forward

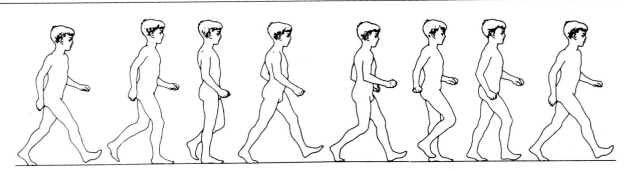

Fig. 1   The gait cycle begins with initial contact and ends with initial contact of the same foot. The period of stance constitutes the first 60% of the cycle and can be subdivided into five subperiods: initial contact, loading response, midstance, terminal stance, and preswing. Swing phase constitutes the last 40% of the cycle and can be subdivided into initial swing, midswing, and terminal swing.

and toward the unsupported side. During this period of acceleration, steady-state walking is achieved by adding back into the the cycle an amount of energy equivalent to that lost earlier in the gait cycle.

In swing phase, the swinging limb behaves as a compound pendulum, and, therefore, the duration of swing is determined by the mass moment of inertia of its segments.[1,2] If the pendulum's speed could not be altered, it would be impossible to vary cadence during gait. To accelerate cadence, the leg must be accelerated early in swing and then decelerated in the latter part of swing. As such, the swing phase of gait can be divided into three periods: a period in which the rate of swing can be altered (accelerated or decelerated) a transition period, and a final period in which the swing rate is reversed. These three periods are known as initial swing, midswing, and terminal swing (Fig. 2).

Running differs from walking in that the two periods of double support are replaced by periods referred to as double float, when neither foot is on the ground. During running, therefore, stance time must always be less than the time of swing to accommodate the periods of double float.

Further characterization of the gait cycle can be done with linear measurements such as walking velocity, cadence, step length, and stride length. Step length is defined as the longitudinal distance between the two feet. Thus, the right step length is measured from the point of contact of the trailing left foot to the point of contact of the right foot. One stride length is the distance covered during a complete gait cycle and represents the sum of the right and left step lengths, or, stated another way, extends from the initial contact of one foot to the following initial contact of the same foot. Walking velocity is usually expressed in centimeters per second or meters per minute and is equal to step length times cadence.

Necessities of Normal Gait

There are three prerequisites for normal ambulation: stability in stance, a means of progression, and the conservation of energy. Standing stability is challenged by two factors: (1) the body is top-heavy, as the center of gravity, located anterior to the S-2 vertebra, is situated above the base of support; and (2) walking continually alters segment alignment, which means that the body must constantly balance the trunk over the base of support.

Progression results from the forward fall of the body from its high point at midstance to its low point at double support, during which time potential energy is converted to kinetic energy. To raise the center of gravity back to its zenith at midstance, kinetic energy must be supplied. This kinetic energy is provided by the inertia of the swinging limb, which in turn derives its energy from the acceleration supplied by the plantar flexors and hip flexors of that limb. In normal walking, it has been hypothesized, 85% of the necessary energy comes from the plantar flexors and 15% from hip flexors.[3]

Forward momentum is not constant during the gait cycle. The body slows down and speeds up during each step. This occurs because the support provided by the lower limbs is not directly under the body at all times. When the supporting foot is in front of the trunk, the center of gravity must be lifted over the base of support, and the body slows down. As the center of gravity passes over the base of support, gravity accelerates forward momentum so that forward velocity peaks during double support when the center of gravity is at its lowest point.[4]

A person walking at a steady pace is in dynamic equilibrium; that is, during each gait cycle the sum of the forces and the sum of the moments around the joints are equal to zero. The external moments around the joints are produced by the ground-reaction forces. The internal moments that balance the ground-reaction forces are produced by muscle action (Fig. 3). Three types of muscle action occur during gait—concentric, eccentric, and isometric. In concentric contraction a muscle shortens while performing work. Accelerators always work concentrically. An example is the iliopsoas as it works to accelerate the thigh in preswing and initial swing. Eccentric contraction occurs when a muscle, by resisting elongation like a spring, performs work while

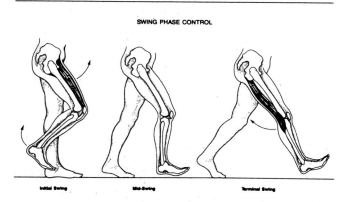

SWING PHASE CONTROL

Initial Swing   Mid-Swing   Terminal Swing

Fig. 2 The leg is essentially a compound pendulum, and each person has a natural cadence dictated by the mass moment of inertia of the shank. Variations in cadence depend on muscles that cross the knee (rectus femoris, hamstrings, and sartorius). Thus, the rate of swing can be accelerated or decelerated in initial swing, and then decelerated or accelerated in terminal swing. Midswing is the switching period during which there is no muscle activity across the knee. This acceleration or deceleration is accomplished by muscles that cross two joints and act to transfer energy between nonadjacent segments. For example, during rapid walking the rectus femoris prevents excessive knee flexion through an eccentric contraction at its distal end, and simultaneously augments hip flexion at its proximal end via a concentric contraction. Thus, the muscle remains more or less isometric as it transfers energy from the shank to the pelvis.

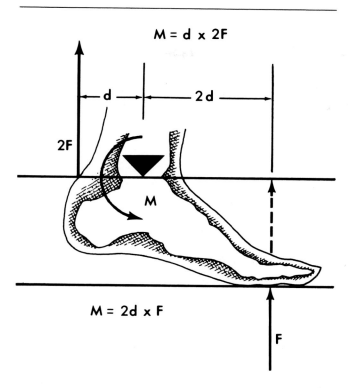

$$M = d \times 2F$$

$$M = 2d \times F$$

Fig. 3 A moment is defined as the product of a force times the distance of the force from the center of an axis of rotation. The unit is Newton-meters (N·m). An unopposed moment produces an angular acceleration about its axis. During walking the joints serve as axes of rotation. External moments created by the ground-reaction forces are balanced by internal moments created by muscle action or by stabilizing ligaments.

being lengthened. Decelerators (including shock absorbers) work eccentrically. The hamstrings, which act to slow the swinging thigh in terminal swing, are an example of this type of contraction. During isometric contraction, a muscle resists a load with little or no change in length. Postural stabilizers such as the gluteus medius work in this mode. Eccentric contraction is the most efficient and the most common type of muscle action during normal walking.

To make gait efficient, energy must be conserved. Energy is conserved in three ways: (1) by minimizing the excursion of the center of gravity, (2) by controlling momentum, and (3) by active or passive transfer of energy between segments. Movement of a wheel is highly efficient because the center of mass remains at a constant level. By contrast, it has been shown that if we walked with stiff limbs and no pelvic rotation, our center of mass would have to be lifted 9.5 cm with each step.[5] By using three planes of pelvic movement—rotation, tilt, and obliquity—and coordinated knee and ankle motion, the vertical excursion can be reduced by 54%, to 4.4 cm. Winter[3] pointed out that during normal walking the vertical and horizontal displacements of the center of mass are almost sinusoidal and are, therefore,

equal and opposite. That is, the peak of vertical movement occurs at the point of minimal horizontal movement, and vice versa. Mechanical gait analysis shows that this pattern of movement conserves energy.[4] If there is interference with these mechanisms, energy costs rise quickly. For example, even with optimal fitting of an above-knee prosthesis, the energy cost of walking is approximately doubled.

Controlling momentum also conserves energy during walking. For example, by maintaining the ground-reaction force in front of the knee during the last half of stance, an extension moment occurs at the knee, which allows it to remain stable without using the quadriceps muscle (Fig. 4). During this movement, the body makes major use of an eccentric, or lengthening, contraction of the soleus muscle to control excessive ankle dorsiflexion. Electromyographic studies show that for a given load, electrical activity of muscles is lower during a lengthening contraction, which suggests that less motor-unit activity is required.[5]

The third method of energy conservation is active or passive transfer of energy between body segments. It is very difficult to estimate the mechanism and magnitude of these transfers. However, methods of mechanical power analysis have been devised that enable an investigator to determine which muscle groups are absorbing and which are generating energy. The assumption inherent in this calculation is that each joint has a torque generator that acts independently of what is happening at adjacent joints.[6,7] On the basis of these calculations, it has been shown that passive flow of energy across joints accounts for most of the energy changes occurring at the distal segments during initiation and termination of swing.[8] In addition, active energy transfers across muscles are significant as adjacent segments rotate in the same direction. Biarticulate muscles probably play a large part in the transfer of energy between segments. For example, during rapid walking the rectus femoris is used as a concentric accelerator to augment hip flexion power during preswing and initial swing. However, distally this muscle is acting simultaneously as an eccentric decelerator of the shank by limiting knee flexion via its patellar insertion. In this way, the rectus absorbs energy at the knee and generates energy at the hip. As it transfers energy from the shank to the thigh, the resultant muscle contraction may be nearly isometric (Fig. 2). It has been shown that this transfer of energy between nonadjacent segments is the major role of two-joint muscles and that performing this function gives an energy savings of 8% to 22%.[9]

Subdivisions of the Gait Cycle

Stance phase is made up of five events or phases: initial contact, loading response, midstance, terminal

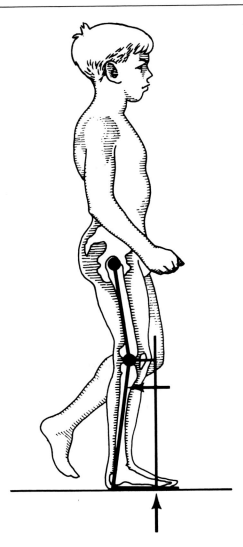

Fig. 4 During midstance, an eccentric contraction of the triceps surae controls the forward progression of the tibia and hence the position of the ground-reaction force relative to the ankle, knee, and hip. Hyperextension of the hip and knee is prevented by ligaments; by maintaining the ground-reaction force anterior to the knee and posterior to the hip, the stability of both joints can be maintained without muscle action. With respect to the knee, this is referred to as a plantar-flexion/knee-extension couple.

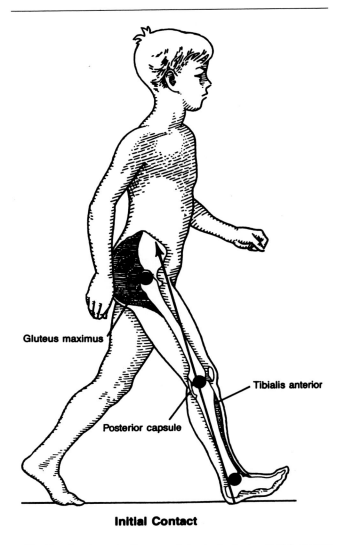

Initial Contact

Fig. 5 A schematic diagram of the body during initial contact. The external moments around the joints produced by the ground-reaction forces are balanced by internal muscle forces.

stance, and preswing. Swing phase has three phases: initial swing, midswing, and terminal swing. Moments produced by the ground-reaction forces are referred to as external; those produced by the action of the muscles are called internal.

Initial Contact

The principal objective of the body at initial contact (0% of cycle double support) is to position the foot correctly as it comes into contact with the floor. The body is about to begin deceleration. The external moment produced by the ground-reaction force is posterior to the ankle, at or just in front of the knee, and anterior to the hip joint (Fig. 5). This produces a plantar flexor moment at the ankle, a zero to slight extensor moment at the knee, and a flexor moment at the hip. These moments are resisted by internal moments created by the ankle dorsiflexors, posterior knee capsule, and hip extensors. This is the beginning of the first rocker (Fig. 6), as the foot, under the control of the pretibial musculature, rocks down from the point of contact at the heel. Electromyographic studies indicate that despite a null or nearly null knee moment, both hamstrings and quadriceps are active, probably to aid in hip extension. In the coronal plane, the hip abductors act eccentrically to resist the adduction moment created by the body's mass acting on the hip joint. The adductor magnus acts to produce an internal moment that extends the hip and externally rotates the pelvis on the femur on the stance side (Fig. 7).

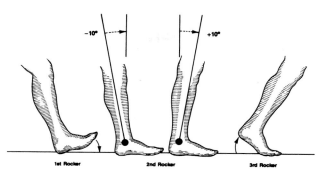

Fig. 6 The three foot rockers create a rolling action, much like the circumference of a wheel. The first two rockers are periods of deceleration controlled by eccentric muscle action of the anterior tibial muscles and the triceps surae, respectively. During third rocker, concentric action of the triceps surae, tibialis posterior, and long toe flexors prevents further dorsiflexion of the ankle, and the axis of rotation moves forward to the metatarsal heads. Thus, the third rocker is a period of acceleration that maintains the steady state.

Loading Response

The principal objective of the body during loading response (0% to 10% of cycle, double support) is to maintain smooth progression while decelerating the body's mass as it travels downward from its zenith at midstance. Forceplate studies indicate that this deceleration amounts to 20% to 30% of body weight during normal gait, and the ground-reaction force increases to approximately 130% of body weight as it resists the combined forces of body mass and inertia (Fig. 8). Ideally, this kinetic energy would be completely converted to potential energy and stored in muscles and ligaments. It could then be reconverted to kinetic energy during the acceleration phase of gait in terminal stance. Although the degree of efficiency of these transfers in normal gait is not known, they are not 100% efficient. Furthermore, with gait deviations, such as occur in cerebral palsy, the efficiency of these transfers drops precipitously.

During loading response, the body weight is decelerated by controlling the rate of knee flexion and ankle plantar flexion. At the end of loading response, the knee is flexed about 15 degrees and the ankle is plantar flexed about 10 degrees. As first rocker is completed and second rocker begins, the external moment produced by the ground-reaction force moves anterior to the ankle (Fig. 9). At that point, anterior tibial muscle action ceases and triceps surae, tibialis posterior, and peroneal action begin. At the knee, there is a large, external, flexor moment that must be resisted by quadriceps contraction. This extensor moment is produced primarily by the three vasti, because the hip flexor motion of the rectus femoris would work against the extending hip. As the ground-reaction force moves posteriorly through the hip, it acts to extend rather than flex the hip joint. Therefore, the hip extensors, which

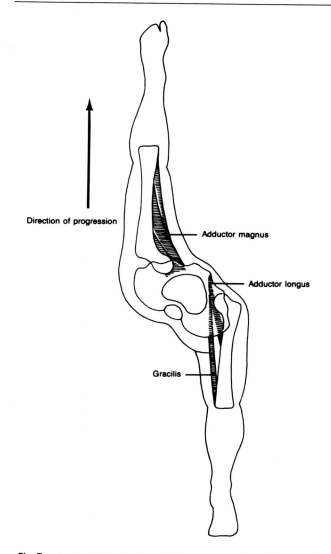

Fig. 7 A schematic drawing of the transverse plane. Because the front foot is fixed, concentric action of the adductor magnus would produce internal rotation of the pelvis and extension of the hip. Concentric action of the superficial adductors on the trailing side would advance the trailing limb along the line of progression.

are no longer required to stabilize the joint, cease being active at the end of this phase.

In the coronal plane, hip abductors are required as weight is transferred to the stance limb. In addition to the abductors, the fascia lata serves as a tension band to resist the external adductor moment at the hip and the varus moment at the knee. At the foot, the ground-reaction force, being lateral to the ankle joint at heel-strike, creates an eversion moment of the heel. As the calcaneus everts, the head of the talus loses its medial support and and rotates medially in the transverse plane. This produces internal rotation of the tibia and fibula via traction on the deltoid and fibulotalar ligaments. Internal rotation travels from the ankle upward

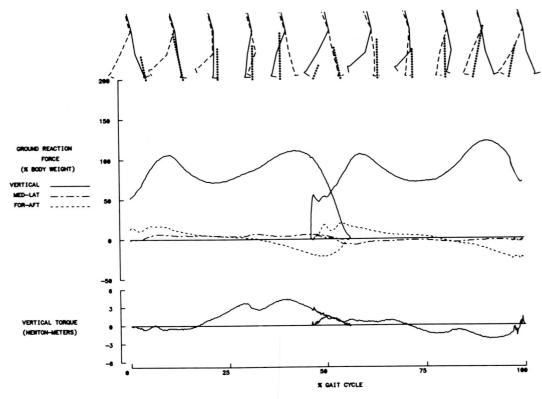

Fig. 8 A computer output illustrating normal ground-reaction forces during walking. Percent of gait cycle is on the abscissa and percent of body weight is on the ordinate. Note that during loading response and terminal stance, the vertical component of the ground-reaction force is about 130% of body weight. Loading response represents deceleration, and terminal stance acceleration of the body's inertia.

as the femur also rotates internally on the tibia via traction through the collateral ligaments of the knee. Internal rotation of the hip is controlled by the adductors, medial hamstrings, and anterior gluteals on the stance side, and acts to bring the pelvis forward on the contralateral side as it moves through preswing and toward toe-off (Fig. 7).

Midstance

Midstance (10% to 30% of cycle, single support) marks the onset of the second foot rocker. The main goal of midstance is to utilize momentum to maintain stability at the hip and knee while advancing the body over a stationary foot.

The onset of midstance is marked by opposite toe-off. Initial swing has begun on the opposite side. The body is in single support. The knee is now in full extension and extension is continuing at the hip. The center of mass has reached its zenith and forward velocity is at its minimum.

In the sagittal plane there is an external dorsiflexor moment at the ankle as the ground-reaction force moves anteriorly along the length of the foot. As the ground-reaction force passes anterior to the knee and posterior to the hip, extension moments are created at

both joints (Fig. 10). Because hyperextension of both joints is prevented by ligaments (iliofemoral ligament at the hip and posterior capsule and cruciates at the knee), no muscle action is necessary at either joint to resist the external moments, and so the gluteus maximus, hamstrings, and quadriceps cease their activity. Therefore, eccentric contraction of the soleus in second rocker, by controlling the sagittal-plane position of the ground-reaction force, stabilizes all three joints. This mechanism for controlling knee extension by means of the ground-reaction force rather than the quadriceps is generally referred to as a plantar-flexion/knee-extension couple (Fig. 10). Because the soleus is a type 1, slow-twitch muscle, it is well suited to this steady, deceleration action.

In the coronal plane, the pelvis has dropped about 5 degrees on the unsupported side (Fig. 11). Because the body's mass is eccentric to and supported solely by the stance limb, there is an external, adductor moment at the hip and a varus moment at the knee on the stance side. To counteract this, the hip abductors and tensor fascia lata are active and the iliotibial band is under tension. At the ankle, the tibialis posterior and peroneals maintain the stability of the foot in stance as the

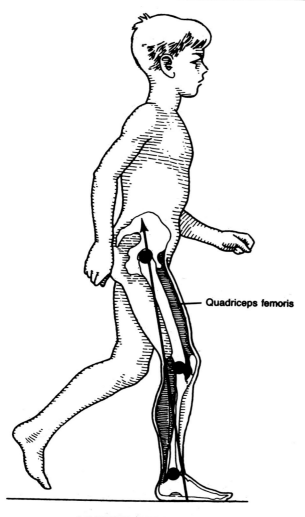

LOADING RESPONSE

Fig. 9 Loading response is a period of shock absorption controlled by eccentric contraction of the anterior tibial musculature at the ankle and the quadriceps at the knee. This is the period of first rocker.

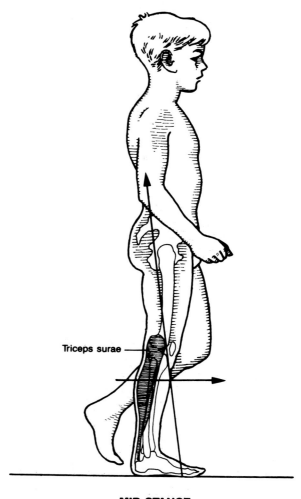

MID-STANCE

Fig. 10 A diagram of the body in midstance. This is the period of second rocker. Eccentric contraction of the soleus maintains the ground-reaction force anterior to the ankle and knee and posterior to the hip. Thus, this one muscle controls the sagittal-plane stability of all three joints.

ground-reaction force progresses along its lateral margin.

In the transverse plane, internal rotation of the shank continues. The thigh rotates internally until full knee extension is reached. At midstance the pelvis reaches a neutral position as the two limbs pass each other. The shoulders are also neutral at this point but rotate in a direction opposite to that of the pelvis as the upper trunk acts as a counterweight. Because the various segments rotate by means of inertia at this point, no muscle action is required.

Terminal Stance

The main goals of terminal stance (30% to 50% of cycle, single support) are to provide acceleration and to ensure an adequate step length. Acceleration is pro-

vided by the forward fall of the body's center of mass and the concentric action of the triceps. Winter[3] referred to this acceleration moment as the A2 power burst, and stated that in normal adults it constitutes about 80% to 85% of the total energy generated during the gait cycle.

Terminal stance begins as the center of mass moves in front of the base of support in such a way that the body falls anteriorly and toward the unsupported side (Fig. 12). In the sagittal plane, the gastrocnemius, a fast-twitch muscle, has now joined the slow-twitch soleus with sufficient power to stop further dorsiflexion of the ankle. The triceps surae now contracts concentrically, and the heel leaves the ground. This marks the onset of the third rocker, as weight is transferred forward, moving the fulcrum of rotation to the meta-

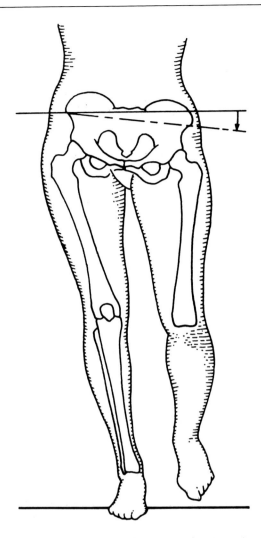

Fig. 11 The coronal plane of the body at midstance. Because the ground-reaction force passes medial to the hip and knee joint, isometric action of hip abductors and the tensor fascia lata is necessary to stabilize the pelvis and knee.

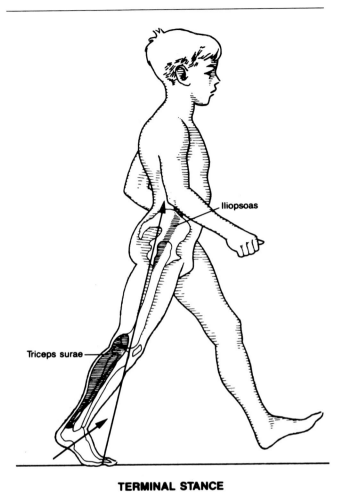

TERMINAL STANCE

Fig. 12 Terminal stance is marked by the onset of third rocker. The triceps surae now contracts concentrically, producing an acceleration force.

tarsal heads. The axis of the metatarsal bases is approximately 30 degrees to the coronal plane. As rotation about this axis begins, inversion of the hindfoot locks the subtalar joint complex. Acceleration and forward propulsion are produced by the combination of triceps action and forward fall of the trunk. The knee reaches full extension and by the end of terminal stance the hip reaches full extension as well. The opposite limb is now in terminal swing. The ground-reaction force remains anterior to the knee and posterior to the hip, which allows both joints to be stabilized by ligaments rather than muscles. At the end of terminal stance, the metatarsophalangeal joints are dorsiflexed to approximately 20 degrees and the body is ahead of the sagittal plane by approximately the same amount.

In the coronal plane, there is an ongoing adductor

moment, and an internal moment must be generated by continued action of the hip abductors and tensor fascia to maintain equilibrium.

In the transverse plane, the unsupported side of the pelvis continues to rotate forward with the swinging limb. By partially interposing the pelvic width into the line of progression, this increases step length. The knee is fully extended and the thigh and shank rotate externally as a unit. Because the foot is not rotating on the floor, the rotation of the limb is absorbed by the joints at its upper and lower ends—the hip and subtalar joints. At the subtalar joint this external rotation causes hindfoot supination (inversion), raising the arch. This is reinforced by the winching action of the plantar fascia as it is pulled around the metatarsal heads during third rocker to create a bowstring effect on the arch. During initial contact and loading response the foot functioned as a shock absorber, but the foot now functions as a rigid cam, thereby ensuring an adequate moment arm for the acceleration force of the triceps. In addition to the triceps, the tibialis posterior, peroneals, and long toe flexors are also active.

Preswing

The principal goal of preswing (50% to 60% of cycle, double support) is to prepare the limb for swing. The initial contact of the opposite limb marks the beginning of double support and of preswing. The joint movements and powers indicate that the hip flexors are now firing concentrically as accelerators, or flexors, of the thigh, which also creates a flexor force at the knee. As weight unloads onto the contralateral limb and the stance limb moves forward, the ground-reaction force passes behind the knee. Thus, the external dorsiflexor moment created by the ground-reaction force falls precipitously as both the force and the moment arm disappear (Fig. 13). At this point, the internal muscle moment powered by the ankle plantar flexors becomes predominant and, therefore, knee flexion is also enhanced. At normal cadence, inertial and gravitational forces are balanced and the knee flexes in preswing and initial swing, and then passively extends again in terminal swing without additional muscle action. However, because the lower extremity behaves as a compound pendulum, knee flexion would be excessive during fast walking, except for the action of the rectus femoris. A faster cadence is achieved by putting more plantar flexion force at the ankle and more flexion force at the hip. The rectus femoris provides additional flexion force at the hip and, at the same time, prevents excessive flexion of the knee. In this way, the muscle eccentrically decelerates knee flexion, preventing excessive heel rise. Similarly, during a slower-than-normal cadence, knee flexion is augmented because inertial forces are insufficient. In this case the sartorius, the gracilis, and the short head of the biceps augment knee flexion during preswing and initial swing.[10]

It should be noted that ankle plantar flexion in preswing lengthens the trailing limb. This prevents excessive drop of the center of mass and conserves energy. At normal cadence, ankle plantar flexion is approximately 27 degrees, knee flexion 45 degrees, and hip flexion 5 degrees at the time of toe-off.

In the coronal plane, the hip abductors become inactive as weight transfers rapidly to the opposite side, lessening the external adduction moment. The hip adductors, particularly the gracilis and adductor longus, now become active. Because of the position of the trailing limb relative to the pelvis (Fig. 7), these muscles assist the hip flexors in accelerating the thigh. As mentioned earlier, the gracilis can also augment knee flexion if required.

In the transverse plane, the pelvis reaches its maximum rotation backward by the end of terminal stance. With the onset of preswing it rotates forward with the trailing limb. As the trailing limb comes forward, the

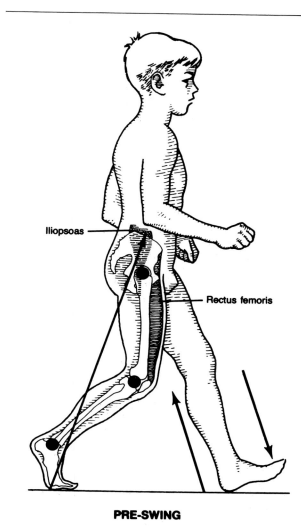

PRE-SWING

Fig. 13   Preswing is marked by the onset of double support. As weight is unloaded onto the contralateral foot, concentric action of the iliopsoas accelerates the thigh. Meanwhile the ground-reaction force has fallen behind the knee, creating a strong flexion moment at that joint. Excessive knee flexion is controlled by the rectus femoris, which transfers superfluous kinetic energy from the shank to the pelvis.

thigh rotates externally relative to the pelvis. The shank and foot also rotate externally relative to the thigh at this time. Under the foot, the center of pressure moves from lateral to medial, and by toe-off the center of pressure is located under the first and second metatarsal heads.

Initial Swing

The critical goals of initial swing (50% to 70% of cycle) are to allow foot clearance and variable cadence. Variable cadence requires complex central nervous system control and precise timing of two-joint muscles. Thus, it is not surprising that these abilities are commonly lost in such neuromuscular conditions as cerebral palsy.

Initial swing begins with toe-off (Fig. 14). Because the foot is in the air, ground-reaction forces are absent, and the only external forces acting on the limb are inertia and gravity. At the ankle these forces produce a plantar-flexor moment that is counterbalanced by the ankle dorsiflexors. The pretibial muscles work as concentric accelerators at this time to bring the foot out of its plantar-flexed attitude.

To vary cadence, the body must have a mechanism to alter the natural period of the limb, which acts as a compound pendulum, as it swings. At the knee a flexion moment is usually present, depending on the balance between the inertial flexion moment created in pre-swing and the extension moment created by gravitational forces. At normal cadence these forces are in relative balance and so no muscle action is necessary. During fast gait, the moment flexing the knee is excessive and must be counterbalanced by the rectus femoris. With slow cadence the flexor moment created by the inertial forces is inadequate to counterbalance the gravitational forces, and knee flexion is augmented by action of the sartorius, the gracilis, and the short head of the biceps femoris. The limb is still in a trailing position with the toes pointing at the floor, so about 60 degrees of knee flexion is required to obtain adequate clearance for the foot. The hip flexors act to accelerate the swinging limb and to counterbalance the extensor moment created by gravity. In normal cadence this internal muscle moment is generated mainly by the iliopsoas. When a more rapid gait is required, the rectus femoris augments the hip flexor moment and at the same time restrains the excessive external flexor mo-

ment created at the knee. This is an example of the isometric action of a two-joint muscle during normal gait. Flexion at the hip lessens the distance between the origin and insertion points of the rectus, but flexion of the knee increases the distance by roughly the same magnitude. Thus, the muscle remains nearly isometric with respect to length and acts as an elastic band to transfer kinetic energy from the knee to the hip (Fig. 2). The hamstrings, gastrocnemius, adductor longus, and iliopsoas act in a similar manner to transfer energy between nonadjacent segments. Thus, the two-joint muscles work to maximize energy conservation.[9,11] Because the timing and functional control necessary for appropriate action of two-joint, as compared to single-joint, muscles are more complex, it is not surprising that their function is compromised in cerebral palsy

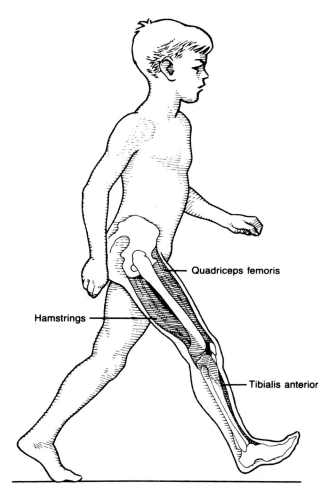

TERMINAL SWING

Fig. 15   The critical goals of terminal swing are deceleration of the shank and correct prepositioning of the foot for contact. In the sagittal plane, complete knee extension and neutral position of the foot are critical for heelstrike and the onset of the next gait cycle.

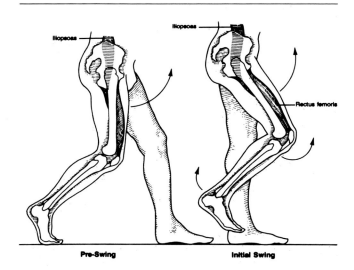

Fig. 14   The foot is still in relative equinus in initial swing, and the knee must flex maximally (approximately 62 degrees) to clear the foot. The iliopsoas still acts concentrically to accelerate the thigh. During slow gait, the short head of the biceps, gracilis, and sartorius augment knee flexion. In rapid gait, excessive knee flexion is prevented by the rectus femoris.

and other conditions that affect central nervous system control.

In the coronal plane, the adductors assist the flexors in advancing the limb. The swing side of the pelvis drops to its maximum point of 5 degrees below the horizontal. While this reduces the vertical excursion of the center of mass and thus conserves energy, it increases the amount of knee flexion required for foot clearance.

In the transverse plane the pelvis rotates forward, acted on by the adductor magnus on the stance side. The thigh, shank, and foot rotate external to the segment above.

Midswing

The critical goal of midswing (70% to 85% of cycle) is to maintain foot clearance. As the knee extends, foot clearance depends on maintaining a relatively level pelvis, sufficient hip flexion, and adequate ankle dorsiflexion. In normal gait, foot clearance is only 0.87 cm in midswing, leaving almost no room for error.[3]

In the sagittal plane the limb behaves as a compound pendulum during swing, and any acceleration of the pendulum that occurs during initial swing must be compensated for by a corresponding deceleration in terminal swing. Midswing then, is a transition period during which there is minimal muscle activity. At the onset of midswing, the thigh is relatively vertical as it passes under the trunk and by the stance limb. By the end of midswing the hip reaches its maximum flexion and the shank is in a relatively vertical position as extension continues at the knee.

Motion at the hip and knee is generated solely by

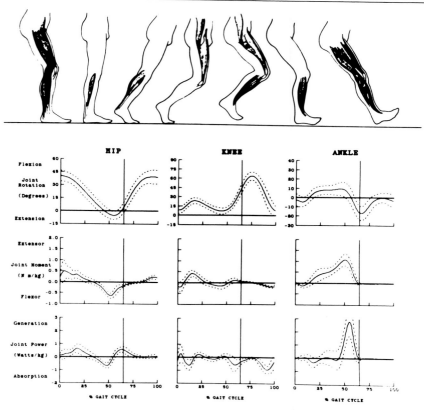

Fig. 16 The sagittal plane of the five subdivisions of stance are shown in the upper part of the figure. In the lower part of the figure are the kinematics (joint rotations) and kinetics (joint moments and powers) of the sagittal plane. These data are used to gain precise information regarding the joint rotations and the magnitude of the external moments produced by the ground-reaction force. The moment graphs also provide a great deal of information about the net muscle function acting across the joint, because the internal moments produced by the muscles must balance those of the ground-reaction force. Therefore, they must be equal in magnitude and opposite in sign. The moment graphs are labeled from the standpoint of the muscles, that is, during an extensor moment, the hip extensors must be active. Thus, by looking at the hip moment graph (first column, second row), it can be seen that the hip extensors are active from the time of initial contact until about 30% of the cycle. At that point, a flexor moment begins, and the hip flexors are active until about 75% of the cycle. The hip extensors become active again in terminal swing to decelerate the thigh and leg. The mechanical power of the muscles can be assessed by multiplying the moment times the joint angular velocity. The sign convention is such that a positive power indicates concentric (acceleration) action of the muscle, whereas a negative power indicates eccentric (deceleration) action of the muscle. Therefore, by looking at the hip power graph (first column, third row), it can be determined that the hip extensors are acting as accelerators during the first 30% of the cycle. At that point, the extensors cease action and eccentric contraction of the hip flexors begins. In preswing, the hip flexors begin to act as accelerators, which continues until midswing.

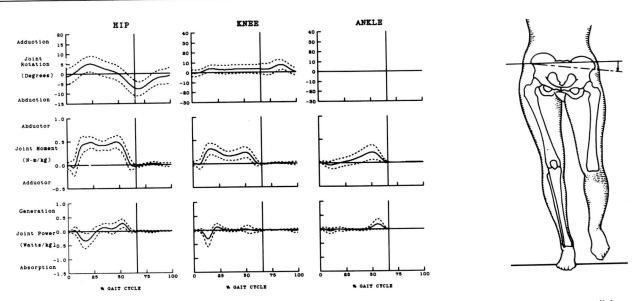

Fig. 17 The coronal-plane kinematics and kinetics are illustrated. Because the ground-reaction force in stance passes medial to the hip, knee, and ankle, it creates an adduction or varus moment at each of these joints. As the hip moment graph (first column, second row) indicates, to balance this moment the abductors must be active throughout stance. This moment begins during loading response and runs through preswing (both periods of double support). The hip joint power curve (first column, third row) reveals that the abductors contract eccentrically (a deceleration) during the first half of stance as the unsupported side of the pelvis is allowed to drop down 4 to 5 degrees, and concentrically during the latter half of stance as the abductors lift the unsupported side of the pelvis back up. No muscle power is generated at the knee and ankle (third row, second and third columns) despite the fact that a moment is present at both joints (second row, second and third columns). Mechanical power is defined as moment times the joint angular velocity; the knee and ankle joints have little or no coronal-plane motion. In both cases the ground-reaction force moments are resisted by ligaments rather than muscles.

inertial forces. At the ankle, the pretibial musculature functions in a concentric acceleration mode to bring the foot from the plantar-flexed position. At the end of midswing, hip flexion reaches its maximum of 35 degrees, flexion at the knee is reduced from 65 degrees to 30 degrees, and the foot regains a neutral position.

In the coronal plane, the hip adductors are inactive and the lower limb moves by inertial action. In the transition between hip adductors and hip abductors, the pelvis returns to a neutral position with respect to the horizontal or transverse plane. As the two limbs pass each other in space, external rotation of the thigh and shank continues with respect to the segment above.

Terminal Swing

The critical goals of terminal swing (85% to 100% of cycle) are deceleration of the shank and correct prepositioning of the foot for contact. In the sagittal plane, complete knee extension and neutral position of the foot relative to the shank are critical for heelstrike and the onset of the next gait cycle (Fig. 15).

An analogy can be made between the foot and a landing airplane. In the case of the aircraft, its position must be appropriate in all three planes as it approaches the runway. If the aircraft's nose is too low (sagittal-plane deviation), it will crash, with the nose making the

initial impact. Deviations in the coronal plane (one wing too low) or transverse plane (malrotation of the plane with respect to the runway) would also mar the landing. In walking, as in flying, appropriate prepositioning of the foot at impact is critical to effective function.

In the sagittal plane, the hip reaches maximum flexion and the foot obtains neutral position by the end of midswing. The knee is in approximately 30 degrees of flexion at the onset of terminal swing and close to full extension at initial contact. The hamstrings decelerate the thigh and shank, preventing excessive hyperextensive force at the knee. Their activity is maximal during this phase of gait. The hip extensors, quadriceps, and pretibial musculature also prepare to resist the moments produced by the ground-reaction force at foot contact.

In the coronal plane, the hip abductors act just before initial contact to resist the impending large adduction moment. Foot position is critical in the coronal plane at this stage of gait because varus and/or valgus prepositioning of the foot at impact would generate large inversion or eversion moments at a time when the muscles required to resist them are normally inactive.

In the transverse plane, the pelvis rotates forward with the swinging limb, reaching maximal rotation as terminal swing ends with initial contact. External rotation of the thigh, shank, and foot relative to the segment above continues until early stance. These rotations probably occur ballistically via inertial forces, but may be secondary to muscle action required in other planes, for instance, the medial hamstrings.

Conclusions

Normal gait is extremely complex, and deviations from normal that occur in abnormal conditions such as cerebral palsy are even more complex. The overall picture of normal joint kinematics and joint kinetics in the sagittal and coronal planes is summarized in Figures 16 and 17. Normal walking has four major attributes that are frequently lost in abnormal gait. These are: (1) stability in stance; (2) sufficient foot clearance during swing; (3) appropriate swing-phase prepositioning of the foot; and (4) an adequate step length. In neuromuscular conditions such as cerebral palsy there is excessive vertical displacement of the center of mass, poor use of body momentum, and marked inefficiencies in the transformations between kinetic and potential energies. As such, energy requirements for walking increase significantly. Using physiologic cost indices, it has been shown that children with cerebral palsy use three to four times the normal amount of energy during walking.[12]

References

1. Hicks R, Tashman S, Cary JM, et al: Swing phase control with knee friction in juvenile amputees. *J Orthop Res* 1985;3:198–201.
2. Tashman S, Hicks R, Jendrejczyk D: Evaluation of a prosthetic shank with variable inertial properties. *Clin Prosthetics Orthotics* 1985;9:23–25.
3. Winter DA: *The Biomechanics and Control of Human Gait.* Waterloo, Ontario, Canada, University of Waterloo Press, 1987.
4. Winter DA, Quanbury AO, Reimer GD: Analysis of instantaneous energy of normal gait. *J Biomech* 1976;9:253–257.
5. Inman VT, Ralston HJ, Todd F: *Human Walking.* Baltimore, Williams & Wilkins, 1981, pp 89–104.
6. Winter DA: Use of kinetic analyses in the diagnostics of pathological gait. *Physiother Can* 1981;33:209–214.
7. Winter DA: Energy generation and absorption at the ankle and knee during fast, natural, and slow cadences. *Clin Orthop* 1983;175:147–154.
8. Winter DA: Kinematic and kinetic patterns in human gait: Variability and compensating effect. *Human Movement Sci* 1984;3:51–76.
9. Yack JH, Winter DA, Wells R: Economy of two-joint muscles. *Proc Can Soc Biomech* 1988;5:180–181.
10. Perry J: Normal and pathologic gait, in American Academy of Orthopaedic Surgeons *Atlas of Orthotics,* ed 2. St. Louis, CV Mosby, 1985, pp 76–111.
11. Hoshizaki TB, Vardaxis V: Intersegment coordination characteristics as defined by joint tendon power flow patterns. *Proc Can Soc Biomech* 1988;5:82–84.
12. Butler P, Engelbrecht M, Major RE, et al: Physiological cost index of walking for normal children and its use as an indicator of physical handicap. *Dev Med Child Neurol* 1984;26:607–612.

The Biomechanics of Running: A Kinematic and Kinetic Analysis

Sylvia Ounpuu, MS

Introduction

Running is a natural extension of walking. The critical velocity at which walking changes to running for normal adults is approximately 2.5 m/s.[1] This transition is a function of leg length and, for this reason, children break into a run at lower velocities than adults. In speed walking, however, velocity greater than minimal running speed is made possible by increased movement in the spine.[1] Because of this, the critical factor that differentiates running from walking is not velocity, but is instead the percentage of stance, or ground contact, in the gait cycle. In walking, there is always contact with the ground either in the form of single support, when one foot is on the ground, or double support, when both feet are touching the ground. During a single stride—the period from initial contact of one foot to the following initial contact with the same foot—there are two periods of double and single support. In running, however, there are times when neither foot is on the ground. These times, termed double float, occur only if the stance phase totals less than 50% of the entire stride time.

A fundamental knowledge of the kinematics and kinetics of normal running is necessary in evaluating and treating running disorders.[2,3] Temporal and stride measures and ground-reaction-force analysis have been studied, but kinematic and kinetic analyses of running are limited. The only extensive works include two-dimensional kinematic and kinetic analyses of sprinting by Mann[4] in 1981 and of jogging by Winter[5] in 1983. For this reason, researchers at the Newington Children's Hospital kinesiology laboratory undertook a three-dimensional analysis of running, including joint rotations and kinetics.

Methods

Twelve children, nine girls and three boys, ranging in age from 5 to 11 years and with no history of injury, took part in the study. A description of the subject population is given in Table 1. For each subject, the study included collection of anthropometric measures, motion analysis and force-plate data collected during walking and running at a self-selected cadence, and surface electromyographic recordings from the quadriceps, hamstrings, tibialis anterior, and triceps surae during walking and running. Results of multiple trials were collected and averaged for each subject.

Running differs from sprinting. In sprinting, the initial contact is made with the toe, energy absorption is less during early stance because the stance limb is used

Table 1
Summary of the subject data

Subject	Age (yrs)	Weight (kg)	Height (cm)	Leg Length (cm)
1	5	21	119	60
2	7	26	127	66
3	7	22	130	63
4	11	44	145	74
5	6	20	122	60
6	7	23	122	61
7	10	27	132	66
8	9	27	135	67
9	9	29	135	67
10	5	20	114	57
11	6	20	117	57
12	9	24	135	71

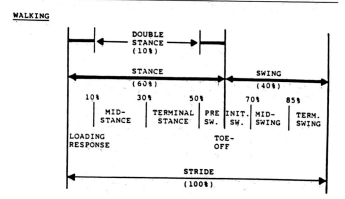

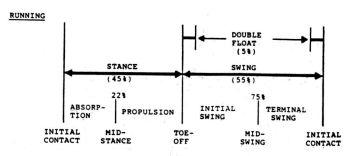

Fig. 1 A summary and comparison of the phase divisions used to describe walking and running.

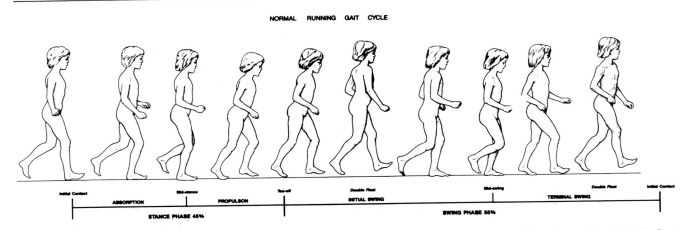

NORMAL RUNNING GAIT CYCLE

Fig. 2 A sagittal-view illustration of one subject running with the corresponding phases included below. Note the periods of double float at the beginning and end of swing phase.

Table 2
Comparison between walking and running temporal and stride parameters

Parameters	Walking*	Running*
Stance (% of stride)	59	43
Swing (% of stride)	41	57
Step length (cm)	53	63
Stride length (cm)	106	126
Cycle time (sec)	0.9	0.6
Cadence (step/min)	134	213
Velocity (cm/sec)	117	223

*Average values for 12 subjects.

much like a pivot, and velocity is greater. The progression from running to sprinting is marked by an increase in step length followed by an increase in cadence.[6] In running, initial contact is made with the heel, and, in our study, whenever initial contact was made with the foot flat or with the toe, that trial was eliminated.

Although the motion analysis system used has already been described in detail,[7] it may be helpful to summarize some important factors. Retroreflective balls marked specific anatomic locations. Three markers, forming a plane, were used on each segment to allow three-dimensional reconstruction. Two embedded force plates, used simultaneously, collected force-plate data. Trials continued until two consecutive force-plate hits were obtained. Surface electrodes were used to collect electromyographic data from the quadriceps, hamstrings, tibialis anterior, gastrocnemius, and soleus muscles during walking and running. Data from a minimum of six strides were linearly enveloped and ensemble averaged by a process described by Yang and Winter.[8] Although electromyographic amplitudes were not calibrated, the gain was not adjusted between the walk-

ing and running trials, so that amplitude as well as phasic activity could be compared. Three-dimensional joint kinematics, kinetics, force-plate data, and electromyographs were averaged across all subjects for both walking and running.

Results

Temporal and Stride Parameters

Running can be divided into segments or phases like those used to describe walking (Fig. 1). The walking stride is typically subdivided into five periods during stance: initial contact, loading response, midstance, terminal stance, and preswing. In running, there are two divisions in stance: absorption and propulsion. During absorption, the knee and ankle joints of the supporting leg flex. During propulsion, all the joints of the supporting limb are extending. The duration of the absorption and propulsion phases depends on running velocity. In slow running, the two equal approximately 40% and 60% of stance, respectively. As running velocity increases, the absorption phase decreases, and the propulsion phase remains about the same. The instantaneous point in time between these phases is midstance. Midstance represents the point of reversal between flexion and extension or absorption and propulsion.

In running, the swing phase is divided into initial swing, which begins at the initiation of first double float, and terminal swing, which terminates at the end of the second double float. These two phases are separated by the instantaneous event of midswing, at which point a reversal between joint flexion and extension occurs.

Thus, running gait can be divided into four phases separated by the instantaneous events of initial contact, midstance, toe-off, and midswing. The phase divisions

LINEAR ENVELOPE EMG

WALKING ————
RUNNING — — — — —

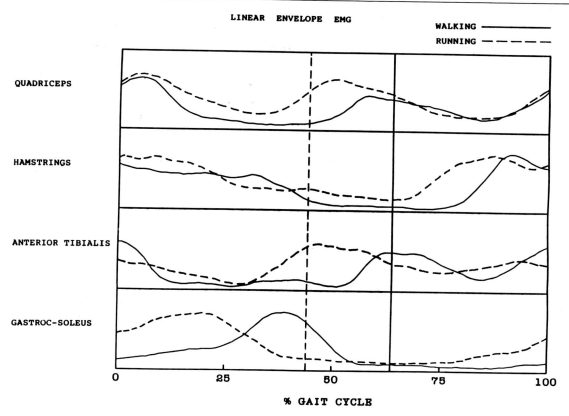

% GAIT CYCLE

Fig. 3 A comparison of linear envelope electromyographic findings for walking (solid line) and running (dashed line). Each linear envelope signal represents multiple strides from each individual subject, which were averaged and than averaged again across all subjects (No. = 12).

Table 3
Increase in selected muscle activity in running compared with walking

Muscle	% Increase (Mean ± 1SD)	P Value
Quadriceps	172 ± 65	<.001
Hamstrings	86 ± 64	<.001
Anterior tibialis	56 ± 44	<.01
Gastrocsoleus	95 ± 41	<.001

in running with respect to the position of the body are illustrated in Figure 2. The periods of double float at the beginning and end of the swing phase are of particular importance.

Table 2 compares the temporal and stride parameters found in running and walking. In walking, the ratio of stance to swing is typically 60:40. While running, the children tested in this study averaged 43% of stride in stance and 57% in swing. Stride, step lengths, and cadence all showed an increase in running over walking. The time for each stride decreased on average by 0.3 second. The average velocity when running was 1.9 times faster than that when walking.

It has been established that initial increases in velocity during running result primarily from increased stride length, after which further changes in velocity up to maximum speed are primarily a function of increased cadence.[9] As velocity increases, there is an increase in nonsupport, or float, time. Horizontal velocity is expressed by the equation $HV = SL \times SR$, in which HV indicates horizontal velocity, SL indicates stride length, and SR indicates stride rate. Most of these temporal parameters are interrelated. Stride length, for example, is a function of leg length and height, as well as running ability.[10,11] Grieve and Gear[3] studied the relationships among length of stride, step frequency, and speed of walking for children and adults. They concluded that by the age of 4 to 5 years a child can walk, run, carry loads, and climb stairs much like an adult.

Electromyography

There is a general consensus that electromyographic activity increases with increasing velocity.[12,13] This study's findings support this conclusion and are presented in Figure 3. Comparisons of walking and running showed significant increases in electromyographic activity during running in all muscles tested (Table 3).

Kinematics

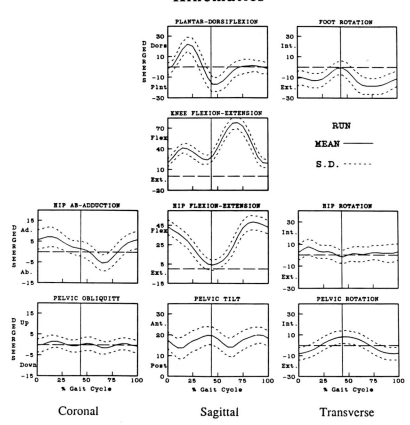

Fig. 4 The average joint rotations in the coronal (first column), sagittal (middle column), and transverse (third column) planes of the ankle, knee, hip, and pelvis are plotted. Average running trials from all 12 subjects are presented. The pelvic motions are in relation to the laboratory space. The foot rotation in the transverse plane only is in relation to the direction of progression. All hip motions are in relation to the pelvis. The ankle and knee sagittal-plane motion represents the relative motion of the adjacent segments. All data are normalized to 100% of stride, and toe-off, indicated by the vertical line in the middle of each plot, separates the stance (first 45%) and swing (last 65%) phases.

Table 4
Comparison of average walking and running joint kinematics (No. = 12 subjects)

Measures	Walking (Mean ± SD)	Running (Mean ± SD)
Ankle		
Plantar flexion (stance)	−8 ± 5	−3 ± 5
Dorsiflexion (stance)	11 ± 5	24 ± 7
Plantar flexion (swing)	21 ± 8	19 ± 7
Dorsiflexion (swing)	0 ± 5	4 ± 6
Range of motion	40 ± 6	50 ± 7
Knee		
Flexion (stance)	25 ± 6	40 ± 5
Flexion (initial contact)	3 ± 4	16 ± 5
Flexion (swing)	65 ± 6	79 ± 9
Range of motion	62 ± 6	63 ± 8
Hip		
Flexion (initial contact)	42 ± 6	50 ± 7
Flexion (toe-off)	−5 ± 5	4 ± 5
Range of motion	47 ± 4	46 ± 6
Foot rotation		
External (stance)	11 ± 7	14 ± 7

Quadriceps During running, the quadriceps muscle shows two peaks of activity. The first, which occurs during absorption, is mainly a vasti component. The sec-ond, which starts just before toe-off and extends into initial swing, is mainly a rectus femoris component. The initial burst is an eccentric, or lengthening, contraction to prevent collapse. The second phase of quadriceps activity is a concentric, or shortening, contraction that flexes the hip to ensure clearance during swing. In terminal swing, there is moderate activity in preparation for initial contact.

Hamstrings The hamstrings are active during terminal swing, at which point they contract eccentrically to slow the forward movement of the thigh. They also act during absorption, contracting concentrically to produce hip extension and bring the upper body over the support limb.

Anterior Tibialis The function and activity of the anterior tibialis are similar during walking and running. The only difference is that it demonstrates less activity at initial contact and early stance in running, probably because there is decreased dorsiflexion at the ankle at initial contact when running. During absorption, the anterior tibialis contracts eccentrically to control the lowering of the foot to the ground. The anterior tibialis is also active at the end of propulsion and throughout

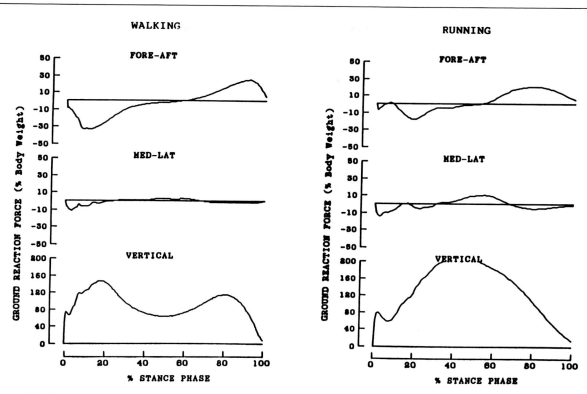

Fig. 5 A comparison of the three-component ground-reaction forces produced during walking and running. The data presented here are from a single subject during a typical walking and running trial at self-selected velocities. The vertical ground-reaction component is the largest and assumes a very different form during running.

swing phase. Concentric contraction during this time provides foot clearance.

Gastrocnemius and Soleus The gastrocnemius and soleus muscles contract eccentrically during absorption to prevent collapse and concentrically during propulsion to produce plantar flexion. Peak activity occurs at 25% of the running cycle, after which activity decreases sharply until toe-off. Brandell[12] used electromyographic readings in combination with film data to study the details of the coordination between limb movement and muscular contraction during walking and running. His results supported previous findings that peak electrical energy precedes maximum mechanical force of muscle contractions by an interval of 40 to 80 msec. This may help to explain why electromyographic readings peak before maximum plantar flexion. These two muscles also show a small increase in activity in terminal swing.

Joint Kinematics

In this study, joint kinematic data were calculated in the coronal, sagittal, and transverse planes for the ankle, knee, hip, and pelvis. The joint angular rotations are presented in Figure 4. Mean values were plotted for the 12 subjects. A description of joint kinematics by plane of motion follows.

Table 5

Comparison between the average walking and running ground-reaction forces (No. = 12 subjects)

Gait	Fore-Aft Component* (% of Body Weight)			Vertical Component† (% of Body Weight)	
Walking	A		B	A	B
Mean	−22		23	122	109
SD	7		4	15	13
Running	A1	A2	B	A	B
Mean	−24	−20	20	134	195
SD	12	5	4	34	17

*In the fore-aft direction, A refers to the breaking force and B to the propulsion force. (During running the breaking force is divided into two peaks: A1 represents the initial impact; A2 represents the main impact.)
†In the vertical direction, A and B refer to the first and second peaks respectively.

Coronal Plane In the coronal plane, the pelvis remains essentially neutral with respect to the horizontal. The hip, however, is slightly adducted (approximately 6 degrees) with respect to the pelvis from initial contact to about midstance. From midstance to midswing, the hip abducts approximately 6 degrees to aid forward progression of the body and clearance of the swinging limb.

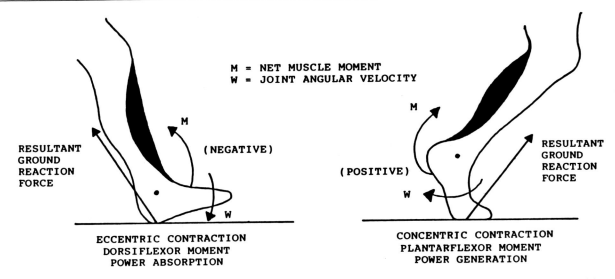

M = NET MUSCLE MOMENT
W = JOINT ANGULAR VELOCITY

RESULTANT
GROUND
REACTION
FORCE

(NEGATIVE)

(POSITIVE)

RESULTANT
GROUND
REACTION
FORCE

ECCENTRIC CONTRACTION
DORSIFLEXOR MOMENT
POWER ABSORPTION

CONCENTRIC CONTRACTION
PLANTARFLEXOR MOMENT
POWER GENERATION

Fig. 6 An illustration of how joint moments and powers are calculated at initial contact (left side) and during the propulsion phase (right side). At initial contact, the external moment produces plantar flexion, which is resisted by a dorsiflexor muscle moment. There is a net power absorption because the angular velocity of the foot segment is in the opposite direction of the muscle moment, resulting in an eccentric contraction.

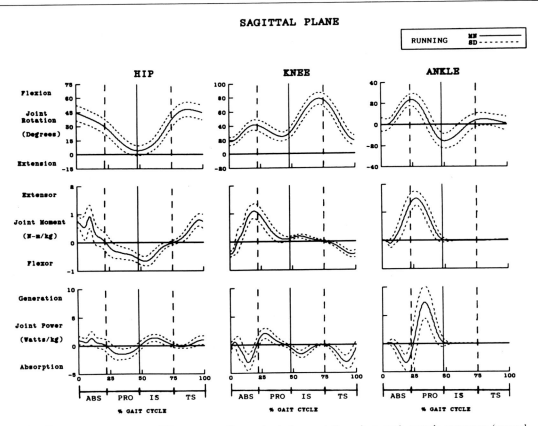

SAGITTAL PLANE

RUNNING
MN
SD

HIP   KNEE   ANKLE

Fig. 7 The average (No. = 12) corresponding sagittal-plane rotations (top row), muscle moments (second row), and powers (bottom row) of the hip, knee, and ankle joints during running. Absorption (ABS), propulsion (PRO), initial swing (IS), and terminal swing (TS) phases are indicated below the plots. The ABS and PRO and the IS and TS phases are separated by the instantaneous event of midstance and midswing respectively (vertical dotted lines), marking the reversal between flexion-extension rotations, extensor-flexor moments, and generation-absorption powers at each joint.

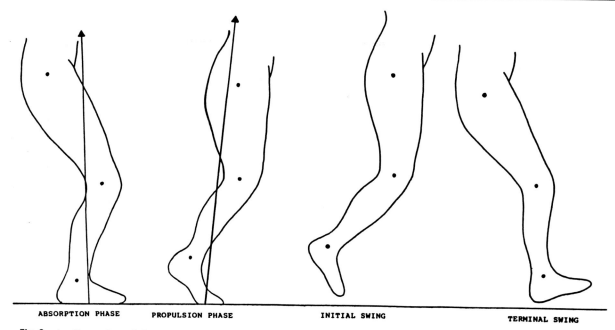

ABSORPTION PHASE   PROPULSION PHASE   INITIAL SWING   TERMINAL SWING

Fig. 8   An illustration of the lower extremity position and muscle activity during the four phases of running. The estimated location of the resultant ground-reaction force (line with arrow) is indicated during the stance phase.

In terminal swing, the hip returns to adduction in preparation for a stable initial contact.

Sagittal Plane   In the sagittal plane, the pelvis shows a biphasic curve with increasing lordosis from midstance to toe-off and from midswing to terminal swing of each limb. The range of motion is approximately 10 degrees. At initial contact, the hip is flexed approximately 45 degrees, after which it continually extends to 5 degrees of flexion at toe-off. During the first half of swing phase, the hip flexes to slightly more than 45 degrees, after which the knee only extends to increase step length. In terminal swing, the hip flexion decreases to approximately 40 degrees, thereby reducing the velocity of the foot relative to the ground, which lessens the shock of initial contact and subsequent braking impulse.[14] Skilled runners achieve this more effectively than unskilled runners.

Both the knee and ankle flex during the absorption phase. At initial contact, the knee is flexed to 15 degrees and the ankle is approximately neutral. The knee reaches a maximum of 40 degrees of flexion and the ankle 20 degrees of dorsiflexion at midstance—the end of the absorption phase. At midstance, motion at the knee and ankle reverses and both begin to extend simultaneously during the propulsion phase. Ankle plantar flexion continues later than knee extension, and maximum plantar flexion of 15 degrees is achieved at toe-off. Until midswing, both the knee and ankle flex concentrically to aid clearance of the swing limb. In terminal swing, the ankle returns to neutral and the

knee extends to 15 degrees of flexion in preparation for initial contact.

Transverse Plane   Transverse plane rotations are shown in Figure 4. These pelvic rotations show the relationship of the pelvis with respect to the direction of progression. An internally rotated left hemipelvis indicates that the left side is toward the direction of progression. Foot rotations are presented in the same way. Hip rotations, however, are shown in relation to the position of the pelvis. Therefore, an internally rotated hip may appear straight if the ipsilateral pelvis is rotated externally or away from the direction of progression.

The pelvis demonstrates 8 degrees of external rotation at initial contact and progresses to 8 degrees of internal rotation at toe-off. Neutral position is achieved at midstance of each limb. During periods of double float, the pelvis is in maximum rotation. The hip shows corresponding rotations with a small internal rotation referable to the pelvis during most of stance. In swing, the hip is essentially in a neutral position. The foot is externally rotated by 10 degrees from initial contact to midstance, after which there is progressive internal rotation to neutral at toe-off. During midswing, the foot shows maximum external rotation of 15 degrees, a position most likely to aid in clearance.

There are no major differences between walking and running kinematics in the coronal and transverse planes. The majority of the kinematic differences occur in the sagittal plane (Table 4). Because increases in sagittal plane motion contribute most effectively to in-

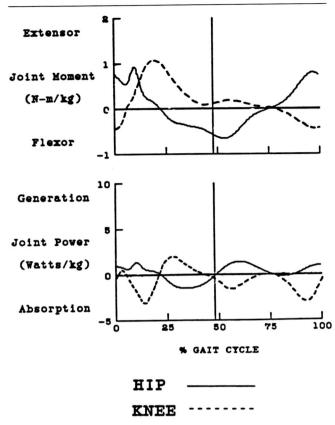

Fig. 9 The consistent reversal of power generation and absorption between the hip (solid line) and the knee (dashed line) is plotted. The zero crossings occur simultaneously for both joints throughout the gait cycle.

creases in velocity in the direction of progression, it is logical that the greatest changes occur in this plane.

Joint Kinetics

Kinetics involves the study of forces that produce movement, such as ground-reaction forces, joint moments, and powers. Compared with kinematics, which are purely descriptive, joint kinetics provide more insight into the cause of movement and movement abnormalities. Unfortunately, joint kinetics are not easy to visualize.

Ground-Reaction Forces Ground-reaction forces are the forces exerted by the ground on the foot when the foot contacts the ground. The ground-reaction force has three component forces: fore-aft, medial-lateral, and vertical. Its point of action is at the center of pressure on the bottom of the foot. The vertical component—the largest component—resembles the resultant ground-reaction force in shape and magnitude. These forces are measured with a device such as a force plate.

The shape and magnitude of the component forces are characteristic of the type of ambulation. In walking, for example, the vertical ground-reaction force takes

on a double bump shape, with magnitudes that are 1.3 to 1.5 times body weight, during loading response and again at push-off (Fig. 5). A comparison of ground-reaction-force parameters in walking and running is given in Table 5. In running, the characteristic double bump shape changes to a small impact force peak during the first 20% of stance and a larger active force or propulsive peak during the rest of stance. The magnitude of this force—from two to three times body weight—is significantly greater during running than walking. Similar results were found by other investigators.[2,8,15]

The fore-aft ground-reaction forces during walking demonstrate braking during the first 50% of stance followed by a propulsive generation during the last 50%. During running, an additional peak braking force occurs at approximately 10% of stance. The braking-propulsion ratio is approximately the same in running, with average magnitudes of 20% of body weight. Magnitudes of the fore-aft ground-reaction force are similar in walking and running.

Medial-lateral forces are of minimal magnitude in both running and walking and represent only 10% of body weight in the subjects tested. Roy[9] also found that medial-lateral forces represented only 10% to 25% of body weight in adults.

Intersubject variability seen in ground-reaction-force measures may result in part from variability in the way each individual's foot hits the ground,[9,15] and in the temporal and kinetic measures obtained in a specific running style.[2] Initial contact during running in this study was made with the heel. The path of the center of pressure, which depends on the type of initial contact, moved from the rear lateral border along the lateral side of the foot to the center of the forefoot where it remained for approximately two thirds of the entire support phase. For midfoot strikers, the center of pressure path begins at the lateral midfoot and progresses posteriorly as the rear of the foot makes contact with the ground. It then moves rapidly to the forefoot, where it remains for most of the support phase.[2,16]

Although not assessed in this study, there is evidence that running velocity affects the magnitude but not the timing of ground-reaction forces.[8,15,17] It is generally agreed that all vertical ground-reaction-force variables increase with running speed.

Joint Moments Joint moments are derived from the principles of newtonian mechanics. A moment, or torque, is the product of the force and its perpendicular distance from the center of rotation. In the human body, the force is produced by the muscle at a certain distance from the estimated joint center of rotation. Thus, each time a muscle contracts it produces a moment at the joint it crosses. Most joints have muscles, tendons, and ligaments crossing on all sides. A muscle moment represents the net activity about a joint and

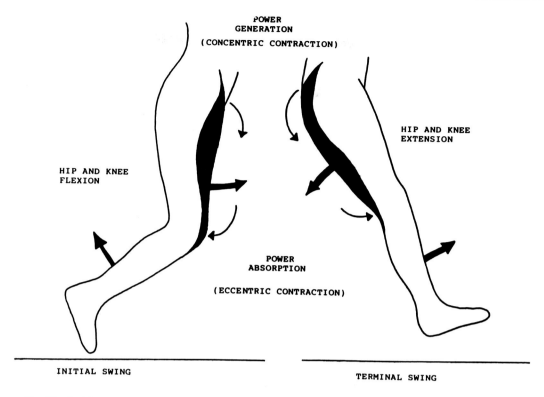

Fig. 10 An illustration of the function of the rectus femoris and hamstrings during swing. In each phase, the double-joint muscle is contracting concentrically at the hip and eccentrically at the knee. The larger arrows indicate the absolute motion of the segment; the smaller arrows indicate the transfer of energy. Energy is being absorbed by the knee and generated by the hip.

thus indicates which muscle group is dominant. Moments produced by the muscles are termed internal moments. These produce motion and resist the external moments exerted on the body by the ground. The ground-reaction force exerted on the foot when it makes contact with the ground acts at a distance from the ankle joint and thus creates an external moment.

As an example, the ankle moments generated during stance will be discussed (Fig. 6). Ankle moments are represented as plantar flexor when the posterior tibial muscles are dominant, or dorsiflexor when the anterior tibial muscles are dominant. At initial contact, the resultant ground-reaction force passes posterior to the ankle center of rotation. If a dorsiflexor muscle moment is not produced, a foot-slap occurs instead of a controlled lowering of the foot. During midstance to terminal stance, a plantar-flexor muscle moment is dominant at the ankle. This muscle moment counteracts the external moment created by the resultant ground-reaction force, which now passes anterior to the ankle-joint center of rotation. Initially this muscle moment eccentrically controls the forward motion of the tibia and then concentrically produces ankle plantar flexion.

Joint Powers A second common measure used to describe locomotion kinetically is joint power. Mathematically, joint power is the product of joint moment and angular velocity. If no joint angular motion is present, angular velocity is equal to zero, and there is no power. A joint moment, however, may still exist. Power is represented either as generation, when the muscle contracts concentrically, or as absorption, when the muscle contracts eccentrically. Power generation occurs when a muscle produces a motion in the same direction as its pull, that is, when the muscle is shortening. Power absorption occurs when motion occurs opposite to the direction of the muscle pull, that is, when the muscle is lengthening. Therefore, it is helpful to interpret powers with the corresponding joint kinematics. Power generation occurs at the third rocker, when the ankle is plantar flexing, and the posterior tibial group is contracting concentrically or shortening (Fig. 6).

Joint kinetics can be calculated by combining joint angular velocity and acceleration data, segment mass and inertial characteristics, and force-plate data. The joint kinetics presented here includes joint moments and powers at the hip, knee, and ankle joints with corresponding joint rotations. Joint kinetic amplitudes are

CORONAL PLANE

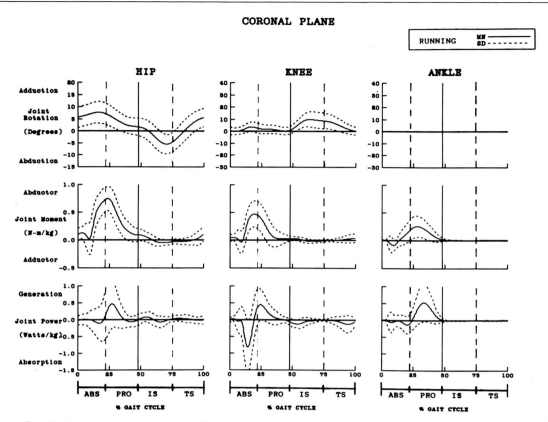

Fig. 11 Explanation of the coronal-plane moments during stance. During absorption, the support hip abductors are contracting eccentrically to control pelvic drop on the contralateral side. Thus, an abductor moment and a power absorption are produced. During propulsion, the support hip abductors are lifting the opposite pelvis and thus contracting concentrically and generating power.

sensitive to body weight[18] and, to control for this effect, the data for each subject were normalized by body weight before averaging. All data were time-base averaged to 100% of the gait cycle. The average sagittal-plane joint kinematics and kinetics for the hip, knee, and ankle are presented in Figure 7. To aid in interpreting these data, knowledge of the approximate location of the resultant ground-reaction force with respect to the joints is useful (Fig. 8).

Sagittal-Plane Results

At initial contact, the body begins absorption. Electromyographic analysis at this time indicates that the quadriceps, hamstrings, tibialis anterior, and gastrocnemius and soleus muscles are all active. The ankle is in neutral position and the resultant ground-reaction force passes just posterior to the estimated ankle-joint center of rotation. As a result, there is a minimal ankle dorsiflexor moment and power absorption as the anterior tibialis contracts eccentrically to control the lowering of the foot. At the knee, there is 20 degrees of flexion, a flexor moment, and minimal power. The flexor moment reverses quickly to an extensor moment that works to prevent collapse. The hip averages 48

degrees of flexion and produces an extensor moment while generating power.

Absorption During the absorption phase, the body's center of gravity reaches its lowest point. Again, the electromyographic output indicates that all muscles tested are active during this phase. The ankle and knee demonstrate rapid dorsiflexion and flexion, respectively. These joints and the muscles that cross them are the prime absorbers. The only power generation during this phase occurs at the hip joint. To absorb the impact, the ankle and knee both absorb energy through eccentric contractions. At the knee, the quadriceps contract eccentrically, producing an extensor moment to prevent collapse. The posterior tibial group also contract eccentrically, producing a plantar-flexor moment to control the forward motion of the shank. The hip-joint muscles contract concentrically, producing an extensor moment and extension of the joint itself. The sharp extensor burst found at 15% of the stride is a result of the impact peak seen in the vertical ground-reaction force.

Midstance During running, the midstance is the point at which absorption stops and generation begins. All muscles tested except the anterior tibialis showed activity. The knee and ankle show a maximum extensor moment and zero power generation at this time, the result of the zero angular velocity produced when both these joints achieve their maximum flexion. The hip continues to extend at this time but the moment and powers are zero. Muscle activity at midstance changes from concentric to eccentric at the hip and eccentric to concentric at the knee and ankle.

Generation During the generation phase, the body propels itself forward for double float. All muscles tested showed activity during this phase. The knee and ankle extend from maximum flexion to maximum extension at toe-off. The resultant ground-reaction force falls in front of the ankle's center of rotation, generating an external flexor moment. The resulting muscle moment is plantar flexor, generated by a concentric muscle contraction or power generation. The knee-joint muscles generate an extensor moment because the resultant ground-reaction force still lies posterior to the knee joint. There is power generation, indicating concentric contraction of the quadriceps. The hip reaches maximum extension at toe-off. This movement is resisted by an eccentric contraction of the hip flexors, causing power absorption and a net hip-flexor moment, which functions to maintain erect trunk position over the supporting limb. Joint kinetics at the knee and ankle show a sharp decrease as support progresses from foot-flat to toe-off.

Toe-off At toe-off, the body prepares to go into double float. The hip, knee, and ankle are at maximal extension. Joint kinetic values at the knee and ankle are approximately zero. At the hip, however, a large flexor moment controls trunk position, but, because there is no joint angular velocity, there is no net power generation. The hip flexor and extensor muscles at this time must be balanced to maintain a stable trunk.

Initial Swing The beginning of initial swing incorporates the period of double float. The ankle dorsiflexes to clear the foot. This is confirmed by anterior tibialis muscle activity. Minimal joint moments and powers are generated because there is no ground contact and the foot has minimal mass. During this phase, the rectus femoris, which is a double-joint muscle, fires concentrically at the hip joint, producing a hip-flexor moment and hip flexion, and eccentrically at the knee joint, to limit knee flexion by generating a small knee-extensor moment. The significance of this point will be discussed in the next section. No hamstring or plantar-flexor activity is present.

Midswing Midswing occurs when the knee reaches maximum flexion and begins extension. At this time, the knee kinetic value is zero because the shank is essentially weightless and there is no angular velocity. The hip shows continuing hip flexion, minimal hip moment,

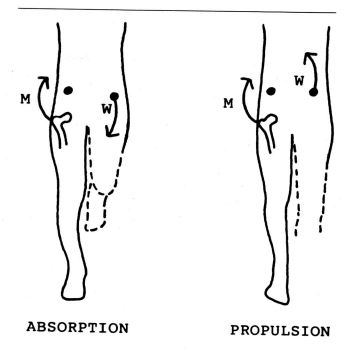

ABSORPTION   **PROPULSION**

M = NET MUSCLE MOMENT
W = ANGULAR VELOCITY

Fig. 12 The average (No. = 12) corresponding coronal-plane rotations (top row), moments (second row), and powers (bottom row) of the hip, knee, and ankle joints during running. The absorption (ABS), propulsion (PRO), initial swing (IS), and terminal swing (TS) phases are indicated below the plots. The ABS and PRO and the IS and TS phases are separated by the instantaneous events of midstance and midswing, respectively (vertical dotted lines), marking the reversal between abduction and adduction and generation and absorption.

and diminishing hip power generation because the hip is close to maximum flexion. Muscle activity during midswing is minimal.

Terminal Swing The end of terminal swing incorporates the second period of double float. No joint moments are seen at the ankle because there is no contact with the ground and the foot mass is minimal. The knee extends to approximately 20 degrees of flexion by initial contact. The velocity of this extension is decreased just before initial contact by a flexor moment generated by an eccentric contraction of the hamstrings. This decreases the forward velocity of the shank in preparation for initial contact. The hip, which reaches a maximal degree of flexion and extends just before initial contact, performs much the same function. To prepare for initial contact, an extensor moment is generated concentrically by the hamstrings. Thus, for the second time in the swing phase, a double-joint muscle contracts concentrically at the hip and eccentrically at the knee.

Power Generation and Absorption Figure 9 shows the consistent reversal of power generation and absorption at the hip and knee. During absorption, initial swing, and

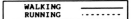

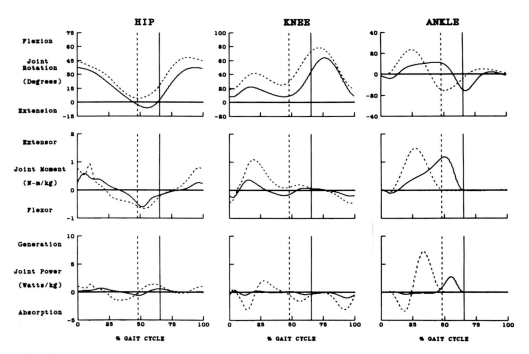

Fig. 13   Comparison between walking (solid line) and running (dashed line) of the average (No. = 12) sagittal-plane joint rotations and kinetics. Differences in magnitudes are evident at all three joints.

terminal swing, the hip generates energy at the same time the ipsilateral knee absorbs energy. Thus, the double-joint muscles that cross these two joints—the rectus femoris and hamstrings—contract concentrically at one end and eccentrically at the opposite, allowing efficient energy transfer between joints. The dual role of the hamstring muscles during swing phase has been described by Mann[4] and Winter.[5] A schematic view is shown in Figure 10.

Coronal-Plane Results

Figures 11 and 12 show the coronal-plane joint rotations and kinetics. The magnitudes of coronal-plane motion and kinetics are much less than those found in the sagittal plane. As a result, the variability with respect to the maximum signal amplitude is higher.

Absorption Phase   During absorption, the support hip demonstrates progressive adduction. Collapse is prevented by the hip abductors, which, in the majority of subjects tested, contract eccentrically and thus absorb power. The knee and ankle function in much the same way, but there the majority of moment and power production is a result of tendinous and ligamentous restraint.

Propulsion Phase   During propulsion, a concentric contraction of the hip abductors progessively abducts the support hip. In the majority of subjects, this produces power generation. Again, the pattern at the knee and ankle is similar but is less marked.

Swing Phase   Joint kinetic values are minimal during swing, because no ground-reaction forces are acting on the lower limb. Because of the segment mass and inertial characteristics, minimal kinetic values are generated at the hip and knee.

Walking vs Running

Figure 13 and Table 6 compare the joint kinetics in the sagittal plane in walking and in running. Greater joint moment amplitudes are produced during running than during walking. In the knee, the maximum extensor moment during the absorption phase in running is three times as great and lasts twice as long as in walking. The consequent increase in patellar-femoral force could increase the potential for injury.[19,20] The ankle shows an increased maximum plantar-flexor moment over shorter duration. Joint powers also show greater magnitudes at all three joints in running, and these differences are more significant in the more distal joints. The ankle demonstrates statistically significant increases in peak generation (3.36 to 9.10 N·m/kg·s) and peak absorption (0.88 to 4.48 N·m/kg·s) values. The larger power generation found when running may also be a causative factor in the Achilles tendon injuries commonly found in runners. The sharp hip extensor moment burst, seen at approximately 15% of stride when running, has been related to the incidence of hamstring injury.[4] In the coronal plane, differences also occurred in the shape and maximum values obtained.

Energy

Although this study did not focus on energy, the topic does warrant a brief discussion. The metabolic costs of running have been studied by many groups.[1,10,12,21] Walking, like running, involves alternate braking and accelerating, with a resulting rise and fall of the center of gravity. During walking, the body is highest when moving slowly and lowest when moving fastest. Therefore, as in a swinging pendulum, the potential energy is highest when the kinetic energy is lowest. As a result the energy cost of walking is reduced. In running, however, during the period of early stance, the body's center of gravity slows and drops, and kinetic and potential energy are lost (Fig. 2). From midstance to midswing, the kinetic and potential energy increase. Running gains efficiency because energy is not wasted as heat during braking but is converted to elastic-strain energy and is rereleased during push-off.[1] Cavagna and associates[21] determined that during running this elasticity contributes about 50% of the total work performed. In running, external positive work is always immediately preceded by negative or eccentric work (Fig. 7). Also, as discussed previously, the double-joint muscles about the hip and knee contribute significantly to the energy efficiency of running.

Table 6

Comparison between walking and running of peak and total joint moments and powers in the sagittal and coronal planes.

Moments/Powers	Walking	Running
Sagittal Plane		
Maximum extensor moment (N·m)		
Hip*	0.83	1.28
Knee*	0.47	1.22
Ankle*	1.14	1.61
Maximum flexor moment (N·m)		
Hip	−0.65	−0.75
Knee	−0.36	−0.51
Ankle	−0.13	−0.20
Maximum generated power (N·m/kg·s)		
Hip*	0.88	2.22
Knee*	0.67	2.57
Ankle*	3.36	9.10
Maximum absorbed power (N·m/kg·s)		
Hip*	−0.78	−2.20
Knee*	−1.28	−4.57
Ankle*	−0.88	−4.46
Total generated power (N·m/kg·s)		
Hip*	0.19	0.30
Knee*	0.05	0.21
Ankle*	0.34	0.64
Total power absorbed (N·m/kg·s)		
Hip*	−0.09	−0.22
Knee*	−0.25	−0.57
Ankle*	−0.10	−0.21
Coronal Plane		
Maximum abductor moment (N·m/kg)		
Hip*	0.46	0.82
Knee*	0.28	0.56
Ankle*	0.12	0.18
Maximum generated power (N·m/kg·s)		
Hip*	0.24	0.77
Knee*	0.24	0.87
Ankle*	0.15	0.40

*Significant at P<.01

Summary

This paper discusses the biomechanics of running and emphasizes three-dimensional joint kinematics and kinetics. To summarize the major points: (1) the major power generator—the ankle—generates three and two times the power of the knee and hip, respectively; (2) the large eccentric action of the ankle plantar flexors illustrates the ankle's secondary role as an absorber of the vertical velocity during absorption; (3) the hip is a secondary power generator, with generation occurring during absorption, initial swing, and terminal swing; and (4) the knee—the primary power absorber—has three periods of absorption that occur during absorption, initial swing, and terminal swing in phasing opposite that of the hip. The knee muscles absorb almost three times the power of the hip and ankle. Comparisons between running and walking data emphasize the higher peak forces found in running, and these may play a significant role in injury.

In this day of high-performance athletics, it is important for physicians who treat sports injuries to increase their knowledge of the mechanisms behind injuries. This requires an understanding of the mechanics of locomotion, which will allow more accurate diagnosis and ultimately better treatment of injuries.

References

1. Alexander RM: Walking and running. *Am Scientist* 1984;72:348–354.
2. Cavanagh PR, Lafortune MA: Ground reaction forces in distance running. *J Biomech* 1980;13:397–406.
3. Grieve DW, Gear RJ: The relationships between length of stride, step frequency, time of swing and speed of walking for children and adults. *Ergonomics* 1966;9:379–399.
4. Mann RV: A kinetic analysis of sprinting. *Med Sci Sports Exerc* 1981;13:325–328.
5. Winter DA: Moments of force and mechanical power in jogging. *J Biomech* 1983;16:91–97.

6. Miller DI: Biomechanics of running: What should the future hold? *Can J Sport Sci* 1978;3:229–236.

7. Gage JR: Gait analysis for decision-making in cerebral palsy. *Bull Hosp Joint Dis Orthop Inst* 1983;43:147–163.

8. Yang JF, Winter DA: Electromyographic amplitude normalization methods: Improving their sensitivity as diagnostic tools in gait analysis. *Arch Phys Med Rehabil* 1984;65:517–521.

9. Roy B: Caracteristiques biomecanique de la course d'endurance. *Can J Appl Sports Sci* 1982;7:104–115.

10. Atwater AE, Morris AM, Williams JM, et al: Kinematic aspects of running in 3- to 6-year-old boys and girls. *Int J Sports Med* 1981;4:282–283.

11. Fenn WO: Work against gravity and work due to velocity changes in running: Movements of the center of gravity within the body and foot pressure on the ground. *Am J Physiol* 1930;93:433–462.

12. Brandell BR: An analysis of muscle coordination in walking and running gaits. *Med Sport* 1973;8:278–287.

13. Mann RA, Hagy J: Biomechanics of walking, running, and sprinting. *Am J Sports Med* 1980;8:345–350.

14. Dillman CJ: A kinetic analysis of the recovery leg during sprint running, in Cooper JM (ed): *Selected Topics on Biomechanics: Proceedings of the C.I.C. Symposium on Biomechanics, Indiana University, Oct 19–20, 1970.* Chicago, The Athletic Institute, 1971, pp 137–165.

15. Munro CF, Miller DI, Fuglevand AJ: Ground reaction forces in running: A reexamination. *J Biomech* 1987;20:147–155.

16. Rodgers MM: Dynamic biomechanics of the normal foot and ankle during walking and running. *Phys Ther* 1988;68:1822–1830.

17. Hamill J: Variations in ground reaction force parameters at different running speeds. *Human Movement Sci* 1983;2:47–56.

18. Winter DA: Kinematic and kinetic patterns in human gait: Variability and compensating effects. *Human Movement Sci* 1984;3:51–76.

19. Perry J, Antonelli D, Ford W: Analysis of knee-joint forces during flexed-knee stance. *J Bone Joint Surg* 1975;57A:961–967.

20. Cox JS: Patellofemoral problems in runners. *Clin Sports Med* 1985;4:699–715.

21. Cavagna GA, Saibene FD, Margaria R: Effect of negative work on the amount of positive work performed by an isolated muscle. *J Appl Physiol* 1965;20:157–158.

Gait Analysis in Sports Medicine

Jacquelin Perry, MD

Visual analysis of athletic performance has been practiced for centuries. As photography and, later, video became available, these techniques have been used to document actions that happen too fast for the eye to perceive. Interpreting these records, however, still depends on the observer's skill. In the last few years, instrumented gait analysis has been applied to sports for more precise definition of the motion patterns, muscle action, and forces involved.

Medically, sport-oriented gait analysis identifies the forces imposed on joints and soft tissues and the required muscle control. It is also used to identify the limitations and adaptations that result from injuries and to determine the effectiveness of various therapeutic measures.

This brief review focuses on the knee and includes the results of studies defining the functional demands imposed by running and cutting, the consequences of cruciate ligament tears, and the therapeutic effectiveness of knee bracing.

Running

Compared with walking, running requires greater muscular effort, larger arcs of joint motion, and tolerance of higher ground-reaction forces.[1-4] Speed dictates the magnitude of these parameters in these three classes of running: jogging, distance running, and sprinting.[2,3] These rates range from two to 5.5 times the speed of walking, which is approximately 1.4 m/s.

Motion

Knee flexion during running is greater, is more persistent, and occurs faster. Mann and Hagy[3] found that the basic knee position during stance is 40 degrees of flexion in running, compared with 7 degrees in walking, and that the knee experiences the same additional 20 degrees of flexion during limb loading. Also, the knee motion for ground clearance (to 100 degrees of flexion) occurs during the float-swing period, because there is no double-support period. The amount of knee movement (60 degrees) is the same as in walking, but is faster and occurs at a more extreme angle. In preparing for the next floor contact, knee extension occurs with equal rapidity. Although loading the limb with the knee flexed provides optimum shock absorption, it also creates a high quadriceps demand.

Forces

The peak vertical force registered on the forceplate in stance during jogging or long distance running is 2.5 times that in walking (Fig. 1).[2,3] By relating vertical force and knee position to determine joint moments, Andriacchi and associates[1] found that the greatest increase in functional demand occurred at the knee. The flexor moments imposed on the knee during running are 7.7 times those imposed during walking. At the hip and ankle, the flexor demands merely double. These values represent the increase in muscular effort that is required.

Muscular Control

The stance phase muscles—hip extensors, quadriceps, and ankle plantar flexors—begin action during terminal swing in preparation for the rapid loading imposed on each joint. The hamstrings begin first, as they aggressively reverse swing-phase flexion toward extension. This activity continues halfway through the brief stance period and may provide a flexor action at the knee that restrains forward tibial shear, helping to protect the anterior cruciate ligament. Quadriceps support of the knee continues through peak flexion and early reversal toward extension. This timing is comparable to that of the hamstrings. Thus, there is considerable co-contraction about the knee during running that is not present in walking. Tibial stability for improved quadriceps function is gained by the early and persistent action of the soleus and gastrocnemius throughout the ankle dorsiflexion period in stance.

Cutting

Cutting, defined as a quick turn while running over an abruptly stabilized foot, imposes high torsional and loading forces on the knee. The two techniques used are (1) turning away from the pivot limb, called straight cut (Fig. 2), and (2) turning across the planted leg, called cross cut (Fig. 3). Forceplate measurement showed that the vertical force of a straight cut exceeds that registered during running by nearly 71% (254 vs 180 kgf). The straight cut's vertical force was also 1.4 times greater than that of the cross cut. Conversely, the external torque impulse, which includes magnitude and time, was 2.6 times higher in the cross cut than in the straight cut. Arnold and associates[5] likened the cross cut to the diagnostic pivot shift maneuver.

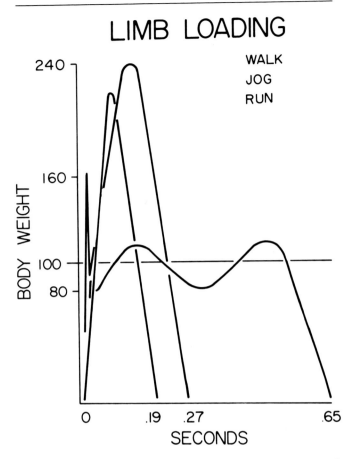

Fig. 1   Vertical ground-reaction forces of walking, running, and jogging. (Adapted from Mann, RA, Hagy J: Biomechanics of walking, running, and sprinting. *Am J Sports Med* 1980;8:345–350.)

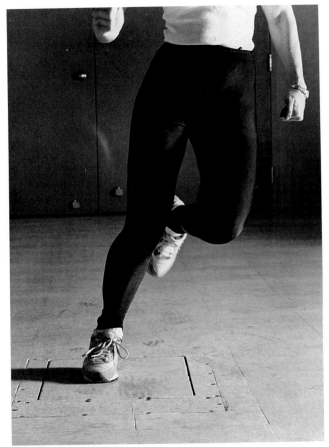

Fig. 2   Straight cut, running turn away from support limb.

Functional Effects of Cruciate Ligament Tears

Today the clinical diagnosis of a cruciate ligament tear is readily made, but it is difficult to define the functional limitation. Observing patients as they walk and run may not reveal any abnormality. Cutting is a more severe functional demand and is avoided by some patients, but others accomplish this maneuver despite their injury.

Investigators, looking for better functional criteria, are using gait analysis. Several studies of athletes with cruciate ligament tears have investigated the functional limitation of athletes with chronic impairment, and the therapeutic effectiveness of surgical management and of bracing.

Anterior Cruciate Ligament

Functional changes resulting from anterior cruciate ligament tears were assessed in 20 athletes whose lesions were subsequently confirmed at surgery. The subjects, whose walking patterns were normal, showed reduced knee flexion in running. Flexion was 16 degrees at initial floor contact and 43 degrees with loading.[6] Only 11 of the 20 were able to do a cutting maneuver.

During running, the involved knee, when compared with the sound extremity, registered several subtle differences in function. Electromyelography showed premature activation of the vastus medialis oblique. Some of the athletes also had premature contraction of the lateral hamstring, or biceps femoris. A more consistent finding, also reported by Branch and associates,[7] was prolonged action of the medial hamstrings. A lower peak vertical force (F3) was registered on the forceplate (Fig. 4). The body vector remained anterior to the joint during limb loading.[1] The loading-response knee flexion of the involved limb was also less than normal.

These findings all represent attempts to reduce the extra shear resulting from the absent anterior cruciate ligament. Biomechanical studies of the anterior cruciate ligament have demonstrated that this ligament resists the anterior displacement of the tibia on the femur that is caused by a quadriceps contraction when the knee is flexed less than 30 degrees.[8-10] Premature activation of the vastus medialis oblique (representative of the total quadriceps) allows patients with anterior cruciate ligament injuries to make floor contact with less knee flexion. This, combined with persistence of an anterior vector, reduces the intensity of the quadriceps action required to control the knee during limb loading. The decrease in vertical force also lessens the flexion torque presented to the quadriceps. Isokinetic strength of the quadriceps of the involved knee averaged 13% less than in the sound limb.

Leaning forward, to move the body vector anteriorly, also stimulates greater hip extensor action by the hamstrings. At the same time, it induces a flexion pull at the knee, which restrains anterior tibial displacement within the knee joint. As the semimembranosus is the largest hamstring muscle (1.4 times larger than the biceps), it is the best hip extensor. This accounts for its prolonged action in stance, even though medial hamstring pull might accentuate internal rotation. For this reason, the primary role of the hamstring is at the hip rather than at the knee. The premature biceps femoris action seen in some patients supports the assumption that this muscle aids knee stability by setting the knee in flexion and external rotation, but this response is not automatic. This finding supports Albright's program of teaching his patients to accentuate biceps femoris action. He advised athletes with anterior cruciate ligament tears to contract their biceps femoris voluntarily to block a pivot shift maneuver. This method's clinical effectiveness seems limited to athletes who undergo daily, intense training, which suggests that the technique may be difficult to learn. Gait studies indicate that some patients learn this substitution spontaneously.

Gait analysis of cutting further defined anterior cruciate ligament disability. The 11 patients who were able to do the tests registered several differences in involved limb function. In the straight cut, both vertical force and aft shear were reduced. In the cross cut, reductions were in lateral and aft shear. A recent, unpublished study showed that the external torque was also reduced. The patients used a flatter, 30-degree angle instead of the normal 41-degree angle for the cross cut. The cutting constant, which relates the product of the ground-reaction forces and cutting angle to time on the force-plate and approach time, was also less. The need to combine these factors implies that despite physical impairment there are several ways to accomplish a quick turn, a multiplicity of approaches that obscures the significance of single measurements. Despite the many protective maneuvers identified in Tibone's patients, all continued to experience disability sufficient to merit surgical reconstruction.

Surgical reconstruction of the torn anterior cruciate ligament has been debated both in terms of need and of timing. Functional outcome two to five years after surgery, as measured by cross-cut gait analysis, has been used to assess the optimum time for surgery. Reconstruction undertaken within one week of injury in five patients was compared to repair undertaken six months or more after injury. Both patient groups were able to perform the cuts normally, both in timing and cutting

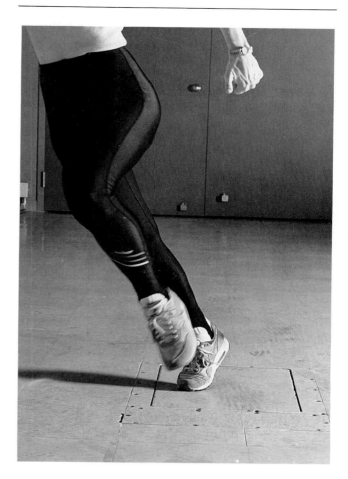

Fig. 3 Cross cut, running turn across the support limb.

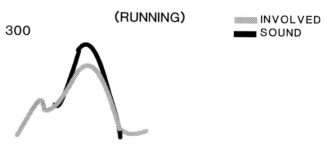

ANTERIOR CRUCIATE TEARS VERTICAL FORCE

(RUNNING)

300

INVOLVED
SOUND

Fig. 4 Bilateral peak vertical ground-reaction forces during running by athletes with confirmed anterior cruciate ligament deficiencies. Solid line, involved limb; broken line, sound limb.

angle. Total, external, and internal cross-cut torsional forces also showed no significant difference, either between the two surgical groups or in comparison to normal values. This performance correlated with postoperative clinical findings of (1) a marked reduction in instability, and (2) muscle strength within 90% of the sound side, except for the acute group's quadriceps, which was 82%. On the negative side, a majority of the patients showed early radiographic changes in the abnormal knee.

Posterior Cruciate Ligament

The functional ability of two groups of athletes, with ten in each group, was assessed by gait analysis.[11] The untreated group had mild to moderate posterior cruciate ligament instability. The second group showed similar signs after postoperative reconstruction for severe instability, using the medial head of the gastrocnemius. Clinically, the treated patients differed from the untreated group by having 13% less hamstring strength in the involved limb. Several subjects also showed radiographic signs of osteoarthritis.

Gait analysis showed several functional differences. Free walking speed for the untreated group was 8% slower, and terminal-swing knee extension was less during fast walking than in those with reconstructed ligaments. Knee flexion at initial ground contact was only 13 degrees compared with 40 degrees in normal runners, and a flexion arc of only 42 degrees, rather than the normal 60 degrees, occurred during limb loading.

The average pattern of muscle action paralleled normal function, although several patients in both groups exhibited additional muscle action. Premature soleus activity, the most common variation, occurred in 62%, and early gastrocnemius activation occurred in 50%. There was a comparable pattern of prolonged action by the knee muscles, involving the semimembranosus in 56%, the vastus lateralis in 44%, and the vastus medialis oblique in 38%.

Vertical (F3) and aft (F6) floor-reaction forces were consistently lower for the involved limb than for the sound side. For the untreated group, this difference was statistically significant during free walking, with the vertical decreased by 10%, and the aft by 15%. In the reconstructed group these forces dropped by a significant 17% during running.

The functional deviations identified by gait analysis imply two protective mechanisms. The more extended knee position at the time of floor contact during running and the reduced vertical floor reaction force demonstrate accommodation to quadriceps weakness. The decrease in aft shear force on the involved side implies a guarding of the posterior joint structures from stretch.

While this study was not intended to judge surgical effectiveness, it did indicate that severe impairment could be reduced to a moderate or mild limitation. Normal function, however, was not restored.

These studies of cruciate ligament injuries serve as an example of the contributions of laboratory gait analysis toward defining patients' functional limitations, substitutive mechanisms, and the effectiveness of therapy.

Knee Bracing for Anterior Cruciate Ligament Deficiency

Although numerous braces have been designed to protect the athlete's knee, their indications and relative effectiveness remain obscure. Cadaveric testing of mechanical restraints of various designs has shown some significant differences. Brace effectiveness for patients with anterior cruciate ligament deficiencies has been tested during a wide variety of activities. These tests have not identified any functional gain.[12]

Recently, a series of gait studies were used to measure the effectiveness of knee bracing. Both functional and rehabilitative designs were assessed. A variety of brace designs were tested both on normal athletes and on patients with anterior cruciate ligament deficiencies.

The effect of bracing on patients with verified, unrepaired, torn anterior cruciate ligaments was assessed in two clinical groups. Fifteen athletes were tested for their ability to perform straight and cross cuts both without a brace and while wearing a custom knee brace. The patients' subjective sense of greater stability with the brace was partially supported by the gait findings. The cutting data identified improved function with the brace. This was supported with moderate statistical significance ($P < .07$).[13] All three factors—total force for the straight cut, cross cut, and cutting index—were greater with the brace than with the knee unprotected.

Another study of bracing for the unrepaired anterior cruciate ligament-deficient knee compared the cross-cut torsional forces of normal individuals and recreational athletes while using a placebo brace, a commercial off-the-shelf design, and no brace. The placebo brace was a simple elastic sleeve with unrestrained metal hinges. The normal subjects registered a 20% reduction in external and total torque values while wearing the commercial compared with the placebo brace. Values with no brace fell in between. The deficient limb, when compared with the sound limb, had 33% lower total torque values in all three brace conditions. The differences in normal performance were significant for the unbraced and commercial brace tests but not for the placebo brace. In the limb with anterior cruciate ligament deficiences there were no statistically significant differences among brace effects.[14]

Extending the analysis of bracing to well-rehabilitated recreational athletes with substantiated anterior cruciate ligament tears, 15 subjects with hamstring muscle strength at least 90% of that of the sound limb were studied. Two custom designs, two off-the-shelf braces, and the no-brace state were compared. No functional differences were found in any of the cross-cut forces.

One can interpret the effectiveness of the placebo brace from two viewpoints. If it is assumed that such a simple design offers no significant restraining force, the clinical effect may be merely proprioceptive, the result of a false sense of security. It is also possible that anteroposterior restraint by a single-axis hinge attached to wide elastic bands and mediolateral limitation imposed by the metal hinges sufficed to decelerate intra-articular shear. Although the placebo brace was preferred for its comfort, the commercial braces were identified as providing the best stability. A third characteristic common to all of these studies was the absence of fatigue. Endurance studies might show that protective bracing is needed to counter fatigue. The better stability gained from a rehabilitation program that restored function of the involved limb's hamstrings to approximately 90% and the quadriceps to 80% of that of the contralateral sound limb was also substantiated.

The effectiveness of a brace in limiting knee motion during early postoperative rehabilitation was evaluated by measuring knee motion during walking.[14] Three off-the-shelf rehabilitation braces were tested for their ability to maintain the desired degree of protective flexion after anterior cruciate ligament repair. The test included five normal subjects and ten patients who had undergone anterior cruciate ligament reconstruction approximately 7.5 weeks earlier. Each brace was set to allow knee motion from 30 to 90 degrees. The motion data demonstrated three significant facts. None of the braces limited knee extension to the desired 30 degrees during walking. All three designs were much less effective on the normal subjects, maintaining only 20% to 35% of the prescribed extension. Among the patients, peak knee extension was limited to 17 to 15 degrees of flexion, or 43% to 50% of the desired position.

Although the braces failed to maintain the prescribed knee position, what did happen may have been preferable. Static stance measurements[15] showed that weightbearing on a knee flexed at 30 degrees presented a 50% quadriceps demand, compared with 20% at 15 degrees of flexion. Supplementing the current bracing capability by teaching the patients to lean slightly forward to lessen quadriceps demand may be a realistic means of providing clinically effective protection.

Bracing the knee is difficult because of the pliability of the soft tissues around the knee. Well-developed thigh musculature interposes several inches of fluid-filled tissue. There is also a layer of subcutaneous fat and a highly elastic skin layer between the brace and the bones to be stabilized. The similarity of results from testing several types of carefully designed braces suggests that these soft-tissue layers limit the use of bracing to correct a patient's disability. Reports by patients that custom-contoured braces provide the greatest sense of security may mean that these braces restrain intrinsic joint shear in some way that cannot easily be measured during dynamic events.

Cross-cutting creates the greatest torsional strains on the knee. More seriously disabled patients avoided the action, and those who could perform the task demonstrated significantly reduced turning forces. Braces improved function but the style of brace did not influence the degree of improvement. It is important to note that all the patients had received intense rehabilitation, and had hamstring strength equal to 90% and quadriceps strength equal to 80% that of the sound limb.

Acknowledgment

To provide current information concerning the contribution of instrumented gait analysis to sports medicine, unpublished data from several Centinela Hospital biomechanical studies done by the Sports Medicine Orthopedic Fellows of the Kerlan Jobe Orthopedic Clinic have been included. J. Bradley, MD, R.S. Kvitne, MD, R. Sellers, MD, D.V. Stevenson, MD, and J.C. Vailas, MD, all contributed important information.

References

1. Andriacchi TP, Goldflies ML, Galante JO, et al: Moments exerted on the lower extremities during running. *Orthop Trans* 1981;5: 228–229.
2. Cavanagh PR, Lafortune MA: Ground reaction forces in distance running. *J Biomech* 1980;13:397–406.
3. Mann RA, Hagy J: Biomechanics of walking, running, and sprinting. *Am J Sports Med* 1980;8:345–350.
4. Payne AH: A comparison of the ground forces in race walking with those in normal walking and running, in Asmussen S, Jorgensen K (eds): *Biomechanics VI-A: International Series on Biomechanics.* Baltimore, University Park Press, 1978, pp 293–302.
5. Arnold JA, Coker TP, Heaton LM, et al: Natural history of anterior cruciate tears. *Am J Sports Med* 1979;7:305–313.
6. Tibone JE, Antich TJ, Fanton GS, et al: Functional analysis of anterior cruciate ligament instability. *Am J Sports Med* 1986;14: 276–284.
7. Branch TP, Hunter R, Donath M: Dynamic EMG analysis of anterior cruciate deficient legs with and without bracing during cutting. *Am J Sports Med* 1989;17:35–41.
8. Hoffer MM, Perry J, Melkonian GJ: Dynamic electromyography and decision-making for surgery in the upper extremity of patients with cerebral palsy. *J Hand Surg* 1979;4:424–431.
9. Cabaud HE, Rodkey WG: Philosophy and rationale for the management of anterior cruciate injuries and the resultant deficiencies. *Clin Sports Med* 1985;4:313–324.
10. Kärrholm J, Elmqvist L-G, Selvik G, et al: Changes of the rotational laxity of the anterior cruciate deficient knee due to anterior or posterior tibial displacements. *Orthop Trans* 1988;12: 462.
11. Tibone JE, Antich TJ, Perry J, et al: Functional analysis of untreated and reconstructed posterior cruciate ligament injuries. *Am J Sports Med* 1988;16:217–223.
12. Tegner Y, Lysholm J: Derotation brace and knee function in

patients with anterior cruciate ligament tears. *Arthroscopy* 1985; 1:264–267.

13. Cook F, Tibone JE, Redfern NF: A dynamic analysis of a function brace for anterior cruciate ligament insufficiency. *Am J Sports Med* 1989;17:519–524.

14. Stevenson DV, Shields CL Jr, Perry J, et al: Rehabilitative knee braces control of terminal knee extension in the ambulatory patient. *Trans Orthop Res Soc* 1988;34:517.

15. Perry J, Antonelli D, Ford W: Analysis of knee-joint forces during flexed-knee stance. *J Bone Joint Surg* 1975;57A:961–967.

Pathologic Gait

Jacquelin Perry, MD

Normal walking depends on a continual interchange between mobility and stability. Free passive mobility and appropriate muscle action are the basic elements. Any abnormality that restricts passive joint mobility below the range used in walking or alters either the timing or intensity of muscle action creates a gait abnormality. The patient's ability to compensate determines the amount of function retained.

Treatment is indicated when the compensations are inadequate or when they introduce penalties in energy cost, joint strain, or muscle overuse. In determining appropriate treatment, gait analysis is used to identify subtle, but significant, gait errors and to differentiate between primary errors and useful substitutions.

Gait errors can be identified by eye or by instrument. With either system, the sequence of events expected in the eight gait phases is the model against which the patient's performance is judged. Observational analysis requires considerable practice and a systematic approach to train the mind and eye to see deviations from normal. Identifying the multiple actions that occur within the stride is made easier if the analysis focuses on one segment at a time. A serial horizontal analysis is used to obtain basic data. Beginning at the foot, the pattern of floor contact is identified. Then, in turn, the actions throughout the stride of the ankle, knee, hip, pelvis, and trunk are noted. Instrumentation records action more consistently and in greater detail, but defining the abnormalities requires that the physician compare the printed data with normal function. The results obtained either by eye or by instrument are interpreted through a vertical correlation of the actions at all the joints, again using the expectations of each gait phase as the model. The final step relates the actions of the two limbs. Determining the cause of the dysfunction depends on a knowledge of the muscles' action. In observational analysis, inferences are made from the patient's muscle test, passive range of motion, and basic diagnosis. Dynamic electromyography provides a printed record of muscle action. If filtered wire electrodes are used, the actions of individual muscles can be differentiated.

Disability Classification

While every diagnosis has some unique characteristics, their effect on walking causes four basic types of physical impairment: contracture; muscle weakness, resulting from disuse or paralysis; pain; and spasticity. Classifying the patient's impairment will aid in identifying the error in gait.

Contractures

These can be elastic or rigid depending on the density of the fibrous tissue changes. With elastic contractures, a vigorous push, rather than the force of two fingers, is required to extend the joint to its full range. Elastic contractures yield under body weight during stance but obstruct motion in swing. Rigid contractures resist the examiner's greatest effort. Their functional effects are constant throughout the stride.[1]

Muscle Weakness

Muscle weakness is judged by manual testing. The amount of the examiner's resistance the muscles will accept determines the strength grade. Beasley's[2] quantification of manual test results showed that the patient's ability is often overestimated. For example grade 4, suggesting four fifths of normal, actually equals only 40% of true normal strength (Table 1). While this amount of strength is sufficient to allow normal movement, the patient will have less endurance. To meet the demands of daily activity, a greater percentage of the muscle must be used with each effort. As a result, the muscle fibers have less opportunity between contractions for refueling and repair (Table 2).

Table 1
Correlation of the manual muscle test and normal strength

Grade	% True Normal	Resistance
5 (normal)	75%	Maximum resistance
4 (good)	40%	Moderate resistance
3 (fair)	15%	No resistance
2 (poor)	5%	No gravity

Table 2
Endurance related to strength

Effort Level	Duration Tolerated
100% of maximum	2 seconds
50% of maximum	10 to 15 minutes
20% of maximum	Indefinite activity

Pain

Pain of musculoskeletal origin generally is related to joint swelling, which causes deformity and muscle weakness. Experimental distension showed the position of minimal pressure for each joint. For the ankle, this position is 15 degrees of plantar flexion; for the knee and for the hip, it is 30 degrees of flexion.[3] All are obstructive for walking. A second joint distension study demonstrated the inhibition of muscle action.[4]

Spasticity

Spastic impairment inhibits motion by its overactive stretch response. Spastic patients also move stiffly, because primitive synergies have replaced normal selective control.[5] The result—premature and prolonged muscle action—obstructs passive mobility. The patient's inability to activate the muscles when needed also causes weakness.

Gait Deviations

Patients limp when they lose one or more arcs of normal motion. They also compensate with extra motion or posturing at adjacent joints. Hence an identified motion error can either be primary error or a deliberate substitution. Each joint has characteristic gait deviations with varying functional significance. The error may be in exaggerated or reduced magnitude of motion or in timing.

Ankle

The gait errors at the ankle are excessive plantar flexion and excessive dorsiflexion. These are caused by equinus contracture (or spasticity), soleus weakness, tibialis anterior weakness, or deliberate posturing to protect a weak quadriceps.

Excessive Plantar Flexion

Excessive plantar flexion indicates either an increase in the normal arc of plantar flexion or inadequate dorsiflexion. An equinus contracture causes a fixed restraint throughout the stride. Soleus or gastrocnemius spasticity, or a primitive extensor synergy, creates premature plantar flexion that is present in terminal swing and persists into preswing.[6] Deliberate posturing because of a weak quadriceps also starts in terminal swing, but the ankle reduces its plantar flexion as the body advances over the foot. The phasic deviations are as follows.

Initial Contact There are two patterns of dysfunction related to excessive ankle plantar flexion. In one, heel contact is reduced; in the other, it is absent.

Low Heel Contact The common 15-degree plantar-flexion posture places the foot almost parallel to the floor.

Heel rocker action is limited because the foot has so little distance available to fall. As a result, the usual loading-response knee-flexion thrust is reduced. The desired shock absorption by knee flexion is lost, but the weak quadriceps is protected.

Forefoot Contact The combination of ankle plantar flexion and knee flexion directs the foot to the floor. If the plantar flexion is caused by spasticity or contracture, the knee is thrust backward (recurvatum).

Midstance Ankle rocker action is inhibited by tension of the plantar-flexor tissues. Advancement of the tibia over the foot is blocked.[7] Progression of the body is retained only to the extent that the patient can substitute. Several mechanisms are used (Fig. 1). Vigorous walkers have early heel rise and roll prematurely to the forefoot. Less able persons rely on knee hyperextension, if the range is available, or, if not, the tissues yield progressively. Forward trunk lean is used to advance the body vector onto the foot. To the extent these substitutions limit advancement of the body, the contralateral step is shortened.

Terminal Stance The vigorous walker who had early heel rise can use forefoot rocker action. Other patients usually lack the needed momentum. Having no heel rise in terminal stance, they lack the advantages of a forefoot rocker, and progression is correspondingly limited. Knee hyperextension may develop in this phase if it has not occurred earlier.

Preswing Passive initiation of knee flexion by the forefoot rocker mechanics is lost. Either there is persistent contact, which leads to a loss of progression, or the heel rises as the unloaded limb moves forward.

Mid-swing Unless the plantar flexion is extreme, this impairment does not interfere with floor clearance until the tibia is approximately vertical. Increased hip flexion is used to lift the foot above the floor, an action commonly noted as increased knee flexion because this is more visible. If excessive plantar flexion is caused by tibialis anterior weakness, the abnormality will be seen only from mid-swing through loading response.

Excessive Dorsiflexion

Excessive dorsiflexion is related either to an increased arc of normal dorsiflexion or to failure to accomplish the expected plantar flexion. There are two primary causes of excessive dorsiflexion: soleus muscle weakness and a locked ankle-foot orthosis.

Loading Response An orthosis with the ankle locked at neutral prevents the normal loading-response of plantar flexion. Instead, the tibia rolls forward as the foot drops to the ground. Knee flexion, increased by the magnitude and rate of motion, stresses a subnormal quadriceps.

Mid-stance Soleus weakness causes excessive ankle

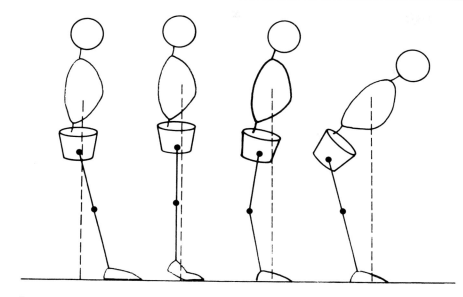

Fig. 1 Ankle plantar flexion: Interference with standing balance and the postures used to realign the body vector over the foot. Early heel off. Knee recurvatum. Forward trunk lean. Dotted line indicates body vector.

rocker action because the muscle is incapable of decelerating the advancement of the tibia.[8,9] As a result, the tibia moves forward faster than the femur, leading to increased and persistent knee flexion, and the quadriceps lacks a stable base for its action. The resultant increased demand on the quadriceps may be poorly tolerated (Fig. 2).

Terminal Stance Forefoot rocker action is unavailable because the weak soleus cannot lock the foot to the tibia. The result is continued heel contact, and progression of the body is reduced.

Foot (Subtalar Joint)

Varus

Excessive inversion of the foot has its greatest significance in stance because the area of support is made less secure. In swing, varus is only a cosmetic problem so long as the foot drops promptly into a neutral posture after contact with the floor.

Varus directs body weight onto the lateral side of the foot. The basic weightbearing areas are the head of the fifth metatarsal and the heel. Equinovarus may make the fifth metatarsal the sole source of support.

Varus can be caused by a contracture, but more commonly this gait deviation is a dynamic deformity caused by overactivity of the muscles on the medial side of the foot. The gait phase in which varus begins varies with the strength of the inverting muscles and the timing of their activation, deviations that are very individualized. Five muscles can contribute to a varus foot posture in stance: the soleus, the tibialis anterior, the tibialis posterior, the flexor hallucis, and the flexor digitorum longus.

Tibialis anterior or tibialis posterior activity can be premature, prolonged, or out of phase.[10] There is no correlation between the foot-support pattern and the relative activity of the two tibial muscles. The toe flexors are contributing forces but not primary sources of varus. They are significant in stroke hemiplegia but not in cerebral palsy.

Soleus muscle overactivity or contracture causes equinovarus because its plantar flexion leverage is greater than that available for inversion. The size of this muscle makes it a dominant inverter.

Peroneal muscle weakness is not a cause of a varus gait. These muscles are essential for lateral support of the inverted, weightbearing foot.

During swing, the primary cause of subtalar varus is tibialis anterior activity associated with weak or absent participation by the long toe extensors and peroneus tertius. The extensor digitorum hallucis, although often prominent, is too small a muscle to be a significant force except at the toe.

Valgus

In both stance and swing, valgus is most commonly a sign of weak inverters. In stance, it may be caused by hypermobility within the foot.

Stance There are two static causes of weightbearing valgus. During loading response, excessive eversion may occur as a passive response to heel loading in the hypermobile foot. Also, subtalar mobility can be substituted for equinus contracture. Subtalar eversion is naturally accompanied by dorsiflexion. When the range

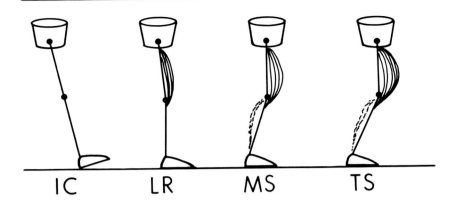

Fig. 2 Excessive dorsiflextion: Soleus weakness allows excessive advancement of the tibia in mid-stance (MS) and terminal stance (TS). Quadriceps demand persists because of the associated knee flexion.

is lost at the ankle, forward travel of the foot can occur in the subtalar joint and unlocked midfoot.

Dynamic causes of weightbearing valgus are generally weakness of the soleus and/or tibialis posterior. The timing of heel rise may differentiate these two causes. A third cause is poor support by the tibialis anterior during loading response.

Swing Valgus in swing results from imbalance between a weak tibialis anterior and strong common toe extensors. During swing the foot everts as the strong toe extensors act to dorsiflex the ankle.

Knee

The alternation of flexion and extension that occurs in both stance and swing makes the classification of gait deviations complex. In phases in which flexion normally occurs, functional errors are classified either as inadequate flexion, when motion is limited, or as excessive flexion, when the arc is greater than the natural arc. The terms inadequate and excessive are also applied to extensor arcs of motion. Excessive extension is subdivided into extensor thrust and hyperextension.

Excessive Flexion

Flexion beyond the normal range is a primary gait deficit in stance. It is common in loading response but not preswing. In swing it is usually a substitutive action and occurs during mid-swing.

Loading response displays increased knee flexion when there is a posterior mechanism acting to hold the tibia back. The causes are hamstring spasticity and knee-flexion contracture. Excessive knee flexion inhibits progression and imposes added demands on the foot and ankle. In mid-swing, knee flexion is greater than normal when floor clearance is impaired by a plantar-flexed ankle. The cause of the ankle posture may be an equinus contracture or a weak tibialis anterior muscle. The increased knee flexion is a carry-over effect of the

greater hip flexion required to lift the foot to clear the floor.

Inadequate Extension

The same mechanisms that cause excessive flexion lead to inadequate extension. This problem arises in terminal swing and, during stance, at initial contact, mid-stance, and terminal stance. In stance the functional penalty is increased quadriceps demand as well as the need for complementary posturing by the hip and ankle-foot complex.[11] Inadequate extension in swing fails to prepare the limb for stance.

In initial contact, mid-stance, and terminal stance the normal trend towards full extension is lost when there is hamstring spasticity or a flexion contracture. Without compensation, the flexed knee aligns the body behind the supporting foot during mid-stance (Fig. 3). Hence, there must be either increased ankle dorsiflexion or a premature heel-off posture during mid-stance. In terminal stance, forward progression of the limb and body will be stopped unless the effective substitution, either heel rise or ankle dorsiflexion, increases.

An added cause of inadequate knee extension in stance is soleus muscle weakness. The lack of an adequate ankle plantar-flexor force to prevent excessive advancement of the tibia allows the knee to flex.[12]

Inadequate Flexion

Limited or absent knee flexion may occur in selected phases of either stance or swing. In stance, the sensitive phases are loading response and preswing. In swing, they are initial and mid-swing.

Loading Response Three types of abnormality limit knee flexion at this time: voluntary substitution for quadriceps weakness, quadriceps spasticity, and fixed ankle plantar flexion. These differ in their effects later in the stride.

Substitution for quadriceps weakness leads to absent loading-response knee flexion, leaving no mechanism to absorb the shock of initial impact. Knee flexion is

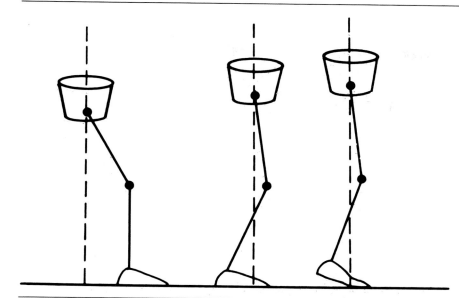

Fig. 3 Excessive knee flexion: Interference with standing balance and the postures used to realign the body vector over the foot. Increased ankle dorsiflexion. Premature heel off.

prevented by using premature ankle plantar flexion to avoid the heel rocker. Usually there is also strong hip extensor muscle action in loading response and mid-stance.

Quadriceps spasticity limits knee flexion by the muscle's overreaction to stretch. The spastic response generally persists into or through the single stance period.

Fixed ankle plantar flexion may represent a contracture or soleus spasticity. Loading the limb after initial contact with the forefoot drives the tibia backward. Loading-response knee flexion is inhibited. More vigorous muscle activity can cause an extensor thrust or knee hyperextension.

Preswing Knee flexion fails to occur during preswing when excessive plantar flexion or extension of the ankle deny the patient an effective forefoot rocker sequence. Persistence of the spastic quadriceps (primitive extensor synergy) directly inhibits preswing knee flexion.

Swing Any mechanism that limits preswing knee flexion also reduces the action in initial swing unless the patient has normal motor control and the strength for rapid motion.

Quadriceps spasticity that continues into swing obstructs knee flexion in initial swing and mid-swing. Prolonged and excessively intense rectus femoris muscle action is the most common obstructing force.[13,14] Continuing or out-of-phase vastus intermedius action is a second discreet cause. The whole quadriceps can also be active in swing.

Hip flexor weakness inhibits swing-phase knee flexion through the loss of femoral advancement. The substitutions for inadequate knee flexion include contralateral vaulting, circumduction, and contralateral trunk lead.

Excessive Extension

Extension beyond neutral, called hyperextension, is posterior angulation of the knee. If the knee is driven backward, but the joint lacks a hyperextensive range, the action is called extensor thrust.

These actions can occur in loading response when the mechanisms inhibiting flexion are strong. More commonly, both the extensor thrust and hyperextension of the knee begin in mid-stance or terminal stance. Substitution for quadriceps weakness, quadriceps spasticity, and rigid ankle plantar flexion are the causes.

Coronal Plane Deviations

Valgus (abduction) and varus (adduction) of the knee can be determined only in stance. During swing, knee flexion and limb rotation commonly create artificial impressions of medial or lateral malalignment. Alignment of body weight over the knee determines the coronal deviation within the knee joint. The tissues yield to the strain.

Valgus is induced by excessive lateral deviation of the trunk in stance. Knee deformity commonly develops secondary to postural substitution for hip abductor-muscle weakness. A second cause is valgus instability at the foot. Both situations place the body vector lateral to normal alignment, and the knee molds in response to the forces experienced. This is a common development in rheumatoid arthritis. There are no intrinsic forces within the knee to induce coronal plane deviations.

Varus deformity within the knee follows excessive medial alignment of the body vector. As normal alignment places the vector medial to the knee joint center, a secondary factor leads to excessive malalignment. This can be a developmental malalignment, progressive osteoarthritic degeneration within the knee, or postural locking for an absent quadriceps.

Hip

Because of its ball-in-socket configuration, the hip can present gait deviations in any of the three planes. Of the many possibilities, three major patterns of dysfunction are discussed here. Gait errors relating to flexion, extension, and abduction are well defined; their causes are identified; and they are major sources of dysfunction. In contrast, deviations such as excessive adduction and transverse rotation, while visible, lack diagnostic clarity.

Inadequate Extension

The normal pattern of continuous hip extension during stance depends on the joint having passive mobility. Three conditions limit this action. Two of these—flexion contracture and flexor muscle spasticity—are related to intrinsic hip abnormalities. The third cause is forward lean to advance the body vector over the supporting limb in the presence of rigid ankle equinus. Single-limb-support phases are sensitive to a loss of hip extension.

Mid-stance and Terminal Stance Inadequate extension at the hip keeps the thigh forward. This impedes advancement of the body over the supporting foot. The duration of single limb support and stride length are reduced. Several substitutions are used (Fig. 4).

Lumbar lordosis is the most common postural adaptation to a lack of hip extension. Anterior tilt of the pelvis to place the thigh in a more vertical, or trailing,

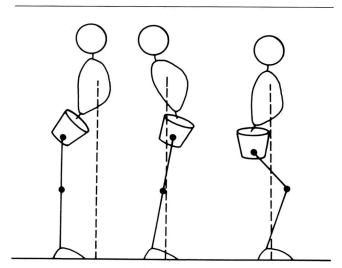

Fig. 4 Excessive hip flexion: Interference with standing balance and the postures used to realign the body vector over the foot. Lordosis sufficient to place trunk center posterior to hip joint. Knee flexion to restore a level pelvis.

posture, combined with upright alignment of the trunk, creates lumbar lordosis.[15] Strain on the posterior facets is likely.

Forward trunk posture, seen in patients with limited lumbar spine mobility, requires some form of manual support such as canes, crutches, or a walker to support the malaligned trunk. Back muscle stress is a common complication of this standing posture.

Knee flexion, or crouch gait, preserves neutral alignment of the pelvis and allows the femur to roll forward. The increased demand on the quadriceps limits the patient's endurance.

Inadequate Abductors

The three abductor muscles (the gluteus medius and gluteus minimus complex, the upper gluteus maximus, and the tensor fascia lata) may lack sufficient strength or adequate bony leverage to stabilize the unsupported pelvis. Reduced muscle action to avoid hip pain is another stimulus. Three possible gait deviations are related to insufficient abductor muscle activity.

In contralateral pelvic drop, the unsupported side drops as body weight shifts to the ipsilateral limb at the onset of loading response. This occurs in patients with equal leg lengths. Ipsilateral limb shortening places the hip in a protective position of slight abduction.

In ipsilateral trunk lean, demand on the hip abductors is lessened by shifting the trunk towards that limb. The body vector may be moved over to the center of the hip joint. To use this substitution, the weight-accepting limb must have good intrinsic stability. Persons use this motion subconsciously to gain postural stability or to reduce joint compression from abductor muscle action.

Contralateral trunk fall represents a lack of postural compensation for the inadequate abductors. Two situations contribute to this lack of adaptability. One cause, often overlooked, is insufficient leg muscle strength to accept the accentuated load. In hemiplegia, a poor body image leads to side neglect, and the patient loses awareness that there is an unsupported side.

Inadequate Flexion

Both stance and swing have an interval in which reduced hip flexion is significant. Generally the cause is dynamic.

Swing Limited ability to flex the hip in initial and midswing blocks limb advancement. It also leads to a lack of knee flexion and thus causes toe drag. Step length is reduced in proportion to the lack of active hip flexion. The cause of the gait deviation may be weak hip flexor muscles or out-of-phase action of the hip extensors, usually the hamstrings.

Substitutions commonly used are ipsilateral pelvic hike combined with circumduction to lift and swing the limb forward using the trunk muscles. Contralateral vaulting is another means of lifting the inadequately flexed limb clear of the floor.

Stance Stability during stance with inadequate hip-extensor muscle strength necessitates keeping the body vector behind the hip-joint axis. In terminal swing, hip flexion is limited to lessen postural instability at initial contact. In addition, the body, rather than being behind the foot, is quickly moved forward to lie over the limb as it is loaded. Both situations lead to inadequate hip flexion at initial contact and loading response.

Excessive Adduction

The adductor longus normally acts with the adductor brevis in preswing to decelerate hip abduction as weight drops rapidly onto the other limb. The activity of these two muscles commonly continues during initial swing to recover the limb from its abducted position. Excessive adductor activity secondary to spasticity can cause the limb to cross the midline, leading to an unwanted gait action. If this action persists into loading response, the excessively adducted limb creates an obstacle for the other limb as it initiates its swing phase. These adductors can also substitute for inadequate iliacus muscle action. Although the action may be excessive, it is also useful.

Pelvis and Trunk

The eye perceives any deviation of the trunk from its normal vertical alignment as abnormal. Displacement of the trunk can occur in any of the three planes. Motion may be backward, forward, to either side, or rotational. In stance, a substitution is judged to be unwanted or useful according to the value of the body vector created at the lower joints, whether it adds stability or creates an additional load to be controlled. In swing, the determining factor is whether or not the motion assists limb advancement.

As the pelvis normally moves only five degrees in each direction, its visible motion is inconspicuous and fluid in nature. For this reason, all obvious deviations from neutral alignment represent abnormal motion. Interpretation uses the same gross criteria cited for the trunk.

Summary

The diagnosis of gait deviations and their causes requires three levels of knowledge. First is an awareness of the functional limitations caused by each type of abnormality (contracture, muscle weakness, pain, and spasticity). Second is familiarity with normal function. Third is having a trained eye or gait analysis system that is capable of identifying the gait deviations. Once diagnosis is complete, a fourth requirement is the ability to use the findings to set up an appropriate treatment regimen.

References

1. Perry J: Normal and pathologic gait, in American Academy of Orthopaedic Surgeons *Atlas of Orthotics*, ed 2. St. Louis, CV Mosby, 1985, pp 76–111.
2. Beasley WC: Quantitative muscle testing: Principles and applications to research and clinical services. *Arch Phys Med Rehabil* 1961;42:398–425.
3. Eyring EJ, Murray WR: The effect of joint position on the pressure of intra-articular effusion. *J Bone Joint Surg* 1964;46A:1235–1241.
4. deAndrade JR, Grant C, Dixon AS: Joint distension and reflex muscle inhibition in the knee. *J Bone Joint Surg* 1965;47A:313–322.
5. Knutsson E, Richards C: Different types of disturbed motor control in gait of hemiparetic patients. *Brain* 1979;102:405–430.
6. Perry J, Hoffer MM, Giovan P, et al: Gait analysis of the triceps surae in cerebral palsy: A preoperative and postoperative clinical and electromyographic study. *J Bone Joint Surg* 1974;56A:511–520.
7. Peat M, Dubo HIC, Winter DA, et al: Electromyographic temporal analysis of gait: Hemiplegic locomotion. *Arch Phys Med Rehabil* 1976;57:421–425.
8. Perry J: Kinesiology of lower extremity bracing. *Clin Orthop* 1974;102:18–31.
9. Sutherland DH, Cooper L, Daniel D: The role of the ankle plantar flexors in normal walking. *J Bone Joint Surg* 1980;62A:354–363.
10. Wills CA, Hoffer MM, Perry J: A comparison of foot-switch and EMG analysis of varus deformities of the feet of children with cerebral palsy. *Dev Med Child Neurol* 1988;30:227–231.
11. Perry J, Antonelli D, Ford W: Analysis of knee-joint forces during flexed-knee stance. *J Bone Joint Surg* 1975;57A:961–967.
12. Perry J, Hislop HJ (eds): *Principles of Lower-Extremity Bracing*. Washington, DC, American Physical Therapy Association, 1967, p 67.
13. Waters RL, Garland DE, Perry J, et al: Stiff-legged gait in hemiplegia: Surgical correction. *J Bone Joint Surg* 1979;61A:927-933.
14. Perry J: Distal rectus femoris transfer. *Dev Med Child Neurol* 1987;29:153–158.
15. Edberg E: Paralytic dysfunction: IV. Bracing for patients with traumatic paraplegia. *Phys Ther* 1967;47:818–823.

Gait Analysis in Neuromuscular Diseases

David H. Sutherland, MD

Introduction

Why should orthopaedic surgeons who care for patients with neuromuscular diseases concern themselves with gait analysis? Through observation and clinical experience they have already gained an excellent understanding of gait abnormalities in neuromuscular diseases. Most experienced orthopaedic surgeons,

pediatricians, neurologists, physiatrists, and physical therapists are skilled in recognizing movement disorders. However, observational gait analysis alone cannot provide sufficient data for scientific progress. The need for objectivity is obvious, but, at the same time, it is necessary to justify the considerable cost, dedicated personnel, and time required for quality gait analysis. Four simple questions will help focus this discussion:

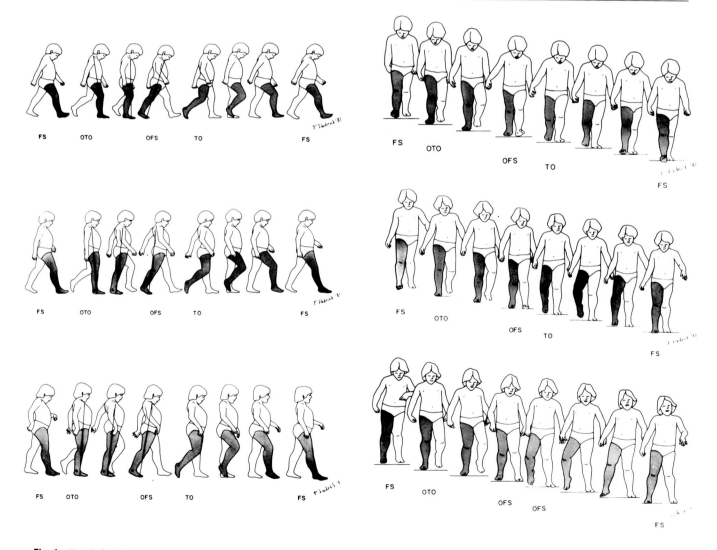

Fig. 1 **Top left** and **top right**, Side and front film tracings of 5-year-old subject with Duchenne's muscular dystrophy—early stage. **Center left** and **center right**, Side and front film tracings at 7 years 6 months—transitional stage. **Bottom left** and **bottom right**, Side and front film tracings in late stage. Note force line, lordosis, and wide-based gait. (Reproduced with permission from Sutherland DH: *Gait Disorders in Childhood and Adolescence*. Baltimore, Williams & Wilkins, 1984.)

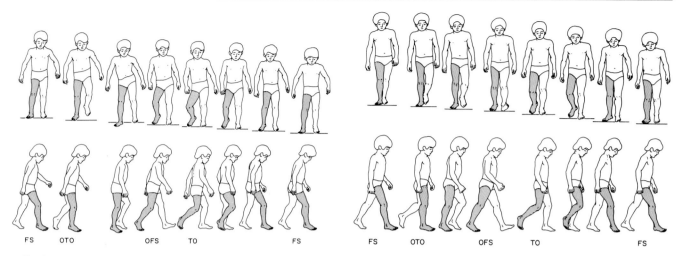

Fig. 2 **Left**, Front and side film tracings of polio patient. Note pelvic obliquity and forward trunk lean. **Right**, Front and side film tracings of patient after surgery.

What is gait analysis? Why is it important? When should it be used? How can patients profit from its use?

What Is Gait Analysis?

In addition to visual observation, gait analysis involves the scientific measurement of movements (joint angles and time and distance parameters), muscle action (dynamic electromyography), force (force-plate recordings), and energy (oxygen consumption or work of walking, derived from force calculations). If the process involved only the collection of the various measurements, it would have little value. All the measurements must be correlated, interpreted, and applied to the individual patient or to a group of homologous patients. At the time of this writing, the tools for measurement are very sophisticated, but persons trained to correlate, interpret, and apply the findings are scarce. Orthopaedic surgeons must be well informed in this discipline or risk losing responsibility for making treatment decisions.

Why Is Gait Analysis Important?

Rational treatment requires an understanding of the functional disorder. This means that normal function must be thoroughly understood to delineate pathologic function accurately. Also, primary errors in walking must be distinguished from compensatory changes because failure to do so can cause errors in treatment planning.

Because muscle action is largely invisible, accurate information about muscle function requires dynamic electromyograms. Normal walking appears to be almost effortless, but this apparent ease depends on a normal motor control system regulating a large number of muscles, each with a brief period of action and a specific task. There are 35 muscles in each lower extremity (excluding the intrinsic muscles of the foot), and each has a defined role in gait. When muscle actions are weak, absent, or out of phase, complex gait changes occur. Although it is not possible to carry out dynamic electromyography of even a small number of these muscles in a single recording session, it is possible to obtain vital information by sampling selected critical muscles.

Measurements allow for comparison. Changes that occur with time or as a result of treatment can be accurately assessed. This unique capability of gait analysis is enough to justify its use. In this time of expanding medical-care costs and competition for healthcare dollars, physicians are being asked to evaluate objectively the outcome of treatment. In assessing gait changes following treatment, there is no substitute for gait analysis.

When Should Gait Analysis Be Used?

Ideally, gait should be analyzed before any major treatment change. Although at present there are not enough facilities to handle all potential patients, there is steady expansion of available laboratories, and accessibility for patients is improving.

How Can Patients Profit From Gait Analysis?

Treatment planning is improved when abnormal movements, functional deficits, and electromyography are correlated. For example, a patient with cerebral palsy who lacks extension of the hip in stance phase is well served by electromyography of the iliopsoas to corroborate abnormal stance-phase activity before undergoing surgical lengthening of the iliopsoas. Failure to verify abnormal muscle activity can result in unnecessary surgery on muscles that are acting normally.

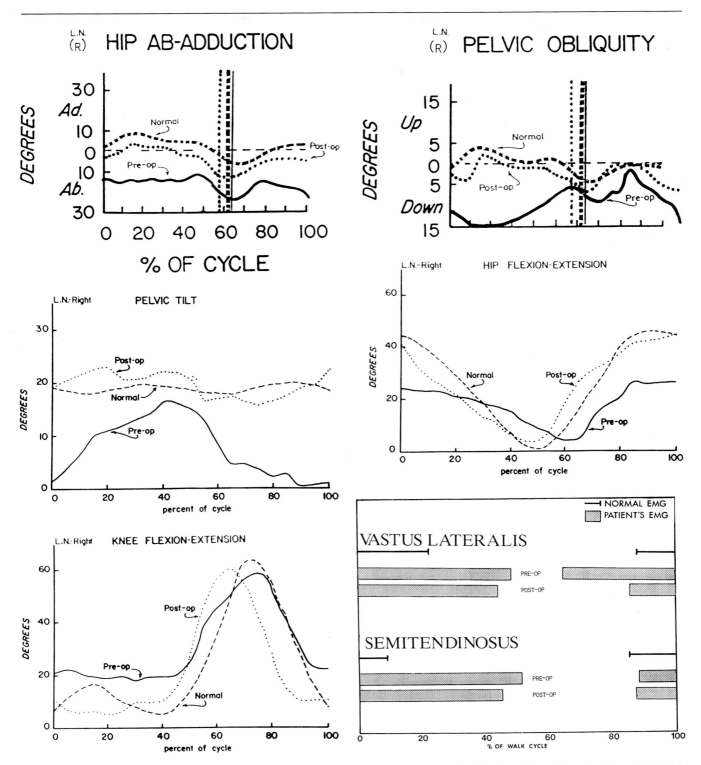

Fig. 3 **Top left,** Hip abduction-adduction (coronal plane) shows increased abduction the hip throughout the cycle. **Top right,** Pelvic obliquity (coronal plane) shows the right iliac crest very low throughout much of the gait cycle. **Top right, Center left,** Pelvic tilt (sagittal plane) shows excessive dynamic range of movement with decreased anterior pelvic tilt. Peak anterior pelvic tilt occurs shortly after 40% of the cycle (which precedes opposite foot strike). **Center right,** Hip flexion-extension (sagittal plane) shows normal extension in late stance but limited flexion of the hip. **Bottom left,** Knee flexion-extension (sagittal plane) shows exaggerated knee flexion in stance and absent early stance-phase knee flexion wave. **Bottom right,** Preoperative and postoperative dynamic electromyography. Vastus lateralis shows premature onset in swing phase and prolongation in stance phase. Semitendinosus shows stance-phase prolongation with cessation at 50% of the cycle. The postoperative vastus lateralis recording now shows normal swing-phase activity and no significant change in the stance phase. Semitendinosus is not significantly changed.

Table 1
Time and distance data for Case 1

Data	Preoperative Right	Postoperative Right	Preoperative Left	Postoperative Left
Opposite toe-off (% cycle)	16	14	8	12
Opposite foot strike (% cycle)	54	47	47	53
Single stance (% cycle)	38	33	39	41
Toe-off (% cycle)	62	58	62	67
Step length (cm)	32	45	36	48
Stride length (cm)	68	93	68	93
Cycle time (sec)	0.9	0.93	0.9	0.93
Cadence (steps/min)	133	129	133	129
Walking velocity				
cm/sec	76	100	76	100
m/min	45	60	45	60

Changes with time and treatment are assessed. There are both individual and collective benefits because the results of these studies are being presented in national and international meetings. Patients profit from the pooling of data and from the possibilities of rapid dissemination of the results of treatment. In the past, efforts at evaluating treatment were largely subjective and confusing. The ability to measure function objectively has brought in a new era.

Gait Laboratory Functions

There are a wide variety of neuromuscular disorders for which gait analysis may be appropriate. General categories include nonprogressive spinal cord and peripheral nerve disorders, disorders of motor control, myopathic disorders, and progressive spinal cord and peripheral nerve disorders.[1]

The functions of gait analysis for this disparate group of patients can include pretreatment or preoperative planning, posttreatment or postsurgical assessment, long-term follow-up, evaluation of orthotics, comparison of treatment methods, and studies of the pathomechanics and natural history of individual diseases. Disorders of motor control, including cerebral palsy, head injury, and stroke, provide the greatest possibility for pretreatment and posttreatment assessment and for comparison of treatment methods. Progressive spinal cord and peripheral nerve disorders and myopathies are particularly appropriate for studies of natural history and pathomechanics. All of these afford the possibilities of evaluation of orthotics and long-term follow-up with objective documentation of function.

Pathomechanics and Natural History of Duchenne's Muscular Dystrophy

A study was carried out, in my laboratory, of the progressive alterations of gait that characterize Duchenne's muscular dystrophy.[2] Three stages of ambulation, early, transitional, and late, can be differentiated, on the basis of gait variables. Although eight significant gait parameters were identified, three of these—cadence, anterior pelvic tilt in stance, and ankle dorsiflexion in swing—are sufficient to establish the stage of progression with 91% accuracy. I found that quadriceps insufficiency, which necessitates maintenance of the body weight force line in front of knee center during single limb support, is the key functional deficit. When this degree of impairment is present, the patient has already progressed into the transitional stage. The application of long leg braces during the transitional or late stages can prolong ambulation, but there can be problems in patient compliance if the bracing is attempted before the child and parents are convinced of the need.

One representative subject will serve to illustrate the adaptive changes in posture necessitated by progressive muscle weakness. Tracings have been made of movie film taken from front and side cameras. The force line, derived from force-plate measurements, has been superimposed over sagittal tracings during single-limb stance (Fig. 1). Figure 1, *top left* and *top right*, is early stage at 5 years of age. Figure 1, *center left* and *center right*, is transitional stage at age 7 years 6 months, and Figure 1, *bottom left* and *bottom right*, is late stage at age 8 years 2 months. Notice that the force line becomes more vertical with increasing impairment, and hip and knee joint centers are brought closer to the force line. This example illustrates the use of gait analysis to characterize the pathomechanics and natural history of a specific disease.

Comparison of Treatment Results in Cerebral Palsy

One of the most important functions of gait analysis is to compare the outcome of various treatment methods and surgical procedures that are in use. Development of this function has been slowed by significant problems in standardization of measurements and in selecting patients with cerebral palsy who have reasonably similar function. Collaborative studies are underway in a number of centers, and it has been demonstrated that some gait measurements, specifically sagittal plane measurements of normal subjects, are

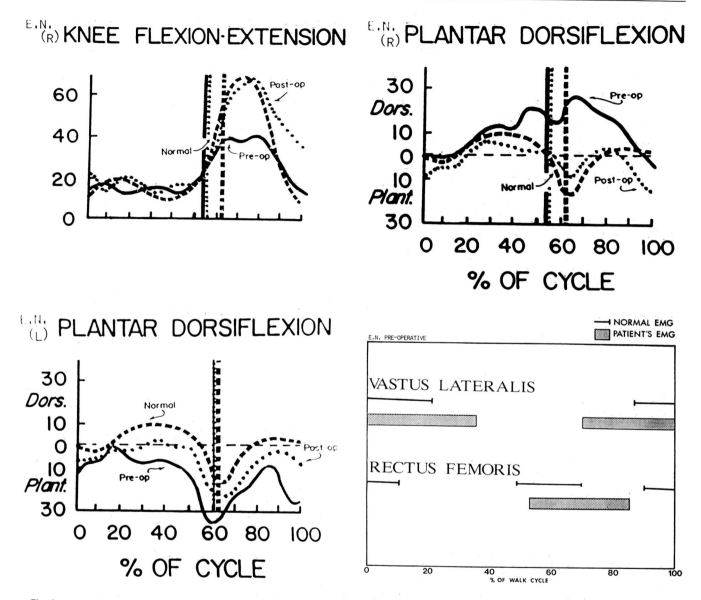

Fig. 4 **Top left,** Shows the measurement of knee flexion-extension. Peak swing-phase flexion of 40 degrees occurs at approximately 80% of the gait cycle. **Top right,** Right plantar-dorsiflexion graph shows exaggerated dorsiflexion in stance with absence of any plantar flexion at toe-off. **Bottom left,** Left plantar-dorsiflexion of patient shows equinus in stance phase with excessive plantar flexion at toe-off. This abnormal movement of the contralateral ankle was considered to be a compensatory vaulting to aid in clearance of the right foot in swing phase. **Bottom right,** Dynamic electromyography of the vastus lateralis shows premature onset in swing phase and stance prolongation. The rectus femoris shows prolongation into swing phase.

quite comparable.[3] This comparison was made by having the same individuals walk in each of the cooperating gait laboratories. The similarity of sagittal measurements taken in the various laboratories opens the possibility of future prospective randomized clinical studies comparing different treatment techniques. The following example compares two surgical methods used to treat stiff-knee gait in cerebral palsy. Although the study was neither prospective nor randomized, it combined the experience of two institutions using the same

measurement technique. The subjects underwent gait studies before and after one of two procedures—proximal rectus release (No. = 14) and distal rectus transfer (No. = 16). The study confirmed the effectiveness of both proximal release and distal transfer of the rectus femoris in relieving stiff-knee gait (D.H. Sutherland, M. Santi, and M.F. Abel, unpublished data). Improvements in maximum knee flexion in swing phase, dynamic range of knee motion, and earlier peak flexion in swing were statistically significant in the rectus transfer

Table 2
Time and distance data for Case 2

Data	Preoperative Right	Postoperative Right	Preoperative Left	Postoperative Left
Opposite toe-off (% cycle)	8	7	9	8
Opposite foot strike (% cycle)	47	49	55	53
Single stance (% cycle)	38	42	46	45
Toe-off (% cycle)	54	53	61	61
Step length (cm)	31	36	40	43
Stride length (cm)	72	78	72	78
Cycle time (sec)	0.66	0.96	0.66	0.96
Cadence (steps/min)	183	136	183	136
Walking velocity (cm/sec)	109	91	109	91

group. Maximum knee flexion in swing and dynamic range of movement were significantly improved in the proximal rectus release group. There was a trend favoring the transfers over proximal release.

Case Studies

Case 1

The patient in this case was an Asian-American boy who contracted polio at the age of 15 months while living in Southeast Asia. Examination showed him to be an independent ambulator with a significant weakness in the right lower extremity and a contracture of the right iliotibial band. In addition to the hip abduction contracture, there was a right knee flexion contracture of 20 degrees. Iliopsoas strength was rated 3, gluteus maximus 4−, quadriceps 1, medial and lateral hamstrings 4+, tibialis anterior 3, extensor hallucis longus 4, extensor digitorum longus 4, peroneals 4, and gastrocsoleus 4.

Film tracings of front and side views (Fig. 2, *left*) graphically depict the movement abnormalities produced by a fixed abduction contracture. Leg-length inequality produced excessive vertical oscillation of the trunk. The side view shows forward lean of the trunk during single-limb stance. This trunk lean was required to stabilize the knee. Treatment was sought to correct the right abduction contracture and stabilize the right knee. The surgery selected was release of the right iliotibial band at the hip and knee and transfer of the semitendinosus and semimembranosus to the patella.

The patient returned for gait assessment nine months after the surgery. Tracings of film from the front and right side cameras (Fig. 2, *right*) show improved trunk and hip alignment and a smoother gait pattern. Improvements are also shown in the joint angles and in the postoperative dynamic electromyelogram of the patient as compared with the preoperative findings (Fig. 3). Measurement of time and distance parameters showed that stride length increased from 68 cm to 93 cm and velocity increased from 76 cm/sec to 100 cm/

sec after surgery (Table 1). The conclusion, based on objective criteria, was that the goals of surgery were reached and the surgery was successful.

Case 2

The patient in this case was a boy, 5 years 7 months old, with cerebral palsy, referred for study of right-sided stiff-knee gait. He was an independent walker. Previous surgery included bilateral distal hamstring lengthenings and lengthening of the right Achilles tendon.

Examination revealed a positive rectus test on the right side. The remaining range-of-motion tests showed no evidence of other muscle contractures. The patient's gait was asymmetric, characterized by circumduction of the right hip and impaired flexion of the right knee in swing phase. The functional deficit was determined to be right-sided stiff-knee gait interfering with foot clearance. Compensatory vaulting on the opposite side was required to clear the foot. The treatment goals were to restore swing-phase knee flexion to facilitate foot clearance.

The options for surgical treatment of rectus spasticity include proximal release,[4] distal release, and distal transfer.[5,6] The surgeon elected to carry out distal rectus release.

Gait assessment carried out one year after the surgery showed that knee flexion-extension was now normal, with peak flexion of nearly 70 degrees occurring early in swing phase. This represents an improvement of nearly 30 degrees in knee flexion (Fig. 4, *top left*). The excessive dorsiflexion of the right ankle was completely corrected (Fig. 4, *top right*). The compensatory vaulting in the left ankle was improved (Fig. 4, *bottom left*). This is an example of correction of a compensatory movement by elimination of the primary gait deficit, right-sided stiff-knee gait. Vaulting is no longer required for foot clearance.

Table 2 shows improvement in stride length, reduction in cadence, and a slight reduction in velocity. Preoperative cadence was abnormally high, thus the postoperative time and distance parameters represent a

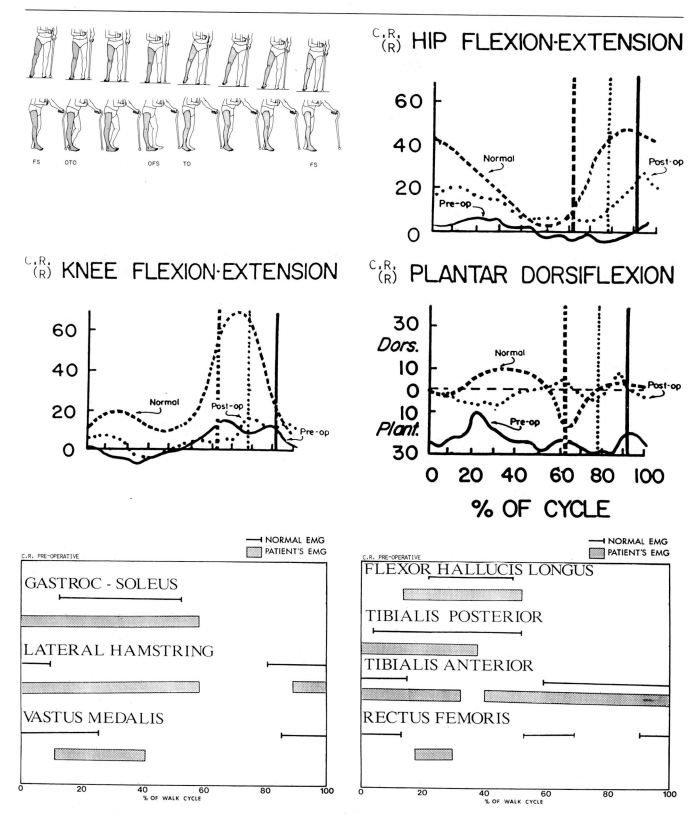

Fig. 5 **Top left,** Front and side film tracings before surgery. **Top right,** Hip flexion-extension preoperative data compared with data after surgery. **Center left,** Knee flexion-extension. Preoperative data compared with postoperative data. **Center right,** Ankle plantar flexion-dorsiflexion data. Presurgical data compared with postsurgical data. **Bottom,** Presurgical dynamic electromyographic tracings.

Table 3
Time and distance data for Case 3

Data	Preoperative Right	Postoperative Right	Preoperative Left	Postoperative Left
Opposite toe-off (% cycle)	24	21	50	56
Opposite foot strike (% cycle)	32	27	67	72
Single stance (% cycle)	8	6	17	16
Toe-off (% cycle)	83	77	88	92
Step length (cm)	16	21	14	9
Stride length (cm)	30	30	30	30
Cycle time (sec)	2.80	3.26	2.80	3.26
Cadence (steps/min)	43	37	43	37
Walking velocity				
cm/sec	11	9	11	9
m/min	6	5	6	5

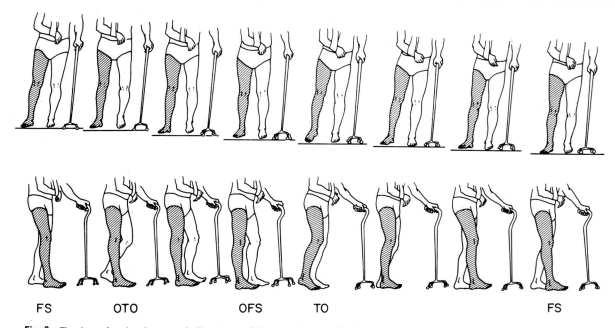

FS   OTO   OFS   TO   FS

Fig. 6   Tracings showing improved alignment of the right foot and ankle.

normalization. Longer follow-up will be necessary to evaluate the permanence of the correction, but at present the knee flexion in swing phase has been corrected to normal. Overall improvement in gait was reflected by a reduction in the abnormally high cadence and an improvement in stride length.

Case 3

The patient in this case was a 57-year-old man who had suffered a head injury in a motorcycle accident ten years before the first gait study. The accident left him with a right-sided spastic hemiparesis necessitating the use of a polypropylene ankle-foot orthosis. His right arm was an impediment, particularly if unrestrained, and he found it necessary to support the arm in a sling.

He walked with great difficulty, stabilizing precariously with a cane in the left hand. Voluntary muscle control on the right side was very poor. An equinovarus deformity was present with dorsiflexion limited to −15 degrees.

Tracings from front and right-side cameras graphically depict right equinovarus instability and limited walking ability (Fig. 5, *top left*).

Sagittal-plane joint-angle measurements of the right hip, knee, and ankle joints permitted analysis of the severe impairment of movement (Fig. 5, *top right, center left,* and *center right*). The hip remained fully extended throughout the entire walk cycle with a dynamic range of no more than 10 degrees (Fig. 5, *top right*). The knee remained in full extension during stance; peak knee flexion during swing was only 15 degrees (Fig. 5, *center left*). The ankle was in plantar flexion throughout the gait cycle, varying between 10 and 30 degrees (Fig. 5, *center right*).

Dynamic electromyography revealed absent swing-phase activity of the rectus femoris, relatively normal activity of the flexor hallucis longus and tibialis posterior, premature onset of the gastrocsoleus, and full-cycle activity of the tibialis anterior (Fig. 5, *bottom*).

The functional deficits were determined to be: (1) a serious balance disorder, (2) stiffness of the knee, not produced by swing-phase activity of the rectus femoris, and (3) equinovarus instability of the right ankle and foot. The treatment goal was limited to improving ankle and foot stability. The surgical treatment selected was split anterior tibial transfer,[7] percutaneous lengthening of the Achilles tendon, tibialis posterior lengthening, and tenotomies of the flexor digitorum longus and flexor hallucis longus.

A gait study was carried out ten months after the surgery. Tracings from right and front cameras show the improved alignment of the right foot and ankle (Fig. 6). The changes in joint angles included some restoration of hip flexion and marked improvement in ankle alignment throughout the gait cycle (Figs. 5, *top right* and *center right*). Knee motion remained unchanged (Fig. 5, *center left*). There was very little change in time and distance parameters (Table 3). There was slight improvement in cadence and velocity.

The postoperative assessment was that there was improvement in stability and that brace wearing was no longer required. There was minimal improvement in walking velocity; nonetheless, the patient was quite satisfied with the outcome.

Acknowledgment

James Moitoza, MD, and J. Michael Casey, MD, treated Patient 3.

References

1. Sutherland DH: *Gait Disorders in Childhood and Adolescence.* Baltimore, Williams & Wilkins, 1984.
2. Sutherland DH, Olshen R, Cooper L, et al: The pathomechanics of gait in Duchenne muscular dystrophy. *Dev Med Child Neurol* 1981;23:3–22.
3. Biden E, Olshen R, Simon S, et al: Comparison of gait data from multiple labs. *Orthop Trans* 1987;11:419.
4. Sutherland DH, Larsen LJ, Mann R: Rectus femoris release in selected patients with cerebral palsy: A preliminary report. *Dev Med Child Neurol* 1975;17:26–34.
5. Perry J: Distal rectus transfer. *Dev Med Child Neurol* 1987;29:153–158.
6. Gage JR, Perry J, Hicks RR, et al: Rectus femoris transfer to improve knee function of children with cerebral palsy. *Dev Med Child Neurol* 1987;29:159–166.
7. Hoffer MM, Reiswig JA, Garrett AM, et al: The split anterior tibial tendon transfer in the treatment of spastic varus hindfoot of childhood. Orthop Clin North Am 1974;5:31–38.

Evaluation of Surgical Procedures and/or Joint Implants With Gait Analysis

Thomas P. Andriacchi, PhD

Introduction

Clinical gait analysis has great potential for evaluating and treating musculoskeletal diseases and injuries.[1-7] To date, quantitative gait analysis has had limited clinical application, and much remains to be learned about functional or gait changes associated with an injury or disease. Although some gait abnormalities are a direct result of a mechanical change brought on by disease or injury, in many cases they represent an adaptation to the pathologic condition.[8-10]

Because some adaptations appear only during locomotion, a functional evaluation must be used to identify and quantify abnormalities. An example of such an adaptation is the characteristic antalgic gait. The stimulus is joint pain; the adaptation is a complex set of movements that, when analyzed, demonstrate reduced load

at the joint. Pathologic stimuli—pain, instability, neuromuscular disability, or muscular weakness—can cause dynamic adaptations. Often, a biomechanical analysis of the adaptation does more than conventional clinical measures to reveal the nature of the underlying abnormality.

Clinical use of gait analysis requires an understanding of the cause and effect of functional adaptations. Proper use of clinical gait analysis is important for planning appropriate treatment and rehabilitation of functionally impaired individuals. These methods can establish the level of disability, aid in diagnosis and treatment planning, allow objective evaluation of treatment, and provide a rationale for modifying treatment on the basis of early functional testing. The goal of the treatment of most musculoskeletal disabilities is to improve function, reduce pain, or both, and a quantitative

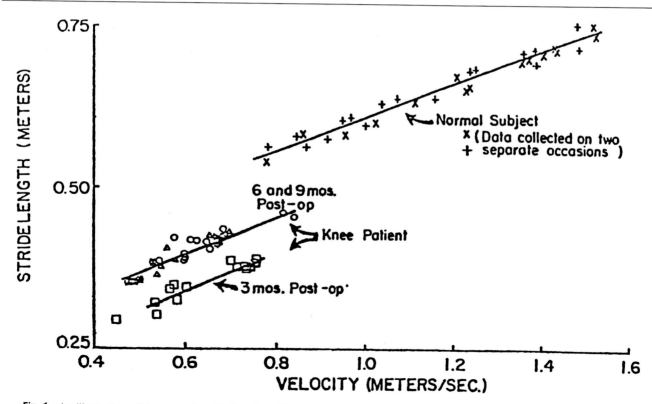

Fig. 1 An illustration of the normal stride length-walking speed relationship in comparison with the measurements taken from a postoperative patient with total knee replacement. (Reproduced with permission from Andriacchi TP, Ogle JA, Galante JO: Walking speed as a basis for normal and abnormal gait measurement. *J Biomech* 1977;10:261–268.)

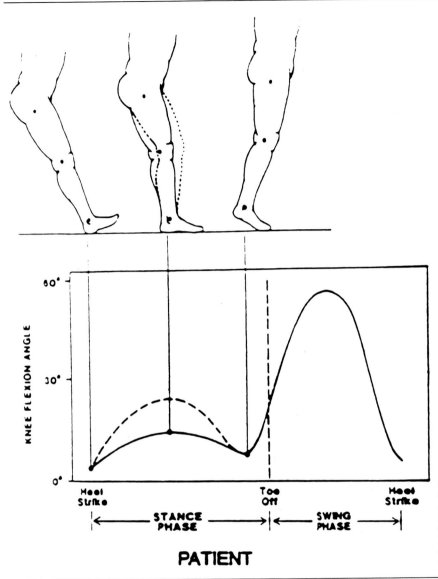

Fig. 2 An illustration of the change in mid-stance knee flexion moment following total knee replacement. (Reproduced with permission from Andriacchi TP, Galante JO, Draganich LF: Relationship between knee extensor mechanics and function following total knee replacement, in Dorr L (ed): Proceedings of the First Annual Meeting of the Knee Society. Baltimore, Maryland, University Park Press, 1985, pp 83–94.)

means of describing the level of disability and the recovery of function should be available to set standards for treatment. This chapter illustrates aspects of our current knowledge of clinical gait analysis, using several examples, and discusses how these methods are used in evaluating and treating individuals with musculoskeletal injuries and disease.

Functional Evaluation of Patients After Total Knee Replacement

Replacement

An analysis of function in patients after total knee replacement illustrates how various parameters are used to evaluate and analyze function. Many parameters can be measured during walking. These gait measures range from fundamental time-and-distance measurements, to motion (kinematics), to joint kinetics.[11,12] The choice of which gait parameters to use depends on the intended application. This example explores the use of three general classes of gait measurements—time-distance, kinematics, and kinetics—and their use in evaluating patients with total knee replacement. Time-distance measurements include measures of stride length, walking speed, and cadence, three important measures of normal and abnormal walking.[7]

Stride length, the distance between consecutive unilateral heel strikes, is a simple and sensitive indicator of walking abnormalities. Stride length varies with walking speed,[1,13,14] and in comparing measurements among individuals with and without walking disabilities, it is important to take differences in walking speed into account. For example, the relationship between stride length and walking speed in normal individuals is relatively linear and reproducible. It has also been shown that recovery of function after surgical reconstructions, such as total knee replacement, can be evaluated by comparing the relationship between stride length and walking speed over a range of walking speeds. Gait evaluations showing that the stride length-walking speed relationship approached normal between three and six months after surgery indicated an improvement in walking ability (Fig. 1). It is important to note that the speeds selected by the patients were substantially slower than normal. Without examining the relationship of stride length to speed, it would have been difficult to compare patients with nonpatients or the patients' abilities at three months with those at six months.

Time-distance parameters are effective in evaluating quantitative changes in the overall characteristics of walking, but they do not provide specific information regarding the cause of the walking abnormality. For example, it has been shown[1] that the stride length-walking speed relationship does not return completely to normal after total knee replacement (Fig. 1). Taking into account differences in walking speed, the patients' stride lengths remain shorter than normal, suggesting that patients with total knee replacement, despite a successful clinical result, do not recover normal function during level walking. The cause of these functional differences cannot be obtained from simple stride-length measurements.

Joint kinematic measurements can help quantify specific joint involvements in walking disability.[2,5,15] In particular, relative segmental angles, which are joint-specific, have been used to quantify changes in patterns of motion and timing related to specific joints. Consider again the example of the gait of patients with total knee replacement. In addition to the shorter-than-normal stride lengths, these patients have reduced knee flexion[2,15] during the midportion of stance phase (Fig. 2). Normal midstance knee flexion is approximately 20 degrees at normal speed. After total knee replacement, patients, despite a pain-free clinical result, tend to walk with less than 10 degrees of midstance knee flexion.

The gait abnormality after total knee reconstruction occurs during the midstance of the gait cycle and involves subtle adaptations that inhibit the midstance knee flexion that normally occurs during the walking cycle. Although kinematic analysis shows where and when the adaptation occurs, at present it cannot explain why it occurs.

Quantification of joint moment during locomotion can aid in identifying the nature and cause of functional abnormality. The moments at the joints provide meaningful measures of function, because the magnitude

PATTERNS OF KNEE FLEXION - EXTENSION MOMENT

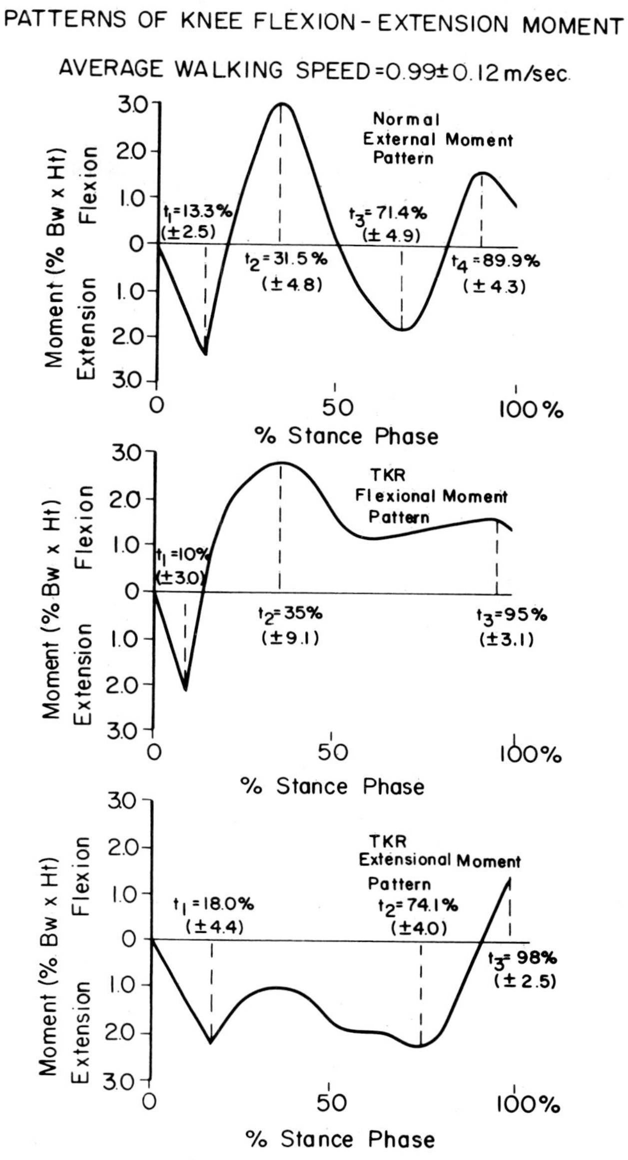

Fig. 3 An illustration of the three patterns of knee moments observed in patients following total knee replacement.[4] (Reproduced with permission from Andriacchi TP, Galante JO, Fermier RW: The influence of total knee-replacement design on walking and stair-climbing. *J Bone Joint Surg* 1982;64A:1328–1335.)

and direction of the components of the joint moment relate to muscular function and joint loading. The normal pattern of flexion-extension at the knee joint (Fig. 3) is biphasic and tends to oscillate about a zero point. In normal gait, duration and magnitude of extreme flexion and extension moments at the knee joint are minimized. More than 75% of patients with knee replacements are reported to have abnormal patterns of flexion-extension moments during stance.[2] The patients tended to deviate from the normal biphasic pattern during midstance (Fig. 3).[4,16] The two abnormal pat-

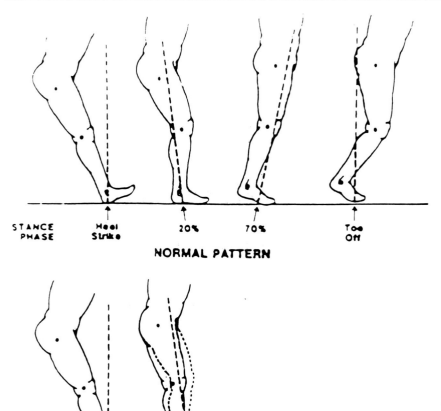

STANCE PHASE   Heel Strike   20%   70%   Toe Off

NORMAL PATTERN

Heel Strike   20%

EXTENSIONAL PATTERN

Fig. 4 An illustration of the mechanism by which the ground-reaction-force vector and the limb position can be used to depict the influence of the moments at the joints. (Reproduced with permission from Andriacchi TP, Galante JO, Draganich LF: Relationship between knee extensor mechanics and function following total knee replacement, in Dorr L (ed): Proceedings of the First Annual Meeting of the Knee Society. Baltimore, Maryland, University Park Press, 1985, pp 83–94.)

terns tended to maintain either joint flexion (flexional moment pattern) or joint extension (extensional moment pattern) throughout stance phase.

A useful way to visualize the joint reaction moment with regard to limb position is to superimpose the ground-reaction-force vector on an image of the leg during walking (Fig. 4). In the normal biphasic flexion-extension moment pattern, the ground-reaction force passes anterior to the knee joint at heel strike, producing an extension moment. At midstance, the ground-reaction-force vector passes posterior to the knee, producing a flexion moment. The cycle then reverses again at approximately 70% of stance, followed by a final reversal just before toe-off. The abnormal gait seen in total knee replacement is associated with a nonoscillatory moment pattern. Typically, after total knee replacement, patients walk either with a pattern that maintains the ground-reaction-force vector anterior to the knee joint (extensional pattern) as illustrated

in Figure 4, or with a pattern that maintains the ground-reaction-force vector posterior to the center of the knee joint (flexional pattern).

The correspondence between the flexion-extension moments and the phasic on-off patterns of the flexor and extensor muscle group suggests that there is abnormal phasing of the extensor muscle group in patients after total knee replacement. As previously noted, these abnormal gait characteristics occur despite pain-free gait and excellent clinical results. It has been suggested[2] that a loss of proprioceptive control alters the patient's ability to control joint position during walking, causing the deviation from normal oscillatory moment patterns. This explanation, although still hypothetical, demonstrates the insight gained by examining joint reaction moments in attempting to interpret abnormal characteristics during locomotion.

In contrast to walking on level ground, function during stair-climbing clearly depends on the design of the

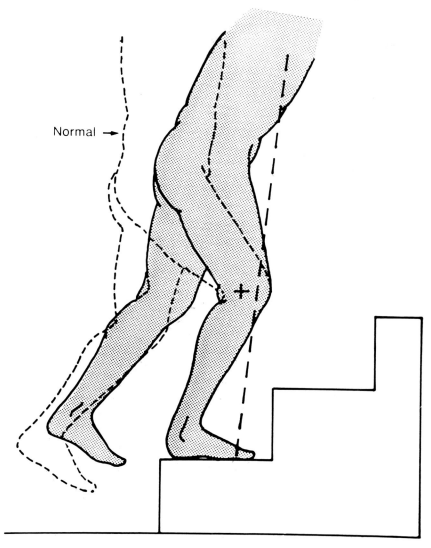

Normal →

Comparison Between Normal and Abnormal Body Positions During Stair Climbing

Fig. 5 The shaded torso represents the configuration of patients climbing up the stairs. By leaning the body forward, the ground-reaction force can be moved anterior to the joint center, reducing or eliminating the moment that tends to flex the joint. This abnormal pattern of stair-climbing was seen in patients with cruciate-sacrificing designs of total knee replacement. (Reproduced with permission from Andriacchi TP, Galante JO, Draganich LF: Relationship between knee extensor mechanics and function following total knee replacement, in Dorr L (ed): Proceedings of the First Annual Meeting of the Knee Society. Baltimore, Maryland, University Park Press, 1985, pp 83–94.)

prosthesis. It has been reported[2] that prosthetic designs that retain the posterior cruciate ligament allow normal function during stair-climbing, while those that remove or attempt to substitute for the posterior cruciate ligament reduce function. These observations suggest that care must be taken to select appropriate tests when attempting to identify abnormal patterns of gait, and that these tests are also useful in determining the causes of functional changes.

Patients with total knee replacement, of whatever design, are characterized by a reduced range of motion while climbing stairs. These functional differences apparently do not stem from a limited passive range of

motion, because close examination has shown that patients in all design groupings had a passive range of motion sufficient to climb stairs (approximately 85 degrees of flexion).

Analysis of the flexion-extension moment during stair-climbing provides a basis for explaining functional differences. Patients and nonpatients who ascended the stairs in a normal manner reached maximum flexion moment during midsupport. This pattern of moment can be visualized by superimposing the ground-reaction-force vector on the limb position during stair-climbing. During normal stair-climbing, the direction of vector passes posterior to the knee, producing a

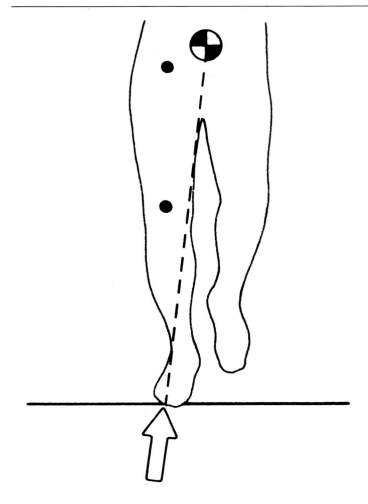

Adduction Moment During Walking

Fig. 6 An illustration of the mechanism that produces the adduction moment during level walking. (Reproduced with permission from Andriacchi TP: Biomechanics of gait analysis in total knee replacement. *Orthop Rev* 1988;5:470–473.)

maximum moment that occurs between 60 and 70 degrees of knee flexion. This flexion moment requires a large quadriceps muscle force for ascending stairs. In the abnormal pattern of stair climbing (Fig. 5), the body tilts forward from the normal position, which moves the line of action and the ground-reaction-force vector anterior to the knee joint, effectively minimizing the demand for extensor force.

Functional Evaluation in High Tibial Osteotomy

An analysis of function in patients with varus gonarthrosis provides an example in which dynamic adaptation to the abnormality can be beneficial when used in conjunction with an osteotomy. The high tibial osteotomy reduces the stress on the medial compartment associated with a varus deformity. High level of medial compartment stress is, in theory, responsible for the symptoms and also accelerates the degenerative process. The high tibial osteotomy is relatively attractive for the younger patient, because it is more conservative than such treatment modalities as total joint arthroplasty. The results, however, have been somewhat variable and unpredictable. It has been assumed that the amount of stress on the medial compartment is proportional to the degree of varus deformity measured on standing radiographs.[17–19] Recent studies[17] have suggested that static varus malalignment may be less significant than the dynamic loads during walking.

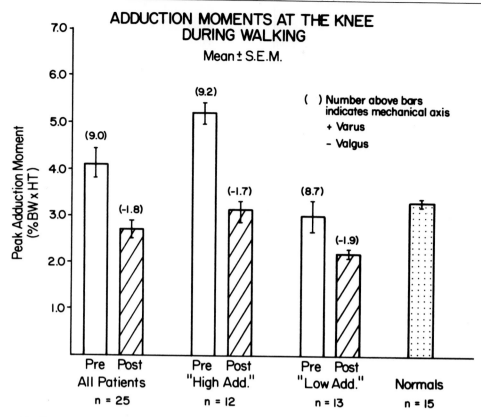

Fig. 7   The relative magnitudes of the adduction moments before and after high tibial osteotomy. (Reproduced with permission from Prodromos CC, Andriacchi TP, Galante JO: A relationship between gait and clinical changes following high tibial osteotomy. *J Bone Joint Surg* 1985;67A:1188–1194.)

This observation was based on a study of patients tested in the gait laboratory before treatment and at yearly intervals after treatment.[17] The investigation, which focused on the dynamic peak adduction moment at the knee (Fig. 6), studied the relationship between the adduction moment and the stress on the medial side of the knee. From static analysis one would expect patients with a large varus deformity to have an adduction moment higher than normal and, thus, more stress on the medial compartment. However, preoperative gait analysis indicated that only about one half of the patients had an adduction moment higher than normal (group 1) during walking, while in the remainder the adduction moment was slightly less than normal despite the varus deformity at the knee joint.

At one year after surgery, the varus deformity was corrected in all patients. Similarly, the adduction moment was reduced in all patients (Fig. 7). Patients originally assigned to group 1 still had a higher adduction moment than the patients in group 2. Patients originally assigned to group 2 now had an even lower adduction moment than that found in normal healthy subjects. Group 2 also had better clinical results than did group

1. Using the Hospital for Special Surgery Knee Rating Form, group 2 had an average clinical score of 92 out of a possible 100, while group 1 scored only 70, a statistically significant difference. In addition, the varus deformity recurred in some patients in group 1.

The results of this analysis suggest that preoperative peak adduction moments during walking can be used to predict the clinical results of surgery. This finding suggests that some patients used dynamic adaptation to reduce the peak adduction moment on the knee with the varus deformity. If this dynamic compensation does not take place, the varus deformity increases the adduction moment and the resulting force on the medial compartment of the knee. The mechanism of dynamic compensation continues after the varus deformity is surgically realigned, because patients with a lower adduction moment before surgery also have a lower adduction moment afterward. It may be that proprioception, subconscious pain, or some other neural control mechanism triggers this compensatory unloading gait in some patients but not in others. The dynamic factors associated with walking appear to be more critical than static alignment measured radiographically.

References

1. Andriacchi TP, Ogle JA, Galante JO: Walking speed as a basis for normal and abnormal gait measurements. *J Biomech* 1977; 10:261–268.
2. Andriacchi TP, Galante JO, Fermier RW: The influence of total knee-replacement design on walking and stair-climbing. *J Bone Joint Surg* 1982;64A:1328–1335.
3. Andriacchi TP, Kramer GM, Landon GC: The biomechanics of running and knee injuries, in Finerman G (ed): American Academy of Orthopaedic Surgeons *Symposium on Sports Medicine: The Knee.* St. Louis, CV Mosby, 1985, pp 23–32.
4. Andriacchi TP, Strickland AB: Gait analysis as a tool to assess joint kinetics, in Berme N, Engin AE, Correia Da Silva KM (eds): *Biomechanics of Normal and Pathological Human Articulating Joints: NATO Advanced Science Series. Series E: Applied Sciences, No 93.* Dordrecht, Martinus Nijhoff, 1985, pp 83–102.
5. Chao EY, Laughman RK, Stauffer RN: Biomechanical gait evaluation of pre and postoperative total knee replacement patients. *Arch Orthop Trauma Surg* 1980;97:309–317.
6. Elftman H: Forces and energy changes in the leg during walking. *Am J Physiol* 1939;125:339–356.
7. Perry J: Clinical gait analyzer. *Bull Prosthet Res* 1974;74:188–192.
8. Murray MP, Drought AB, Kory RC: Walking patterns of normal men. *J Bone Joint Surg* 1964;46A:335–360.
9. Murray MP, Brewer BJ, Zuege RC: Kinesiologic measurements of functional performance before and after McKee-Farrar total hip replacement: A study of thirty patients with rheumatoid arthritis, osteoarthritis, or avascular necrosis of the femoral head. *J Bone Joint Surg* 1972;54A:237–256.
10. Prodromos CC, Andriacchi TP, Galante JO: A relationship between gait and clinical changes following high tibial osteotomy. *J Bone Joint Surg* 1985;67A:1188–1194.
11. Bresler B, Frankel JP: The forces and moments in the leg during level walking. *Trans Am Soc Mech Eng* 1953;48A:62.
12. Cappozzo A, Figura F, Marchetti M: The interplay of muscular and external forces in human ambulation. *J Biomech* 1976;9:35–43.
13. Grieve DW: Gait patterns and the speed of walking. *Biomed Engin* 1968;3:119–122.
14. Lamoreux LW: Kinematic measurements in the study of human walking. *Bull Prosthet Res* 1971;10:3–84.
15. Rittman N, Kettelkamp DB, Pryor P, et al: Analysis of patterns of knee motion walking for four types of total knee implants. *Clin Orthop* 1981;155:111–117.
16. Simon SR, Trieshmann HW, Burdett RG, et al: Quantitative gait analysis after total knee arthroplasty for monarticular degenerative arthritis. *J Bone Joint Surg* 1983;65A:605–613.
17. Insall JN, Joseph DM, Msika C: High tibial osteotomy for varus gonarthrosis: A long-term follow-up study. *J Bone Joint Surg* 1984;66A:1040–1048.
18. Kettelkamp DB, Johnson RJ, Smidt GL, et al: An electrogoniometric study of knee motion in normal gait. *J Bone Joint Surg* 1970;52B:775–790.
19. Maquet P: The biomechanics of the knee and surgical possibilities of healing osteoarthritic knee joints. *Clin Orthop* 1980;146:102–110.

Amputation and Prosthetic Management of the Lower Limb

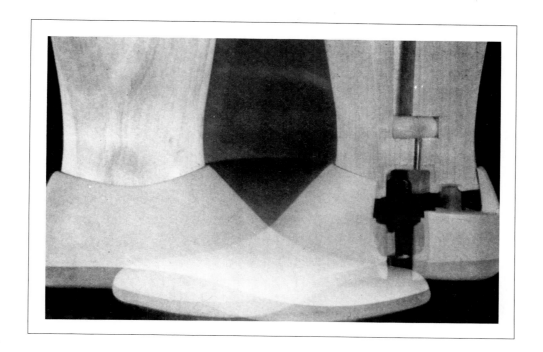

The Orthopaedist as Prosthetic Team Leader: Getting the Best for Your Patient From the Team

Bertram Goldberg, MD

Introduction

The magnitude of the task of treating amputees is considerable. It is estimated that there are at least 300,000 amputees in the United States,[1] with approximately 58% of cases secondary to peripheral vascular disease and 33.2% secondary to trauma. A study by Holbrook and associates[2] estimated that 2.5% of nursing home patients at any one time were amputees, whose care costs almost $289 million per year. Kostuik and Gillespie,[3] in a thorough study of the Canadian amputee population, found that the primary amputation rate in the population is about 0.16 per thousand, with vascular disease being the most common cause. Congenital defects, the most common cause of amputations in children, pose additional and unique problems for the pediatric orthopaedic surgeon.[4]

The care of the amputee, whether juvenile or adult, is an ongoing process. It begins with the first meeting between patient and physician and continues through the performance of the amputation to prescribing and fitting the prosthesis and subsequent prosthetic training. In addition to the patient, a closely knit and coordinated group of people, the amputee clinic team, is involved. The word "team" must be emphasized, because no single individual has the wide range of knowledge and expertise needed to provide complete care for the patient. However, like any team, the amputee clinic team must have a leader, and the orthopaedic surgeon, an individual schooled not only in the performance of the surgical procedure, but also in the biomechanics of the human body before and after the amputation, is uniquely qualified to carry out that role.

History

Amputations were mentioned in the fifth century BC by Hippocrates in his treatise, *On Joints.*[5] Artificial limbs for the upper and lower extremities were first described by Paré in 1575.[5] The care of the amputee, however, really came of age in the middle of this century when the large numbers of amputees among soldiers wounded during World War II made it apparent that some sort of directed approach was needed to treat these amputees and to deal with the problems they faced. At that time, Norman T. Kirk, who was Surgeon General of the Army, established amputee clinics in major army medical centers. Directed by orthopaedic surgeons, these clinics gave rise to the team concept as we know it.

The clinic team approach was refined by the Veterans Administration in 1948, after the introduction of the suction socket above-knee prosthesis. This led to the formation of clinics at the University of California at Berkeley, at Northwestern University, and at New York University for the care of the amputee and for basic research. The clinic team concept next moved into the area of care for the pediatric and juvenile amputee, and centers started in Florida under the direction of McCollough,[6] and in Michigan at the Mary Free Bed Rehabilitation Center directed by Frantz and Aitken.

Specific Amputee Considerations

The clinic team approach is unique in that it provides, in one setting, a method for evaluating the total milieu of the amputee, at the same time taking into consideration unique problems that each amputee may have. The dysvascular diabetic amputee, if a prosthetic candidate, will have energy expenditures that might make the prolonged use of a prosthesis unrealistic.[7] For this reason, if patients are to be considered by the clinic team for a primary amputation or revision of an existing amputation, their vascular and nutritional status must be determined.[8] In fact, prescribing a prosthesis for the dysvascular amputee can be totally unrealistic. It has been stated that "the goal for dysvascular bilateral above-the-knee amputees is wheelchair ambulation."[9]

The pediatric amputee population also requires the knowledge and expertise of people aware of their unique problems, one of the most significant being stump overgrowth and how to treat it. And, in addition to their medical and surgical problems, their psychological problems and those of their parents are also important and must be dealt with. The clinic team can be of great help in this situation.

Other special situations that the team may face and in which they can provide direction include the care of phantom-limb symptoms, fractures in limb stumps, and total joint replacements in joints proximal to amputated parts.

Prosthetic Considerations

In addition to systemic factors, the amputee clinic team must also consider the amputation itself and its potential prosthesis. What will be the length of the residual limb? Will it pose a problem in fitting and/or suspension? Will the skin covering the limb be able to bear the pressure that the prosthesis will transmit, or are neuromas present that will defeat any fitting that may be attempted? How will the amputee power the upper-extremity prosthesis and terminal device, and will an alternate source of power be necessary? Can the limb use standard suspension systems or will alternate systems be necessary? What type of foot-ankle assembly will be of greatest benefit, the standard solid ankle, cushion heel foot, the multiaxis foot, or one of the newer stored-energy feet? And lastly, will the amputee be able to carry the weight of the prosthesis or will newer space-age materials be needed? All of the above are questions that the amputee clinic team can address in an efficient and professional manner.

Amputee Clinic Team

The makeup of the clinic team obviously can vary from situation to situation, but since its inception it has evolved into a more or less specific group of persons, each of whom provides knowledge and suggestions in order to get the best for and out of each patient.

The patient, around whom the entire concept functions, must always be treated professionally and caringly and, without question, should be considered an integral part of the decision-making process. The patient should never be made to feel secondary to any discussion that may be going on about the amputated limb or its potential prosthesis.

The orthopaedic surgeon, by virtue of training, is well suited to be the chief and director of the clinic team, the person to whom the patient and other team members can look for direction and final decision-making. But, the orthopaedist should not be autocratic and should take into full consideration the recommendations of all team members.

Other members of the team[10] include the prosthetist, ideally a graduate of an accredited university-based prosthetic program, who can offer advice and educate all the members of the team and the patient on potentially beneficial developments. The physical therapist provides invaluable assistance by working with the patient in a total rehabilitation program, before and after surgery and after prosthetic fitting. The occupational therapist does the same, working particularly with the upper-extremity amputee in the workplace to effect a return to gainful employment. The nurse assists the amputee with stump care and provides other services for inpatient or outpatient care. The vocational counselor, like the occupational therapist mentioned above, assists the amputee in returning to work or arranges retraining for some other occupation. The social worker helps the amputee and family by providing information regarding funding and home transition and by contacting other agencies that can help promote the amputee's well-being. Finally, the secretary keeps records of the patient's history and progress through the clinic and sees that all appointments are made when necessary.

In order for the team to work together smoothly and efficiently, an overall plan must be in effect. Clinic teams vary from institution to institution and so do the methods by which they operate. A plan developed at New York University has proven to work well. The procedure includes a preprosthetic examination, at which one or more of the team members may be present, followed by the writing of the prosthetic prescription, prefitting treatment, prosthetic fabrication, initial evaluation, prosthetic training, final evaluation, and follow-up. At any of the above steps, one or more or all of the members may be present, but at some point in the process each plays an important part.

Summary

In summary, care of the amputee is an ongoing process, from evaluation and treatment of the initial disease or traumatic event, through fabrication and fitting of the prosthesis, to the amputee's return to as normal a lifestyle as possible. It is a process that has evolved over the years into a distinct approach designed to get the best for the patient from the team.

References

1. Glattly HW: A statistical study of 12,000 new amputees. *South Med J* 1964;57:1373–1378.
2. Holbrook TL, Grazier K, Kelsey JL, et al: *The Frequency of Occurrence, Impact and Cost of Selected Musculoskeletal Conditions in the United States.* Park Ridge, Illinois, American Academy of Orthopaedic Surgeons, 1984.
3. Kostuik JP, Gillespie R (eds): *Amputation Surgery and Rehabilitation: The Toronto Experience.* New York, Churchill Livingstone, 1981.
4. Krebs DE, Fishman S: Characteristics of the child amputee population. *J Pediatr Orthop* 1984;4:89–95.
5. Vasconcelos E, Kirk NT: *Modern Methods of Amputation.* New York, Philosophical Library, 1945.
6. McCollough N: Conception, birth, infancy and adolescence of the juvenile amputee program in North America. *J Assoc Child Prosthet-Orthot Clin* 1988;23:50–56.
7. Waters RL, Perry J, Antonelli D, et al: Energy cost of walking of amputees: The influence of level of amputation. *J Bone Joint Surg* 1976;58A;42–46.
8. Pinzur M, Kaminsky M, Sage R, et al: Amputations at the middle level of the foot: A retrospective and prospective review. *J Bone Joint Surg* 1986;68A:1061–1064.
9. Volpicelli LJ, Chambers RB, Wagner FW Jr: Ambulation levels of bilateral lower-extremity amputees: Analysis of one hundred and three cases. *J Bone Joint Surg* 1983;65A:599–605.
10. Thompson RG, Kramer S: The amputee clinic team, in American Academy of Orthopaedic Surgeons *Atlas of Limb Prosthetics: Surgical and Prosthetic Principles.* St. Louis, CV Mosby, 1981, pp 63–66.

Surgical Techniques for Conserving Tissue and Function in Lower-Limb Amputation for Trauma, Infection, and Vascular Disease

John H. Bowker, MD

Introduction

In lower-limb amputation, the primary objective of the surgeon is to create a residual limb that will interface comfortably with a prosthesis and provide the most efficient gait possible. The realization of that goal has been made more complex by the rapid evolution in prosthetic design seen in the past decade. Creative prosthetists and engineers, spurred by patients desirous of an active, even athletic, life-style, have developed an array of new functional designs. These are based on thermosetting plastics; improved reinforcing materials, such as carbon fiber; and lighter metals, such as titanium.[1]

Definition of a Good Amputation

Good amputation surgery includes the conservation of all tissue commensurate with the diagnosis. Certainly, amputation must be done above the level of a tumor, gangrenous tissue, or an irreparable body part, but once these basic requirements have been met, an effort should be made to save maximum length to enhance future prosthetic usage.

The next consideration is the creation of an adequate soft-tissue envelope that will move easily over the bone and absorb the shear forces at the limb-socket interface. The ideal soft-tissue envelope is formed of skin, sub-

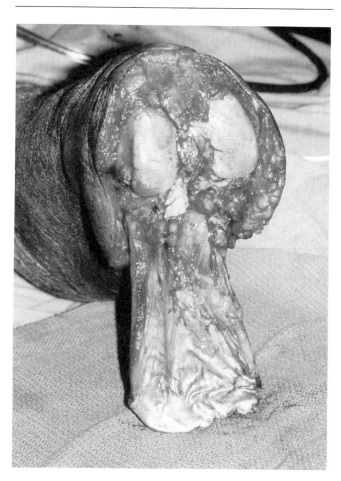

Fig. 1 Progressive closure of through-knee amputation illustrating tenodesis of quadriceps tendon to cruciate ligaments.

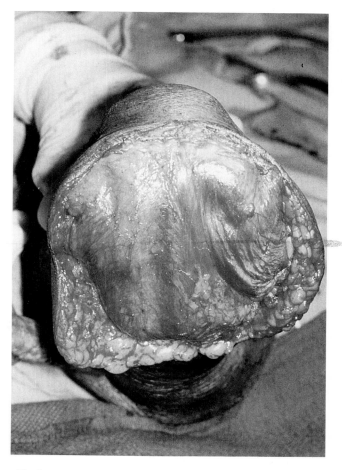

Fig. 2 Further closure of wound in Figure 1 showing myodesis of gastrocnemius muscle to quadriceps retinaculum to prevent adherence of skin flaps to femoral condyles.

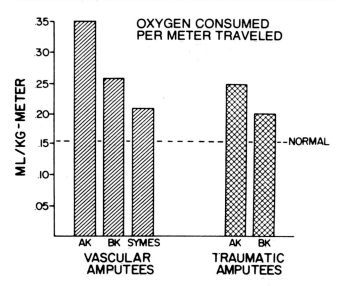

Fig. 3 Energy cost per meter walked in dysvascular and traumatic amputees at selected amputation levels compared to normal. (Reproduced with permission from Waters RL, Perry J, Antonelli D, et al: Energy cost of walking of amputees: The influence of level of amputation. *J Bone Joint Surg* 1976;58A:42–46.)

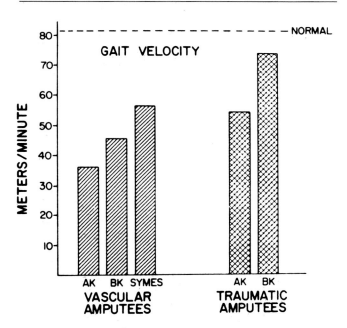

Fig. 4 Gait velocity for dysvascular and traumatic amputees at selected amputation levels, compared to normal. (Reproduced with permission from Waters RL, Perry J, Antonelli D, et al: Energy cost of walking of amputees: The influence of level of amputation. *J Bone Joint Surg* 1976;58A:42–46.)

cutaneous tissue, and investing fascia and muscle, and is well secured by tenodesis, myoplasty, or myodesis (Figs. 1 and 2). If no underlying soft tissue is present,

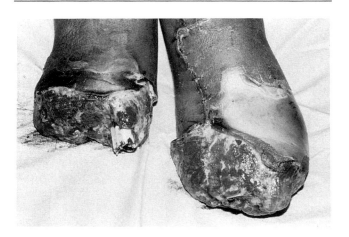

Fig. 5 Bilateral traumatic below-knee amputations after several days of skin traction. Note large areas of skin necrosis that were not originally present.

the skin will adhere directly to the bone. Resultant ulceration and interruptions in prosthetic wear can then be anticipated. Proper shaping of the cut shaft of the bone is also important. If the bone end has sharp edges, the soft-tissue envelope can be damaged from within as the bone compresses the soft tissues between itself and the hard prosthetic socket.

Another aspect of a good amputation is retention of a full range of motion of residual joints. This begins at surgery with proper muscle tensioning during myoplasty or myodesis and continues with short-term rigid immobilization of joints during the painful postoperative phase.[2,3] Thereafter, active range-of-motion exercises will prevent contracture. On occasion, a very short trans-segmental amputation is associated with severe, noncorrectable loss of joint muscle motion resulting in a nonfunctional residual limb. In this situation, disarticulation at the next higher level should be considered.

Advantages of Tissue-Conserving Amputations

A residual limb in which maximum tissue has been conserved has several advantages. A number of studies have proven the inverse relationship between length of the residual limb and energy consumption and the direct relationship between length and gait velocity and cadence.[4,5] Expressed another way, the oxygen consumed per meter walked increases as the level of amputation rises, while the gait velocity and cadence decrease (Figs. 3 and 4). A longer residual limb requires less excess energy. This results in less cardiopulmonary stress, an important factor when dealing with dysvascular individuals.

With a longer limb segment, a more even distribution

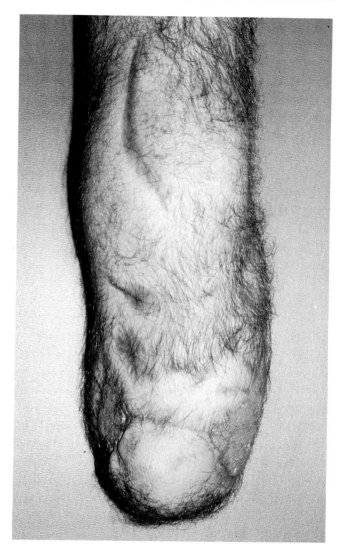

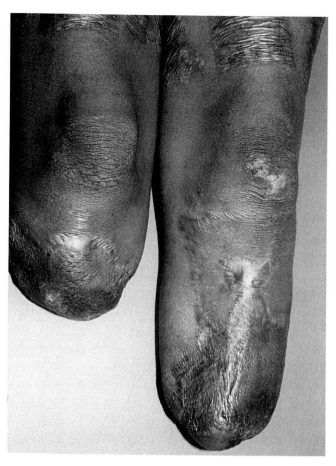

Fig. 7 Bilateral below-knee amputations nine months after split-thickness skin grafting. (Same patient shown in Figure 5). Grafts are well incorporated and have now matured to allow fitting with below-knee prostheses with thigh corsets and knee joints to minimize weight-bearing stress through patella-tendon bearing sockets.

Fig. 6 Traumatic below-knee amputation illustrating delayed closure with a posterior skin flap originally ankle-length. It covers the tibia in areas of greatest prosthetic stress. Coverage medially and laterally is with split-thickness skin graft.

Specific Tissue Conservation Techniques

of weightbearing forces is allowed over the broader residual limb-socket interface. This becomes important with the development of new socket designs in which total surface bearing replaces patellar-tendon and ischial weightbearing.[6,7] Joint contractures are also less likely with longer limb segments. For example, knee-joint contracture is extremely rare after Syme's amputation, whereas it is quite common in short below-knee amputations. Amputations that preserve greater residual limb length also result in less alteration of body image. Not only are the mutilating effects of amputation less evident, but the amputee has a better opportunity to mask the loss and its accompanying impairment through achievement of a more normal gait pattern.

In a trauma case requiring amputation, it is mandatory that all tissues, soft and bony, be carefully evaluated for their possible use in secondary reconstruction. This approach is preferred to guillotine amputation, in which considerable additional bone shortening is required to effect wound closure. Meticulous cleansing and debridement of the wound are of primary importance, both to prevent infection and to determine the viability of the muscle and skin that will form the soft-tissue envelope for the bony residuum. Electric stimulation of muscle helps determine what tissue is viable, and evaluation of capillary refill will help to determine the level of skin viability. All wounds should be left open to facilitate secondary debridement, if needed, and to minimize the risk of abscess and resultant tissue necrosis. All viable soft tissue should be retained, but allowed to contract. This approach is pref-

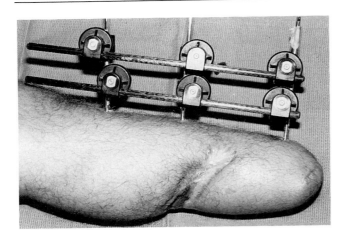

Fig. 8 Comminuted tibia fracture treated by external fixation. Patient initially had open ankle disarticulation. Delayed skin closure combined with conversion to a long below-knee amputation preserved maximum limb length. External fixation facilitated fracture management.

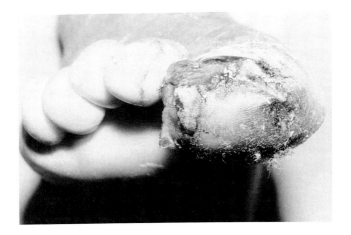

Fig. 9 A 49-year-old diabetic with necrosis of great toe and adequate web-space Doppler pressures.

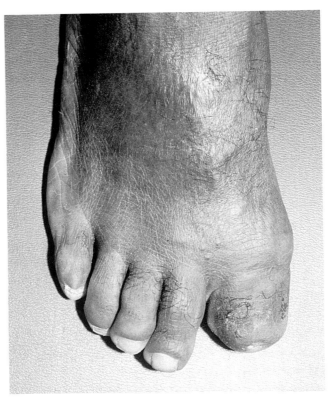

Fig. 10 Same case shown in Figure 9 showing interphalangeal joint amputation resulting from conservative debridement and closure over Kritter irrigation system.

erable to the use of skin traction, which can compromise the viability of already traumatized skin by applying uncontrolled shear forces on blood vessels that supply the skin (Fig. 5).

Reconstruction following trauma can be accomplished by using flaps of muscle and skin in a variety of ways. The only major requirement is that sufficient soft tissue covers those portions of the bone that take a significant amount of direct pressure as they support body weight or move the prosthesis. For example, if there is sufficient muscle to cover the bone, but not enough skin to cover the entire residual limb, the available skin should be used to cover the crucial areas, and split-thickness skin graft used to provide the remaining

coverage (Fig. 6). If no skin is available to cover any of the muscle, split-thickness skin graft can be used alone, and the weightbearing pressures are decreased by prosthetic alterations. In the case of a below-knee amputation, this would be a thigh corset and joints (Fig. 7).

In segmental shaft fracture, a significant distal bone fragment should be saved if there is sufficient soft-tissue coverage available. This may be accomplished by judicious use of internal or external fixation devices, thereby avoiding amputation through the more proximal fracture. Minor changes in position of the external fixator will allow easy closure (Fig. 8).

Infection and Dysvascularity

The majority of lower-limb amputations are done as a result of limb infection and/or vascular impairment in persons with diabetes mellitus (J.H. Bowker, unpublished data). These patients manifest both atheromatous disease, which obstructs arteries, and small vessel disease, which impairs capillary perfusion of the oxygen, leukocytes, and antibiotics needed to combat infection and promote wound healing.[8] To conserve residual limb tissue without putting the patient at unreasonable risk of reamputation, limb circulation should be assessed, especially if ablation at the foot or

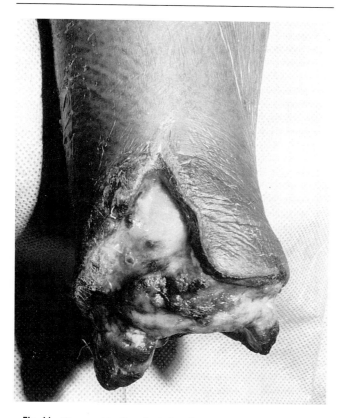

Fig. 11 Open ankle disarticulation for severe diabetic infection of entire foot. Note debridement of necrotic skin and tendons.

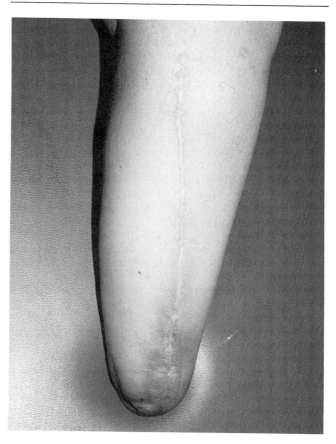

Fig. 12 Lateral view of below-knee limb salvage in case of infection ascending from foot. Complete debridement of lateral and posterior compartments allowed significant preservation of residual limb length. Note long lateral incision used for complete debridement of lateral compartment of leg.

Syme levels is contemplated. Of the numerous techniques described, Doppler evaluation is available to most surgeons. Healing can be reliably expected if the systolic pressure at the desired level of amputation is 50% of brachial pressure and no lower than 70 mm Hg, all pressures being obtained with the patient in the supine position.[9] Evaluation of the proper amputation level, in cases of dry gangrene, can easily be achieved by this method. In cases of wet gangrene, however, determining the best level is more difficult. When the vascular evaluation indicates that a toe or partial foot amputation might be carried out, a careful debridement of necrotic infected tissue often reveals more viable tissue than was anticipated (Figs. 9 and 10). At the other extreme, if a diabetic is very ill from a wet gangrenous foot, an open ankle disarticulation can be carried out with the patient under local anesthesia in a few minutes (Fig. 11). This will allow rapid reversal of the infection, enhance control of diabetic ketoacidosis, and permit later closure at a long below-knee level. This is preferable to freezing procedures for control of severe foot infection, which, despite appropriate insulation, will often cause thermal necrosis of normal calf tissues. If severe foot infection is associated with ascending leg infection, the appropriate compartments can be incised longitudinally, debrided, and packed

open, often preserving considerable tibial length (Fig. 12). After this procedure, the soft tissues can recover from the ascending cellulitis, indicating that it is not mandatory initially to go proximal to all evident cellulitis. The alternative is a short below-knee amputation, if primary closure is the only goal of the amputation surgeon.

In many long-term diabetics, neuropathy results in significant loss of sensation, sometimes to just below the knee level. In my opinion, it is not necessary to amputate insensate, but viable, portions of a limb, because they function very well as long as an adequate prosthetic fit is achieved and maintained.

Summary

Certain factors regarding amputation level, such as the level of traumatic amputation, the position of a malignant tumor in a limb, or the level to which gangrene has progressed, cannot be changed. More important, in this regard, is the attitude of the surgeon toward amputation. This attitude determines the care with which the final level is selected, the manner in which the amputation is performed, and the way in which postoperative management, including prosthetic care, is handled. To achieve the desired long-term result for the amputee, the surgeon should view amputation as a reconstructive procedure rather than a destructive one, should be willing to do staged procedures to preserve potentially functional tissue, should be ready to consider and plan innovative surgical approaches, and should keep abreast of prosthetic advances as they affect surgical technique and postoperative management.

References

1. Michael JW, Gailey RS, Bowker JH: New developments in recreational prostheses and adaptive devices for the amputee. *Clin Orthop*, in press.
2. Burgess EM: General principles of amputation surgery, in American Academy of Orthopaedic Surgeons *Atlas of Limb Prosthetics: Surgical and Prosthetic Principles*. St. Louis, CV Mosby, 1981, pp 14–18.
3. Burgess EM: Postoperative management, in American Academy of Orthopaedic Surgeons *Atlas of Limb Prosthetics: Surgical and Prosthetic Principles*. St. Louis, CV Mosby, 1981, pp 19–23.
4. Waters RL, Perry J, Antonelli D, et al: Energy cost of walking of amputees: The influence of level of amputation. *J Bone Joint Surg* 1976;58A:42–46.
5. Gonzalez EG, Corcoran PJ, Reyes RL: Energy expenditure in below-knee amputees: Correlation with stump length. *Arch Phys Med Rehabil* 1974;55:111–119.
6. Staats TB, Lundt J: The UCLA total surface bearing suction below-knee prosthesis. *Clin Prosthet Orthot* 1987;11:118–130.
7. Redhead RG: Total surface bearing self suspending above-knee sockets. *Prosthet Orthot Int* 1979;3:126–136.
8. Levin ME, O'Neal LW: Peripheral vascular disease, in Ellenberg M, Rifkin H (eds): *Diabetes Mellitus: Theory and Practice*. New Hyde Park, New York, Medical Examination Publishing, 1983, pp 803–828.
9. Wagner FW Jr: Orthopedic rehabilitation of the dysvascular lower limb. *Orthop Clin North Am* 1978;9:325–350.

New Concepts in Lower-Limb Amputation and Prosthetic Management

Michael S. Pinzur, MD

Amputation Level Selection

The metabolic cost of walking is increased and self-selected walking speed decreased with more proximal level amputations[1] (M.S. Pinzur and associates, unpublished data). These factors become critical in the rehabilitation of elderly, dysvascular amputees whose concomitant cardiopulmonary and cerebral vascular diseases limit their metabolic reserves and ultimate rehabilitation potential. To optimize function and independence in this patient population, it is essential to perform amputations at the most distal level feasible in patients with the potential for walking.

The rehabilitation team should take into account the patient's preamputation level of ambulatory function and cardiopulmonary capacity. Volpicelli and associates[2] outlined seven functional levels, ranging from level 0, for patients confined to bed, to level VI, for patients able to move about the community independently. Cognitive, motivational, and psychosocial attributes necessary for a patient to learn how to use a lower-limb prosthesis have been identified through objective psychological testing.[3] When the rehabilitation potential for the prospective amputee has been determined, the next step is to determine the "biologic level," which is the most distal amputation level with a reasonable potential to support wound healing. I have modified Wagner's criteria for the performance of the two-stage Syme's amputation,[4,5] and use the following prerequisites, together with careful clinical examination, in selecting patients to undergo amputations in the foot and ankle. (1) The patient must have the potential for using a prosthesis. (2) The heel pad must be free of open lesions. (3) The ankle-to-arm ratio of systolic blood pressures (ultrasound Doppler ischemic index, ankle-brachial index) must be at least 0.5. (4) There should be no gross pus at the amputation site. (5) There should be no ascending lymphangitis. (6) The serum albumin must be at least 3 g/dl. (7) The total lymphocyte count must be at least 1,500/mm.[3]

If the patient with peripheral vascular insufficiency and gangrene does not meet these criteria, amputation surgery should be performed at the below-knee or through-knee level. In the nonwalker, the surgical morbidity and risk of wound failure is not adequately offset by any functional benefits afforded by distal amputation.[4,6]

Healing of an amputation wound appears to be closely related to the arterial blood flow at the site of amputation. The instrument commonly used to measure segmental blood pressure and flow in the dysvascular limb is the ultrasound Doppler. The techniques of impedance plethysmography,[7] the laser Doppler, and photoplethysmography used by vascular surgeons to evaluate arterial pressure and flow may also be used to select amputation levels.[7,8] Segmental pressures used to predict wound healing for amputation surgery are taken at the dorsalis pedis and posterior tibial arteries for amputations in the foot and ankle, the popliteal for below-knee and through-knee, and femoral for above-knee amputations. Yao and Bergan[9] have shown an increase in the rate of wound healing when the absolute Doppler pressure is 70 mm Hg at the level in question. Wagner[4,5] popularized the use of the ankle-to-arm ultrasound Doppler arterial pressure ratio (ischemic index, ankle-brachial index, or ABI), and states that one can obtain a better than 90% wound-healing rate if the ischemic index is greater than 0.45 in nondiabetics and 0.5 in diabetics. Scintigraphic techniques and fluorescein have also been used,[10,11] with varying degrees of success, but only the segmental Doppler, because of its ease of operation and reproducibility, has gained widespread use.

The Doppler and plethysmographic techniques rely on the measurement of a pressure wave in the wall of the artery, and measure flow as a function of that pressure curve. In patients with atherosclerosis, the vessel walls become less pliant and transmit a pressure wave without corresponding blood flow. In these patients, the pressure measurements are falsely elevated and are not related to the true blood flow. Measurement of transcutaneous oxygen tension at the projected level of amputation may well improve our capacity to understand and predict wound healing by measuring the oxygen-delivering capacity to the skin. Transcutaneous oxygen tension is measured by sealing a small, heated sensor to the surface of the skin at the level of interest, and heating the skin to 44 to 46 C to maximize blood flow. Several investigators[12,13] have shown a high correlation between wound healing and a threshold oxygen tension of between 20 and 30 mm Hg. While not absolute, it may be the first step in understanding wound-healing potential as opposed simply to blood flow in a dysvascular limb. Recent work using transcutaneous carbon dioxide tension in addition to oxygen tension may further our capacity to understand this complex problem.[14]

While vascular inflow is essential for amputation

wound healing, it is only one of several factors that can influence the outcome after an amputation. Dickhaut and associates[15] were able to improve their wound-healing rate with the Syme's two-stage amputation by setting a minimum criteria of 3.5 g/dl for serum albumin as a measure of tissue nutrition, and a total lymphocyte count of 1,500 mm³ as a measure of immunocompetence. I have had similar success in midfoot amputations by following similar guidelines, and, working with patients who initially did not meet the criteria, have achieved these same results by using preoperative oral or, occasionally, parenteral hyperalimentation to raise the patients to the minimum criteria.[16]

Once the biologic levels have been determined, rehabilitation potential must also be assessed before determining the appropriate surgery. Amputations in the foot and ankle should be reserved for those patients who will at least become limited household walkers. If the patient has not walked for a prolonged period of time before amputation, it is generally unrealistic to expect independent walking after surgery.

Ray resections are limited to a single medial or lateral ray that has an infected neurotrophic ulcer. When performed for apparently localized gangrene, there is an unacceptably high rate of wound failure. Excision of more than one ray frequently leaves a very narrow forefoot with an equinus deformity that is difficult to accommodate in a shoe. Central ray resections leave a large wound that must be managed over a long period of time. Neither the narrow forefoot after multiple ray resection nor the foot with a central ray resection outperforms the midfoot amputation.[17] Midfoot amputations performed at the proximal transmetatarsal or tarsometatarsal (Lisfranc) levels allow patients to walk wearing standard oxford shoes. High-topped shoes are rarely necessary. Late equinus deformity after Lisfranc amputation can be prevented by performing a percutaneous Achilles lengthening at the time of amputation. While hind-foot amputees can be fitted with footwear,[18,19] the related difficulties do not warrant recommending these amputations over the two-stage Syme's.[4,5]

Below-knee amputation should be reserved for patients who can reasonably be expected to be walkers.[1,4] Nonambulatory below-knee amputees can develop knee-flexion contractures from prolonged sitting, with the subsequent development of terminal residual limb pressure ulcers from contact with their bed. Because these patients do not require a prosthesis for wheelchair transfer, they are better served with through-knee amputation.[4,6]

The dysvascular below-knee amputee who is predicted to be a minimal walker does not appear to use the extensor power of his quadriceps during walking (M.S. Pinzur and associates, unpublished data). Ground-reaction forces in a series of patients amputated at the below-knee level on one limb and through-

knee level on the other limb actually revealed that walking stability, as measured by temporal monitors and the progression of the center of foot pressure during gait, was greater on the through-knee limb (M.S. Pinzur and associates, unpublished data), while propulsion power was similar in the two limbs.

The small increase in the metabolic cost of walking may well be offset by the intrinsic stability afforded by the four-bar linkage prosthetic knee joint used in the through-knee prosthesis.[2,20] In addition, the end bearing of this level may provide proprioception, which, by adding to patient confidence, enhances walking stability. In some elderly patients, those on renal dialysis, or those with venous disease, there is a great deal of fluctuation in residual limb volume. This fluctuation can make it difficult to function with a below-knee prosthesis, which requires an intimate socket fit for optimum function and prevention of stump ulcers. These patients may also be better served with through-knee amputation, which allows end bearing and does not require an intimate prosthetic socket fit for reasonable function.

Above-knee and hip disarticulation amputations are performed only when a more distal amputation cannot reasonably be performed. Walking and even sitting function in these patients does not approach that of patients with more distal amputations.

In summary, amputation level selection cannot be accomplished by a single test. Testing techniques assist the rehabilitation team once the functional rehabilitation potential for the patient has been determined. The biologic amputation level is the most distal amputation level with a reasonable potential to heal. This is determined by combining careful clinical examination with the tools previously discussed. Information gleaned from the assessment of rehabilitation potential and from the determination of the biologic level is combined to determine the most appropriate amputation level for the individual patient.

Immediate Postsurgical Prosthetic-Limb Fitting

Older patients with peripheral vascular insufficiency benefit greatly from early ambulation and weightbearing to decrease the potential for aerobic deconditioning or the development of pressure ulcers or disabling joint contractures. While immediate postsurgical prosthetic limb fitting (IPSF) has been successful in the young traumatic or tumor amputee, it has been fraught with an unacceptably high rate of complications in the older peripheral vascular insufficiency population, probably because of the fragility of the terminal skin and muscle. We have been taught that residual limb wounds break down and fail because of direct pressure from the prosthetic socket. In fact, as the residual limb shrinks during the early postoperative period, the intimate fit, or total

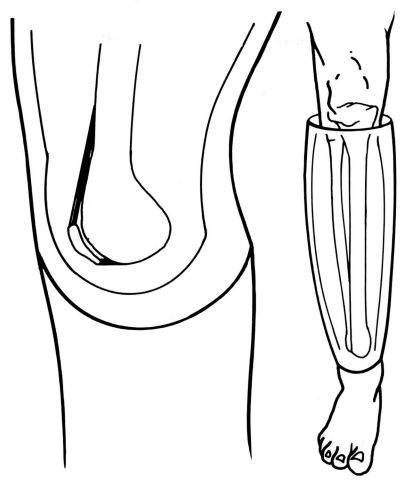

Fig. 1   Direct load transfer is accomplished in the (**left**) through-knee and (**right**) Syme's ankle disarticulation amputations.

contact, between the limb and prosthetic socket is lost. This leads to pistoning of the residual limb within the socket, the creation of a shearing force across the fresh, dysvascular surgical wound, and eventual wound break-down. The ideal IPSF prosthetic socket retains its intimate fit, which eliminates the pistoning and shearing of the fresh surgical wound and allows weightbearing. For this reason, most centers delay weightbearing until the residual limb has shrunk, and they use early post-surgical prosthetic limb fitting (EPSF) during a period of time when the shrinkage of the residual limb is more gradual. The failure of IPSF may be related more to the nonadaptability of the systems employed than to limitations of the technique itself.

Weightbearing and Load Transfer

The prosthetic socket in the lower-extremity amputee

acts as an interface between the hard bone of the patient's residual limb and the hard plastic of the socket. The transfer of weight between the patient's limb and the prosthesis can be accomplished by direct or indirect means.

Through-knee or Syme's ankle disarticulation amputations allow weightbearing through the end of the residual limb (Fig. 1). This direct load transfer, or end bearing, requires bone and a soft-tissue envelope that will accommodate a concentration of weightbearing pressure over the small surface area of the residual limb.

When the tissues of the residual limb cannot tolerate this concentration of pressure, the load must be distributed over the entire surface of the residual limb (Fig. 2). This indirect load transfer, or total-contact weightbearing, largely unloads the end of the residual limb. The intimate contact between the residual limb and the prosthetic socket then acts as a friction interface between the socket and the sides of the residual

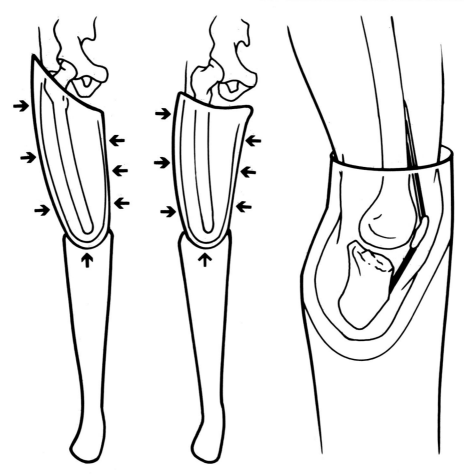

Fig. 2   Indirect load transfer is accomplished in above-knee amputations with either (**left**) a standard quadrilateral socket or (**center**) an adducted narrow medial-lateral socket. The below-knee amputation (**right**) transfers weight indirectly with the knee flexed approximately 10 degrees.

limb, in effect, by grasping the sides of the residual limb to hold it aloft (Fig. 3).

Soft-Tissue Envelope

The muscle and skin of the amputee's residual limb is the interface between the remaining bone and the prosthetic socket (Fig. 4). Good amputation surgery should provide an adequate soft-tissue envelope composed of a mobile, nonadherent muscle mass, and full-thickness skin. Adherent muscle or split-thickness skin graft may not tolerate the inherent pistoning of the residual limb within the prosthetic socket that occurs during walking. When a skin graft is necessary, it should be placed in areas that do not transfer appreciable load or shear.

IPSF in the amputation that allows direct load transfer is relatively simple. Weight is transferred through the bone and soft-tissue envelope at the end of the residual limb. Because there is relatively little shear force present, intimate prosthetic socket fit is less essential as the volume of the residual limb decreases during the early postoperative period. Standard rigid plaster-of-paris dressings with materials to make up for lost limb length can be used confidently with only occasional refabrications of the temporary socket. With indirect load transfer in below-knee and above-knee amputation levels, however, intimate prosthetic socket fit is critical in order to minimize the shear forces produced by pistoning within the socket as the residual limb decreases in volume.

Several attempts have been made to develop socket systems that can adjust to this rapid change in residual-limb volume, a change accelerated by early weight-bearing. Both Kerstein[21] and my co-workers and I[22] have been successful with an inflatable temporary plastic limb that fits inside a metal cylinder. This system is

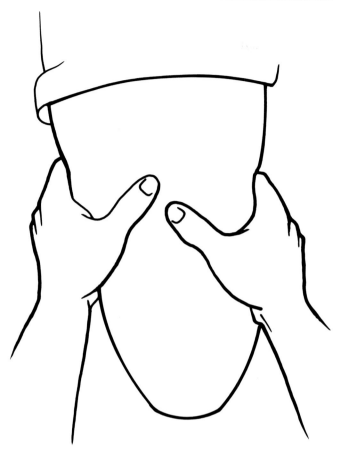

Fig. 3 Indirect load transfer is accomplished by a "friction" fit. Intimate prosthetic socket fit unloads the end of the residual limb, much as if the limb were suspended aloft by hands tightly grasping the sides.

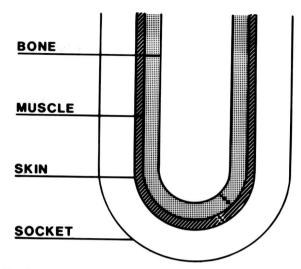

Fig. 4 The soft-tissue envelope acts as an interface between the bone of the residual limb and the prosthetic socket. Ideally, it should be composed of a mobile, nonadherent muscle mass, and full-thickness skin that will tolerate the direct pressures and pistoning within the prosthetic socket.

used until the shape and volume of the residual limb stabilize. Mooney and associates[23] have successfully used a two-piece rigid plastic socket, available in several prefabricated sizes, that can be made smaller by tightening Velcro straps. Several investigators are using flexible, adjustable plastics that are adaptable and stable enough for weight transfer in a fresh amputation wound.

In summary, the system is not the answer. Careful supervision is essential with a system that can accommodate changes in volume and shape of the residual limb. I recommend that allowing patients early weight-bearing be reserved to rehabilitation teams with appropriate experience and expertise. This expertise can be gained initially by postoperative wound management in a rigid plaster-of-paris dressing[24] and nonweight-bearing ambulation for 14 to 21 days, by which time the size and shape of the residual limb will be more stable. As the team gains experience and expertise, the delay to weightbearing can be shortened.

References

1. Waters RL, Perry J, Antonelli D, et al: Energy cost of walking of amputees: The influence of level of amputation. *J Bone Joint Surg* 1976;58A:42–46.
2. Volpicelli LJ, Chambers RB, Wagner FW Jr: Ambulation levels of bilateral lower-extremity amputees: Analysis of one hundred and three cases. *J Bone Joint Surg* 1983;65A:599–605.
3. Pinzur MS, Graham G, Osterman H: Psychologic testing in amputation rehabilitation. *Clin Orthop* 1988;229:236–240.
4. Wagner FW Jr: Management of the diabetic-neurotrophic foot: Part II. A classification and treatment program for diabetic, neuropathic, and dysvascular foot problems, in American Academy of Orthopaedic Surgeons *Instructional Course Lectures, XXVIII.* St. Louis, CV Mosby, 1979, pp 143–165.
5. Wagner FW Jr: Amputations of the foot and ankle: Current status. *Clin Orthop* 1977;122:62–69.
6. Pinzur MS, Smith DG, Daluga DJ, et al: Selection of patients for through-the-knee amputation. *J Bone Joint Surg* 1988;70A:746–750.
7. Raines J: Segmental plethysmography, in Rutherford RB (ed): *Vascular Surgery*, ed 2. Philadelphia, WB Saunders, 1984, pp 1157–1173.
8. van den Broek TAA, Dwars BJ, Rauwerda JA, et al: Photoplethysmographic selection of amputation level in peripheral vascular disease. *J Vasc Surg* 1988;8:10–13.
9. Yao JS, Bergan JJ: Application of ultrasound to arterial and venous diagnosis. *Surg Clin North Am* 1974;54:23–38.
10. Moore WS, Henry RE, Malone JM, et al: Prospective use of xenon X[133] clearance for amputation level selection. *Arch Surg* 1981;116:86–88.
11. Tanzer TL, Horne JG: The assessment of skin viability using fluorescein angiography prior to amputation. *J Bone Joint Surg* 1982;64A:880–882.
12. Wyss CR, Harrington RM, Burgess EM, et al: Transcutaneous oxygen tension as a predictor of success after an amputation. *J Bone Joint Surg* 1988;70A:203–207.

13. Oishi CS, Fronek A, Golbranson FL: The role of non-invasive vascular studies in determining levels of amputation. *J Bone Joint Surg* 1988;70A:1520–1530.

14. Malone JM, Anderson GG, Lalka SG, et al: Prospective comparison of noninvasive techniques for amputation level selection. *Am J Surg* 1987;154:179–184.

15. Dickhaut SC, DeLee JC, Page CP: Nutritional status: Importance in predicting wound-healing after amputation. *J Bone Joint Surg* 1984;66A:71–75.

16. Pinzur M, Kaminsky M, Sage R, et al: Amputations at the middle level of the foot: A retrospective and prospective review. *J Bone Joint Surg* 1986;68A:1061–1064.

17. Pinzur MS, Sage R, Schwaegler P: Ray resection in the dysvascular foot: A retrospective review. *Clin Orthop* 1984;191:232–234.

18. Roach JJ, Deutsch A, McFarlane DS: Resurrection of the amputations of Lisfranc and Chopart for diabetic gangrene. *Arch Surg* 1987;122:931–934.

19. Rubin G: Indications for variants of the partial foot prosthesis. *Orthop Rev* 1985;14:688–695.

20. Greene MP: Four bar linkage knee analysis. *Orthot Prosthet* 1983;37:15–24.

21. Kerstein MD: An improved modality in lower extremity amputee rehabilitation. *Orthopedics* 1985;8:207–209.

22. Pinzur MS, Littooy F, Osterman H, et al: A safe pre-fabricated immediate post-operative prosthetic limb system for rehabilitation of below-knee amputees. *Orthopedics*, in press.

23. Mooney V, McClellan B, Cummings D, et al: Early fitting of the below knee amputee. *Orthopedics* 1985;8:199–202.

24. Burgess EM, Romano RL, Zettl JH: The Management of Lower Extremity Amputations. United States Government Printing Office, 1969.

Overview of Prosthetic Feet*

John W. Michael, MEd, CPO

Innovative technology in prosthetic feet has long been an American tradition. The modern era began in 1861, when amputee-prosthetist J. E. Hanger substituted rubber bumpers for the tendon-like cords of earlier inventors.[1] Over the next hundred years this single-axis design (Fig. 1) became the predominant choice for amputees worldwide, and in the United Kingdom it is still the foot most frequently prescribed.[2]

In the 1950s, researchers at the University of California at Berkeley developed the solid ankle cushion heel, or SACH foot (Fig. 2), resurrecting the concept that a prosthesis without moving mechanical parts could restore foot function.[3] Because it is light in weight, reliable, and inexpensive, the SACH foot gradually supplanted the mechanically articulated versions. By the 1970s, it had become the most commonly prescribed prosthetic foot in North America.[4]

Studies comparing the function of these two competing designs have found few significant differences between them.[2,5,6] The general conclusion has been that the SACH foot offers the smoothest transition from heel strike to midstance while the single-axis type slightly enhances prosthetic knee stability.[2] Widespread patient acceptance of both types clinically confirms that local custom has been as much a factor as scientific evidence in determining which of these prosthetic feet was prescribed.

Until recently, the only other foot design to gain any widespread clinical acceptance was the multi-axis type (Fig. 3). Similar in weight and reliability to the single-axis version, the multi-axis offers additional mediolateral motion and transverse rotation and tends to be used for the more active individual, particularly for activities on uneven ground.[7]

Until 1980 these three types described virtually all the prosthetic feet available. Each could be categorized according to its characteristic function. Once the function was determined, the choice among alternatives followed logically. The state of the art before 1980 is summarized in Table 1.

Since 1980, at least 18 new prosthetic feet have been introduced to the American market. Some, such as Ryan's Superfoot or Cope's Bionic Ankle, had design problems and were quickly abandoned. Others have become increasingly popular and represent genuine advances in prosthetic restoration.

The stationary ankle flexible endoskeleton, or SAFE, foot initiated the first wave of innovative contemporary designs. Substituting a flexible rubber keel for the rigid hardwood of previous designs allowed a smoother roll-over than ever before. Dacron bands simulated the windlass effect of the plantar fascia and permitted fore-

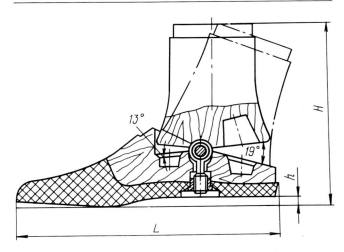

Fig. 1 Civil War-era design of the single-axis foot enhances prosthetic knee stability and is widely used in the United Kingdom to this day.

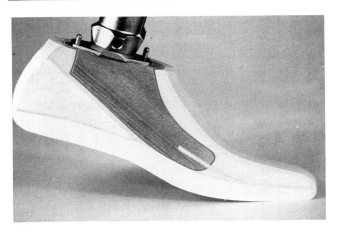

Fig. 2 The solid ankle cushion heel, or SACH, foot is widely prescribed in the United States because it is simple and reliable.

*The discussion and evaluation of various manufacturers' products present solely the views of the author and are in no way meant to be an endorsement by the American Academy of Orthopaedic Surgeons of any product or products.

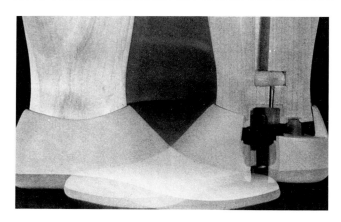

Fig. 3 The multi-axis foot offers three-dimensional motion, making it particularly well suited for activities on uneven ground.

foot pronation and supination as well as some transverse rotation.[8]

The SAFE foot inaugurated a new functional class of feet grouped as flexible-keel designs (Fig. 4). Its characteristic is smoother rollover; its general indication is to permit easier ambulation. Kingsley Manufacturing's STEN foot, another member of this class, has been joined recently by Otto Bock's 1D10 Dynamic foot. These three feet are characterized by smoothly increasing anterior resistance during rollover, which makes this phase of gait less abrupt and jarring than does the SACH design. In my experience, the flexible-keel group has been well accepted by most unilateral amputees and by selected bilateral amputees. Patients, particularly those who previously used a SACH foot, often comment favorably on the easier rollover.

Although some manufacturers claim an energy-storing function for these feet, others do not. I believe that, in fact, the flexible-keel feet dissipate most of the bending moment as heat and do not actively return energy to the gait cycle. However, they may require less effort or energy expenditures in walking than earlier designs. Preliminary findings in this regard will be discussed shortly.

The final functional group includes the dynamic-response designs (Fig. 5). Although they, too, permit smoother rollover, the characteristic that distinguishes them from the flexible-keel type is that these feet provide a measure of active push-off. Although this may be of some value during walking, the dynamic-response foot is particularly useful during more vigorous activities. Thus, the indication for this class of feet is to permit an increased activity level. Members of this class include various spring-keel designs such as the Seattle foot, Carbon Copy II, the Quantum foot, and the resilient pylon assembly of the Flex-Foot. Characteristics of currently available prosthetic feet are summarized in Table 2.

Beyond these broad distinctions, how is the choice made among specific available feet? By understanding the factors of cost, weight, reliability, ability to propel the patient forward, and the effort required to walk, the orthopaedic surgeon and prosthetist can select the optimal foot for the individual patient.

Weight and cost are summarized in Figures 6 and 7. In general, cost increases directly with the complexity of the design. Weight is more interesting: although the majority of sophisticated feet are heavier than the standard SACH, some are significantly lighter.

Reliability is also variable. Some designs had significant difficulties when first introduced, but have been modified for greater durability now. Both Flex-Foot and Carbon Copy II have enjoyed excellent reliability records from the outset. In general, all the sophisticated prosthetic feet discussed above have a failure rate within the first year of less than 4%.[9]

There is a dearth of published data to assist in discriminating further among these components, but some intriguing findings are just beginning to appear. Wagner and associates[10] published the first detailed motion analysis comparing the Flex-Foot and SACH designs. Although many similarities were noted, one of the key findings was that the Flex-Foot pylon had increased range of motion at the ankle during late stance phase. In essence, the flexibility of the component allowed the body to glide forward and measurably eased the impact of the sound heel on the ground. In contrast, the SACH foot forced the amputee to develop enough momentum to ride over the rigid keel, then

Table 1
Traditional prosthetic feet (1861–1980)

Characteristics	SACH	Single-Axis	Multi-Axis
Characteristic function	Simplicity	Rapid foot-flat	Hindfoot inversion-eversion
General indication	General utility	To enhance prosthetic knee stability	To accommodate uneven terrain
Examples	Various manufacturers	Various manufacturers	Greissinger, Multi-Flex
Cost	Low	Moderate	Moderate
Weight	Medium	Heavy	Heavy
Reliability	Very high	Moderate	Moderate
Apparent efficacy	Low	Low	Moderate

free-fall until the opposite heel struck the ground. Murray and associates[11] recently reported similar improvement in ankle motion with the Seattle foot. One implication for our geriatric and dysvascular patients is that a more sophisticated prosthetic device may result in less stress on the other foot, which is also at risk.

A simple test of vertical leap, using a modified pogo stick (Fig. 8), resulted in the ground-clearance ranking illustrated in Figure 9. In this parameter, the feet fell neatly into flexible-keel and dynamic-response categories, with Flex-Foot emerging as clearly the most resilient.

Nielsen and associates[12] published a preliminary report comparing the gait efficiency of the Flex-Foot with that of the SACH design. At velocities of less than 2 mph, little difference could be detected. However, using the Flex-Foot, subjects tended to choose a faster walking speed than when using the SACH. As the pace increased from 3 to 4 mph, a decrease in the oxygen consumed per kilogram of bodyweight was documented with the Flex-Foot. At 4 mph, the advantage represented a 10% reduction.

In an effort to investigate different manufacturers' claims of energy efficiency, a pilot study is underway comparing the SACH foot with many of the more sophisticated designs. Using a single subject wearing a well-fitted supracondylar soft socket plus neoprene sleeve, parameters such as oxygen consumption and heart rate are measured during ambulation on a powered treadmill.

Each foot component is individually aligned to the patient's and prosthetist's satisfaction. The optimum alignment is verified by independent examination by another certified prosthetist. The patient is then permitted a minimum of three weeks of full-time ambulation on each component prior to the treadmill testing. Because all other factors are held constant, and the only variable is the foot, any decrease in oxygen consumption should indicate a more efficient component.

To simulate normal brisk walking, the protocol calls for six minutes of ambulation on a level surface at a constant pace of 3 mph. To simulate a slight incline, the treadmill is elevated to a 2-degree grade and the patient walks another six minutes. Finally, to simulate a mild hill, the grade is increased to 4 degrees for the last six minutes.

Blood gases are collected and analyzed, and blood pressure is measured throughout the entire 18-minute test. Heart rate is measured constantly via remote telemetry. The patient's subjective rate of perceived exertion is also recorded. The results are shown in Table 3.

Although statistical analysis has not been performed, it is highly unlikely that the closely clustered scores will prove significant, particularly in a single-subject experiment. For the level grade, the SACH foot does require more oxygen consumption by the patient than

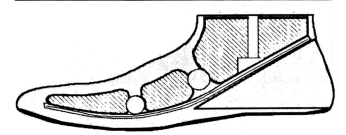

Fig. 4 Cutaway of one type of flexible-keel foot. Round rubber plugs permit the forefoot to bend, allowing a smoother rollover.

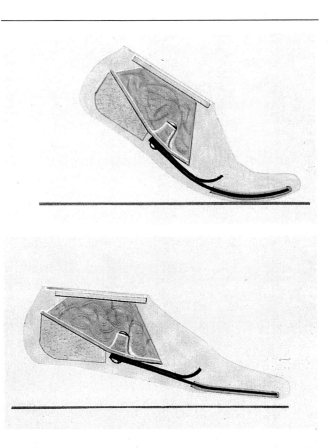

Fig. 5 Schematic of a dynamic-response foot. Dual carbon fiber deflection plates function as plastic leaf springs to simulate active pushoff.

any others tested, and it may indeed make walking more difficult. These data are corroborated by clinical experience, because virtually every amputee given a choice between the SACH and any of the contemporary designs has rejected the SACH.

For the slight (2%) grade, the clusters are again rather close, and once again the SACH seems to be clearly the least efficient. On slight grades, it appears that the more flexible Seattle and Dynamic foot designs require less effort.

Table 2
Contemporary prosthetic feet (1980–1988)

Characteristics	Flexible-Keel	Dynamic-Response
Characteristic function	Smooth rollover	Active push-off
General indication	Easier ambulation	Increased activity level
Examples	SAFE II Sten Dynamics	Seattle, Carbon Copy II, Flex-Foot, Flex-Walk, Quantum
Cost	Moderate	High to very high
Weight	Moderate to light	Heavy to very light
Reliability	Moderate	Moderate to very high
Apparent efficacy	Moderate to high	High to very high

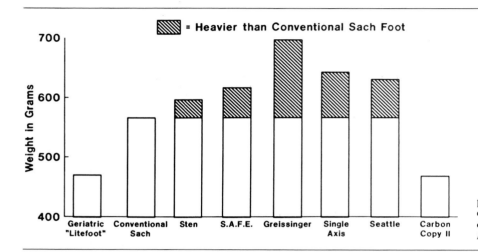

Fig. 6 Weight of men's size 10 foot components, not including ankle block. (Reproduced with permission from Michael JW: Energy storing feet: A clinical comparison. *Clin Prosthet Orthot* 1987;11:154–168.)

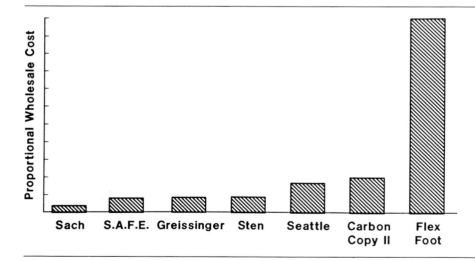

Fig. 7 Relative wholesale costs for prosthetic foot mechanisms. (Reproduced with permission from Michael JW: Energy storing feet: A clinical comparison. *Clin Prosthet Orthot* 1987;11:154–168.)

For the mild (4%) slope, the ranking is the same as for the lesser grade, with the Seattle and Dynamic feet being relatively efficient, and the SACH design appearing to consume the most energy.

One must be extremely cautious in interpreting such preliminary single-subject results, particularly without corroboration by other investigators. However, my per-

sonal assessment of the state of sophisticated prosthetic feet at this time is as follows.

The SACH foot apparently consumes more energy than any of the more sophisticated options, both on level and on sloping ground. This is particularly true at higher cadences. If this continues to be corroborated, it will be increasingly difficult to justify widespread clinical application of "energy-consuming" conventional prosthetic feet. The more flexible the forefoot, the better the foot seems to perform when going up mild inclines.

The strong showing by the rubber-keel Dynamic foot suggests that a major mechanism for conserving energy (at least for ordinary walking) may be the softer roll-over, presumably because this minimizes the vertical oscillation of the body's center of gravity.

For ordinary level walking, it is extremely difficult to discriminate between the various sophisticated designs in terms of energy consumption. However, preliminary evidence is emerging suggesting that the higher the cadence, the better the performance of the dynamic-response group.

New variations are coming onto the prosthetic market almost monthly, and accepted feet are being redesigned and improved. The following dynamic-response designs were announced in 1988. The Flex-Shank, a machined aluminum analogue to the Flex-Foot, is intended for short-term use in a diagnostic or evaluation prosthesis. The Flex-Walk, a low-profile version from the manufacturers of Flex-Foot, seeks to offer most of the function of its predecessor at a significantly lower cost. The Quantum Foot, developed by Hanger of England, offers independent heel and keel springs, a removable cosmetic outer shell, and an electric light-emitting diode apparatus to facilitate dynamic alignment. These new prosthetic feet appear to represent a significant improvement over those available a few years ago, but, like those, the new ones can be understood by placing them in the five functional classes discussed previously.

Initial prescription decisions can be based on the characteristics and indications for each functional class,

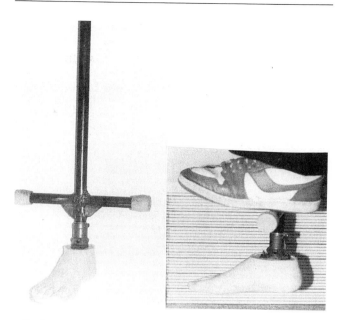

Fig. 8   Pogo stick device used to test vertical spring capabilities of various feet. (Reproduced with permission from Michael JW: Energy storing feet: A clinical comparison. *Clin Prosthet Orthot* 1987;11:154–168.)

Table 3
Oxygen consumption (Vo$_2$ in ml/min/kg) during ambulation with various prostheses

Prostheses	Level	2% Grade	4% Grade
Seattle	14.0	14.8	16.6
Dynamic	14.1	15.1	17.0
Flex-Foot	14.4	16.2	18.0
Carbon copy II	13.9	16.4	18.2
SACH	15.4	16.7	19.0

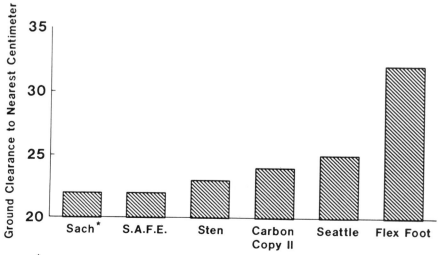

* **Note: Sach keel fractured upon impact**

Fig. 9   Ground clearance after vertical leap using pogo stick apparatus: 175-lb male subject, men's size 10 foot. (Reproduced with permission from Michael JW: Energy storing feet: A clinical comparison. *Clin Prosthet Orthot* 1987;11:154–168.)

after which specific selection is made based on cost, weight, reliability, and effectiveness of individual designs.

These sophisticated feet represent a significant advance in prosthetic technology. As our experiences are documented and shared, indications for each prosthetic foot will become more and more precise.

References

1. American Academy of Orthopaedic Surgeons: *Orthopaedic Appliances Atlas.* Ann Arbor, JW Edwards, 1960, vol 2, p 10.
2. Goh JC, Solomonidis SE, Spence WD, et al: Biomechanical evaluation of SACH and uniaxial feet. *Prosthet Orthot Int* 1984;8:147–154.
3. Radcliffe CW, Foort J: *The Patellar-Tendon-Bearing Below-Knee Prosthesis.* Berkeley, University of California, 1961.
4. Fishman S, Berger N, Watkins D: A survey of prosthetics practice: 1973–74. *Orthot Prosthet* 1975;29:15–20.
5. Doane NE, Holt LE: A comparison of the SACH and single axis foot in the gait of unilateral below-knee amputees. *Prosthet Orthot Int* 1983;7:33–36.
6. Culham EG, Peat M, Newell E: Below-knee amputation: A comparison of the effect of the SACH foot and single axis foot on electromyographic patterns during locomotion. *Prosthet Orthot Int* 1986;10:15–22.
7. Michael JW: Prosthetic feet for the amputee athlete. *Palaestra* 1986;2:37–41.
8. Campbell JW, Childs CW: The S.A.F.E. foot. *Orthot Prosthet* 1980;34:3–16.
9. Michael JW: Energy storing feet: A clinical comparison. *Clin Prosthet Orthot* 1987;11:154–168.
10. Wagner J, Sienko S, Supan TJ, et al: Motion analysis of SACH vs. Flex-Foot in moderately active below-knee amputees. *Clin Prosthet Orthot* 1987;11:55–62.
11. Murray DD, Hartvikson WJ, Anton H, et al: With a spring in one's step. *Clin Prosthet Orthot* 1988;12:128–135.
12. Nielsen DH, Shurr DG, Golden JC, et al: Comparison of energy cost and gait efficiency during ambulation in below-knee amputees using different prosthetic feet: A preliminary report. *J Prosthet Orthot* 1988;1:24–31.

Current Concepts in Above-Knee Socket Design

John W. Michael, MEd, CPO

Before 1950, there was no widespread agreement as to the most effective socket design for above-knee amputees. Numerous idiosyncratic variations existed in the United States and throughout the world.

Under the leadership of Charles Radcliffe, M.S., Professor of Mechanical Engineering at the University of California (Berkeley), scientific research has brought a more explicit understanding of the principles necessary for successful prosthetic fitting. Radcliffe[1] described a three-dimensional rigid receptacle that simultaneously provides weight-bearing, suspension, and control of residual limb motion. A key component of this design is an area of pronounced vertical weightbearing beneath the ischial tuberosity and gluteal musculature (Fig. 1). This approach dictated a characteristic shape for the proximal portion of the socket, a shape known as the quadrilateral brim (Fig. 2).

From 1964 until very recently, this concept enjoyed almost universal acceptance in the United States and throughout much of the world. Although the quadrilateral-brim socket remains the most widely prescribed design in above-knee prosthetics to this day, it is being increasingly challenged by alternate approaches.[2-9]

I contend that these new designs represent evolutionary rather than revolutionary advances, notwithstanding the strident claims of some of the more partisan proponents, and that the long-term success of some of the more radical departures remains to be

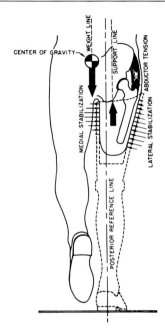

Fig. 1 Biomechanical conception of the quadrilateral socket, per Radcliffe. Note pronounced vertical loading at ischial tuberosity. (Reproduced with permission from Radcliffe CW: Functional considerations in the fitting of above-knee prostheses. *Orthot Prosthet* 1955; 2:35–60.)

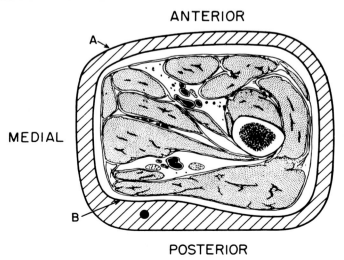

Fig. 2 Socket cross section, at ischial level, illustrating quadrilateral shape as originally proposed by Radcliffe in 1955. (Reproduced with permission from Radcliffe CW: Functional considerations in the fitting of above-knee prostheses. *Orthot Prosthet* 1955;2:35–60.)

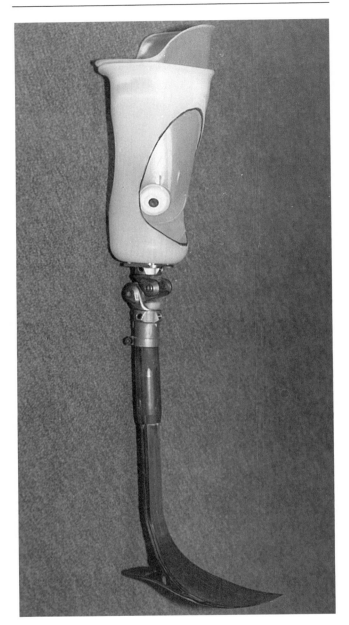

Fig. 3 Example of a flexible-frame socket, as originally proposed by Kristinsson of Iceland. (Reproduced with permission from Jendrzejczyk D: Flexible socket systems. *Clin Prosthet Orthot* 1985;9:27–30.)

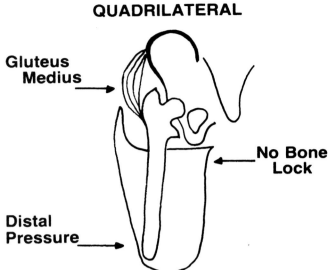

Fig. 4 Socket migration can compromise femoral mediolateral stability, as originally proposed by Long. (Reproduced with permission from Sabolich J: Contoured adducted trochanteric-controlled alignment method. *Clin Prosthet Orthot* 1985;9:15–26.)

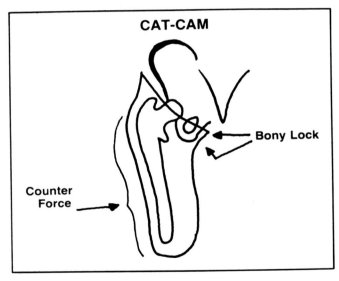

Fig. 5 Encapsulating the ischium within the socket may reduce socket migration. (Reproduced with permission from Sabolich J: Contoured adducted trochanteric-controlled alignment method. *Clin Prosthet Orthot* 1985;9:15–26.)

proven. However, I also believe that there is a great deal of merit in this new wave of prosthetic thought, and that most amputees can be successfully fitted with virtually any of the designs proposed. The question of which specific approach is optimum has no definitive answer at this time and must await additional collective experience, more impartial field testing, and more objective scientific evaluation.

The essence of all the recent controversies in above-knee prosthetic design can be summarized by considering two basic issues dealt with in this chapter. First, should the socket walls be rigid, flexible, or a combination thereof, and second, to what degree should the ischial tuberosity be contained within the confines of the socket?

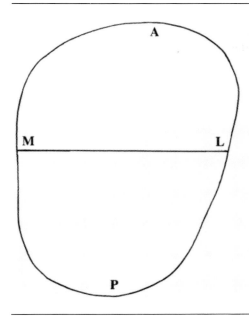

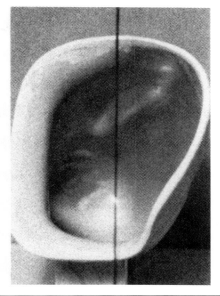

Fig. 6 Typical brim shape of Long's normal shape-normal alignment (NSNA) socket. (Reproduced with permission from Long IA: Normal shape-normal alignment (NSNA) above-knee prosthesis. *Clin Prosthet Orthot* 1985;9:9–14.)

Flexibility

Kristinsson[4] of Iceland should be credited with sparking the current interest in developing progressively more flexible socket designs. Before 1983, when his report was published, almost all above-knee sockets were rigid plastic receptacles, reflecting the philosophy initiated by Radcliffe. Kristinsson observed that when he converted a bilateral above-knee amputee from primitive leather sockets to modern plastic ones, the patient rejected them because of sitting discomfort, even though walking was more comfortable and secure in the plastic sockets. In collaboration with Scandinavian colleagues, he developed a more comfortable, flexible polyethylene socket, which was connected to a rigid weightbearing frame for skeletal support (Fig. 3). An initial series of 300 cases demonstrated the feasibility of this approach.

This report triggered a flurry of creative developments worldwide. It must be understood that, although flexible, none of these sockets are expansile: a key distinction. Although Volkert[10] of Germany had reported preliminary results with an expansile frame socket in 1982, it never achieved widespread clinical acceptance. An expansile socket fails to contain the soft tissue effectively because its volume varies, increasing skeletal weightbearing and discomfort.

A flexible nonexpansile socket, on the other hand, accommodates the changing contours of functioning muscles within the socket. It also contributes effectively to peripheral weightbearing because of its fixed volume, even more, in some instances, than a rigid socket of the same contours.

The middle portion of an above-knee socket has a roughly circular cross-sectional area. If formed of a flexible, nonexpansile material, it will deform under the forces of the remaining musculature into a more ovoid cross section. Although the perimeter remains constant, the less circular shape contains a smaller cross-sectional area. In effect, the flexible socket becomes functionally smaller under weightbearing conditions, and the increased hydrostatic pressure increases the weight-bearing support. Kawamura and Kawamura[3] of Japan reported laboratory confirmation in 1986 that this deformation did, in fact, occur. They also documented that the femoral adduction angle at midstance was virtually identical in rigid and flexible sockets formed over the same mold.

Following Kristinsson's report, numerous other centers reported similarly favorable results, and advocated a variety of socket shapes and frame contours.[2,3,7,9] Both upper-limb and lower-limb applications have been successful.[11] Although not yet the majority design in the United States, flexible frame sockets have been widely accepted and are now part of this country's mainstream prosthetic practice.

A recent international conference listed the following advantages of the flexible-frame socket: improved sitting comfort; improved proprioception because the environment can be felt through the socket walls; better heat dissipation through thin, often transparent walls; and better accommodation of functioning muscles because the shape can be altered under pressure.

The major drawbacks to flexible designs have been decreased durability (because of tearing of the material over time) and imprecise fit because of linear shrinkage

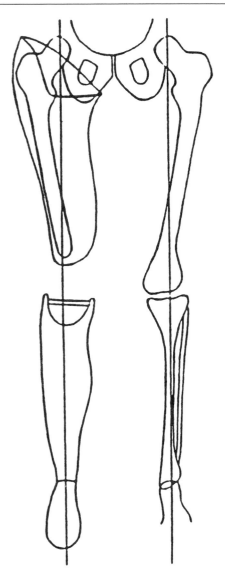

Fig. 7 Static socket alignment, based on skeletal anatomy, as proposed by Long. (Reproduced with permission from Jendrzejczyk D: Flexible socket systems. *Clin Prosthet Orthot* 1985;9:27–30.)

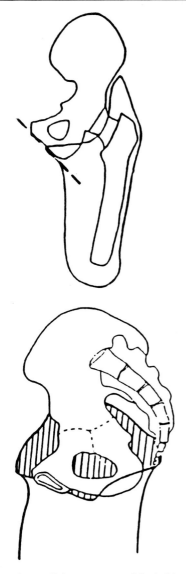

Fig. 8 Aggressive medial encasement of the ischium, as advocated by CAT-CAM proponents. (Reproduced with permission from Schuch CM: Modern above-knee fitting practice (a report on the ISPO workshop on above-knee fitting and alignment techniques May 15–19, 1987, Miami, USA). *Prosthet Orthot Int* 1988;12:77–90.)

of thermoplastic materials.[4] These are somewhat counterbalanced by the ease with which a flexible socket can be replaced.[7] Further acceptance of flexible designs awaits improvements in the durability and reliability of the materials available.

Ischial Containment

Long[6] initiated the current movement away from classic quadrilateral contours. In 1975, he published a brief technical note observing that many quadrilateral sockets failed to stabilize the femur in the desired amount of adduction, and proposed using the anatomic axis of the lower limb as the foundation for above-knee alignment.[12] For the next decade, Long pursued greater control of the femur by progressively narrowing the mediolateral dimension of the above-knee socket. He noted that, with this narrowing, the socket tended to displace laterally until the ischium was no longer resting on the flat quadrilateral shelf. He then increased the slope of the posteromedial shelf, partially enclosing the ischial tuberosity within the socket (Figs. 4 and 5).[6]

Because soft tissue has limited compressibility, a tighter mediolateral dimension dictated a larger anteroposterior diameter within the socket. A roughly oval brim shape evolved that more closely resembles the

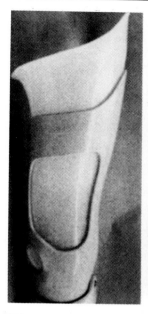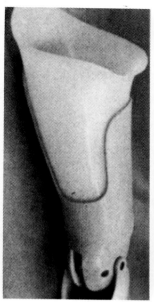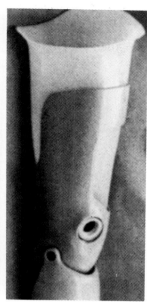

Fig. 9 Flexible proximal brim is a prerequisite for comfort if the ischium is fully contained within the socket. (Reproduced with permission from Sabolich J: Contoured adducted trochanteric-controlled alignment method. *Clin Prosthet Orthot* 1985;9:15–26.)

normal cross section of a thigh than does the squared-off quadrilateral design (Fig. 6). To emphasize this humanoid shape and his views on anatomic skeletal alignment, Long calls his technique NSNA, for normal shape-normal alignment (Fig. 7).[6]

I believe that the concept of ischial containment is Long's most significant contribution. Subsequent developments differ primarily in the degree to which they encapsulate the ischiopubic ramus. These developments include the contoured adducted trochanteric-controlled alignment method (CAT-CAM) above-knee socket proposed by Sabolich.[9] This device has been associated with undocumented claims but, despite this, I believe the concept has genuine merit. In terms of socket design, members of the CAT-CAM group advocate two key characteristics: (1) maximum ischiopubic enclosure (Fig. 8), and (2) a totally flexible proximal brim (Fig. 9).

These are intimately related. Long's NSNA socket is a completely rigid receptacle, with mildly sloping walls that enclose the tip of the ischial tuberosity. The CAT-CAM concept implies full ischial enclosure (particularly medially) and requires the flexibility of a resilient brim to accomplish this comfortably.

One factor limiting wider use of either the NSNA or the CAT-CAM approach is the difficulty some experienced prosthetists have reported in applying the techniques. At the present time, although a substantial number of clinical prosthetists use one or both techniques in their practices, many do not. At this stage of development, it often takes repeated costly modifications, involving multiple check sockets, to achieve a satisfactory clinical result.

One effort to simplify the process is the casting technique developed by Shamp. Instead of using a hand-formed plaster impression of the residual limb, Shamp argues that a preformed brim can allow more accurate preliminary evaluation and simplify the fitting protocol. This results in a socket that reflects Shamp's vision of the proper brim contour, which may be arguable, but indeed permits reliable production of a socket that encloses much of the ischium. Shamp recommends a flexible brim and walls, but states that this technique will also work with rigid walls (D. Shamp, personal communication, 1988). The Ohio Willow Wood Company, of Mount Sterling, Ohio, in 1987 prepared a "Manual for use of the Shamp brim."

Current Trends

How is the clinician to choose among all these competing philosophies? In an effort to provide more global weightbearing, greater comfort, and increased femoral stability, the concept of ischial containment is making wider inroads into mainstream prosthetic practice every day. However, the difficulty in achieving consistently comfortable results with perineal trimlines, the increased costs associated with fitting such intimate contours, and the decreased reliability of flexible thermoplastics tend to inhibit greater application of these concepts. It is hoped that all of these factors will diminish as clinicians disseminate and refine these techniques.

I concur fully with the recent conclusion of an international panel of medical, prosthetic, and engineering experts, who stated that there are "no specific contraindications noted for any socket design."[13] The panel went on to add that it may be unwise to convert satisfied previous wearers to any new design, and that the quadrilateral design seems most successful on long, firm residual limbs with good muscle tone. They further proposed that the shorter or fleshier residual limb often does marginally well with the quadrilateral socket, and is more likely to benefit from one of the nonquadrilateral designs. The highly active individual will often, but not always, find ischial containment more comfortable than quadrilateral ischial weightbearing.

Summary

To review the fundamental tenets of above-knee socket design proposed by Radcliffe nearly 40 years ago, sockets must be designed to achieve vertical support of body weight, stabilization of the residual skeleton in both the coronal and sagittal planes, accommodation of functioning muscles, voluntary control of the prosthetic knee, individualized design, and an optimum balance of comfort, function, and appearance, both statically and dynamically. Contemporary approaches represent enhancements and refinements toward these ends, but each of these fundamental goals must be satisfied no matter what socket design is selected.

References

1. Radcliffe CW: Functional considerations in the fitting of above-knee prostheses. *Orthot Prosthet* 1955;2:35–60.
2. Jendrzejczyk D: Flexible socket systems. *Clin Prosthet Orthot* 1985; 9:27–30.
3. Kawamura I, Kawamura J: Some biomechanical evaluations of the ISNY flexible above-knee system with quadrilateral socket. *Orthot Prosthet* 1986;40:17–23.
4. Kristinsson O: Flexible above-knee socket made from low density polyethylene suspended by a weight-transmitting frame. *Orthot Prosthet* 1983;37:25–27.
5. Lehneis HR: Beyond the quadrilateral. *Clin Prosthet Orthot* 1985; 9:6–8.
6. Long IA: Normal shape-normal alignment (NSNA) above-knee prosthesis. *Clin Prosthet Orthot* 1985;9:9–14.
7. Pritham CH, Fillauer C, Fillauer K: Experience with the Scandinavian Flexible Socket. *Orthot Prosthet* 1985;39:17–32.
8. Redhead RG: Total surface bearing self suspending above-knee sockets. *Prosthet Orthot Int* 1979;3:126–136.
9. Sabolich J: Contoured adducted trochanteric-controlled alignment method. *Clin Prosthet Orthot* 1985;9:15–26.
10. Volkert R: Frame type socket for lower limb prostheses. *Prosthet Orthot Int* 1982;6:88–92.
11. Fornuff DL: Flex-frame sockets in upper extremity prosthetics. *Clin Prosthet Orthot* 1985;9:31–34.
12. Long I: Allowing normal adduction of femur in above-knee amputations, technical note. *Orthot Prosthet* 1975;29:53–54.
13. Schuch CM: Modern above-knee fitting practice (a report on the ISPO workshop on above-knee fitting and alignment techniques May 15–19, 1987, Miami, USA). *Prosthet Orthot Int* 1988;12:77–90.

Skeletal Dysplasia

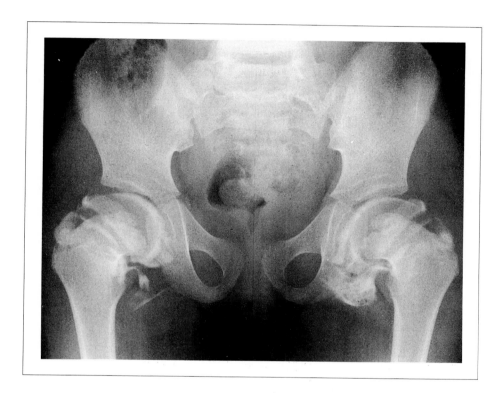

Orthopaedic Aspects of Skeletal Dysplasias

George S. Bassett, MD

Skeletal Dysplasias

Skeletal dysplasias are a heterogeneous group of disorders that result in a myriad of orthopaedic abnormalities that affect the spine and extremities. Although most of the skeletal dysplasias cause dwarfism, in which the standing height is below the third percentile, with disproportionate length of the limbs, trunk, or both, the resultant skeletal deformities, their natural history, and other associated findings differ widely for the different skeletal dysplasias. Furthermore, more than 120 specific dysplasias have been characterized by clinical, radiographic, and histologic criteria. However, as a group the frequency of occurrence of these disorders ranges from uncommon to extremely rare. For these reasons, and because the majority of skeletal dysplasias are heritable, consultation with a geneticist familiar with these disorders is important for the patients, their families, and the orthopaedic surgeon planning to treat the associated abnormalities.

This section will describe the characteristic features of six of the more common skeletal dysplasias encountered by the orthopaedic surgeon. Subsequent sections will emphasize the evaluation and treatment of spinal deformities and lower-extremity abnormalities for this group of patients.

Achondroplasia

Achondroplasia, the most common type of short-limb disproportionate dwarfism, is transmitted as an autosomal dominant trait. The majority of cases represent a random new mutation. A paternal age effect has been recognized with many fathers older than 36 years of age at the time of conception.[1] For average-size parents with one affected child, there is virtually no increased risk that subsequent children will have achondroplasia nor will the offspring of average-size siblings be affected. An achondroplastic parent has a 50% chance of transmitting the single gene responsible for achondroplasia to each child.[1]

Achondroplasia is recognizable at birth. Because intramembranous ossification is normal, the calvarium is relatively enlarged, with apparent frontal bossing. The midface, including the nasal bridge, is flattened, and there is a prominent mandible. The limbs are disproportionately shortened in a rhizomelic distribution, but the trunk is relatively normal in length. The thorax is

flattened and the abdomen protuberant. A significant thoracolumbar kyphosis is usually present. Typically, spontaneous resolution of the kyphosis occurs once independent ambulation begins. Hyperlordosis of the lumbar spine and associated hip flexion contractures

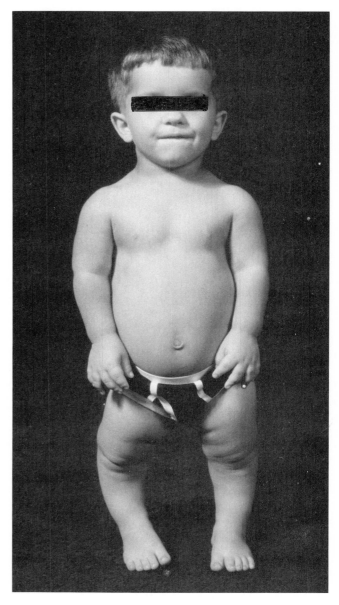

Fig. 1 Achondroplasia (14 years): Enlarged calvarium, rhizomelic shortening, and genu varum deformities.

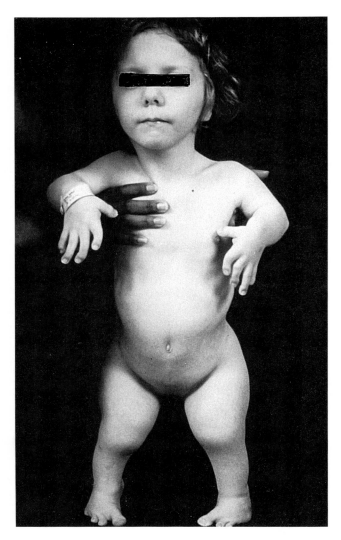

Fig. 2 Diastrophic dysplasia (7 years): Typical facies, "hitchhiker" thumb, severe hip-knee flexion contractures, and equinovarus foot deformities. (Reproduced with permission from Bassett GS, Scott CI Jr: The osteochondrodysplasias, in Morrissy RT (ed): *Pediatric Orthopaedics*, ed 3. Philadelphia, JB Lippincott, 1990.)

magnum. Characteristic radiographic features include an enlarged calvarium with mid-face hypoplasia and prominence of the mandibular and frontal regions. There is interpedicular narrowing in the lumbar spine on the anteroposterior view. Lateral radiographs of the spine reveal shortened pedicles, posterior scalloping of the vertebral bodies, and a thoracolumbar kyphosis of varying severity. Standing projections of the spine demonstrate excessive lordosis of the lumbar spine and a horizontally oriented sacrum. The pelvis is broad and short with horizontal acetabular roofs. Although the femoral neck is shortened, with mild overgrowth of the greater trochanter, true coxa vara does not exist. The hips generally remain spherical and premature osteoarthritis is unusual. The long bones are short and thick with flaring of the metaphyses. The distal femoral physis is V-shaped during childhood. Genu varum is frequently present, often in association with varus deformities of the ankles. The fibulas are elongated relative to the tibias.

Medical considerations include progressive hydrocephalus, recurrent otitis media, hearing deficits, malocclusion, and obesity. Many patients will have stenosis of the foramen magnum which, in some instances, may lead to respiratory compromise, quadriplegia, or sudden death.[3-5]

Diastrophic Dysplasia

Diastrophic dysplasia is a rare short-limb disproportionate dwarfing condition characterized by severe limb and spinal deformities. Adult height averages 118 cm. The probability of having a second child with diastrophic dysplasia, which is transmitted as an autosomal recessive trait, is 25% for average-size parents.

This disorder is also recognizable at birth. There is no cranial enlargement in diastrophic dysplasia, although a distinctive facial appearance exists. The nasal bridge is narrow with broad, flared nostrils and there is a characteristic circumoral fullness to the mouth. More than one half of the patients have a cleft palate. Feeding and respiratory problems may develop during infancy. The so-called "cauliflower ear" is not present at birth. Swelling and acute inflammation of the pinnae occur by 6 weeks of age with subsequent calcification in more than 80% of cases.

There is a rhizomelic pattern of extremity shortening with significant contractures of the elbows, hips, and knees. A hitchhiker-thumb deformity and symphalangism of the proximal interphalangeal joints are typically present (Fig. 2). Dislocated hips develop during adolescence in at least 20% of individuals with diastrophic dysplasia, and the disorder is associated with severe epiphyseal involvement of the femoral heads. Extremely rigid equinovarus deformities are present at birth. Severe cervical kyphosis is not infrequent and

are evident. The muscles appear bulky for the length of the extremities. In the upper extremities, the elbows lack full extension and a trident hand deformity is apparent. There is typically a varus deformity of the lower extremities (Fig. 1).

Motor milestones are usually later than in children of average size. Independent head control, sitting, standing, and walking are three to six months behind in achondroplastic children.[2] These delays have been related to the enlarged head, the discrepancy in proportion between the limbs and trunk, hypotonia, and ligamentous laxity. Further developmental delays occur in children with neurologic compromise secondary to progressive hydrocephalus or stenosis of the foramen may lead to quadriplegia if allowed to progress untreated. Significant thoracolumbar kyphoscoliosis develops in more than 80% of cases.[6,7]

Typical radiographic features include a cervical kyphosis with hypoplasia of the third, fourth, and/or fifth anterior cervical vertebral bodies. This is frequently associated with dysraphism of the posterior elements and instability during forward flexion.[7] Congenital segmentation abnormalities of the thoracolumbar spine may exist, leading to spinal deformities. Other patients without segmentation defects develop kyphoscoliosis because of irregular vertebral growth as a consequence of the underlying dysplasia. In the extremities, the epiphyseal centers of ossification appear late, leading to joint deformities. A peculiar saucer-shaped defect occurs in the central weightbearing portion of the femoral head. The long tubular bones are shortened, with marked metaphyseal flaring. The fibulas are disproportionately short with respect to the tibias. A valgus angulation is frequent at the knee. Radiographs of the feet reveal severe equinovarus deformities in addition to marked changes in the tubular and tarsal bones.

Pseudoachondroplastic Dysplasia

Pseudoachondroplastic dysplasia is a heterogeneous group of disorders characterized by epiphyseal and metaphyseal changes in the tubular bones with spinal involvement. Originally considered a subgroup of spondyloepiphyseal dysplasia, pseudoachondroplasia is now considered a separate and specific skeletal dysplasia. Both autosomal dominant and autosomal recessive forms have been identified. Four types have been proposed, based on inheritance patterns and the severity of skeletal involvement.[8]

In most patients, the disease is not detected at birth because the growth disturbance is usually not manifest until 2 or 3 years of age when the rhizomelic shortening becomes evident. This disorder results in a short-limb disproportionate dwarfism. Adult height ranges from 106 to 130 cm. The cranium and face have a normal appearance. A thoracolumbar kyphosis or increased lumbar lordosis may be present and so may scoliosis. However, trunk involvement is generally less marked than in achondroplasia. The digits of the hands and feet demonstrate severe shortening and have a fat, stubby appearance. Pes planus is common and may be related to a marked ligamentous laxity that involves most joints. Varus, valgus, or windswept angular deformities occur at the knees (Fig. 3).

Platyspondyly is generally mild in pseudoachondroplasia. There is frequently anterior beaking of the vertebral bodies secondary to delayed ossification at the attachment of the annulus fibrosis. The interpedicular distances are not narrowed in the lumbar spine. Odontoid hypoplasia with resultant atlantoaxial instability

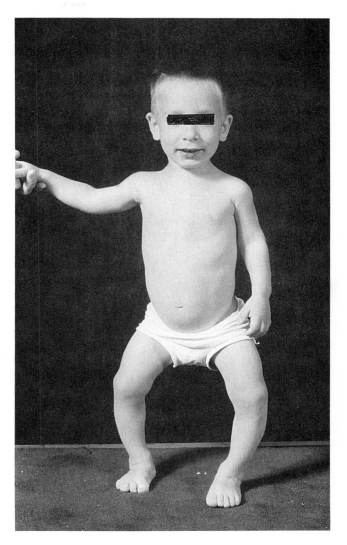

Fig. 3   Pseudoachondroplastic dysplasia (3.5 years): Normal cranium, rhizomelic shortening, and severe genu varum deformities.

may be present. Radiographic changes in the metaphyseal and epiphyseal regions of the tubular bones is characteristic of this disorder. The delayed ossification of the epiphyses leads to deformation of the articular surfaces, particularly in the weightbearing joints. There is rhizomelic shortening of the long bones with flaring of the metaphyses. The short tubular bones of the hands and feet, as well as the tarsal and carpal bones, are similarly involved. Subluxation, lateral extrusion, or hinge-abduction of the hip may occur, leading to premature osteoarthritis.

Spondyloepiphyseal Dysplasia Congenita

Spondyloepiphyseal dysplasia congenita is a specific skeletal dysplasia resulting in a short-trunk disproportionate dwarfism. Spondyloepiphyseal dysplasia congenita is transmitted as an autosomal dominant trait. However, most cases are the result of a new random mutation. As infants, these children have a normal head circumference with flattening of the midface. The eyes may be wide set, with retinal detachment and severe myopia present in more than one half of the patients. Cleft palate is not uncommon. There is disproportionate shortening of the trunk with pectus carinatum, a barrel-shaped chest, a short neck, and increased lumbar lordosis. The abdomen is protuberant and hip flexion contractures are present. There is marked rhizomelic and mesomelic shortening, with relatively less involvement of the hands and feet. A valgus deformity of the knees is more common than genu varum (Fig. 4).

Two clinical subtypes have been described on the

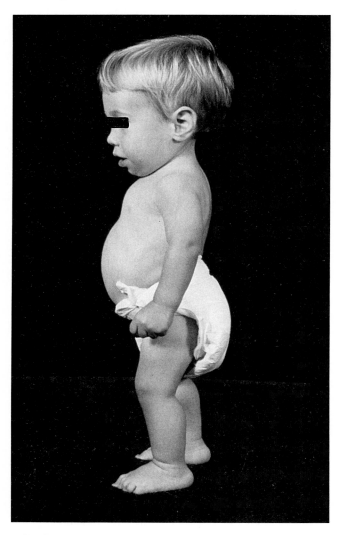

Fig. 4 Spondyloepiphyseal dysplasia congenita (4 years): Short-trunk disproportionate dwarfism with pectus carinatum, increased lordosis, protuberant abdomen, hip flexion contractures, and genu valgum.

basis of the severity of skeletal involvement, particularly coxa vara.[9] Differentiating between patients with mild and those with severe coxa vara is frequently not possible until the age of 3 or 4 years. Patients with spondyloepiphyseal dysplasia congenita and severe coxa vara have significantly short stature. Adult height ranges from 90 to 120 cm. Those with the milder form of coxa vara may reach nearly the third percentile for height.

Radiographically, there is a generalized delay in the appearance of the primary ossification centers of the carpal and tarsal bones as well as the secondary ossification centers of the short and long tubular bones. Platyspondyly of varying severity is present and progressive kyphoscoliosis is a frequent occurrence in childhood or adolescence. Odontoid hypoplasia or os odontoideum with associated atlantoaxial instability is common. Coxa vara may be mild or severe and is frequently associated with femoral head deformity as a natural consequence of the epiphyseal dysplasia. Subluxation and even dislocation may occur in those patients with ligamentous laxity. The coxa vara may be progressive and lead to discontinuity of the neck. Premature osteoarthritis of weight-bearing joints is typical of patients with spondyloepiphyseal dysplasia congenita.[10]

Spondyloepiphyseal Dysplasia Tarda

Unlike spondyloepiphyseal dysplasia congenita, the clinical manifestations of spondyoepiphyseal dysplasia tarda often go unrecognized until late childhood or adolescence, when a growth disturbance, scoliosis, or complaints of hip pain become a concern to the patient or parents. Many patients are initially referred for bilateral Legg-Calvé-Perthes[1] disease. The most common inheritance is X-linked recessive transmission, although autosomal dominant and recessive forms have been described. True dwarfism may not be present; many patients attain a height greater than the third percentile. However, mild disproportionate trunk shortening develops secondary to the mild platyspondyly or as a result of a kyphoscoliosis and associated exaggerated lumbar lordosis (Fig. 5).[11,12]

As the name of this condition implies, radiographic changes are present both in the spine and in the epiphyseal regions of the extremities. Epiphyseal involvement characteristically is observed only in larger, more proximally located joints. Again, delayed ossification of the epiphyses predisposes to early osteoarthritis. In the hips, coxa magna, flattening, extrusion, or subluxation of varying severity, resembling bilateral Perthes' disease, are typical, but these changes are bilaterally symmetric. Angular deformities about the knees are uncommon and, if present, are generally mild. Atlantoaxial instability may occur in association with abnormalities of the odontoid process. Changes of plat-

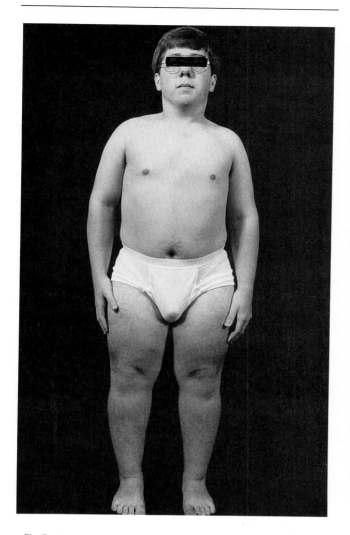

Fig. 5 Spondyloepiphyseal dysplasia tarda (18 years): Mild disproportionate shortening of the trunk.

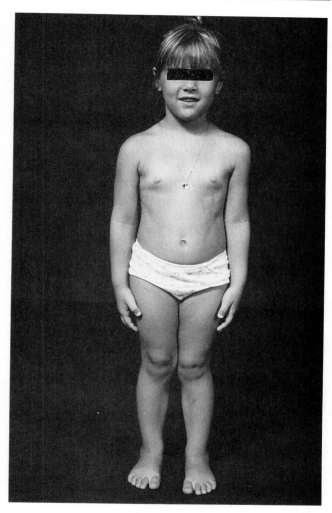

Fig. 6 Multiple epiphyseal dysplasia (7 years): Apart from mild genu valgus deformities, this girl has a normal appearance and is in the tenth percentile for standing height.

yspondyly, with anterior beaking and vertebral end-plate abnormalities, are usually more severe in the thoracic spine.

Multiple Epiphyseal Dysplasia

Multiple epiphyseal dysplasia is characterized by a generalized disturbance of ossification involving many epiphyses. One of the most commonly encountered intrinsic skeletal dysplasias, it has marked heterogeneity in its clinical presentation. A severe form, the so-called Fairbank type, has historically been differentiated from the Ribbing type, a milder form. However, these two types probably reflect the clinical heterogeneity common to many of the skeletal dysplasias.[13] Both are usually transmitted as autosomal dominant traits, although autosomal recessive forms have also been documented (Fig. 6).[14]

Most patients seek medical attention because of lower-extremity pain, deformity, loss of motion, or gait disturbances. Symptoms can develop as early as childhood or may not appear until the adult years. The limbs are mildly disproportionately shortened with respect to the trunk. However, many patients are above the third percentile for standing height and are not truly dwarfed. Involvement tends to be symmetric, with the hips, knees, and ankles predominantly affected. These patients are frequently referred for bilateral Perthes' disease. Valgus or varus deformities of the knees may occur.

As the name of this condition implies, the epiphyseal region of the short and long tubular bones are predominantly affected. Because ossification is delayed, the growing epiphyseal cartilage is poorly supported by bone. Progressive deformities of the joints occur with

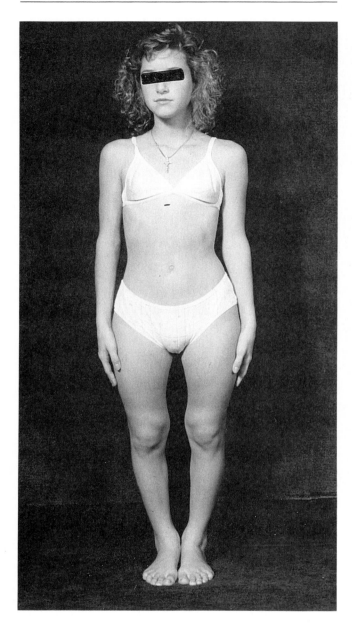

Fig. 7   Schmid-type metaphyseal chondrodysplasia (13 years): Mild shortening of the limbs with bowing of the lower extremities.

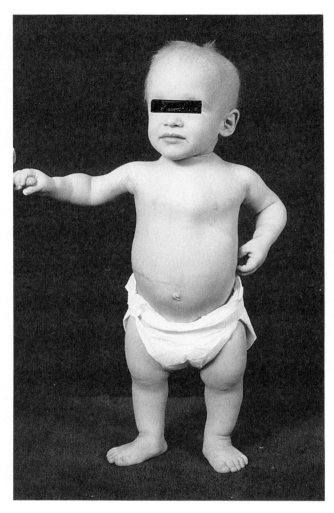

Fig. 8   Cartilage-hair hypoplasia (3 years): Disproportionate short stature with pectus excavatum, increased lumbar lordosis, sparse light hair, and abdominal incisions from previous surgery for megacolon.

loading and with continued growth of cartilage. This is most apparent in the major weightbearing joints of the lower extremities. Sequential radiographs during childhood reveal a decreased volume of the epiphyses and delayed development of the ossific nuclei. The fragmented appearance of the epiphyses stems from a gradual coalescence of multiple ossification centers rather than from resorption of existing bone, as seen in Perthes' disease. However, osteonecrosis of the capital femoral epiphysis has been documented by bone scintigraphy or magnetic resonance imaging in patients with multiple epiphyseal dysplasia.[15] Other radiographic findings include coxa vara, varus or valgus deformities of the knees, and osteoarthritis. Mild endplate abnormalities of the vertebral bodies may occur as well.

Metaphyseal Chondrodysplasia

The metaphyseal chondrodysplasias are a heterogeneous group of disorders characterized by radiographic changes in the metaphyseal regions of the short and long tubular bones. The Schmid type and the McKusick type (cartilage-hair hypoplasia) are the more common metaphyseal chondrodysplasias.[16] Patients are frequently referred to the orthopaedic surgeon because of short stature, excessive lumbar lordosis, gait disturbances, or bowed legs. Historically, many patients have been incorrectly diagnosed and treated for vitamin D-resistant rickets.[17] The Schmid type is transmitted as an autosomal dominant trait; cartilage-hair hypoplasia is inherited as an autosomal recessive.

Patients with Schmid-type metaphyseal chondrodysplasia appear normal at birth. With growth, the clinical features of mild shortening of the limbs, bowing of the legs, and increased lumbar lordosis become more obvious. The face and head are normal. Aside from possible mild expansion of the costochondral junctions of the ribs, the thorax is also normal (Fig. 7).[18,19] Patients with cartilage-hair hypoplasia are frequently Amish and are disproportionately shorter than patients with the Schmid type. Pectus excavatum is common, as are enlargement of the costochondral junctions and symmetric depression of the lower thorax anteriorly. Similarly, these patients have increased lumbar lordosis and varus of the knees and ankles. In contrast to the Schmid type, patients with cartilage-hair hypoplasia have sparse, light-colored hair, a propensity for intestinal malabsorption, megacolon, and an increased susceptibility to viral infections (Fig. 8).[20]

Radiographic findings include widened, scalloped metaphyses of the long and short tubular bones, mild physeal widening and irregularity, and radiolucent areas that project into the metaphyses. There is bowing of the femurs and tibias. Relative distal overgrowth of the fibulas in the McKusick type frequently leads to a varus ankle deformity. Coxa vara is also common. Changes in the vertebral column are generally mild, except for odontoid hypoplasia and associated atlantoaxial instability.

Acknowledgment

Illustrations in this chapter are used courtesy of The Department of Medical Education, Alfred I. duPont Institute, Wilmington, Delaware.

References

1. Scott CI Jr: Achondroplastic and hypochondroplastic dwarfism. *Clin Orthop* 1976;114:18–30.
2. Todorov AB, Scott CI Jr, Warren AE, et al: Developmental screening tests in achondroplastic children. *Am J Med Genet* 1981; 9:19–23.
3. Pauli RM, Scott CI Jr, Wassman ER Jr, et al: Apnea and sudden unexpected death in infants with achondroplasia. *J Pediatr* 1984; 104:342–348.
4. Reid CS, Pyeritz RE, Kopits SE, et al: Cervicomedullary compression in young patients with achondroplasia: Value of comprehensive neurologic and respiratory evaluation. *J Pediatr* 1987; 110:522–530.
5. Yang SS, Corbett DP, Brough AJ, et al: Upper cervical myelopathy in achondroplasia. *Am J Clin Pathol* 1977;68:68–72.
6. Walker BA, Scott CI Jr, Hall JG, et al: Diastrophic dwarfism. *Medicine* (Baltimore) 1972;51:41–59.
7. Bethem D, Winter RB, Lutter L: Disorders of the spine in diastrophic dwarfism. *J Bone Joint Surg* 1980;62A:529–536.
8. Hall JG: Pseudoachondroplasia. *Birth Defects* 1975;11:187–202.
9. Wynne-Davies R, Hall C: Two clinical variants of spondylo-epiphysial dysplasia congenita. *J Bone Joint Surg* 1982;64B:435–441.
10. Spranger JW, Langer LO Jr: Spondyloepiphyseal dysplasia congenita. *Radiology* 1970;94:313–322.
11. Barber KE, Gow PJ, Mayo KM: A family with multiple musculoskeletal abnormalities. *Ann Rheum Dis* 1984;43:275–278.
12. Diamond LS: A family study of spondyloepiphyseal dysplasia. *J Bone Joint Surg* 1970;52A:1587–1594.
13. Spranger J: The epiphyseal dysplasias. *Clin Orthop* 1976;114:46–59.
14. McKusick VA: *Mendelian Inheritance in Man: Catalogs of Autosomal Dominant, Autosomal Recessive, and X-Linked Phenotypes*, ed 7. Baltimore, Johns Hopkins University Press, 1986.
15. MacKenzie WG, Bassett GS, Mandell GA: Avascular necrosis of the hip in multiple epiphyseal dysplasia. *J Pediatr Orthop*, in press.
16. Kozlowski K: Metaphyseal and spondylometaphyseal chondrodysplasias. *Clin Orthop* 1976;114:83–93.
17. Evans R, Caffey J: Metaphyseal dysostosis resembling vitamin-D refractory rickets. *Am J Dis Child* 1958;95:640–648.
18. Dent CE, Normand ICS: Metaphysial dysostosis, type Schmid. *Arch Dis Child* 1964;39:444–454.
19. Rosenbloom AL, Smith DW: The natural history of metaphyseal dysostosis. *J Pediatr* 1965;66:857–868.
20. McKusick VA, Eldridge R, Hostetler JA, et al: Dwarfism in the Amish: II. Cartilage-hair hypoplasia. *Bull Hopkins Hosp* 1965; 116:285–326.

Lower-Extremity Abnormalities in Dwarfing Conditions

George S. Bassett, MD

Introduction

Hip deformity and premature arthritis are frequent sequelae of skeletal dysplasias with epiphyseal involvement, such as pseudoachondroplastic dysplasia, diastrophic dysplasia, multiple epiphyseal dysplasia, and the spondyloepiphyseal dysplasias. In contrast, osteoarthritis of the hip occurs infrequently in achondroplastic dwarfism, in which the predominant defect is in the physeal region rather than in the epiphysis.

With epiphyseal involvement, the cartilaginous femoral head typically deforms early in childhood. One of the earliest radiographic indications of deformation is the sagging rope sign described by Apley and Wientroub[1] (Fig. 1). This is visualized as a thin sclerotic line in the upper femoral metaphysis and has been associated with a disturbance in physeal growth. The sagging-rope sign may be present as early as 4 or 5 years of age, especially if ossification of the capital femoral epiphysis is significantly delayed. Arthrography at this time usually demonstrates a mushroom-shaped femoral head with early flattening (Fig. 2). With flattening of the femoral head, lateral extrusion, subluxation, or hinge-abduction frequently develops. It is likely that both intrinsic and extrinsic factors are involved in the

deformation of the epiphyses. Distinct alterations of the cartilage metabolism and ultrastructure in these skeletal dysplasias may predispose to deformity. Furthermore, the growing epiphyseal cartilage lacks osseous support because of the delayed ossification. Hence, normal mechanical forces across the hip joint are likely to deform the largely cartilaginous femoral head.

Lower-extremity angular deformities also occur frequently in patients with dwarfing conditions. The pattern of abnormality, whether varus or valgus, is often characteristic for the specific skeletal dysplasia. For instance, varus angulation is the most common deformity seen in achondroplasia, whereas valgus angulation is more typical in the patient with diastrophic dysplasia or spondyloepiphyseal dysplasia congenita.

Many clinical factors must be considered when evaluating these patients. Is the patient experiencing pain, instability, difficulty walking, decreased endurance, or progressive angulation? What is the natural history of the deformity for the specific dysplasia? For instance, although premature osteoarthritis commonly occurs in dysplasias with epiphyseal involvement, the risk of degenerative arthritis does not appear to be substantially increased for achondroplastic dwarfs. In addition to determining the magnitude of

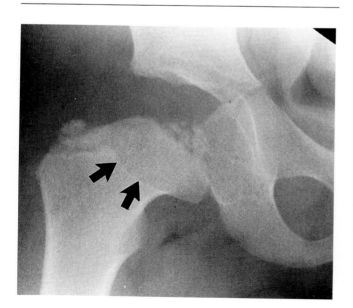

Fig. 1 Multiple epiphyseal dysplasia (7 years): Delayed ossification and a "sagging-rope" sign.

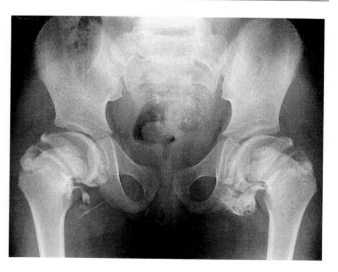

Fig. 2 Multiple epiphyseal dysplasia (7 years): Hip arthrography performed in the same patient shown in Figure 1 reveals mushroom-shaped femoral heads with flattening and mild subluxation.

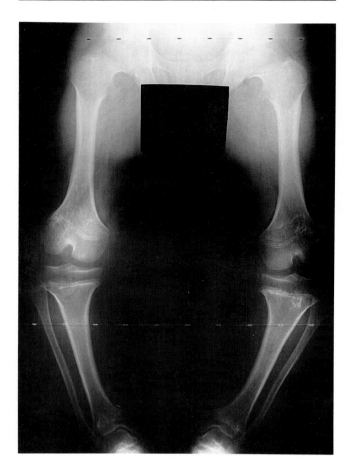

Fig. 3 Achondroplasia (14 years): The fibulas are elongated compared with the tibias, which are bowed throughout their length. The mechanical axis falls medial to the knees and lateral to the ankles.

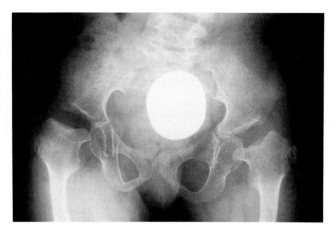

Fig. 4 Diastrophic dysplasia (4 years): Typical saucer-shaped defects of the femoral heads with delayed ossification.

the angular deformity, the physical examination must assess joint motion, ligamentous laxity, and muscle strength, and, at the same time, evaluate coexisting orthopaedic abnormalities.

The goal of treatment is to restore a normal hip-knee-ankle mechanical axis with the plane of the knee and ankle joints oriented parallel to the floor. Standing radiographs should include both lower extremities from hips to ankles on the same film. During presurgical planning, the surgeon determines the primary site of angulation and the effect of a given osteotomy on the alignment of the entire lower extremity. Osteotomies for lower-extremity angular deformities may be required either singly or in combination at the intertrochanteric, supracondylar, proximal tibial, and supramalleolar levels, depending on the location of greatest angulation and the orientation of joint surfaces. For children and adolescents, one-stage single-level osteotomies may be performed through small incisions, followed by cast immobilization. Additional stability may be achieved by performing a spike osteotomy.[2] In my

opinion, this is generally preferable to internal fixation, which requires more extensive exposure and a second procedure for hardware removal. Like other children, pediatric patients with these types of skeletal dysplasia demonstrate rapid healing of osteotomies and rarely have a nonunion.

Achondroplasia

Coxa vara is not generally present in patients with achondroplasia. The illusion of a coxa vara is created by a shortened femoral neck with relative overgrowth of the greater trochanter. The neck is shortened because of diminished physeal growth. However, the growth of the greater trochanter is relatively unimpaired, because appositional growth is not affected in achondroplasia.

Genu varum is the most common malalignment problem seen in achondroplastic dysplasia. Anatomically, the femurs are only mildly bowed and the plane of their condyles is generally parallel to the floor, but the fibulas are relatively long and the tibias are usually bowed throughout their entire length. Hence, ankle varus is frequently found in association with the genu varum deformity. In achondroplastic dwarfs with severe varus malalignment, the mechanical axis frequently falls medial to the knee and lateral to the ankle joint (Fig. 3).[3] Apart from the cosmetic aspects, progressive varus, laxity of the fibular collateral ligament, or symptoms of pain often develop. If there is excessive laxity, the lateral compartment may visibly open during stance phase with a resultant lateral shift of the tibia. However, premature osteoarthritis of the knees is rarely seen in adult patients with persistent untreated varus.

Indications for treatment in children and adolescents include pain, progressive deformity, lateral tibial shift,

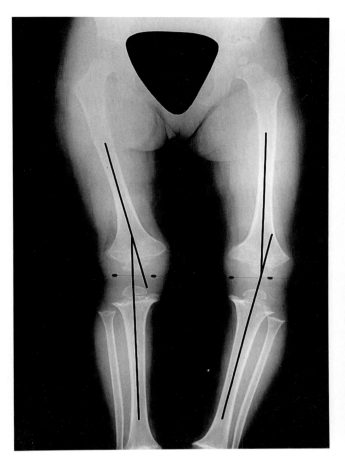

Fig. 5 Pseudoachondroplastic dysplasia (5 years): Genu valgum deformity on the right and contralateral genu varum ("windswept"). This will frequently progress to a subluxated hip on the right.

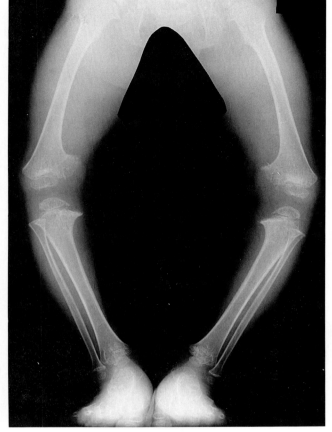

Fig. 6 Pseudoachondroplastic dysplasia (3.5 years): Marked genu varum deformities that have progressed rapidly. In contrast to achondroplasia, bowing is present in both the distal femur as well as the proximal tibia.

and cosmesis. Bracing has not been helpful and can be complicated by peroneal nerve palsies. Surgical intervention is generally accomplished by proximal tibial and fibular osteotomies. The tibial osteotomy is done transversely, through a small anterior incision distal to the tibial tubercle. The fibular osteotomy is done through a separate small lateral incision, and the bone ends are allowed to overlap during correction. Alternatively, a 1- to 2-cm segment of fibula may be removed. Prophylactic fasciotomies are recommended. The extremity is immobilized in a long leg plaster cast for six weeks. Care must be taken to ensure that the desired correction is achieved at the osteotomy site rather than through stressing the medial collateral ligament of the knee. A proximal tibial osteotomy usually corrects both knee and ankle varus simultaneously. For the occasional achondroplastic patient who has more varus at the ankle than at the knee, a single-level osteotomy of the distal tibia is preferred. However, these distal tibial osteotomies usually require longer immobilization.

Other procedures have been proposed that attempt

to diminish the possible adverse influence of the longer fibula on the tibia in producing a varus deformity of the leg. Proximal and distal fibular epiphysiodeses performed when the patient is between the ages of 7 and 10 years have resulted in spontaneous straightening of the bowed tibia and subsequent growth in a small group of patients (IV Ponseti, personal communication). Prophylactic removal of a short segment of fibula or fibular osteotomy has been performed in very young patients in an attempt to prevent development of the varus deformity. There are no published results for these two surgical alternatives.

Diastrophic Dysplasia

Coxa vara is commonly present in diastrophic dysplasia. In addition, these patients typically have a defect of epiphyseal ossification that produces a saucer-shaped depression in the superior aspect of the femoral head

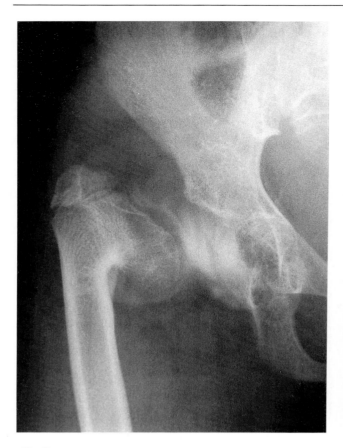 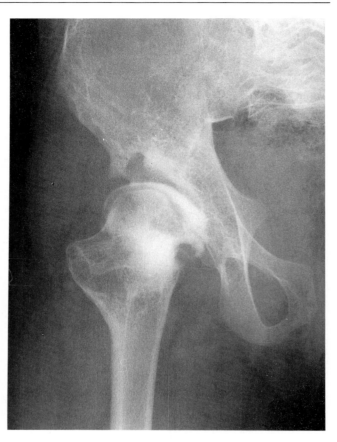

Fig. 7 Spondyloepiphyseal dysplasia congenita (9 years). **Left,** Preoperative arthrogram demonstrating severe coxa vara and dislocation. **Right,** Arthrogram after simultaneous open reduction, Chiari osteotomy, and valgus intertrochanteric osteotomy. (Reproduced with permission from Bassett GS, Scott CI Jr: Hip abnormalities in dwarfism, in Balderston RA, Rothman RH (eds): *The Hip.* Philadelphia, Lea & Febiger, in press.)

(Fig. 4). Marked incongruity of the femoral head and acetabulum results, often in association with subluxation. Hip dislocations develop in 25% of these patients.[4] Treatment of these hip abnormalities is further compromised by severe hip and knee contractures that are present from birth. If there is adequate motion, an occasional patient may benefit from a valgus-extension intertrochanteric osteotomy. However, this usually is not the case. Premature arthritis of the hip is the rule in diastrophic dysplasia and only rarely can this natural history be altered by early surgical intervention.

Patients with diastrophic dysplasia usually have a valgus deformity of the knees in association with flexion contractures of the hips and knees. Recurrence of the flexion deformities has been common after either soft-tissue releases or supracondylar extension osteotomies. The genu valgum has generally been insufficient to warrant surgical intervention. Other skeletal abnormalities, particularly those of the foot and spine, usually take treatment priority in diastrophic dysplasia. Fortunately, the lower-extremity angular and flexion deformities do not ordinarily preclude independent ambulation.

Pseudoachondroplastic Dysplasia

Patients with pseudoachondroplastic dysplasia have epiphyseal, physeal, and metaphyseal involvement of the tubular bones. Although the coxa vara that is present in pseudoachondroplasia is generally mild and non-progressive, delayed epiphyseal ossification frequently leads to deformation of the predominantly cartilaginous femoral head. Incongruity of the hip joint, lateral extrusion, hinge abduction, subluxation, and premature osteoarthritis are frequent sequelae. Symptoms include pain, limp, and decreased range of motion. Arthrography should be performed prior to osteotomy with anteroposterior neutral, abduction, and adduction views. Typically, the deformity is not improved with abduction; instead, this motion causes abnormal hinging and incongruity. Improved congruity and coverage of the femoral head by the acetabulum will typically be demonstrated in adduction. Hence, surgical realignment is accomplished with an intertrochanteric valgus osteotomy. An added benefit of this surgery is a more distal and lateral displacement of the greater trochanter

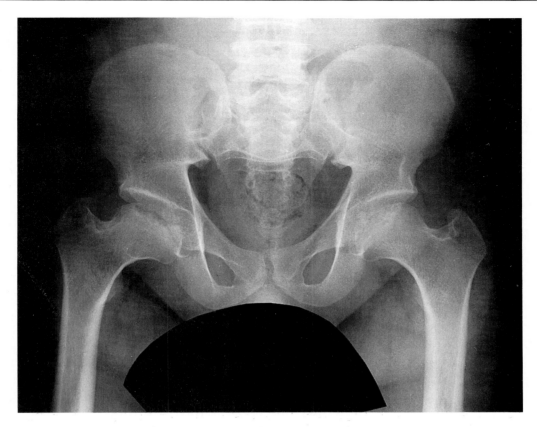

Fig. 8 Spondyloepiphyseal dysplasia tarda (18 years): Patient referred for evaluation of hip pain and bilateral "Perthes'" disease. There is symmetric irregular ossification of the hips. This patient was found to have more than 1 cm of atlantoaxial instability from an os odontoideum. (Reproduced with permission from Bassett GS, Scott CI Jr: Hip abnormalities in dwarfism, in Balderston RA, Rothman RH (eds): *The Hip.* Philadelphia, Lea & Febiger, in press.)

and, therefore, improved abductor function. A flexion contracture may also be corrected by adding a posterior closing wedge to the valgus osteotomy.

Pelvic osteotomy to improve femoral head containment is only occasionally indicated as a reconstructive procedure for the hip affected by skeletal dysplasia. Relative coxa vara and incongruity of the joint is frequently a contraindication for procedures such as the single (Salter), double (Sutherland), or triple (Steel) osteotomy. The Chiari displacement osteotomy or acetabular shelf augmentation procedure can improve anterior and lateral coverage of the femoral head, but these procedures are usually performed in conjunction with intertrochanteric femoral osteotomies.

The hip abnormalities in pseudoachondroplasia have been confused or erroneously compared with those in Legg-Calvé-Perthes disease.[5] The delayed ossification of the capital femoral epiphysis often appears patchy and irregular. This may resemble the fragmentation phase of Perthes'; however, bilateral Perthes' disease is not typically symmetric and does not involve other epiphyses. The patchy irregular ossification of the dys-

plasias shows gradual coalescence associated with gradual enlargement of the epiphyseal ossification centers. Furthermore, the dysplasias do not show a loss of epiphyseal ossification (resorption) once it is present as occurs in Perthes' disease.[5]

Patients with pseudoachondroplasia may have bilateral genu varum, genu valgum, or unilateral genu varum with contralateral genu valgum ("windswept") deformities (Figs. 5 and 6). Treatment of these angular deformities is complicated by associated ligamentous laxity and delay in epiphyseal ossification. Recurrence of the deformity is unfortunately common in the growing child and adolescent.[6]

For patients with genu varum, radiographic assessment before surgery often reveals that bowing is present in both the femur and the tibia. A distal femoral valgus osteotomy should be performed if the plane of the femoral condyles is in varus. Simultaneous osteotomy of the tibia may be required if the femoral osteotomy realigns the ankle into valgus. Arthrography of the knee during surgery may facilitate proper alignment of the hip-knee-ankle mechanical axis. If the plane of

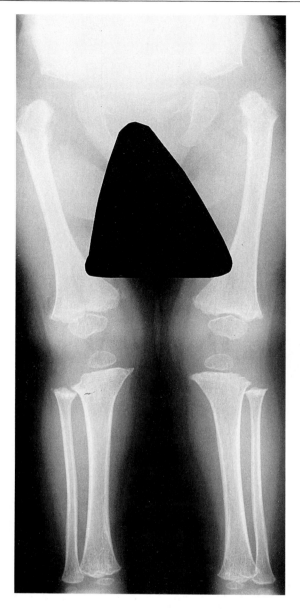

Fig. 9 Spondyloepiphyseal dysplasia congenita (4 years). Valgus alignment of the knee associated with relative shortening of the fibulas. Mild coxa vara is present.

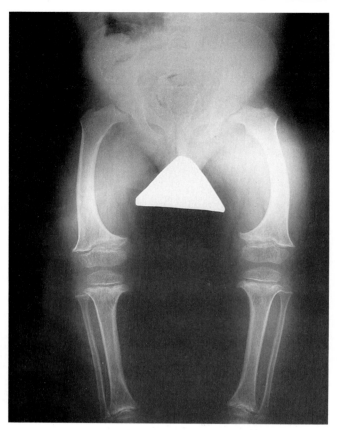

Fig. 10 Cartilage hair hypoplasia (4 years): Bilateral coxa vara, bowed femurs, and metaphyseal changes. (Reproduced with permission from Bassett GS, Scott CI Jr: Hip abnormalities in dwarfism, in Balderston RA, Rothman RH (eds): *The Hip.* Philadelphia, Lea & Febiger, in press.)

the femoral condyles is parallel to the floor, proximal tibial-fibular osteotomies, rather than supracondylar osteotomies, are performed. A valgus deformity of the knee is usually corrected by an opening wedge osteotomy of the distal femur. I prefer to do this through a small incision, using a hip spica cast rather than rigid internal fixation.

Spondyloepiphyseal Dysplasia

Severe coxa vara, with a neck shaft angle of less than 90 degrees, is typically present in spondyloepiphyseal

dysplasia congenita. Discontinuity of the femoral neck may occur, with accentuation of the coxa vara. The epiphyseal disturbance further predisposes these patients to flattening of the femoral head, incongruity of the hip joint, lateral extrusion, and hinge-abduction. Valgus intertrochanteric femoral osteotomy should be considered for coxa vara measuring 100 degrees or less, radiographic demonstration of progressive varus, a Hilgenreiner's epiphyseal angle of more than 60 degrees, or a triangular metaphyseal fragment in the femoral neck.[7,8] In some patients with marked ligamentous laxity, dislocation of the hip may occur in association with the coxa vara. Open reduction with simultaneous valgus intertrochanteric and pelvic osteotomies is one option for these patients (Fig. 7).

Patients with the tarda form of spondyloepiphyseal dysplasia are frequently referred to the orthopaedic surgeon for bilateral Perthes' disease (Fig. 8).[5] For many of these patients, the presence of the underlying skeletal dysplasia has not been previously recognized. However, as previously noted, the femoral heads have a symmetric appearance and there is evidence of gen-

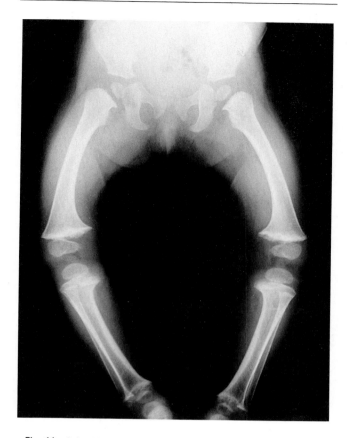

Fig. 11   Schmid-type metaphyseal chondrodysplasia (18 months): Marked genu varum with bowing of the femurs and the tibias.

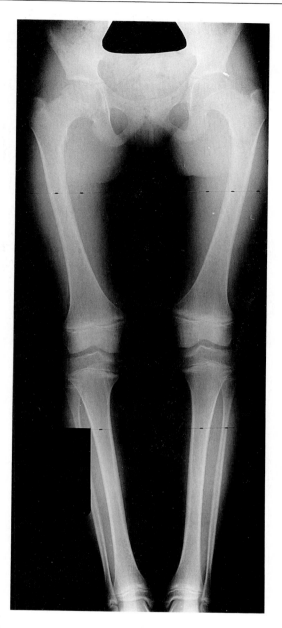

Fig. 12   Schmid-type metaphyseal chondrodysplasia (13 years): Significant spontaneous correction of the bowed legs is evident in the same patient shown in Figure 11.

eralized epiphyseal and spinal involvement. Significant incongruity of the hip joint is uncommon in spondyloepiphyseal dysplasia tarda, and coxa vara is mild. Hence, reconstructive or realignment osteotomies about the hip are generally not required for these patients.

Genu valgum is the most common angular deformity that occurs in spondyloepiphyseal dysplasia. The magnitude of the valgus is variable, generally corresponding to the severity of the coxa vara. Hence, the genu valgum is usually mild in those patients with spondyolepiphyseal dysplasia tarda. Radiographically, valgus angulation may be evident in the femur or the tibia, involving the diaphyses, metaphyses, and/or the epiphyses. Disproportionate shortening of the fibulas often contributes to valgus of the knee or ankle (Fig. 9). Patients with spondyloepiphyseal dysplasia often are predisposed to premature osteoarthritis. Because of the underlying epiphyseal dysplasia, restoring a normal mechanical axis to the lower extremity may not alter the onset of degenerative changes. Careful assessment before surgery is important in order to identify the proper level or levels for osteotomy. In general, significant valgus of the knee will require a varus supracondylar oste-

otomy. If valgus intertrochanteric osteotomies are required for the treatment of coxa vara, these should be completed before correcting the angular deformities of the knee.

Metaphyseal Chondrodysplasia

Coxa vara, in conjunction with generalized bowing of the entire femur, is seen in the metaphyseal chondrodysplasias (Fig. 10). Patients with the Schmid type

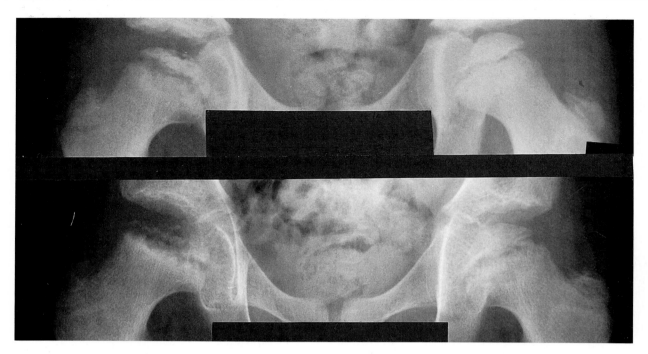

Fig. 13 Osteonecrosis superimposed on multiple epiphyseal dysplasia. This 8-year-old boy had right hip pain. There is a positive family history for multiple epiphyseal dysplasia and the skeletal survey revealed involvement of multiple epiphyses. **Top**, Radiograph (8 years): The left ossific nucleus is small for age. There is a subchondral fracture line visible on the right. **Bottom**, Radiograph (9 years): Progressive resorption on the right side. (Reproduced with permission from Bassett GS, Scott CI Jr: Hip abnormalities in dwarfism, in Balderston RA, Rothman RH (eds): *The Hip*. Philadelphia, Lea & Febiger, in press.)

are generally involved to a greater extent than those with the McKusick type. The varus is generally not progressive unless there is a triangular metaphyseal fragment in the inferior subcapital region of the femoral neck. Valgus intertrochanteric osteotomy should be considered for patients with either this ossification defect or progressive varus.[7,8]

Varus deformities of the knees and ankles are common in the metaphyseal chondrodysplasias. Premature osteoarthritis of the weightbearing joints does not occur as frequently as in those skeletal dysplasias with predominantly epiphyseal involvement. The genu varum is generally mild in cartilage-hair hypoplasia and ordinarily does not require treatment. In those patients with Schmid-type metaphyseal chondrodysplasia, bowing of the legs can be quite marked during infancy and early childhood (Fig. 11) but spontaneous correction often occurs during the first decade of life (Fig. 12).[9] Surgery should be delayed until such time as it becomes evident that full correction will not occur. If surgical correction is indicated, proximal tibial-fibular osteotomies are usually performed. Although many patients will have some residual bowing of the femurs in association with coxa vara, the plane of the distal condyles usually remains parallel to the floor and distal femoral osteotomies are unnecessary.

Distal fibular overgrowth may lead to varus deformity of the ankle in patients with cartilage-hair hypoplasia. Supramalleolar osteotomy is performed if the genu varum is mild.

Multiple Epiphyseal Dysplasia

Many patients with multiple epiphyseal dysplasia first consult a physician for symptoms of hip pain, limp, or decreased range of motion. As is the case with pseudoachondroplasia and spondyloepiphyseal dysplasia tarda, the radiographic appearance of the hips may be confused initially with bilateral Perthes' disease.[5] In patients with multiple epiphyseal dysplasia, a skeletal survey will reveal symmetric involvement of the hips, knees, and ankles. The patchy, irregular ossifications of the involved epiphyses gradually enlarge and coalesce, but, in many of these patients, delayed ossification leads to deformation of the femoral head with flattening, lateral extrusion, or hinge-abduction.

Osteonecrosis of the capital femoral epiphysis does occur in patients with multiple epiphyseal dysplasia and has been documented by various radiographic imaging techniques.[10,11] These patients demonstrate a typical progression of unilateral Perthes'-like changes superis generally contraindicated in these patients, because varus is already present to some degree.

Valgus deformities of the knees or ankles may develop in patients with multiple epiphyseal dysplasia (Fig. 14). These patients frequently have coexisting limitation of motion as a consequence of the epiphyseal involvement leading to incongruity of the joint surfaces. Asymmetric epiphyseal or physeal growth often causes recurrent deformity after corrective osteotomy. For genu valgum, varus osteotomy is performed in the supracondylar region if the plane of the condyles is in valgus with reference to the floor. If the plane of the knee is parallel to the floor, the osteotomy is accomplished through the proximal tibia to avoid disturbing the normal weightbearing position of the knee joint.

It must be emphasized that, in many cases, the treatment of lower-extremity deformities represents only one of the many potential medical problems faced by a patient with a skeletal dysplasia. Accurate diagnosis and an understanding of the natural history of the disorder are essential. The orthopaedic surgeon treating these patients must be involved with their total care.

Acknowledgment

Illustrations in this chapter are used courtesy of The Department of Medical Education, Alfred I. duPont Institute, Wilmington, Delaware.

References

1. Apley AG, Wientroub S: The sagging rope sign in Perthes' disease and allied disorders. *J Bone Joint Surg* 1981;63B:43–47.
2. Dietz FR, Weinstein SL: Spike osteotomy for angular deformities of the long bones in children. *J Bone Joint Surg* 1988;70A:848–852.
3. Kopits SE: Genetics clinics of The Johns Hopkins Hospital: Surgical intervention in achondroplasia. Correction of bowleg deformity in achondroplasia. *Johns Hopkins Med J* 1980;146:206–209.
4. Walker BA, Scott CI, Hall JG, et al: Diastrophic dwarfism. *Medicine* 1972;51:41–59.
5. Crossan JF, Wynne-Davies R, Fulford GE: Bilateral failure of the capital femoral epiphysis: Bilateral Perthes disease, multiple epiphyseal dysplasia, pseudoachondroplasis, and spondyloepiphyseal dysplasia congenita and tarda. *J Pediatr Orthop* 1983;3:297–301.
6. Kopits SE: Orthopedic complications of dwarfism. *Clin Orthop* 1976;114:153–179.
7. Schmidt TL, Kalamchi A: The fate of the capital femoral physis and acetabular development in developmental coxa vara. *J Pediatr Orthop* 1982;2:534–538.
8. Weinstein JN, Kuo KN, Millar EA: Congenital coxa vara: A retrospective review. *J Pediatr Orthop* 1984;4:70–77.
9. Rosenbloom AL, Smith DW: The natural history of metaphyseal dysostosis. *J Pediatr* 1965;66:857–868.
10. MacKenzie WG, Bassett GS, Mandell GA, et al: Avascular necrosis of the capital femoral epiphysis. *J Pediatr Orthop*, in press.
11. Mandell GA, MacKenzie WG, Scott CI Jr, et al: Identification of avascular necrosis in the dysplastic proximal femoral epiphysis. *Skeletal Radiol* 1989;18:273–281.

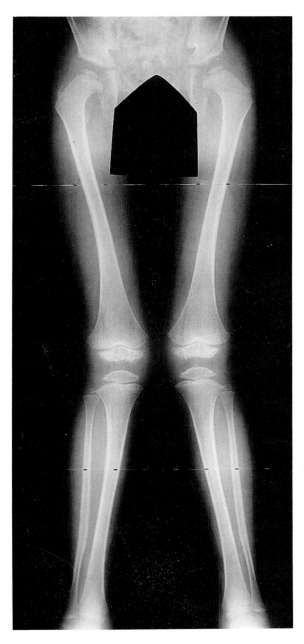

Fig. 14   Multiple epiphyseal dysplasia (7 years): Mild genu valgum and delayed ossification of the epiphyses.

imposed on the underlying dysplasia. These include subchondral fractures, increased radiodensity of the ossific nucleus, resorption of previously ossified cartilage, reossification, head-at-risk signs, and asymmetric images by magnetic resonance imaging or bone scintigraphy (Fig. 13). The combination of osteonecrosis and multiple epiphyseal dysplasia often results in a greater deformity for the involved hip than for the side without necrosis. Whether containment will improve the natural history of these hips is not known. Varus osteotomy

Spinal Deformity in Short-Stature Syndromes

Vernon T. Tolo, MD

Achondroplasia

Achondroplasia, the most common form of short-limbed dwarfism, is associated with the greatest frequency of clinically relevant spinal abnormalities among the skeletal dysplasias. Spinal problems in the achondroplastic patient may occur in the foramen magnum, the cervical spine, the thoracolumbar area, and the lumbar spine. Each patient may have one or several of these areas involved, which makes it difficult to diagnose precisely the area of abnormality.

At birth, the clinical diagnosis of achondroplasia can be further substantiated by the radiographic finding of interpediculate narrowing in the lumbar spine, even though neurologic findings related to this narrowing are not present at this early age. The principal spinal physical finding in infancy is a kyphotic projection of the thoracolumbar spine, especially when the child is placed in a sitting position. Developmental milestones are generally delayed about six months, compared with normal subjects, and whether the hypotonia associated with an infant achondroplastic child is constitutional or at least partly related to foramen magnum compression remains unsettled. There are advocates for both theories. However, because of the possibility of upper cervical cord compression at the foramen magnum level, this is the first area of the spine that may be a problem in these infants. In infancy, many of these children have impaired respiratory function and abnormal sleep studies, with sleep apnea and sudden infant death syndrome reported in association with achondroplasia. The foramen magnum is narrow, the area being reduced by two to three standard deviations below the mean foramen magnum area for age-matched controls.[1]

Foramen magnum narrowing leads to constriction of the upper cervical cord, not the brain stem, and has been reported to be of two major types: the first with posterior indentation at the foramen level and the second with posterior compression at the atlas level with ingrowth of the foramen into the inner space of the atlas ring. Either anatomic variation causes narrowing of the upper cervical cord on magnetic resonance imaging studies, and the spinal cord compression has been thought to lead to respiratory difficulties. One must, however, differentiate the breathing difficulties caused by the characteristic mid-face hypoplasia from those of neurologic cause. This differentiation can usually be made by sleep-monitoring studies and somatosensory evoked potential monitoring.[2]

If it is determined that foramen magnum compression is present, two options for treatment are available. The first is to continue to observe the child, using apnea monitors at home, because some children outgrow this problem, with gradual resolution of the apneic episodes as the foramen magnum enlarges with growth. The other option, probably more widely favored at this time, is to perform a foramen magnum decompression. Supporters of this approach report improvement in their children after decompression, but detractors state that the morbidity and mortality associated with this relatively high-risk decompression are greater than those of monitoring and follow-up without surgery. Undoubtedly, some achondroplastic children require foramen magnum decompression, but the general use of this procedure remains debatable.

Once an achondroplastic child becomes ambulatory, generally at about 18 months of age, the thoracolumbar kyphosis, so apparent in the sitting child, begins to resolve in more than 90% of these children. This kyphosis resolves or improves significantly by the age of 2 years; if it is still present in a 3-year-old, bracing should be strongly considered, although bracing may be poorly tolerated because of the need these children have for pelvic movement because of their short arms and legs.

At all ages, there is a link among the lumbar lordosis, the thoracic kyphosis, and hip-flexion contractures. When the achondroplastic child begins to stand, hip-flexion contractures lead to further development of lumbar lordosis. In most of these children, the thoracolumbar kyphosis resolves with early walking, but in some the increased lumbar lordosis exaggerates the kyphosis above this. In a cadaver study of an achondroplastic child's spine, it was demonstrated that the volume of the spinal canal in full lumbar lordosis is less than half that in the kyphotic lumbar spine.[3] The combination of the decreased capacity of the lordotic lumbar spine and the narrow interpediculate distances in the lumbar area becomes increasingly important as the child becomes a teenager and an adult, at which time neurologic signs and symptoms may appear.

The principal spinal problem between the ages of 5 and 15 years is persistence of excessive thoracolumbar kyphosis. At present, I believe that, if the thoracolumbar kyphosis is not resolved by 5 or 6 years of age, surgical treatment should be considered, particularly if the persistent kyphosis is greater than 40 degrees and

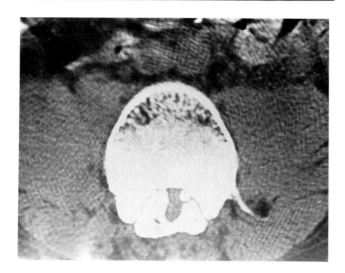

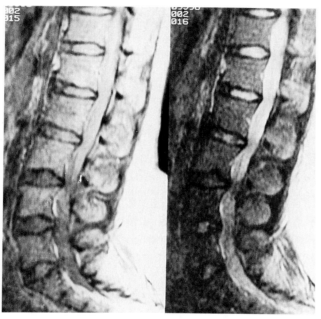

Fig. 1 **Top**, Computed tomographic scan of achondroplastic lumbar vertebra demonstrates marked interpediculate narrowing exacerbated by facet degenerative changes. **Bottom**, Magnetic resonance imaging scan of lumbar spine in achondroplasia demonstrates multiple levels of spinal stenosis, mainly at the disk levels. A laminectomy of the lumbar spine alone is inadequate and would not decompress the T11–12 level.

disks.[4] The first signs and symptoms resulting from this degeneration usually occur in the lumbar spine. Four main neurologic problems can occur: (1) slow, progressive onset of lower-extremity weakness; (2) intermittent spinal claudication; (3) nerve root compression; and (4) acute neurologic deficit, possibly paraplegia, sometimes associated with urinary incontinence.[5] These neurologic problems are rare before the mid-teen years and are almost always associated with at least some lumbar or cervical degenerative changes. These neurologic symptoms generally appear earlier in those patients with associated thoracolumbar kyphosis, because the combination of thoracolumbar kyphosis, increased lumbar lordosis, narrowed interpediculate distances, and degenerative disk protrusions serves to decrease the lumbar spinal canal size and leads to cauda equina or spinal cord compression.

The evaluation of lumbar and cervical spinal stenosis has been aided greatly by the advent of computed tomography and magnetic resonance imaging, particularly when viewed in the transverse plane. If computed tomographic myelography is used for this evaluation, the contrast material should be inserted via cisternal puncture, rather than by lumbar puncture.[6] Particularly if thoracolumbar kyphosis is present, a lumbar puncture may lead to increased neurologic deficit if cerebrospinal fluid leaks or is removed, as the spinal cord becomes subject to increased anterior compression at the apex of the kyphosis. The typical finding with myelography in achondroplasia consists of pooling of dye at the concave posterior aspects of the vertebral bodies with compression most obvious at the intervertebral disk levels. Although the computed tomographic scan and the magnetic resonance imaging are helpful individually, I currently use both tests before attempting surgery, because the combination of the two often shows more widespread compressive changes than are shown by either study alone (Fig. 1).

Aside from the foramen magnum decompression mentioned earlier, surgical treatment in achondroplasia spinal problems is usually indicated for either (1) lumbar or cervical stenosis or (2) persistent thoracolumbar kyphosis.

Kyphosis

If by 5 or 6 years of age the thoracolumbar kyphosis is greater than 40 degrees and is associated with an apical single wedge-shaped vertebra, surgery is advised. In the young child, anterior diskectomy and strut graft fusion is combined with posterior spinal fusion in a single-stage procedure. No instrumentation should be placed within the spinal canal, as iatrogenic neurologic deficits are extremely likely. Neurologic deficits have been reported with the use of Harrington compression instrumentation.[7] Even the use of Drummond interspinous wires attached to a rod, such as a Luque rectangle, with all instrumentation outside the spinal canal,

is associated with a single wedge-shaped apical vertebra at the thoracolumbar junction. In some ways this surgical approach resembles that used to manage congenital kyphosis. For patients of this age, I recommend a combined anterior and posterior fusion of the involved segments, but without the usual spinal instrumentation devices.

As the achondroplastic patient becomes older, degenerative changes begin to occur in the intervertebral is dangerous. If used, this device requires careful intraoperative spinal cord monitoring. I have safely used interspinous wires linked together to provide some posterior support, but casting is always needed after surgery until solid arthrodesis is achieved. In older patients, it may be necessary to use a two-stage procedure, because the blood loss and time required for surgery in larger patients is generally somewhat greater.

Results of surgical treatment of the thoracolumbar kyphosis in achondroplasia were recently reported by Tolo and Kopits.[7] In 18 patients treated with spinal fusion, the median curves measured 85 degrees preoperatively and 67 degrees following surgery, with a median correction of 20%. On the basis of a review of these patients, many with kyphosis greater than 100 degrees, I advise performing early fusion if a wedge-shaped apical vertebra is present by the age of 5 years (Fig. 2). At this age, correction is enhanced and, to date, this early fusion has stopped kyphosis progression. Whether the early fusion will decrease the subsequent stenosis and the need for decompression remains to be answered.

Stenosis

Stenosis may occur in the cervical area, in the lumbar area, or in both.[8] In the cervical area, the onset of symptoms tends to occur in early to mid-adult years. Both upper- and lower-extremity signs and symptoms may occur, with hyperreflexia a common finding. Multiple levels are generally involved. After computed tomographic myelography and a magnetic resonance imaging evaluation, the exact number of vertebrae requiring decompression can be determined, but it is common practice to decompress three levels above and below the most compressed segments.[9,10] Fusion of the decompressed segments is not generally needed in this age group.

In the lumbar spine, symptoms of stenosis generally begin with a slow, progressive weakening of the lower extremities. The weakness is noted in the erect position with walking and is relieved by squatting or bending forward to decrease the lumbar lordosis. Here, as well as in the cervical area, computed tomographic myelography and magnetic resonance imaging will distinguish the areas of compression, but it is not unusual for compression to extend from the lower thoracic spine to the sacrum. Rather than decompress a few middle levels, it is important to decompress all these levels. A limited decompression often leads to incomplete resolution of symptoms and to the need for another operation. If kyphosis is not present in the decompressed areas, fusion is rarely needed, perhaps because of the stability afforded by the partially degenerated disks. Not having to fuse these levels decreases postoperative morbidity and inconvenience considerably.

The type of surgical treatment for spinal cord compression in achondroplasia depends in part on the

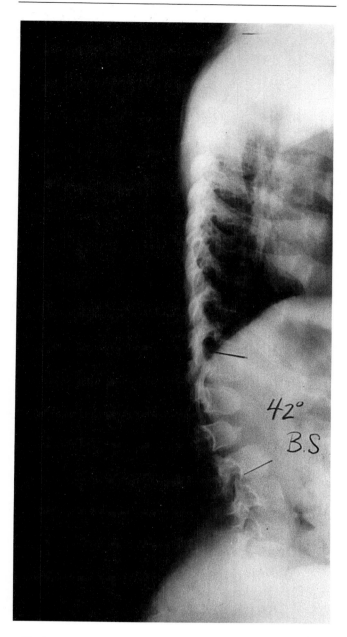

Fig. 2 Lateral radiograph of the spine of a 5-year-old achondroplastic boy demonstrates 42 degrees of thoracolumbar kyphosis. If L-1 or L-2 remains wedged to this degree by the age of 4 or 5 years, anterior and posterior spinal fusion is recommended.

presence or absence of thoracolumbar kyphosis. If spinal stenosis is present without kyphosis, surgical treatment with decompressive laminectomy is sufficient. With lumbar spine involvement, it is also often necessary to include laminectomy of the low thoracic area. Laminectomy is accomplished using a high-speed burr to avoid placing instruments into the small, tight spinal canal. Undercutting, but preserving, the lumbar facets is preferred.

If the thoracolumbar kyphosis is greater than 40 de-

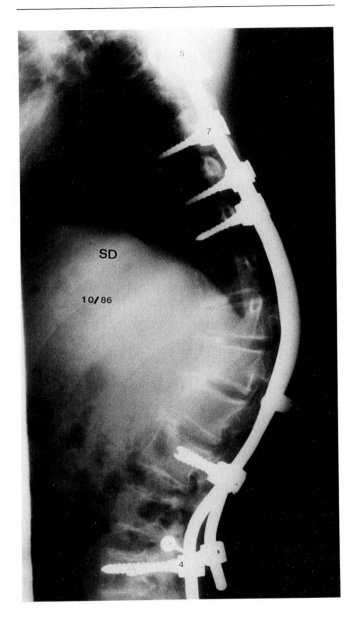

Fig. 3 Lateral radiograph of an achondroplastic spine demonstrates use of Cotrel-Dubousset instrumentation to assist in stabilization after laminectomy from T-8 to S-1 and anteroposterior fusion of T-5 to L-4 for progressive kyphosis.

ment is necessary for fusion. Following posterolateral fusion, immobilization, usually by a body-jacket cast, appears to be required to attain fusion. If 5- or 6-mm pedicle screw fixation, such as the Cotrel-Dubousset system, is used, a brace can be worn to improve spinal stability after laminectomy (Fig. 3). After surgery, patients are allowed to sit and walk as tolerated in the cast or brace.

If neurologic compromise results from a combination of spinal stenosis in the lumbar area and spinal cord compression from a sharply angular thoracolumbar kyphosis, it is necessary to perform both anterior and posterior spinal surgery. In this two-stage procedure, the first stage involves anterior spinal cord decompression by partial vertebrectomy and anterior spine fusion with rib or fibula strut grafts. Approximately one week later, the second stage involves multiple-level laminectomies and posterolateral fusion. It is recommended that the laminectomy include at least three vertebral levels above the apex of the kyphosis. Anterior fusion seldom extends distal to the third lumbar vertebra, and I advocate stopping the posterior fusion at the fourth lumbar vertebra, no matter how severe the lumbar lordosis. This will allow some pelvic movement, a facilitative motion in patients with short arms and legs.

Diastrophic Dysplasia

Diastrophic dysplasia encompasses the classic dystrophic dwarf as well as a more mildly affected variant with radiographs similar but physical changes less severe. The major spinal features are fourfold; (1) cervical spina bifida; (2) cervical kyphosis; (3) thoracic kyphoscoliosis; and (4) lumbosacral and sacral lordosis.

All patients with diastrophic dysplasia have spina bifida.[11] Upper cervical instability does not result from this spina bifida, and, in fact, most patients have limited neck motion. The other common cervical spine abnormality is mid-cervical kyphosis, with an apex at the third or fourth cervical vertebra. This kyphosis, generally present at a young age, often resolves without treatment. However, in a small proportion of diastrophic dwarfs, the kyphosis progresses, leading to marked deformity and anterior cervical cord compression. If the kyphosis does not resolve in childhood, or if it progresses, leading to an apical wedged vertebra, fusion is indicated. While in some instances posterior fusion is sufficient, if the kyphosis is marked, combined anterior and posterior fusion is preferred. Using autopsy materials, histologic findings have confirmed the presence of permanent neurologic damage in the cervical spinal cord of untreated patients.[12]

In the thoracic spine, kyphosis and scoliosis are the most common spinal problems encountered. In one series of 43 patients, 70% had more than 10 degrees

grees, progression of kyphosis following laminectomy has been observed. To prevent this problem, it is recommended that fusion accompany decompression if thoracolumbar kyphosis is present. If there are several vertebrae with mild to moderate anterior wedging without a severely wedged apical vertebra, posterior fusion is generally sufficient. Bone from the laminectomy may be used in part, but additional autologous bone should be added. After laminectomy the only posterior bone elements remaining will be short transverse processes and part of the lateral facet, so lateral bone-graft place-of scoliosis, with about 30% having curves greater than 30 degrees.[13] Treatment is indicated if significant scoliosis is present by the age of 4 years or earlier. Some of these children have severe curves by 2 or 3 years of age, making management extremely difficult. A diminished range of motion is present in the thoracic spine as well as in the cervical and lumbar areas. In addition, in the children with the most rapidly worsening curves, segmentation defects that appear similar to congenital deformities may be seen (Fig. 4).

The scoliosis is usually one of two types: idiopathic-like or sharply angular. If the curve is gradual, management is easier and follows guidelines for bracing and surgery similar to those used for idiopathic scoliosis. However, if the scoliosis is sharply angular, there is virtually always an associated severe mid-thoracic kyphosis at the same or adjacent level. In these more severe curves, bracing is used at an early age, but instrumentation without fusion may be needed, even when the patient is only 2 or 3 years of age. In diastrophic dysplasia, growth seems to be complete by about the age of 9 years. Therefore, definitive instrumentation and fusion can be accomplished earlier than in other scoliotic conditions. Because the kyphoscoliosis is usually quite rigid, spinal cord monitoring and judicious use of spinal instrumentation is essential. I have used various instrumentation systems in this syndrome and for all types the spinal canal has been sufficiently large to allow customary placement. It should be kept in mind that, even in patients with severe kyphoscoliosis, the neurologic problems that occur in these patients generally result from too much surgical correction, rather than from intrinsic spinal cord compression by the instrumentation.

In the lumbar area, a number of features have been noted. Each by itself seldom requires treatment.[13] The characteristic radiographic signs include mild anterior wedging of the first or second lumbar vertebra, posterior wedging of the fifth lumbar vertebra leading to increased lordosis in about 30%, and interpediculate narrowing at the fifth lumbar and first sacral vertebrae. Despite the interpediculate narrowing at the lumbosacral region, spinal stenosis signs and symptoms are rare, and the myelogram does not show the posterior disk bulging seen in achondroplasia. Lumbar laminectomy is rarely necessary in diastrophic dysplasia.

Pseudoachondroplasia

These patients have the same general body proportions found in achondroplasia, but facial features are normal and spinal radiographic features differ from those seen in achondroplasia. In pseudoachondroplasia, the vertebrae have an anterior tongue-like protrusion from the mid-portion of the vertebral body, and

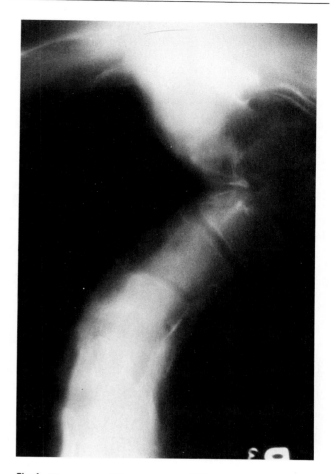

Fig. 4 Tomogram of thoracic spine of diastrophic dwarf illustrates severe thoracic scoliosis apparently caused by lack of segmentation similar to that seen in congenital kyphoscoliosis.

the lumbar spine shows no narrowing of the interpediculate distances.

More than in some of the other skeletal dysplasias, the hip abnormalities have a strong influence on possible spinal abnormalities. Although structural scoliosis may be present at about the same rate seen in the general population, postural scoliosis may be present secondary to the pelvic obliquity caused by asymmetric hip alignment or leg length discrepancy. Scoliosis with balanced hips is usually associated with an increased kyphosis, but the curvature is not sharply angular as is seen in diastrophic dysplasia.

The kyphosis seen in pseudoachondroplasia is of two types: persistent wedging at the thoracolumbar area or additive wedging at multiple levels in the thoracic spine. Increased lumbar lordosis may be secondary to excessive thoracic kyphosis, but is more likely to be caused by hip-flexion deformities. Therefore, extension osteotomies of the proximal femur or pelvis may be the best treatment of excessive lumbar lordosis. With thoracolumbar kyphosis caused by anterior vertebral body wedging, anterior and posterior spinal fusion with instrumentation is needed. Although achondroplasia cannot be treated with intraspinal placement of instrumentation systems, I have safely used the standard instrumentation systems in pseudoachondroplasia deformity surgery, because in this case the spinal canal is not narrowed.

Spondyloepiphyseal Dysplasia Congenita

As the name implies, abnormalities are present in both the epiphyses and the vertebrae in this short-trunk form of dwarfism. The two primary spinal problems involve upper cervical instability and thoracolumbar deformity.

The most important spinal problem to recognize in this condition is atlantoaxial instability secondary to odontoid hypoplasia, at times with an os odontoi-

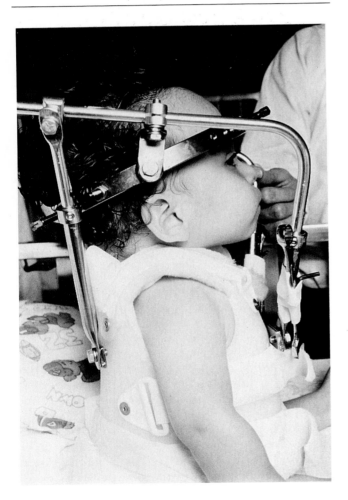

Fig. 5 This 1.5-year-old-child with spondyloepiphyseal dysplasia congenita required upper cervical fusion for C1-2 instability causing delayed motor milestones. Halo-brace can be used for immobilization even in children this young.

deum.[14] Approximately one third of these children develop spinal cord compression caused by upper cervical instability. This compression may occur before the age of 1 year. In general, the cord compromise due to atlantoaxial instability occurs at a younger age in spondyloepiphyseal dysplasia than in Morquio's syndrome, another short-stature syndrome commonly associated with odontoid hypoplasia. In spondyloepiphyseal dysplasia congenita, the diagnosis of cervical instability may be difficult to make at an early age, but delay in motor milestones, sleep studies, and somatosensory evoked potentials help to confirm findings of compression on flexion-extension magnetic resonance imaging studies. If pathologic atlantoaxial instability is diagnosed, the treatment is posterior fusion. The child should be stabilized in a halo-brace both before and after fusion (Fig. 5). In children less than 5 years old, the posterior arch of the first cervical vertebra may not be fully ossified and it may be necessary to wire the second cervical vertebra to the occiput at the time of fusion. If an os odontoideum is present, care should be taken to avoid excessive tightening of the wires and "overreduction" of the atlas. Bone graft may be obtained either from the iliac crest or from the proximal tibial metaphysis, which has a contour similar to that of the upper cervical region.

Scoliosis in the thoracic spine generally can be managed by brace treatment in younger patients, although surgical instrumentation and fusion may be needed later for large curves. The spinal canal in this condition is large enough to accept the standard hooks for spinal instrumentation systems.

In the lumbar spine, the principal abnormality seen is marked lumbar lordosis. The majority of this is secondary to hip-flexion contractures and is usually best managed by hip or pelvic osteotomy, rather than by spinal treatment.

Spondyloepiphyseal Dysplasia Tarda

The tarda form of this condition is inherited in a X-linked recessive manner and varies significantly from the type termed congenita.[15] These children usually reach a height of a little over 5 feet. Atlantoaxial instability may be present, but is less common in the tarda form. Although the trunk is short and vertebrae are flattened on radiographs, spinal deformity is rare. Back pain, presumably resulting from the platyspondyly and degenerated disks, may be present during the teenage years, but the most disabling orthopaedic problem is early-onset degenerative hip disease, which may require total hip arthroplasty in early adult life.

Mucopolysaccharidosis

Although they are not strictly speaking skeletal dysplasias, mucopolysaccharidoses generally lead to a short-trunk form of dwarfism. Patients may exhibit spinal problems, primarily upper cervical spine instability and thoracolumbar kyphosis.[16] Morquio's syndrome, or type 4 mucopolysaccharidosis, is the most common of these syndromes to demonstrate spinal involvement. Odontoid hypoplasia often leads to upper cervical spinal cord compression with resultant myelopathy in this syndrome. This is often first seen as a decrease in endurance at 4 to 6 years of age and may, at first, be incorrectly attributed to the genu valgum deformity often present.[14] Once instability is demonstrated, posterior upper cervical fusion is needed to arrest or reverse the myelopathy. Though less common, upper cervical instability has been also reported in Hurler's syndrome, or type 1 mucopolysaccharidosis.

Thoracolumbar kyphosis may be noted in several types of mucopolysaccharidosis. In Morquio's syndrome, thoracolumbar kyphosis, with deficient anterior ossification at the 12th thoracic or first lumbar vertebral body, is often present in infancy. If the anterior vertebral body projections characteristic of Morquio's syndrome are not recognized, this condition can be confused with congenital kyphosis. Other mucopolysaccharidosis syndromes with thoracolumbar kyphosis include Maroteaux-Lamy, Hunter's, and Hurler's syndromes. The majority of these kyphoses either resolve spontaneously or with early brace treatment, but occasional patients have persistent apical vertebral wedging that requires surgical fusion.

Summary

Although almost any spinal deformity can occur in any skeletal dysplasia, there are specific spinal problems in each disorder that require periodic assessment and a particular awareness.[17] Atlantoaxial instability frequently accompanies spondyloepiphyseal dysplasia congenita and Morquio's syndrome. Severe progressive kyphoscoliosis is found in diastrophic dysplasia. Although scoliosis can be found in many of these syndromes to some degree, it is very rare in achondroplasia. The most common deformity found in skeletal dysplasias as a whole seems to be kyphosis: cervical kyphosis in diastrophic dysplasia and thoracolumbar kyphosis in achondroplasia, pseudoachondroplasia, and many of the short-stature syndromes of metabolic etiology. Spinal stenosis is extremely common in achondroplasia, both

at the lumbar and cervical areas. It is important to establish the correct diagnosis early so that the orthopaedist is able to focus on the areas at highest risk of developing spinal problems, and proceed with efficacious and timely treatment.

References

1. Wang H, Rosenbaum AE, Reid CS, et al: Pediatric patients with achondroplasia: CT evaluation of the craniocervical junction. *Radiology* 1987;164:515–519.
2. Reid CS, Pyeritz RE, Kopits SE, et al: Cervicomedullary compression in young patients with achondroplasia: Value of comprehensive neurologic and respiratory evaluation. *J Pediatr* 1987; 110:522–530.
3. Siebens AA, Hungerford DS, Kirby NA: Curves of the achondroplastic spine: A new hypothesis. *Johns Hopkins Med J* 1978; 142:205–210.
4. Alexander E Jr: Significance of the small lumbar spinal canal: Cauda equina compression syndromes due to spondylosis. Part 5. Achondroplasia. *J Neurosurg* 1969;31:513–519.
5. Lutter LD, Langer LO: Neurological symptoms in achondroplastic dwarfs: Surgical treatment. *J Bone Joint Surg* 1977;59A: 87–92.
6. Suss RA, Udvarhelyi GB, Wang H, et al: Myelography in achondroplasia: Value of a lateral C1–2 puncture and non-ionic, water-soluble contrast medium. *Radiology* 1983;149:159–163.
7. Tolo VT, Kopits SE: Surgical treatment of thoracolumbar kyphosis in achondroplasia. *Orthop Trans* 1988;12:254–255.
8. Morgan DF, Young RF: Spinal neurological complications of achondroplasia: Results of surgical treatment. *J Neurosurg* 1980; 52:463–472.
9. Pyeritz RE, Sack GH Jr, Udvarhelyi GB: Cervical and lumbar laminectomy for spinal stenosis in achondroplasia. *Johns Hopkins Med J* 1980;146:203–206.
10. Pyeritz RE, Sack GH Jr, Udvarhelyi GB: Thoracolumbosacral laminectomy in achondroplasia: Long-term results in 22 patients. *Am J Med Gen* 1987;28:433–444.
11. Herring JA: The spinal disorders in diastrophic dwarfism. *J Bone Joint Surg* 1978;60A:177–182.
12. Kash IJ, Sane SM, Samaha FJ, et al: Cervical cord compression in diastrophic dwarfism. *J Pediatr* 1974;84:862–865.
13. Tolo VT, Kopits SE: Spinal deformity in diastrophic dysplasia. *Orthop Trans* 1983;7:31–32.
14. Kopits SE: Orthopedic complications of dwarfism. *Clin Orthop* 1976;114:153–179.
15. Harper PS, Jenkins P, Laurence KM: Spondylo-epiphyseal dysplasia tarda: A report of four cases in two families. *Br J Radiol* 1973;46:676–684.
16. Tolo VT: Spinal deformity in dwarfs, in Hensinger RM, Bradford DS (eds). *The Pediatric Spine*. New York, Thieme, 1985, pp 338–349.
17. Bethem D, Winter RB, Lutter L, et al: Spinal disorders of dwarfism: Review of the literature and report of eighty cases. *J Bone Joint Surg* 1981;63A:1412–1425.

Thromboembolic Disease

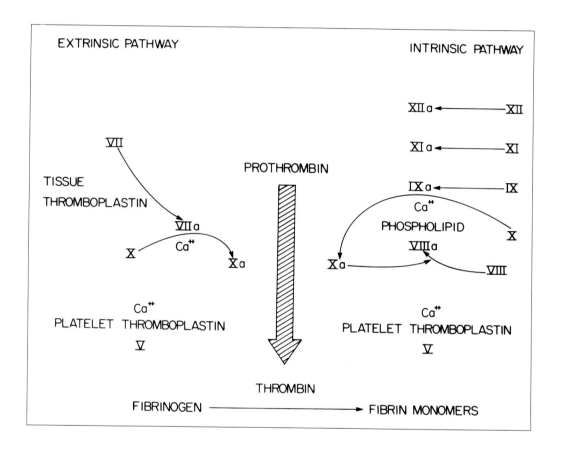

Thromboembolic Disease After Total Knee Surgery: A Critical Review

Paul A. Lotke, MD

Eugene A. Elia, MD

Introduction

Thromboembolic disease, which can result in a fatal pulmonary embolism, remains one of the most serious postoperative problems in reconstructive surgery. Despite numerous reports and studies, considerable controversy continues as to the best methods to protect against this potentially disastrous complication. This chapter focuses on what is known about thromboembolic disease as related to total knee surgery, discusses the problems associated with drawing conclusions from our current database, and attempts to raise questions in the hope that this will stimulate further investigation. The methods of detection of deep venous thrombosis and data on incidence and significance will be discussed first, followed by methods of detection and incidence of pulmonary embolism, and a review of current methods of prophylaxis and treatment.

Deep Venous Thrombosis

Diagnosis

Deep venous thrombosis has long been associated with pulmonary embolism and, as a result, numerous techniques have been developed to identify these clots. These techniques include the widely used and respected venogram, which identifies, visualizes, and allows quantification of the clots.[1] Other studies are less specific and sensitive and are unable to quantify clots. They include [125]In fibrinogen,[2,3] cuff-impedance plethysmography,[4-6] Doppler flow studies,[7] and clinical examination.[1,8-10] Monoclonal antibody tests[11] and real-time B-mode ultrasonography[12] may be of value in the future, but techniques are just now being evaluated. Because venography is so precise, studies that lack this assay as an end point may have significant errors in their analysis. Unfortunately, because many studies reported in the literature did not use venography, their conclusions should be assessed with some skepticism.

Incidence

The incidence of deep venous thrombosis after total knee replacement surgery has been well defined in two independent studies[13,14] and ranges from 50% to 84%. The location and size of the clots varied greatly. Approximately two thirds of the clots, which form in the calf, can be classified as small and scattered. One third are large, multiple, and/or involve the popliteal vein.

There was a 5% incidence of clots in the femoral vein. These were usually small and associated with a valve cusp. Contralateral deep venous thrombosis was noted in 3.2% of total knee patients. This is in contrast to reports of the incidence of deep venous thrombosis after total hip replacement, in which there is an equally high incidence of calf thrombi, but a much higher incidence in the thigh. The occurrence of thigh thrombi has been reported to be as high as 30% after total hip surgery.[3,13]

Despite strong historic prejudices, the incidence of deep venous thrombosis has not been shown to be statistically different in patients previously assumed to be at high risk because of such factors as varicose veins, stasis dermatitis, obesity, diabetes mellitus, or history of smoking or deep venous thrombosis. Neither did perioperative factors, such as tourniquet time, blood loss, and medications, affect the incidence of deep venous thrombosis. The elderly, however, do show a higher incidence of deep venous thrombosis.[13,14]

Critique

The significance of deep venous thromboses in the calf, thigh, or iliac veins remains to be determined. It appears that larger clots and/or more proximal clots create a greater clot burden and, therefore, a greater risk. The size at which a clot should be considered critical remains to be determined. In the past, most studies did not consider size, and, until recently, most studies did not differentiate between proximal and distal thrombi.[15] There is increasing evidence that distal clots (calf) are not associated with symptomatic pulmonary embolism and are not clinically important.[16-18] Because deep venous thromboses in the calf are so common and symptomatic pulmonary embolism so infrequent, it is difficult to determine if calf deep venous thromboses have any clinical significance. The relationship of these thrombi with pulmonary embolism will be discussed later.

In the past, patients with hip fractures, those with carcinoma, those undergoing general surgery, and others were grouped together and conclusions regarding the risk of deep venous thrombosis were generalized to all patients. The risk from a calf clot in patients who have undergone total knee replacement may not be the same as in other patient populations. In reality, the risks from deep venous thrombosis are probably different for different patient populations, and generalizations may lead to inaccurate assumptions. Only recently have studies begun to appear in the orthopaedic literature that differentiate selective populations, such as hip and knee patients.

The surgeon performing total knee replacement is presented with a special dilemma. Some 50% to 84% of these patients will have a deep venous thrombosis but the thrombi will vary in size and location. From the information available today, we cannot determine which clots represent sufficient threat to patients to warrant the risks involved in initiating therapy.

Pulmonary Embolism

Diagnosis

Pulmonary embolism is the major threat to our patients and the focus of our problems with thromboembolic disease. In the past, the diagnosis of this condition was based on clinical examination, ventilation-perfusion scans, and pulmonary angiography. Clinically, patients may have such symptoms as chest pain, hemoptysis, and diminished arterial blood gases.[19] Using clinical criteria alone, only about 20% or fewer of the patients thought to have a pulmonary embolism will have the diagnosis confirmed by further studies.[20,21]

The ventilation-perfusion scan has traditionally been the next step in establishing the diagnosis of pulmonary embolism. In this study, a ^{133}Xe ventilation scan is compared with a ^{99m}Tc perfusion study.[19] Both isotopic scans should have an even distribution throughout the lung fields. A ventilation-perfusion scan mismatch, in which there is a perfusion defect but not a ventilation defect, is considered to make diagnosis of pulmonary embolism likely. Although the sensitivity of this study is good, its specificity is often inaccurate, and only in 20% to 86% of the patients thought to have ventilation-perfusion scan defects is a pulmonary embolism confirmed by pulmonary angiography.[19,22]

Hull and associates,[23] using confirmatory pulmonary arteriography, found that a large sequential ventilation-perfusion scan mismatch was accurate in 86% of the patients but a subsegmental ventilation-perfusion scan mismatch yielded a documented pulmonary embolism in only 27%. Patients with a moderate ventilation-perfusion scan mismatch had a 57% probability of documentation of a pulmonary embolism by angiography. Therefore, small lung-scan abnormalities may be inaccurate in diagnosing pulmonary embolism.

Pulmonary angiography remains the standard for establishing the diagnosis of pulmonary embolism.[1] It is relatively safe and has a very low morbidity in most medical centers today. Because it is more difficult to obtain than a lung scan, it has not been used routinely except in cases in which pulmonary embolism is highly suspected clinically or following a positive ventilation-perfusion quotient scan. Many internists now believe that angiography should be carried out before initiating treatment in order to avoid exposing their patients to the risks of treatment without a confirmed diagnosis.

The incidence of pulmonary embolism after total knee replacement is difficult to quantitate. We now classify pulmonary embolism as asymptomatic (found only on routine postoperative ventilation-perfusion quotient testing), symptomatic, or fatal. Data on these three categories are beginning to evolve. Asymptomatic pulmonary embolisms are more common than previously reported,[24] with the incidence after total hip surgery estimated to be approximately 19%.[25] After total knee replacement, the incidence of asymptomatic pulmonary embolism is 8.2% to 17%.[13,14,22] It must be emphasized that these emboli are completely asymptomatic, and that they are noted on routine postoperative ventilation-perfusion quotient scans. It must also be appreciated that these figures may be high, because the scans have a significant number of false positives. Interestingly, one study noted no correlation between the presence of a deep venous thrombosis in the lower extremity and the incidence of an asymptomatic pulmonary embolism,[14] although another study showed an increase in asymptomatic pulmonary embolism with the presence of larger deep venous thromboses.[22] It is noteworthy that after bilateral total knee surgery, deep venous thromboses occur twice as often in the lower extremity, meaning that each leg has a 50% to 70% probability of developing a deep venous thrombosis. The incidence of asymptomatic pulmonary embolism was not affected in one study.[14] However, the realization that a high percentage of patients do develop real but asymptomatic pulmonary embolism after total knee replacement raises new questions regarding thromboembolic disease. A discussion of these questions follows.

Symptomatic pulmonary embolism occurrence after total knee replacement ranges from 0.5% to 3%.[16,17,22] The exact incidence, because it is low, is difficult to determine. A large series is necessary to avoid errors caused by method of diagnosis. Statistically significant variations are associated with low-incidence problems such as pulmonary embolism. In a group of 1,100 patients undergoing total knee replacement, the overall incidence of symptomatic pulmonary embolism was 0.81%.[26] The incidence of fatal pulmonary embolism after total knee replacement is also difficult to determine precisely because of its low occurrence and because the cause of death is not always clear. The series of 1,100 patients had an incidence of fatal pulmonary embolism of 0.27%.[26]

Critique

Limited knowledge about the incidence of symptomatic and fatal pulmonary embolism makes decisions about prophylaxis and treatment more difficult. Because these decisions are based on the ratio of risk to benefit, accurate data regarding each of these risks must be available in order for an informed decision to be made. Many older studies, in referring to the incidence of fatal pulmonary embolism, quoted figures as high as 3% and 7%,[1,15,19,20,27] figures that are alarming but probably inaccurate, particularly for total knee replacement. As we stratify the patient population, improve diagnostic techniques, and obtain large enough patient populations to develop accurate databases, we should be better able to define the risks of this problem.

The fact that both asymptomatic and symptomatic pulmonary embolisms can occur after total knee replacement is now apparent. Difficult questions remain to be answered. First, we must ask whether an asymptomatic pulmonary embolism should be treated. Because ventilation-perfusion scans are not routinely performed, the vast majority of asymptomatic pulmonary emboli are detected as part of an academic study. Therefore, at present it is difficult to justify treating all asymptomatic pulmonary embolisms. Until more data are available, physicians must therefore decide for themselves if an asymptomatic pulmonary embolism should be treated. The facts on this issue are not fully determined, but, at present, we elect not to treat these patients because they are asymptomatic and do not appear to be at great risk after discharge from the hospital. Furthermore, therapeutic anticoagulation can cause considerable complications.

Prophylaxis for Thromboembolic Disease

We believe that some form of prophylaxis should be considered for all patients undergoing total knee replacement. The best method of prophylaxis has yet to be determined. Currently available methods include low-dose heparin,[5,27,28] low-dose coumadin,[5,16,26,28] aspirin,[3,9,13,16] intermittent pneumatic compression,[19,29,30] dextran,[4] and combined modalities.[4,31] There have been several excellent reviews on all agents, and most appear to have their advocates.[4–9,15,17,19,20,26–29,32–34] We shall not discuss each of the agents in this article. At our institution, aspirin (325 mg) is given twice daily to all patients undergoing total knee surgery, beginning on admission and continuing throughout the period of hospitalization. It should be noted that no agent is perfect in preventing symptomatic pulmonary embolism and that all have some risk.

Critique

Despite numerous studies on prophylaxis after orthopaedic surgery, it is still difficult, for several reasons, to choose the best agents. Because of low incidence, it is difficult to determine statistical significance. It has been calculated that to show reduction in the incidence of pulmonary embolism from 3% to 1.5% would require a population base of 5,000 patients.[28] To show a decrease in the incidence of fatal pulmonary embolism

from 0.8% to 0.4% would require a patient population of 20,000. Few studies to date offer anything approaching these numbers.

To increase the numbers, many authors have used deep venous thrombosis in the calf or thigh to validate the effectiveness of prophylactic regimens. However, it has yet to be shown that calf clots are indeed prodromal to pulmonary embolism. Therefore, the tests used to determine the efficacy of prophylaxis for pulmonary embolism may not be appropriate and may lead to the conflicting results that have been so prominent in the literature. A better definition of the true population at risk is needed, and calf thrombi may not be this marker.

Treatment of Thromboembolic Disease

Treatment of thromboembolic disease includes the use of heparin in the acute phases, followed by a gradual transfer to a long-term agent such as warfarin. In general, all treatment regimens have some associated risks. In this regard, treatment is clearly distinct from prophylaxis. The latter has relatively minimal risks, whereas the former has significant risks. The dangers of anticoagulation therapy have been somewhat diminished by the realization that lower doses can give the same results as the traditional higher doses.[29] Reports in the literature on the management of anticoagulation regimens have shown a 5% to 21% incidence of bleeding complications when therapeutic levels exceed twice control levels. Anticoagulation therapy with heparin, followed by conversion to warfarin with therapeutic levels approximately 1.5 times control, is now generally accepted.[29,30]

The decision as to when to treat remains extremely controversial. Most physicians now realize that a small calf clot by itself does not represent a significant threat to the patient and they would, therefore, avoid the risks of therapy.[5,17,19,25] However, with larger and more proximal clots the decision is more difficult. Current recommendations for therapeutic intervention are as follows: (1) for small calf thrombi we do not treat, but continue routine prophylaxis for two weeks after discharge; (2) for large calf thrombi, including the popliteal vessels, we do not treat but continue routine prophylaxis; (3) for thigh thrombi of less than 2 to 3 cm, we do not treat but continue routine prophylaxis; (4) for thigh thrombi more than 7 cm in length, we initiate treatment; (5) for asymptomatic pulmonary embolism, found on a routine postoperative ventilation-perfusion quotient scan, we do not initiate therapy but continue prophylaxis; and (6) for symptomatic pulmonary embolism, we initiate therapy.

An ongoing prospective, randomized study on prophylactic regimens has not yet been reported. We hope that information from this and similar studies will help establish future recommendations for therapeutic intervention.

Critique

Therapeutic anticoagulation for thromboembolic disease is dangerous, but the risks of fatal pulmonary embolism are intimidating. Balancing these risks will require more accurate data. Because there is no consensus in the literature about how best to balance these therapeutic decisions, each physician must critically review the data and decide what is best for each total knee patient.

Summary

Thromboembolic disease represents a major threat to our patients after total knee surgery. At present, the significance of calf and thigh thrombi is undetermined, the incidence of pulmonary embolism is poorly defined, and the best regimens for prophylaxis and therapy are not yet finalized. Continued open-minded investigation will be needed to resolve these problems.

References

1. Hull RD, Raskob GE: Prophylaxis of venous thromboembolic disease following hip and knee surgery. *J Bone Joint Surg* 1986; 68A:146–150.
2. Adolfsson L, Nordenfelt I, Olsson H, et al: Diagnosis of deep vein thrombosis with ^{99}Tc^m-plasmin. *Acta Med Scand* 1982;211: 365–368.
3. Guyer RD, Booth RE Jr, Rothman RH: The detection and prevention of pulmonary embolism in total hip replacement: A study comparing aspirin and low-dose warfarin. *J Bone Joint Surg* 1982; 64A:1040–1044.
4. Harris WH, Athanasoulis CA, Waltman AC, et al: Prophylaxis of deep-vein thrombosis after total hip replacement: Dextran and external pneumatic compression compared with 1.2 or 0.3 gram of aspirin daily. *J Bone Joint Surg* 1985;67A:57–62.
5. Harris WH, Salzman EW, Athanasoulis CA, et al: Aspirin prophylaxis of venous thromboembolism after total hip replacement. *N Engl J Med* 1977;297:1246–1249.
6. Olsson C-G, Albrechtsson U: A modified ^{125}I-fibrinogen technique in suspected deep vein thrombosis: A comparison with plethysmography and phlebography. *Acta Med Scand* 1980;207: 461–467.
7. Gallus A, Raman K, Darby T: Venous thrombosis after elective hip replacement: The influence of preventive intermittent calf compression and of surgical technique. *Br J Surg* 1983;70:17–19.
8. DeLee JC, Rockwood CA Jr: Current concepts review: The use of aspirin in thromboembolic disease. *J Bone Joint Surg* 1980; 62A:149–152.
9. Harris WH, Athanasoulis CA, Waltman AC, et al: High and low-dose aspirin prophylaxis against venous thromboembolic disease in total hip replacement. *J Bone Joint Surg* 1982;64A:63–66.
10. Huisman MV, Buller HR, ten Cate JW, et al: Serial impedance plethysmography for suspected deep venous thrombosis in outpatients: The Amsterdam general practitioner study. *N Engl J Med* 1986;314:823–828.
11. Alavi A, Gupta N, Berger H, et al: Detection of venous thrombosis with In-111 labelled antifibrin (59D8) antibody imaging, abstract. *J Nucl Med* 1988;29:825.
12. Lensing AWA, Prandoni P, Brandjes D, et al: Detection of deep-

13. Lotke PA, Ecker ML, Alavi A, et al: Indications for the treatment of deep venous thrombosis following total knee replacement. *J Bone Joint Surg* 1984;66A:202–208.
14. Stulberg BN, Insall JN, Williams GW, et al: Deep-vein thrombosis following total knee replacement: An analysis of six hundred and thirty-eight arthroplasties. *J Bone Joint Surg* 1984;66A:194–201.
15. Paiement G, Wessinger SJ, Waltman AC, et al: Low-dose warfarin versus external pneumatic compression for prophylaxis against venous thromboembolism following total hip replacement. *J Arthrop* 1987;2:23–26.
16. Francis CW, Ricotta JJ, Evarts CM, et al: Long-term clinical observations and venous functional abnormalities after asymptomatic venous thrombosis following total hip or knee arthroplasty. *Clin Orthop* 1988;232:271–278.
17. Hull R, Delmore T, Carter C, et al: Adjusted subcutaneous heparin versus warfarin sodium in the long-term treatment of venous thrombosis. *N Engl J Med* 1982;306:189–194.
18. Moser KM, LeMoine JR: Is embolic risk conditioned by location of deep venous thrombosis? *Ann Intern Med* 1981;94:439–444.
19. Hartman JT, Pugh JL, Smith RD, et al: Cyclic sequential compression of the lower limb in prevention of deep venous thrombosis. *J Bone Joint Surg* 1982;64A:1059–1062.
20. Leyvraz PF, Richard J, Bachmann F, et al: Adjusted versus fixed-dose subcutaneous heparin in the prevention of deep-vein thrombosis after total hip replacement. *N Engl J Med* 1983;309: 954–958.
21. Stevens PM, Robin ED, Jackson D: Spurious pulmonary embolism: A nondisease. *Heart Lung* 1979;8:141–147.
22. Lotke PA, Wong RY, Ecker ML: Asymptomatic pulmonary embolism after total knee replacement. *Orthop Trans* 1986;10:490.
23. Hull RD, Hirsh J, Carter CJ, et al: Diagnostic value of ventilation-perfusion lung scanning in patients with suspected pulmonary embolism. *Chest* 1985;88:819–822.
24. Williams JW, Eikman EA, Greenberg S: Asymptomatic pulmonary embolism: A common event in high risk patients. *Ann Surg* 1982;195:323–327.
25. Hanel KC, Abbott WM, Reidy NC, et al: The role of two noninvasive tests in deep venous thrombosis. *Ann Surg* 1981;194: 725–730.
26. Morrey BF, Adams RA, Ilstrup DM, et al: Complications and mortality associated with bilateral or unilateral total knee arthroplasty. *J Bone Joint Surg* 1987;69A:484–488.
27. Harris WH, McKusick K, Athanasoulis CA, et al: Detection of pulmonary emboli after total hip replacement using serial C^{15}O$_2$ pulmonary scans. *J Bone Joint Surg* 1984;66A:1388–1393.
28. Collins R, Scrimgeour A, Yusuf S, et al: Reduction in fatal pulmonary embolism and venous thrombosis by perioperative administration of subcutaneous heparin: Overview of results of randomized trials in general, orthopedic, and urologic surgery. *N Engl J Med* 1988;318:1162–1173.
29. Hull R, Hirsh J, Jay R, et al: Different intensities of oral anticoagulant therapy in the treatment of proximal-vein thrombosis. *N Engl J Med* 1982;307:1676–1681.
30. Francis CW, Marder VJ, Evarts CM, et al: Two-step warfarin therapy: Prevention of postoperative venous thrombosis without excessive bleeding. *JAMA* 1983;249:374–378.
31. Kakkar VV, Fok PJ, Murray WJ, et al: Heparin and dihydroergotamine prophylaxis against thrombo-embolism after hip arthroplasty. *J Bone Joint Surg* 1985;67B:538–542.
32. Hull R, Delmore T, Genton E, et al: Warfarin sodium versus low-dose heparin in the long-term treatment of venous thrombosis. *N Engl J Med* 1979;301:855–858.
33. Stulberg BN, Dorr LD, Ranawat CS, et al: Aspirin prophylaxis for pulmonary embolism following total hip arthroplasty: An incidence study. *Clin Orthop* 1982;168:119–123.
34. Salzman EW, Harris WH: Prevention of venous thromboembolism in orthopaedic patients. *J Bone Joint Surg* 1976;58A:903–913.

Advances in Prevention of Venous Thromboembolic Disease After Elective Hip Surgery

Guy D. Paiement, MD

Norman E. Beisaw, MD

William H. Harris, MD

Sara Jane Wessinger, RN

E. MacKenzie Wyman, MD

Epidemiology and Risk Factors

Thromboembolic disease is a major public health problem in North America. It has been estimated that each year 200,000 people die of pulmonary embolism. Between 60% and 70% of these patients have an otherwise good prognosis; pulmonary embolism, in these cases, is a potentially preventable complication of a nonfatal condition and/or its treatment. It is also remarkable that more than half of these patients die in modern general hospitals while under the care of competent physicians.[1]

Elective lower-extremity surgery exemplifies this problem. It treats essentially nonfatal conditions, such as osteoarthritis of the hip, using total hip replacement and other procedures that carry an important risk of venous thromboembolism. Epidemiologic studies in Sweden have demonstrated that the annual incidence of symptomatic deep vein thrombosis in people over 50 years of age ranges from 0.2% to 0.5% depending on their sex and whether they live in the city or the country.[2] If these same people undergo an elective total hip replacement, their chance of developing an asymptomatic deep venous thrombosis increases to 50% and a symptomatic one to 15% to 20%. Moreover, they expose themselves to a 2% risk of dying of pulmonary embolism during the three months after surgery.[3-6]

Risk factors implicated in postoperative venous thromboembolism include operations in the lower extremities or pelvis, tissue trauma, immobility, age (risk increases beyond 40 years of age), history of previous thromboembolism, varicose veins, congestive heart failure, malignant tumors, obesity, increased blood viscosity, use of oral contraceptives, and inherited factors. The first three of these risk factors are present in all patients undergoing total hip replacement, and the fourth is present in the majority of them. A large number of patients also have one or more of the other risk factors. This explains why an incidence of fatal pulmonary embolism of around 2% has been consistently reported among unprotected patients undergoing total hip replacement in various Western countries in the last 15 years.[3-6] These studies had a 100% follow-up rate at three months and used postmortem examination as their diagnostic end point. The main risk factors for venous thromboembolism in patients undergoing total hip replacement are the same today as in the early 1960s, when Charnley introduced his revolutionary low-friction arthroplasty.

Deep Venous Thrombosis in Hip Surgery: A Unique Disease

Deep venous thrombosis after elective total hip replacement involves special problems. In a review of 537 venograms performed on patients undergoing elective total hip replacement just before their discharge from the hospital, proximal deep venous thromboses were isolated in 40%, with no evidence of more distal thromboses.[7] This is to be contrasted with deep venous thromboses encountered in general or thoracic surgery in which blood stasis in the calves induces a local deep vein thrombosis that propagates proximally. Clinical diagnosis of deep venous thrombosis is notoriously unreliable, especially after hip surgery, because of the pain and swelling induced in the limb by the procedure itself. Another unique characteristic is that pulmonary emboli occur often in these patients after their discharge from the general hospital. In unprotected patients undergoing total hip replacement from one of the Charnley series, 50% of the fatal pulmonary emboli occurred more than 21 days after surgery.[3]

The Orthopaedist's Point of View

Although orthopaedic surgeons are generally aware of the problem, a survey in 1985 of 10% of all American orthopaedists showed that while 84.4% of them used some form of pharmacologic prophylaxis for all patients undergoing total hip replacement, 10.0% used it for high-risk patients only. Another 5.6% used no prophylaxis at all.[8] This is disturbing, because all patients undergoing total hip replacement are at high risk for thromboembolic disease. These figures, however, do show improvement when compared with the situation a decade ago.[9] As shown in Table 1, aspirin is favored by many orthopaedists. The three methods with proven efficacy (intravenous dextran, low-dose warfarin, and adjusted-dose heparin) are much less used.

Table 1
Prophylactic methods used for patients undergoing total hip replacement (percent of practicing surgeons using different methods)

Prophylaxis	High-Risk Patients	Low-Risk Patients
None	—	10.0%
Warfarin	26.3%	11.0%
Aspirin, both sexes	23.3%	44.6%
Aspirin for men only	5.7%	12.7%
Low-dose heparin	17.5%	8.5%
Heparin according to PTT	9.6%	0.7%
Dextran	6.3%	5.0%
External pneumatic compression	6.8%	4.9%
Vena cava filter	1.1%	—
Other	3.6%	2.6%

Aspirin's popularity stems from the fact that it was widely promoted as efficacious in the late 1970s. It is also cheap, is easy to administer and monitor, and rarely involves bleeding. It is, however, noteworthy that one third of the surgeons surveyed reported that at least one of their patients undergoing elective total hip replacement had died of pulmonary embolism during the last five years.

These modes of prophylaxis should change for many reasons. First, in many studies, the efficacy of aspirin was based on isotopic phlebography, mostly fibrinogen scanning, sometimes performed on a small number of patients. This diagnostic method is not accurate in asymptomatic patients. In a review of 537 patients undergoing elective total hip replacement, isotopic phlebography was found to have a 60% sensitivity for distal deep venous thrombosis and cuff impedance plethysmography a 12% sensitivity for proximal deep venous thrombosis when compared with radiologic phlebography.[7] Conclusions from studies using isotopic phlebography as a diagnostic end point must be considered very cautiously.

Second, most studies evaluating prophylactic methods considered reduction of the overall deep venous thrombosis incidence as conclusive proof of efficacy. This can be misleading, because the overall reduction can involve mostly distal reduction. A study comparing low-dose warfarin and external pneumatic compression in 138 patients undergoing elective total hip replacement illustrates this very well (Table 2).[10]

The overall incidence of deep venous thrombosis is similar in both groups but, because the proximal incidence is considerably less in the low-dose warfarin group, this prophylaxis is probably more effective in preventing significant pulmonary embolism.

Pathogenesis of Venous Thrombi

Virchow's triad—hypercoagulability, venous stasis, and endothelial damage—are generally accepted as the main precipitating factors in the generation of venous thrombi.[11] Patients undergoing total hip replacement probably have a high incidence of deep venous thrombosis because during their treatment all three factors occur simultaneously.

The "coagulation cascade" develops intravenous clots by two basic pathways. The intrinsic system, monitored by the prothrombin time, is activated by the release of tissue thromboplastin from bone and soft tissue during surgical dissection. The extrinsic system, monitored by the partial thromboplastin time, is activated by exposure of venous subendothelial collagen and subsequent platelet activation. Both systems lead to thrombin formation and the development of a fibrin clot. The fibrinolytic system acts to prevent clot propagation and allows for clot dissolution as healing takes place. Key elements in fibrinolysis are the plasminogen activators, which convert plasminogen to plasmin. Plasmin in turn breaks up the fibrin stroma of the clot. Hemostasis is not a rigid mechanism, but a constant competition and balance between coagulation and fibrinolysis aimed at keeping the vasculature intact and the blood fluid.

Hypercoagulability exists when coagulation dominates fibrinolysis. This hypercoagulable state is present during the perioperative period. Giercksky and associates[12] measured tissue thromboplastin blood levels at various times during total hip replacement surgery. A significant increase in circulating thromboplastin antigen was noted during reaming of the acetabulum, preparation of the femur, and impaction of the prosthesis. This implicates extrinsic system activation during total hip replacement. In addition, Gitel and associates[13] noted an acute drop in antithrombin III levels during and immediately after total hip replacement surgery. Antithrombin III is a naturally occurring inhibitor of thrombin, activated factor X, and possibly the other activated factors of the intrinsic system. The depletion of antithrombin III during surgery implies activation of intrinsic and extrinsic coagulation cascades, resulting in high levels of thrombin formation during and immediately after surgery.

Prophylaxis of Venous Thromboembolism

Heparin

The concept of using subcutaneously administered heparin for thromboembolic disease prophylaxis[14] was directed at the hypercoagulability portion of of Virchow's triad. Heparin, derived from porcine and bovine lung and intestine, is a heterogeneous mixture of polysaccharide chains of varying molecular weights. As a highly charged anion, heparin binds to antithrombin III, and enzymatically increases its affinity 1,000-fold for factors Xa, thrombin, and possibly all other activated factors in the intrinsic system. Heparin affects factor Xa and thrombin of the common coagulation pathway in both the extrinsic and intrinsic systems. Although heparin does not lyse clots directly, it dampens coagulation, in turn allowing the fibrinolytic system to work more effectively on clot lysis.

Heparin's peak plasma level, which occurs two to four hours after subcutaneous injection, has a highly variable half-life. The partial thromboplastin time, used to monitor heparin's effect on intrinsic system activity, also varies significantly because of laboratory reagent and protocol differences. Precise clinical control of heparin's effects is difficult.

The most common adverse effect of heparin is hemorrhage. Hemorrhage occurs more commonly with high subcutaneous and intravenous doses, probably because of a bolus effect that paralyzes coagulation. Heparin-induced thrombocytopenia[15] occurs in two forms. The frequent mild form, usually not important clinically, is seen as an immediate slight drop in platelet count caused by a temporary heparin-related platelet sequestration.

The severe form, although uncommon, carries a 30% mortality rate. In this form, a severe thrombocytopenia of less than 100,000 platelets/mm^3 occurs seven to ten days after heparin is started and is not related to dose or route of administration. Both arterial and venous thrombi may develop in the syndrome and are probably the result of antibody-related aggregation.

Low-Dose Heparin The objective of fixed, low-dose heparin is to provide a simple protocol to lessen the hypercoagulable state by inactivating factors Xa and thrombin, and at the same time allow normal clotting to take place. This regimen should be effective when started preoperatively because of the small amount of active factors present at that time, when coagulation and fibrinolysis are in balance. Low-dose heparin given after surgical activation of the clotting cascade is less effective, because activated factor Xa has already produced a higher level of thrombin.

The use of low-dose heparin in general surgery has evolved into two standard regimens beginning with 5,000 IU given two hours preoperatively. After surgery, the same dose is given at either eight-or 12-hour intervals. Both regimens are regarded as effective for general surgical procedure as determined by fibrinogen scanning. In most studies, the incidence of deep venous thrombosis is decreased from 25% to 7% when compared with a placebo. The results of general surgical trials, using venography, have been less impressive.[16]

Clinical trials in elective total hip replacement surgery using venography[17-20] or lung scanning[21] have shown low-dose heparin to be an ineffective prophylaxis, probably because the twice-a-day dosage has a subtherapeutic effect and the thrice-daily dosage carries the risk of overanticoagulation.

The difference in effectiveness of heparin prophy-

Table 2

Number of patients with deep venous thrombosis, according to prophylactic regimen and thrombus location

Location	Low-dose Warfarin (72 Patients)	External Pneumatic Compression (66 Patients)
Distal	10	2
Popliteal	0	0
Proximal	5	14
Total	15	16

laxis noted between general surgery and orthopaedic surgery patient populations may be related to the endothelial damage and venous stasis aspects of Virchow's triad. In 1983 Stewart and associates[22] published micrographs of femoral and jugular veins documenting endothelial damage associated with total hip replacement and abdominal surgery. They postulated that the tears were caused by excessive venodilation resulting from venous smooth muscle relaxation brought on by blood-borne vasoactive substances. In addition, Stamatakis and associates[23] demonstrated venographic proof of torsion of the proximal femoral vein during hip dislocation in total hip replacement surgery, which caused almost total occlusion. Routine anesthetics, inactivity, and positioning can also have a vasodilatory effect. During surgery, the patient undergoing total hip replacement is also vulnerable to the development of deep venous thrombosis because of the increase in the intrinsic and extrinsic clotting cascade. Not only does tissue thromboplastin stimulate coagulation, but the vein is probably overdilated, separating the endothelial cells and exposing the subendothelial collagen. The venograms of Kakkar and associates[24] showed frequent filling of the long saphenous vein during hip dislocation, suggesting a pressure differential across the torsioned part of the vein and increasing venodilation distally caused by increased intraluminal pressure. It is true that the operated limb has higher rates of deep venous thrombosis and proximal venous thrombosis.[7]

Heparin-Dihydroergotamine Dihydroergotamine prevents excessive intraoperative venodilation and postoperative venous pooling. Its main action, when given in low subcutaneous doses, is direct stimulation of venous smooth muscle leading to venoconstriction, and it has also been shown to affect platelet inhibition.[22] Kakkar and associates[24] demonstrated that the administration of 0.5 mg of dihydroergotamine subcutaneously produced femoral venoconstriction from 16 to 12 mm and popliteal venoconstriction from 18 to 16 mm.

Three published reports have presented venographically proven deep venous thrombosis results using the combination of 5,000 units of heparin and 0.5 mg of dihydroergotamine. In 1985 Kakkar and associates,[6] in 500 patients, reported a 26% deep venous thrombosis rate and a 5% incidence of wound hematoma. In 1988 Beisaw and associates,[25] in 63 patients, reported a 25% deep venous thrombosis rate and a 5% incidence of wound hematoma, and in 1988 Leyvraz and associates,[26] using twice-daily doses, reported a 20% deep venous thrombosis rate in 52 patients and a 13% incidence of postoperative wound hematoma. Proximal vein clot formation has been shown to be significantly less in treated patients, suggesting that venous dilatation and intimal wall damage was lessened by the venoconstrictive effects of dihydroergotamine.[25] Animal and clinical studies indicate that combined dihydroergotamine and heparin effectively countered the three components of Virchow's triad.

A theoretical drawback to the use of dihydroergotamine has been the risk of arterial vasospasm, causing ischemia or ergotism. This was first reported by van den Berg and associates[27] in 1982. From a review of all known published case reports of arterial vasospasm associated with the use of dihydroergotamine,[27-30] nine cases of ergotism have been reported. Vasospasm seems to be more common in younger trauma patients. The site of vasospasm is usually in the lower extremity. Skin necrosis and anecdotal reports of angina and mesenteric thrombosis have also been documented.[30] It is important to note that fixed-dose dihydroergotamine has a disadvantage in that levels cannot be monitored. Of the nine published cases of vasospasm, no fewer than six doses and an average of 20 doses were given before the onset of vasospasm. This suggests that multiple doses are required before ergotism occurs, even in those who are sensitive to dihydroergotamine. Contraindications to dihydroergotamine prophylaxis include hemodynamic instability, sepsis, compromised hepatic or renal function or perfusion, recent arterial surgery, age less than 40 years, peripheral vascular disease, and coronary artery disease. Proponents of dihydroergotamine report an annual incidence of vasospasm in Europe of 0.003%, possibly because of strict adherence to contraindications in its use.[25] There have been no published reports of ergotism associated with dihydroergotamine in the United States. The American experience has been limited, although dihydroergotamine-heparin treatment is commonly used in Europe.

In summary, dihydroergotamine is effective for deep venous thrombosis prophylaxis when combined with subcutaneous heparin, and there is evidence to suggest that dihydroergotamine administered intraoperatively counteracts endothelial damage and venostasis as well as platelet inhibition. Dislocation of the hip must be done during total hip replacement, and it is specifically at this time that the endothelial cells are most likely to be pushed apart by the combination of increased intraluminal pressure and relaxation of venous smooth muscle. Of the entire hospital course, this is the time of highest risk for clot formation, and dihydroergotamine is currently the only agent available to reduce the

extent of subendothelial collagen exposure. Embolex (heparin-dihydroergotamine) is not presently available, and, if it were, there is strong debate about the risk of using it postoperatively. However, there is no evidence that one subcutaneous injection of dihydroergotamine two hours before surgery has any adverse effect, and there is strong evidence of intraoperative efficacy. Dihydroergotamine is available under the trade name DHE-45 at a concentration of 1 mg/ml.

Adjusted-Dose Heparin Sharnoff and associates,[14] in their original work on prophylactic subcutaneous heparin, adjusted the dose in order to maintain the clotting time in the normal range. When the failure of low-dose heparin became apparent in total hip replacement surgery, the concept of adjusted dose was again explored. In 1982, Poller and associates[31] compared the use of 5,000 units of heparin every eight hours to heparin, also administered every eight hours, but adjusted in order to prolong the partial thromboplastin time to 50 seconds (the normal range is 38 to 45 seconds.) Although fibrinogen scanning revealed less thrombosis in the adjusted-dose group, the difference was not significant.

In 1983, Leyvraz and associates[32] published another adjusted-dose protocol intended to overcome variations in patient response to subcutaneous heparin. By the protocol, patients were admitted to the hospital 48 hours before surgery. On the day of admission, 4,000 units were given subcutaneously at 2 and 10 PM. Thereafter, dosage was based on the partial thromboplastin time drawn one day before surgery, in the recovery room, and on alternate days after surgery. The adjusted-dose heparin schedule was meant to keep the partial thromboplastin time at the upper range of normal. For a partial thromboplastin time less than four seconds above control, the heparin dose was increased by 500 units. No change was made for times between control and 4.5 seconds longer than control. Heparin was decreased by 500 units for times between five and 7.5 seconds longer than control and by 1,000 units for times more than eight seconds longer than control.

Leyvraz and associates[32] have published two trials using adjusted-dose heparin. In 1983, a 13% deep venous thrombosis rate and 17% postoperative bleeding rate was shown in 38 patients. In 1988, an attempt was made to simplify adjusted-dose heparin by checking partial thromboplastin time only on the first, third, and sixth days after surgery.[26] However, in 50 patients, the deep venous thrombosis rate rose to 22%, with a 24% postoperative bleeding rate. In their article, the authors stated that adjusting the dose every day would decrease both the deep venous thrombosis and hematoma rates.

Adjusted-dose heparin appears to be effective in the prophylaxis of deep venous thrombosis. Advantages include immediate onset of action, easy reversal with protamine, and a dose schedule that can be written as a sliding scale. Disadvantages include the fact that one must monitor the partial thromboplastin time daily, a strict protocol for administration, and reports of increased intraoperative and postoperative bleeding.

Low-Molecular-Weight Heparin Standard commercial heparin contains a heterogeneous mixture of polysaccharide chains that vary in molecular weight from 2,000 to 40,000 daltons, averaging 15,000 to 18,000 daltons. Structures larger than 5,000 to 8,000 daltons are not required for factor Xa and thrombin inhibition but are responsible for the platelet interactions that are thought to increase heparin's risk of hemorrhagic side effects.[33,34] Preparations of heparin containing only chains of 5,000 to 8,000 daltons can be made by hydrolyzing standard heparin or through commercial synthesis of small oligosaccharides. Advantages of low-molecular-weight heparin include greater potency, longer half-life, and, theoretically, a more predictable pharmacologic effect than standard heparin. Less platelet interaction should result in lower postoperative hematoma rates.

There have been few studies in the literature using low-molecular-weight heparin in orthopaedic patients, and most have not used venography to detect thromboembolism. In 1986, Turpie and associates[35] published a clinical trial comparing low-molecular-weight heparin with placebo. With venography used as the end point in measuring venous thrombosis, 37 patients who received 1,500 units of low-molecular-weight heparin every 12 hours starting 12 to 24 hours postoperatively were followed up for 14 days or until discharge. Of these patients, 11% developed thrombi, of which 50% were proximal. These rates were significantly better than the placebo group, which had a 50% thrombotic rate in 39 patients, 45% being proximal. There were no differences in bleeding complications between the two groups. Because the authors omitted preoperative dosing in order to reduce intraoperative bleeding, a higher rate of proximal thrombi may have resulted. Further studies are required to determine the efficacy and safety of low-molecular-weight heparin alone or in combination.

Low-Dose Warfarin

Mechanism of Action Warfarin interferes with vitamin K metabolism in the liver. Vitamin K is necessary for the synthesis of clotting factors II, VII, IX, and X; proteins C and S; and other proteins involved in fibrinolysis. More specifically, vitamin K is needed as a cofactor by a liver microsomal enzyme to catalyze the gamma carboxylation of some glutamyl residues on the precursors of these proteins. In order to become a cofactor, vitamin K must be first transformed to a quinone and then to hydroxyquinone. Warfarin blocks these two transformations, probably by noncompetitive inhibition of epoxide reductase, the enzyme responsible. The presence of these gamma-carboxyglutamyl res-

idues on the clotting factors is essential for the normal calcium ion/phospholipid-mediated activation of prothrombin. In patients receiving warfarin, the clotting factors secreted lack this biologic activity and, thus, have a reduced thrombotic potential.

Warfarin counteraction by a massive dose of vitamin K is explained by the NADH-dependent quinone reductases. These enzymes, which are less sensitive to warfarin than epoxide reductase, can transform vitamin K to its active form.[36]

Short-Term Efficacy and Safety After publication of the seminal article by Hull and associates,[37] low-dose warfarin as a prophylaxis against deep venous thrombosis was used in 195 consecutive patients undergoing elective total hip replacement. All patients had a venogram before their discharge from the hospital. The overall deep venous thrombosis incidence was 14.4%; the proximal incidence was 7.2%. There were no fatal pulmonary embolisms and three nonfatal clinical pulmonary embolisms. This regimen was also found to be very safe, with only three (1.5%) major bleeding complications. Major bleeding complications criteria are a decrease in hemoglobin level of 2 g/dL or more after 24 hours postoperatively, transfusion of 2 or more units of blood after 24 hours postoperatively, retroperitoneal bleeding, intercranial bleeding, and bleeding in a major prosthesis joint.[37] There were also five minor bleeds (2.5%). Even in terms of perioperative blood losses, a comparative series of 136 patients showed no significant difference between low-dose warfarin and external pneumatic compression. Overall blood loss for primary procedures was 1,821 ± 721 ml for the external pneumatic compression group vs 1,861 ± 648 ml for the low-dose warfarin group. The values were 3,218 ± 2,076 ml and 3,122 ± 1,700 ml, respectively, for revision procedures.[10] In conclusion, low-dose warfarin is as effective as traditional-dose warfarin and is safer in terms of bleeding complications.

No prophylaxis in use today can eliminate deep venous thrombosis completely. Thromboembolic disease will develop in 15% to 20% of patients undergoing total hip replacement despite skillfully managed antithrombotic protection and aggressive rehabilitation. The question is how to deal with these patients, of whom half have a potentially fatal proximal thrombus.

There are three possible answers to that question. First, during their hospital stay, efficacious prophylaxis can be administered, stopping when the patient leaves the hospital. The risk of developing a fatal pulmonary embolism in such circumstances has been estimated at around 0.8%.[38] A second answer is to perform a routine venogram on all patients before they leave the hospital, in order to diagnose and to treat those in whom deep venous thrombosis develops despite the prophylaxis. This option, while efficacious in terms of lives saved, would be very expensive.[38] A third answer is to assume that all patients have a proximal deep venous thrombosis at the time of discharge and to treat them accordingly, with low-dose warfarin, for 12 weeks. This alternative would treat adequately the 15% to 20% of patients with deep venous thrombosis, but would expose the remaining 80% to the bleeding complications of a 12-week course of low-dose warfarin. Table 3 lists five different strategies for dealing with venous thromboembolic disease in a theoretical group of 1,000 patients undergoing total hip replacement.

Using published figures for deep venous thrombosis, fatal and nonfatal pulmonary embolism incidences, and charges in effect at the Massachusetts General Hospital in August 1985, the theoretical study outlined in Table 3 reached striking conclusions. Using low-dose warfarin (strategy C) is cheaper by $200,000 than using no prophylaxis at all (strategy A). Doing so also spares at least 12 patients per 1,000 a fatal pulmonary embolism. If one adds routine venography to low-dose warfarin (strategy D), the incidence of fatal pulmonary embolism is reduced to 0.2 per 1,000 total hip replacement patients, but at a cost of around $100,000 per extra life saved.

Strategy E (low-dose warfarin for 12 weeks for all patients and no radiologic phlebography) may solve the dilemma of giving high-quality health care at reasonable cost. This strategy reduces the fatal pulmonary embolism incidence from 20 per 1,000 to 0.18 per 1,000, and its cost is the same as using no prophylaxis at all and relying on clinical surveillance of deep venous thrombosis (strategy A).

In order to validate this strategy, 291 consecutive patients undergoing total hip replacement were given low-dose warfarin for 12 weeks after surgery without routine venography. Patients were given 10 mg of warfarin orally the night before surgery, and 5 mg orally the night of surgery. The dosage was reduced for very old patients or if blood losses were excessive. Thereafter, the warfarin dosage was adjusted to keep the prothrombin time between 1.25 and 1.50 times control. The number of patients who completed the full 12-week, low-dose warfarin course was 268.

Patients were discharged on warfarin, and their prothrombin time was monitored twice a week for the first two weeks, once a week for the following two weeks, and once every other week for the remainder of the study, unless otherwise indicated. Each patient was seen at least once between the third and the sixth months after surgery.

There was no fatal pulmonary embolism during the six months after surgery (100% follow-up rate). Symptomatic nonfatal pulmonary embolism developed in two patients during their hospital stay as proven by angiography. During the course of study, 13 patients reported some sort of chest symptoms after discharge. Two were proven to have purely cardiac problems, three had a negative ventilation-perfusion scan, and one had a positive ventilation-perfusion scan but a negative pulmonary angiogram. The remaining seven patients felt that their symptoms were not severe or persistent enough to require medical attention.

There were ten major bleeding complications, all during the hospital stay. Nine were wound bleeds and one was a gastrointestinal bleed. There were also 22 minor bleeding complications, six during the hospital

Table 3
Efficacy and cost effectiveness of various prophylactic strategies in dollars and lives saved for 1,000 patients undergoing total hip replacement

Prophylactic Strategies	Deep Venous Thrombosis (No.)	Deep Venous Thrombosis Diagnosed (No.)	Fatal Pulmonary Embolism (No.)	Symptomatic Nonfatal Pulmonary Embolism (No.)	Cost of Thromboembolism Treatment
A. No prophylaxis, clinical surveillance	450	150	19.91	20	$550,100
B. No prophylaxis, routine venography	450	450	1.45	20	$1,503,879
C. Low-dose warfarin, clinical surveillance	180	60	7.92	7.92	$290,299
D. Low-dose warfarin, routine venography	180	170	0.18	7.92	$1,096,720 ($1,032,613)*
E. Low-dose warfarin for three months for all patients, no venography	180	Not applicable	0.18	7.92	$571,038

*Figure in parentheses is for conservative treatment hypothesis, that is, treatment of proximal thrombi and large calf thrombi only.

stay and 16 after discharge. None of the 22 required specific treatment.

This bleeding complication rate compares favorably with medical patients on mid-length and long-term anticoagulotherapy. This protocol is a feasible solution to the problem of protecting the patient against pulmonary embolism at an expense bearable by the healthcare system. The 12-week, low-dose warfarin regimen, without radiologic phlebography, is cost-effective, efficacious, and safe.

Outpatient Anticoagulation Therapy: Practical Aspects Management of anticoagulation outside the hospital can be a major problem for the busy physician. Management can be done by a general practitioner, an internist, or an anticoagulation unit.

At the Massachusetts General Hospital, patients are referred to the Anticoagulation Unit. This unit was set up to manage anticoagulation for a large volume of outpatients. Patient's names, addresses, telephone numbers, test results, warfarin dosages, and pertinent medical information are logged into a computer database connected to the central processing unit of the hospital.

The computer program sorts patients according to their prothrombin time levels. They are sorted into categories of those who are in-range (1.2 to 1.5 times control), high-range (more than 1.5 times control), low-range (less than 1.2 times control), or unstable. To fall into the unstable group, the last four prothrombin time levels are considered for any fluctuations out of range.

Postcards are printed for those patients who are in-range, high-, or low-range. Patients are notified by mail of test results and any necessary changes in the dosages. For those in the unstable category, the anticoagulation unit telephones the patients to inform them of the warfarin dose and when the next test is to be done.

Warfarin dosages are adjusted according to the total number of milligrams prescribed for one week. Conservative adjustment is preferred. Our routine is a 10% increase or decrease, whichever is needed.

Patients who are not local are asked to locate a laboratory facility in their area to do the prothrombin time and partial thromboplastin time measurements. Any hospital will do these tests. They are usually less expensive, and will often bill the insurance company directly. The only drawbacks in using a hospital laboratory are that it takes longer for the patient to have a blood sample taken, the paperwork may involve registration for each blood test, and the hospital location may be inconvenient.

Commercial laboratories, now available in many areas, have several advantages. One is convenience, because many have readily accessible drawing stations in smaller communities. Moreover, they offer extended in-home services for patients who are unable to go to a laboratory. Although they are often more expensive,

they usually require only a doctor's written order, and waiting time is minimal.

For patients who require in-home laboratory services, visiting nurses are available. Visiting nurses may have difficulty getting insurance payment for patients who require no other care other than obtaining a blood sample. Because this is not considered a skilled nursing need, the patient may not be allowed payment. Written referrals are usually required to obtain a visiting nurse's service. If a patient lives in a different state, a local physician may have to write such a referral. Visiting nurses may be of assistance in locating a commercial laboratory.

Patient Education A detailed teaching program for patients preparing for discharge on warfarin therapy will provide better informed and more cooperative patients. The main goal is safety in patient care along with the best treatment available for the patient.

A teaching program should tell the patient what warfarin is and what it does. Patients receive an identification wallet card and a Medi-Alert bracelet in case of an accident or emergency. They also receive a patient instruction booklet that lists drugs that cannot be taken in conjunction with warfarin and drugs that can be taken with caution. Patients are to notify the Anticoagulation Clinic if they begin taking these or any drug. They are taught to recognize the signs of abnormal bleeding and thromboembolic disease. Dental work is to be avoided during the 12 weeks. They also receive dietary counseling. Written information is supplied for easy reference.

Because safety is a major concern, patients are given only one size of warfarin pill, either 2 mg or 5 mg. A specific point is made of telling them not to make up a dose if they miss one, but to report any missed dose to the clinic the next time they have blood test.

Conclusion

Subcutaneous heparin is still used as prophylaxis against thromboembolism in elective lower-extremity orthopaedic surgery. However, its effectiveness was initially based on clinical studies using nonvenographic testing techniques, and recent studies question the efficacy of low-dose heparin in patients undergoing total hip replacement when venography is used as the diagnostic end point. Presently, if one is to use heparin, the adjusted dose is the only method available that is both effective and safe. Its disadvantages are significant, however, in terms of bleeding complications, cost, and demands on the nursing and medical staff. It is too early to predict whether low-molecular-weight heparin will prove to be an improvement over standard heparin.

Based on data covered in this review, the authors believe there is an excellent scientific and clinical basis for the use of one 0.5-mg dose of dihydroergotamine administered subcutaneously two hours before surgery with or followed by a regimen of a standard periodic dose of low-molecular-weight heparin. This method theoretically addresses two parts of Virchow's triad, and thigh-high sequential compression boots are easily added for patients with additional risk factors, thereby covering the third part of the triad. In addition, such a protocol is cost-effective, easily administered, and well accepted by patients and staff. On the basis of this theory, we intend to study the technique of low-molecular-weight heparin and single-dose dihydroergotamine in future clinical trials, and we encourage others to do the same.

Low-dose warfarin has all the efficacy of traditional higher-dose warfarin without much of its bleeding complication risk. It has a definitive advantage in terms of efficiency, because the 10% to 20% of patients receiving the current recommended prophylaxis in whom deep venous thrombosis has developed at the time of discharge can receive low-dose warfarin for another 12 weeks. If the patient is already receiving low-dose warfarin prophylaxis, anticoagulation is maintained at the same level for three months without a prolonged hospital stay, new monitoring, or medication change.

If, at the time of discharge, one cannot diagnose deep venous thrombosis because of limited availability of radiologic venography or skillfully performed sonography, the 12-week, low-dose warfarin regimen is the prophylaxis of choice. Although it involves administering anticoagulants to the 80% or 85% of patients in whom deep venous thrombosis has not developed, the data presented here show the regimen to be very safe. Serious bleeding complications in patients undergoing total hip replacement tend to occur in the immediate postoperative period, while the patient is still in the hospital under close medical and nursing care. In the present series of almost 268 patients there were no serious bleeding complications after discharge, and the minor ones were negligible in severity.

Judged by data currently available, low-dose warfarin is as safe and efficacious as any other recommended prophylaxis. It is, however, clearly superior in terms of cost-effectiveness when used either for 12 weeks without routine venography or for the postoperative hospital stay with routine venography before discharge.

References

1. Bell WR, Simon TL: Current status of pulmonary thromboembolic disease: Pathophysiology, diagnosis, prevention, and treatment. *Am Heart J* 1982;103:239–262.
2. Kierkegaard A: Incidence of acute deep vein thrombosis in two districts: A phlebographic study. *Acta Chir Scand* 1980;146:267–269.
3. Johnson R, Green JR, Charnley J: Pulmonary embolism and its prophylaxis following the Charnley total hip replacement. *Clin Orthop* 1977;127:123–132.
4. Coventry MB, Nolan DR, Beckenbaugh RD: "Delayed" prophylactic anticoagulation: A study of results and complications in 2,012 total hip arthroplasties. *J Bone Joint Surg* 1973;55A:1487–1492.
5. Bombelli R, Gerundini M, Aronson J: Early results of the RM-isoelastic cementless total hip prosthesis: 300 consecutive cases with 2-year follow-up, in Welch RB (ed): *The Hip: Proceedings of the 12th Open Scientific Meeting of the Hip Society.* St.Louis, CV Mosby, 1984, pp 133–145.
6. Kakkar VV, Fok PJ, Murray WJ, et al: Heparin and dihydroergotamine prophylaxis against thrombo-embolism after hip arthroplasty. *J Bone Joint Surg* 1985;67B:538–542.
7. Paiement G, Wessinger SJ, Waltman AC, et al: Surveillance of deep vein thrombosis in asymptomatic total hip replacement patients: Impedance phlebography and fibrinogen scanning versus roentgenographic phlebography. *Am J Surg* 1988;155:400–404.
8. Paiement GD, Wessinger, SJ, Harris WH: Survey of prophylaxis against venous thromboembolism in adults undergoing hip surgery. *Clin Orthop* 1987;223:188–193.
9. Simon TL, Stengle JM: Antithrombotic practice in orthopedic surgery: Results of a survey. *Clin Orthop* 1974;102:181–187.
10. Paiement G, Wessinger SJ, Waltman AC, et al: Low-dose warfarin versus external pneumatic compression for prophylaxis against venous thromboembolism following total hip replacement. *J Arthrop* 1987;2:23–26.
11. Virchow R: Neuer Fall von todlicher Embolie der Lungenarterien. *Arch Pathol Anat* 1956;10:225–228.
12. Giercksky KE, Bjrøklid E, Prydz H, et al: Circulating tissue thromboplastin during hip surgery. *Eur Surg Res* 1979;11:296–300.
13. Gitel SN, Salvati EA, Wessler S, et al: The effect of total hip replacement and general surgery on antithrombin III in relation to venous thrombosis. *J Bone Joint Surg* 1979;61A:653–656.
14. Sharnoff JG, Kass HH, Mistica BA: A plan of heparinization of the surgical patient to prevent postoperative thromboembolism. *Surg Gynecol Obstet* 1962;115:75–79.
15. Barber FA, Burton WC, Guyer R: The heparin-induced thrombocytopenia and thrombosis syndrome: Report of a case. *J Bone Joint Surg* 1987;69A:935–937.
16. Groote Schuur Hospital Thromboembolus Study Group: Failure of low-dose heparin to prevent significant thromboembolic complications in high-risk surgical patients: Interim report of prospective trial. *Br Med J* 1979;1:1447–1450.
17. Evarts CM, Alfidi RJ: Thromboembolism after total hip reconstruction: Failure of low doses of heparin in prevention. *JAMA* 1973;225:515–516.
18. Harris WH, Salzman EW, Athanasoulis C, et al: Comparison of warfarin, low-molecular-weight dextran, aspirin, and subcutaneous heparin in prevention of venous thromboembolism following total hip replacement. *J Bone Joint Surg* 1974;56A:1552–1562.
19. Moskovitz PA, Ellenberg SS, Feffer HL, et al: Low-dose heparin for prevention of venous thromboembolism in total hip arthroplasty and surgical repair of hip fractures. *J Bone Joint Surg* 1978;60A:1065–1070.
20. Kakkar VV, Stamatakis JS, Bentley PG, et al: Prophylaxis for postoperative deep-vein thrombosis: Synergistic effect of heparin and dihydroergotamine. *JAMA* 1979;241:39–42.
21. Williams JW, Eikman EA, Greenberg SH, et al: Failure of low dose heparin to prevent pulmonary embolism after hip surgery or above the knee amputation. *Ann Surg* 1978;8:468–474.
22. Stewart GJ, Alburger PD Jr, Stone EA, et al: Total hip replacement induces injury to remote veins in a canine model. *J Bone Joint Surg* 1983;65A:97–102.
23. Stamatakis JD, Kakkar VV, Sagar S, et al: Femoral vein thrombosis and total hip replacement. *Br Med J* 1977;2:223–225.
24. Kakkar VV, Welzel D, Murray WJ, et al: Possible mechanism of

the synergistic effect of heparin and dihydroergotamine. *Am J Surg* 1985;150:33–38.

25. Beisaw NE, Comerota AJ, Groth HE, et al: Dihydroergotamine/heparin in the prevention of deep-vein thrombosis after total hip replacement. *J Bone Joint Surg* 1988;70A:2–10.

26. Leyvraz P, Bachmann F, Vuilleumier B, et al: Adjusted subcutaneous heparin versus heparin plus dihydroergotamine in prevention of deep vein thrombosis after total hip arthroplasty. *J Arthrop* 1988;3:81–86.

27. van den Berg E, Walterbusch G, Gotzen L, et al: Ergotism leading to threatened limb amputation or to death in two patients given heparin-dihydroergotamine prophylaxis, letter. *Lancet* 1982;1:955–956.

28. van den Berg E, Rumpf KD, Fröhlich H, et al: Vascular spasm during thromboembolism prophylaxis with heparin-dihydroergotamine, letter. *Lancet* 1982;2:268–269.

29. Cunningham M, de Torrenté A, Ekoé JM, et al: Vascular spasm and gangrene during heparin-dihydro-ergotamine prophylaxis. *Br J Surg* 1984;71:829–831.

30. Monreal M, Foz M, Ubierna MT, et al: Skin and muscle necrosis during heparin-dihydroergotamine prophylaxis, letter. *Lancet* 1984;2:820.

31. Poller L, Taberner DA, Sandilands DG, et al: An evaluation of APTT monitoring of low-dose heparin dosage in hip surgery. *Thromb Haemost* 1982;47:50–53.

32. Leyvraz PF, Richard J, Bachmann F, et al: Adjusted versus fixed-dose subcutaneous heparin in the prevention of deep-vein thrombosis after total hip replacement. *N Engl J Med* 1983;309:954–958.

33. Salzman EW: Low-molecular-weight heparin: Is small beautiful?, editorial. *N Engl J Med* 1986;315:957–959.

34. Salzman EW, Rosenberg RD, Smith MH, et al: Effect of heparin and heparin fractions on platelet aggregation. *J Clin Invest* 1980;65:64–73.

35. Turpie AGG, Levine MN, Hirsh J, et al: A randomized controlled trial of a low-molecular-weight heparin (Enoxaparin) to prevent deep-vein thrombosis in patients undergoing elective hip surgery. *N Engl J Med* 1986;315:925–929.

36. Wessler S, Becker CG, Nemerson Y: The biochemical basis of warfarin, in Suttic JW (ed): *The New Dimensions of Warfarin Prophylaxis.* New York, Plenum Press, 1987, pp 3–16.

37. Hull R, Hirsh J, Jay R, et al: Different intensities of oral anticoagulant therapy in the treatment of proximal-vein thrombosis. *N Engl J Med* 1982;307:1676–1681.

38. Paiement GD, Bell D, Wessinger SJ, et al: New advances in the prevention, diagnosis and cost effectiveness of venous thromboembolic disease in patients with total hip replacement in, *The Hip: Proceedings of the 14th Open Scientific Meeting of the Hip Society.* St. Louis, CV Mosby, 1987, pp 87–119.

Blood and Blood Products

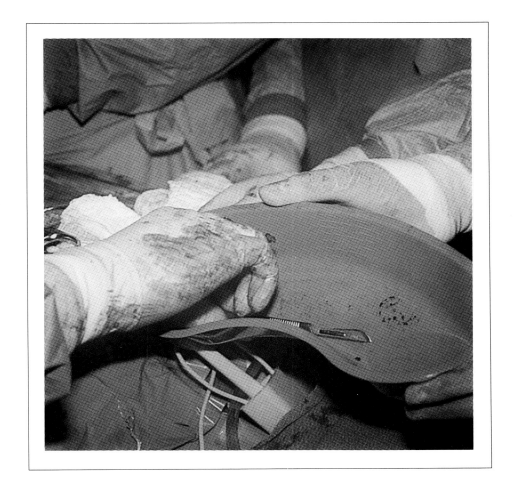

Blood Conservation Techniques in Orthopaedic Surgery

Carl L. Nelson, MD

Ruth L. Nelson, MD

John Cone, MD

Introduction

Because of increasing concern about the use of homologous transfusions, an important goal for orthopaedic surgeons is to reduce the number of such transfusions. Methods to reduce blood loss during surgery and to retrieve blood intraoperatively have been available for many years. These include selective arterial embolization, preoperative and intraoperative autotransfusion, hypotensive anesthesia, hemodilution, preplanned surgery, and meticulous hemostasis. These techniques have long been available, but have not been used routinely until recently, when acquired immune deficiency syndrome (AIDS) became a concern. Fear of acquiring AIDS from homologous transfusions stimulated many patients and orthopaedic surgeons to consider methods of reducing blood loss at the time of surgery and to avoid using homologous transfusions. The purpose of this report is to review the dangers of homologous transfusion, the physiologic indications for transfusion, and the various methods of minimizing blood loss.

Dangers of Homologous Transfusions

How dangerous are transfusions? With present screening techniques, it appears the chance of contracting AIDS from a homologous transfusion is 1 in 40,000. The chance of contracting hepatitis is 1% to 3% and is proportional to the number of transfusions.[1,2] These data alone are enough to encourage one to reduce homologous transfusions.

Attitude Toward Homologous Transfusions

To reduce the use of homologous transfusions, it is necessary to consider blood-conserving techniques, and also the criteria used to determine whether a transfusion is needed.

A question that may be asked is, do physicians use homologous transfusions too often? In 1981, an NIH-sponsored panel concluded that 25% of whole-blood transfusions were unjustified. Although this statement reflects opinion rather than specific irrefutable data, it represents a consensus from a group of experts knowledgeable about blood products and their use. Most unnecessary homologous transfusions were probably given because the traditional guidelines for transfusion are too liberal. It is time to reconsider the general policy that transfusions should be given when the hemoglobin is 10 g/dl or less, or the hematocrit is 30% or less. Basing transfusion policies on the hemoglobin concentration alone is not justified, because shock is rarely caused by anemia alone. In practice, a patient who is acutely or chronically anemic may function well if normal blood volume is maintained.[3] It is clear that tissue perfusion and adequate oxygen tension are the essential determinants, and these factors vary among individuals.[4] The hemoglobin mass of a 70-kg man is capable of delivering 1,000 ml of oxygen per minute to the tissues. Yet, the oxygen needs of a man at rest may only be 250 ml/min.[5] Oxyhemoglobin disassociation permits 60% delivery of bound oxygen, and it is possible for a patient with a hemoglobin of 6.5 g/dl to deliver the required 250 ml/min. In many patients, hematocrit levels in the low twenties and high teens will not cause significant ill effects, and, in general, lower postoperative hematocrits are more acceptable than previously thought.

Preoperative Preparation and Preplanned Surgery

Preplanning of surgery can minimize unexpected occurrences and alert the physician to those aspects of the procedure that have a potential for rapid blood loss and therefore require special precautions. Rehearsal promotes efficiency and reduces the time spent during critical surgical steps. Presurgical planning also insures that appropriate equipment and implants will be available in the operating room. Preparation for joint arthroplasties requires careful measurement of preoperative radiographs to select appropriate acetabular and femoral components. In revision surgery, it is essential that revision components or custom-made prostheses be ready before surgery. Because most fractures are amenable to preoperative implant sizing, many decisions can be made before surgery commences. These preoperative efforts will minimize the constant oozing of blood that occurs when unnecessary delays prolong the operation.

Medications To Reduce Blood Loss

The preoperative administration of drugs to decrease blood loss at the time of surgery is a newer concept.

Kobrinsky and associates[6] reported results of a randomized, double-blind, controlled trial of desmopressin (1-desamino-8-D-arginine vasopressin) in patients having Harrington rod spinal fusion surgery. The study groups comprised 35 patients with normal hemostatic function; 17 patients received desmopressin and 18 received a placebo. Preoperative testing established that desmopressin increased factor VIII coagulant activity, von Willebrand antigen concentration, glass-bead platelet retention, and prothrombin consumption, and decreased the partial thromboplastin and bleeding times. Blood loss at the time of surgery in the desmopressin group decreased by 32.5%. The administration of desmopressin results in fluid shift consistent with the observed decrease in mean platelet volume and hematocrit. However, data are not available regarding the effect of desmopressin on the incidence of deep venous thrombosis and pulmonary embolism. Accordingly, the use of this drug requires further study.

Selective Arterial Embolization

If a surgical procedure has the potential for excessive blood loss, a preoperative arteriogram or venogram can provide critical information.[7] After careful analysis of the vascular network serving the area to be operated on, selective embolization can be used before, during, or even after the surgical procedure. Materials used successfully include sterile absorbable gelatin sponge, lyophilized human dura mater, steel coils, plastic or glass beads, detachable balloons, and rapidly setting polymers such as isobutyl-2-cyanoacrylate (IBC).[8] Selective arterial embolization has proven especially helpful in the management of tumors[9-11] and pelvic fractures.[12-14]

Hypotensive Anesthesia

Multiple studies have shown that hypotensive anesthesia can effectively reduce intraoperative blood loss.[15-19] We have found hypotensive anesthesia to be very helpful in total hip replacement arthroplasty, and have used this technique for patients needing hip arthroplasty who would not accept homologous transfusions because of their religious beliefs. When hypotensive anesthesia was used in 100 Jehovah's Witness patients who underwent primary total hip replacement, the intraoperative blood loss was reduced by 40% as compared with matched controls. In patients who had previous hip surgery before undergoing total hip replacement arthroplasty, a 30% reduction in the intraoperative blood loss was achieved. Eleven of the patients studied were considered unsuitable for hypotensive anesthesia. Therefore, they underwent surgery under normotensive anesthesia, with the use of

preplanning, sponge packing, meticulous hemostasis, and speed. In this group of patients, a 30% reduction in blood loss was achieved. Although surgery was completed more rapidly in those patients who would not accept transfusions of any type, statistical studies showed that only 15% of the reduction in blood loss could be attributed to speed. Therefore, although speed is a factor, hypotensive anesthesia and surgical techniques appear to be more effective in reducing intraoperative blood loss.

Of the 100 patients studied, none was given homologous transfusions. There were no instances of myocardial infarction, cerebrovascular accident, or renal failure that could be attributed to hypotensive anesthesia. Also, there was no increased blood loss after surgery. In all cases, the blood pressure was raised to prehypotensive levels before wound closure.

Patients who were not given transfusions had an average preoperative hematocrit of 40%; after surgery, the hematocrit dropped to the lowest level six days later, averaging 28%. Subsequently, the hematocrit rose to a level of 31% by discharge, usually on the ninth postoperative day. Although the data regarding hematocrit levels after total hip replacement without transfusions are not absolute, it is possible to anticipate with some assurance that the lowest hematocrit level will be reached six days after surgery, and therefore treatment can be planned accordingly.

The usual agents used in the past to provide hypotensive anesthesia were sodium nitroprusside and halothane.[16,18,19] Sodium nitroprusside is administered via an infusion pump that provides the exact dosage required to maintain proper systolic blood pressure and avoid fluctuations. Use of sodium nitroprusside is a refined technique, but must be carefully monitored. If the blood pressure varies during hypotensive anesthesia, a reactive hyperemia results and bleeding can increase. The use of an infusion pump during anesthesia and careful monitoring to maintain a stable low blood pressure are essential. A 35% reduction in pressure is the usual goal.

Presently, anesthesiologists feel control is better achieved using a combination of the narcotic, sufentanil, and the inhalant, isoflurane.[15] The narcotic produces a stable basal analgesia while the isoflurane produces the desired degree of hypotension via vasodilation. Total dosage of sufentanil is limited to 1 to 1.5 μg/kg of body weight.

Epidural anesthesia can also be used to produce hypotension, but epidural anesthesia is not controllable on a minute-to-minute basis and the level achieved by epidural anesthesia cannot be altered during surgery. When a general anesthetic is contraindicated because of medical status or patient choice, epidural anesthesia provides a reasonable alternative. Agents used include lidocaine and bupivacaine.

In addition to hypotensive anesthesia, it is suggested

that the patient be placed in Trendelenburg position of 20 degrees to reduce engorgement of the blood vessels at the surgical site. In total hip arthroplasty, the lateral position appears to be beneficial, allowing gravity to reduce venous engorgement, thus reducing intraoperative blood loss. We have studied the effects of positioning on blood loss by measuring blood loss in patients undergoing total hip replacement in the lateral and in the supine position. In these patients there was less intraoperative bleeding when the lateral position was used, but the difference was not statistically significant.[18]

If, during surgery, the anesthesiologist determines that it is essential that the patient receive a transfusion, it is wise to delay the transfusion until the surgery is nearly complete. It is preferable to maintain the intraoperative blood volume with crystalloids because this results in hemodilution of the intraoperative blood loss, and, subsequently, the patient loses fewer erythrocytes. Also, if the needed transfusion is given with surgical closure, the transfused blood volume will aid in raising the blood pressure to prehypotensive levels.

Blood Loss During Surgery

Using total hip replacement arthroplasty as an example, it is clear that there is an insensible, constant rate of blood loss that occurs once the operation has begun. Although the total amount of insensible blood loss is related to time, there are certain surgical acts that produce the majority of blood loss during surgery. If no attempt is made to minimize blood loss during these specific periods, then large amounts of blood will be lost. In total hip replacement, peak blood losses occur when the femoral neck is cut and when the acetabulum and the femur are reamed. It is, therefore, essential to be prepared to quell bleeding during these peak periods. Packing sponges behind retractors and between fascial planes is a useful adjunct to aid coagulation at all times; however, filling the dead spaces left in the acetabulum and in the femur after reaming is essential. Packing with sponges prevents significant blood loss and also enhances the surgeon's view and efficiency. It has been our policy to soak sponges in adrenaline in a concentration of 1 in 1 million parts; we believe the addition of adrenaline also reduces blood loss. The use of hemostatic agents, such as thrombin-soaked Gelfoam, to cover bleeding bone after it has been cut also appears worthwhile.

A final factor often discussed among surgeons, but rarely recorded, is speed. Blood loss increases as the length of the procedure increases; however, speed should never be at the expense of control. A well-planned surgical procedure that progresses in a step-by-step fashion, in a controlled, efficient manner, is effective in reducing the time spent during a surgical procedure, and thus the amount of blood loss. Conversely, quick but purposeless movements, by increasing the time needed to complete a surgical procedure, actually increase intraoperative blood loss.

Asanguinous Fluid Replacement

After acute blood loss, the body attempts to compensate for diminished oxygen transport by increasing cardiac output. The body increases cardiac output by shifting fluid into the vascular space from the interstitial fluid compartment and, to a lesser extent, from the intracellular fluid compartment. There is obviously a limit to the extent of fluid shift that can be accomplished in a given time. In a normal, healthy individual, it appears that an acute blood loss of 10% of the circulating blood volume is well tolerated. As much as a 25% blood loss may be tolerated if it occurs gradually, over a longer period of time.[20] When cardiac output cannot be increased sufficiently to maintain oxygen delivery, the secondary response is to increase oxygen extraction by the peripheral tissues. With extensive and rapid blood loss, both of these compensatory mechanisms may be exceeded, producing a state referred to as shock.

Initial Therapy

The initial therapy for blood loss is directed to refilling the intravascular compartment. This takes precedence over reestablishing hemoglobin levels. Two basic types of fluid, crystalloids and colloids, are used for such replacement. Crystalloids are essentially isotonic solutions. Crystalloids, while capable of refilling the intravascular space, are not retained there. They distribute freely throughout the intravascular and interstitial fluid compartments. If the osmolality of the administered fluid is low, there will also be distribution into the intracellular compartment. Thus, volume replacement with crystalloid must exceed the volume of blood lost by a factor of two to perhaps as much as three times. Crystalloids, however, have the advantage of being virtually without side effects, are easy to administer rapidly, and are inexpensive and effective.

Colloids represent an alternative to crystalloid fluid administration. Colloids are solutions containing salt but also large molecules such as proteins and starches. Examples of widely used colloids include albumin, dextran, and hydroxyethyl starch. Colloids offer the advantage that so long as the capillary membrane is intact, they are retained within the vascular space to a much greater extent than are crystalloids. Therefore, a smaller volume of fluid is required to replace blood loss. Colloids, on the other hand, have the disadvantages of slower administration (because of their viscosity), greater expense, and higher incidence of complications. Complications seen with routinely available colloids include allergic reactions, coagulation abnormalities, and difficulties with typing and cross-matching for future transfusions. Many studies have been performed comparing the efficacy of crystalloids and colloids in the replacement of acute blood loss. The results are controversial, but it appears at this time that the majority of patients can be successfully managed with crystalloids alone. For patients in whom a problem with soft-tissue edema is foreseen, colloids may offer an advantage.

Transfusion Trigger

Historically, what is referred to as the transfusion trigger has been an arbitrarily defined hemoglobin of 10 g/dl and hematocrit of 30%. The physiologic basis for these numbers is very weak. If we wish to avoid the use of blood products after acute blood loss, we must have more rational guidelines that will still protect the patient's oxygen needs. Low-risk patients, such as the young, healthy adult undergoing elective surgery, may be successfully monitored by following routine vital signs and urine output. High-risk patients may benefit from more invasive and intensive monitoring,[5] including oximetric pulmonary artery catheters, intra-arterial lines, continuous electrocardiographic monitoring, and frequent sampling for hemoglobin levels and arterial blood gases. The distinction between low risk and high risk is not sharp but represents a continuum between the two extremes. Lacking objective criteria to distinguish between low-risk and high-risk patients, it is necessary to rely on good clinical judgment.

Low-Risk Patients

For patients in the low-risk category, hypovolemia may be successfully treated with the infusion of crystalloid. The volume of crystalloid administered can be monitored by the parameters described above. If soft-tissue edema is a problem or is likely to become a problem, there may be an advantage to the use of colloid to reduce the amount of fluid replacement required. If there is to be an automatic transfusion trigger based on hemoglobin and hematocrit in this patient, it should probably be in the range of 7 g/dl of hemoglobin or a hematocrit of 20%.

High-Risk Patients

Patients at high risk will not only require more invasive monitoring but will undoubtedly require higher hemoglobin and hematocrit levels. Such signs as tachycardia, tachypnea, and low mixed venous oxygen saturation may be present despite apparently adequate central venous pressure, pulmonary capillary wedge pressure, and other measurements. If any of these findings exist in the high-risk patient, the patient should be transfused with packed erythrocytes until the offending signs disappear.

Extraordinary Measures

More extreme measures may be necessary when blood is unavailable or when the patient refuses blood transfusions.[21] These include maximizing oxygen delivery by increasing the inspired oxygen concentration, increasing the cardiac output by optimizing the intravascular volume, and perhaps the use of inotropic agents while at the same time reducing oxygen consumption by treating fever, reducing pain, and, in extreme circumstances resorting to muscle relaxants, mechanical ventilation, and external cooling.

Summary

In summary, reduction of blood loss and coincidental decrease in the number of blood transfusions is now of paramount importance in orthopaedic surgery. Methods to reduce blood loss include preoperative planning, hypotensive anesthesia, and meticulous surgical technique. If transfusion is necessary, autologous replacement is always preferable. Overall, the goals in blood conservation in surgery are first to decrease the amount of blood lost, and second to be sensible in replacement of this loss.

References

1. Bove JR: Transfusion-associated hepatitis and AIDS: What is the risk? *N Engl J Med* 1987;317:242–245.
2. Task Force on AIDS and Orthopaedic Surgery: *Recommendations for the Prevention of Human Immunodeficiency Virus (HIV) Transmission in Orthopaedic Surgery Practice.* Park Ridge, Illinois, American Academy of Orthopaedic Surgeons, 1989.
3. Cowell HR: Perioperative red blood-cell transfusion, editorial. *J Bone Joint Surg* 1989;71A:1–2.
4. Wilmore DW: *The Metabolic Management of the Critically Ill.* New York, Plenum Medical Book Co, 1977, p 9.
5. Snyder JV, Carroll GC: Tissue oxygenation. *Curr Prob Surg* 1982; 19:649–720.
6. Kobrinsky NL, Letts RM, Patel LR, et al: 1-Desamino-8-D-arginine vasopressin (desmopressin) decreases operative blood loss in patients having Harrington rod spinal fusion surgery. *Ann Intern Med* 1987;107:446–450.
7. Margolies MN, Ring EJ, Waltman AC, et al: Arteriography in the management of hemorrhage from pelvic fractures. *N Engl J Med* 1972;287:317–321.
8. Allison DJ: Therapeutic embolization. *Br J Hosp Med* 1978;20: 707–715.
9. Channon GM, Williams LA: Giant-cell tumor of the ischium treated by embolisation and resection: A case report. *J Bone Joint Surg* 1982;64B:164–165.
10. Moore JR, Weiland AJ: Embolotherapy in the treatment of congenital arteriovenous malformations of the hand: A case report. *J Hand Surg* 1985;10A:135–139.

11. Murphy WA, Strecker EB, Schoenecker PL: Transcatheter embolisation therapy of an ischial aneurysmal bone cyst. *J Bone Joint Surg* 1982;64B:166–168.

12. Berenstein A, Kricheff II: Neuroradiologic interventional procedures. *Semin Roentgenol* 1981;16:79–94.

13. Saueracker AJ, McCroskey BL, Moore EE, et al: Intraoperative hypogastric artery embolization for life-threatening pelvic hemorrhage: A preliminary report. *J Trauma* 1987;27:1127–1129.

14. van Urk H, Perlberger RR, Muller H: Selective arterial embolization for control of traumatic pelvic hemorrhage. *Surgery* 1978; 83:133–137.

15. Lam AM, Gelb AW: Cardiovascular effects of isoflurane-induced hypotension for cerebral aneurysm surgery. *Anesth Analg* 1983; 62:742–748.

16. Lawson NW, Thompson DS, Nelson CL, et al: Sodium nitroprusside-induced hypotension for supine total hip replacement. *Anesth Analg* 1976;55:654–662.

17. Mandel RJ, Brown MD, McCollough NC III, et al: Hypotensive anesthesia and autotransfusion in spinal surgery. *Clin Orthop* 1981;154:27–33.

18. Nelson CL, Bowen WS: Total hip arthroplasty in Jehovah's Witnesses without blood transfusion. *J Bone Joint Surg* 1986;68A: 350–353.

19. Rosberg B, Fredin H, Gustafson C: Anesthetic techniques and surgical blood loss in total hip arthroplasty. *Acta Anaesth Scand* 1982;26:189–193.

20. Laks H, Pilon RN, Klovekorn WP, et al: Acute hemodilution: Its effect on hemodynamics and oxygen transport in anesthetized man. *Ann Surg* 1974;180:103–109.

21. Nearman HS, Eckhauser ML: Postoperative management of a severely anemic Jehovah's Witness. *Crit Care Med* 1983;11:142–143.

Blood Products:
Optimal Use, Conservation, and Safety

John Cone, MD

Lorraine J. Day, MD

Gregory K. Johnson, MD

David G. Murray, MD

Carl L. Nelson, MD

Introduction

After the introduction of total joint arthroplasty into the United States in 1969 and 1970, the issue of blood loss and fluid management seemed less important than such concerns as prosthetic design, technical considerations, and the impressive results. Even the possibility of revision surgery drew little attention. Very few of the early reports even commented on associated blood loss.[1] Publications on this topic were primarily comparisons of blood loss associated with anterior, posterior, or lateral approaches,[2-5] trochanteric osteotomies, or with various types of anesthesia.[6] For example, Wiesman and associates[7] reported average blood replacement of 4.4 units when using a transtrochanteric approach and 3.1 units when the trochanter was left intact. Sculco and Ranawat[8] reported that blood replacement averaged 2.1 units with spinal anesthesia and 3.1 units with general anesthesia. Specifically, this report stated that of 134 hips done under general anesthesia, three required no blood transfusion. Of 100 hips done under spinal anesthesia, nine received no blood transfusions. Weaver,[9] in 1975, reported an average blood replacement of 4 units with the transtrochanteric approach and 1.6 units with posterior approach. Nelson and associates,[10] in reporting on hypotensive anesthesia in 1977, noted that 32 patients operated on without hypotensive anesthesia received a combined total of 83 units, or more than 2 units per case. In reviewing the rather extensive literature between 1970 and 1980, it becomes obvious that with few exceptions blood loss during surgery was considered a matter of course. Even when discussed in relation to the various approaches, it was presented as more of a peripheral issue than a feature that should influence the decision on surgical technique.[11]

Two major factors have stimulated attention to this matter. The first was the Jehovah's Witnesses, whose beliefs preclude the receipt of blood by any means. In order for them to have the benefit of hip replacement surgery, some attention obviously would have to be paid to the subject of blood loss. This turned out to be a minor factor, because most surgeons solved the dilemma by avoiding surgery in this circumstance. A few took up the challenge and concentrated on techniques to modify blood loss.[12] Although this could be done

successfully, most hip surgery went on more or less as before.

The second factor was the introduction of the acquired immune deficiency syndrome (AIDS) into the United States in the early 1980s. Concern about the risk associated with homologous blood transfusions is encapsulated in the following quotation from an article that appeared in the Jan 23, 1989, issue of *Newsweek* magazine. The article, entitled "AIDS, Blood and Money," begins, "Sabrina Crawford contracted AIDS one night in May 1984 when she received a transfusion supplied by a California blood bank. Now Crawford, 21, is dying..." Unquestionably, the AIDS crisis has brought into focus and highlighted the dangers inherent in taking blood from one person and giving it to another. The public at large is now requesting, and often demanding, that physicians consider alternatives to homologous transfusions.

The primary concern to surgeons is the risk of transmitting disease through the transfusion of blood or blood products. Blood products that are not considered safe include whole blood, packed cells, plasma, platelets, and cryoprecipitate. Blood products that are safe at this point are albumin, gamma-globulin, factor VIII, and factor IX. These later products were not safe early on but currently are treated in such a manner as to render them safe but still effective.

AIDS, caused by human immunodeficiency virus (HIV) is, of course, not the only disease that is transmitted through blood transfusion. It happens to be the one that is 100% fatal if contracted. Other diseases include hepatitis B, non-A, non-B hepatitis, delta hepatitis, and HTLV-I.[13-15]

A separate but related issue involves liability. Up to this point, maloccurrences related to transfusions have generally been assumed to be the responsibility of someone other than the physician. Increasingly, publicity surrounding the potentially adverse effects of blood transfusion, coupled with growing awareness of alternatives, may shift the responsibility for such incidents to the physician or surgeon who ordered the blood transfusion in the first place. The entire subject has, therefore, become one that the medical profession must constantly review and reassess, altering current practices as needed.

In this chapter, the technique and results of two

methods for reducing the need for homologous transfusions are discussed. Both involve autotransfusion. Predonation is done in the week or weeks before surgery and requires the patient's time and effort. With present-day concerns and almost universal cooperation from the Red Cross and other blood centers, this is rarely a problem. Intraoperative cell salvage can be used in emergency or elective surgery, but has certain limitations. It is also possible, in some instances, to use both techniques concurrently.

Predeposit and Intraoperative Autotransfusion

Predonation

Resources for autologous blood collection, processing, and transfusion have been available for years,[16-19] but scant use was made of them until recently. As the demand has risen, both the logistics and the limitations have been clarified.[20,21] The Red Cross program is probably the most widely used resource, and their predonation centers are well distributed throughout the country.

The limitations on autologous donation are not stringent. The Red Cross protocols may vary slightly from one region to another, but generally their guidelines recommend that donors be older than 12 years of age and younger than 70 years. Even outside these limits, exceptions can be made by mutual agreement between the Red Cross and the surgeons. There are reports in the literature of predonations by children less than 2 years old and adults more than 80 years old. Other parameters include a weight base of 110 lbs to qualify for a full unit to be drawn. Smaller amounts will be taken if the weight is less. The hematocrit should be greater than 0.34 (34%). The last donation should be scheduled no closer than four days before the date of the surgical procedure.[22] Units can be drawn at weekly intervals, so long as the hematocrit can be maintained. Supplemental iron is essential. A standard prescription for adults is 320 mg of ferrous sulfate three times a day beginning a week or more before the first donations and continuing to the time of surgery. For children, preparations that provide 5 mg/kg/day of elemental iron are prescribed on a similar schedule. The blood is tested, stored, and supplied by the Red Cross when the surgery is performed.

The risks associated with autologous transfusions are minimal. The chance of mislabeling or substitution of units is extremely remote. The possibility that repeated phlebotomies will result in significant anemia can be resolved by discontinuing phlebotomies, by postponing surgery, or, under unusual circumstances, by reinfusing the donated blood.

The number of units collected is directly related to the type of surgery performed. Most patients do not find the donation of as much as 4 units to be excessively traumatic. The most frequent complaint relates to the need to take iron with its attendant gastrointestinal side effects.

There has been considerable debate regarding the use of autologous blood when it is available, in the absence of other indications for transfusions. Because the patient has given it, should it be given back? Most sources say no, and this is the policy that we endorse. Although the risks associated with the use of autologous blood are minuscule, the risks of not using it when it is not needed are nil. This position may be modified slightly by transfusing autologous blood at hematocrit levels that are low, but not low enough to merit giving homologous blood.

The autologous transfusion program tends to be almost completely trouble-free. The most frequent problem relates to cancelled surgery. Donated autologous blood can be stored for six weeks; if surgery can be rescheduled promptly, the blood will not become outdated, or at least 1 or 2 units will remain usable. Of course, under those circumstances, phlebotomy can be continued so that the required number of units will be on hand when the patient is operated on. Otherwise, the blood can be frozen and held indefinitely, although with some loss of effective red-cell volume.

Intraoperative Autotransfusion

A second method for autologous blood collection is during the actual surgery. Known as intraoperative autotransfusion, this method requires specialized equipment and personnel knowledgeable about the process.

Immediate reinfusion of blood lost at surgery has long been an attractive notion.[23-26] Reports date from the 1800s, but complications associated with collection and reinfusion prevented any significant use of these various techniques.[27,28] In 1970, Klebanoff[29] reported a practical method for collecting and reinfusing blood. The method frequently required systemic anticoagulation, and was associated with reports of air embolism and a variety of coagulopathies.[30,31]

About the same time, the concept of reinfusing washed red cells was introduced by Wilson and associates.[32] This involved centrifuging the aspirated blood to concentrate the cells, washing the cells with saline, and then diluting the cells back to a hematocrit of 0.50 (50%) to 0.60 (60%) before reinfusing. Plasma and most of the platelets are removed during the process. With some refinements, this is basically the process used today. The equipment is easily portable, and the risk of an embolism has been essentially eliminated; however, an operator is required for the equipment. Currently the Red Cross in many areas is equipped to provide whatever is necessary, from complete service, including equipment, disposables, and operator, to simply an operator able to monitor hospital-owned equipment.

The current costs are roughly as follows. The aspiration set, which consists of a double-lumen suction tube, costs $18. The reservoir into which the blood is collected costs $54. The cell-saver pack is $84. The total, $156, may be doubled by the hospital to cover handling and other expenses. It is possible to use the aspiration set and the reservoir independently of the pack so that, if insufficient blood is recovered to reinfuse, the basic costs are reduced to $72.

The cost-effectiveness of the cell saver in much of orthopaedic surgery, particularly hip replacement, is not completely documented. Episodes of major hemorrhage are rare during the average operation. Because at least 2 units of blood must be lost during surgery to justify the involvement of the equipment and operator, routine use for straightforward primary hip replacement is probably not justified. Unfortunately, if blood loss becomes excessive for some unexpected reason, much of the loss will be unavailable for the cell saver if it has not been used from the beginning. As a general rule, the cell saver is not necessary for routine total hip replacement cases if 1 or 2 units of predonated autologous blood are available. For other routine procedures, the aspiration set and reservoir may be used. Then, a decision can be made toward the end of the case as to whether or not the volume is sufficient to process. Approximately one half the cost is saved if collected blood is not reinfused.

Because a significant percentage of blood loss in orthopaedic surgical procedures occurs after surgery, one half or more of the total blood lost may be unavailable for the cell saver. Add to that the blood that is taken up with sponges or drapes during surgery, and it becomes apparent that the cell saver alone is unlikely to eliminate the need for transfusions. In reported series of orthopaedic procedures using the cell saver, the requirements for blood replacement were reduced by approximately 50%. On the positive side, there were no reported complications from the use of reinfused autologous blood. Although the debris, such as fat, bone, and connective fragments, that accumulates in blood during orthopaedic procedures might be expected to have some untoward effects, these have not been reported. Moreover, in experimental procedures on dogs, no tissue emboli were noted on microscopic examination of various tissues post mortem.

Summary

A review of our experience in total joint arthroplasty revealed that the cell saver was not cost-effective in the case of routine primary hip or knee replacement. Its use should be restricted to cases of revision hip and knee surgery in which infection has been ruled out. Preoperative aspiration remains the most reliable method for accomplishing this. However, if the aspiration is negative and the intra-articular fluid obtained at the time of surgery is suspicious for infection, either

in appearance or on Gram stain or cell count, it is best to abandon use of the cell saver.

Predonation should be routine for all hip replacement cases unless there are specific contraindications. In general, there is good acceptance of this program by patients, although a few have specifically indicated they would prefer to run the risk of homologous transfusion. Two units available for primary replacement are more than ample. In cases of revisions, a first revision justifies a minimum of 3 units. For complex revision cases involving patients with three or more previous procedures on the hip, or those requiring significant bone resection or large segment grafting, the maximum possible number of units should be obtained.

Autologous blood reinfusion should be done for essentially the same indications as homologous transfusion even though risks are sharply reduced. The local source for autologous collection will then follow its own specific protocol for the disposition of remaining units. In every case, the surgical technique should be careful and directed toward limiting intraoperative blood loss.

Conclusion

A variety of factors are currently focusing attention on the risks associated with homologous blood transfusion. It is now possible through a variety of methods to limit the use of homologous blood to 10% or less of orthopaedic surgical cases. The underlying essential principle is adequate preplanning. Preparation of the patient by ensuring an adequate hematocrit at the time of surgery and by avoiding medications that increase bleeding will set an appropriate stage. Predonation of an appropriate number of units provides a cushion. Meticulous attention to surgical details, shortened operating time, and hypotensive anesthesia, when practical, will further limit the need for blood replacement by diminishing blood loss. Where considerable blood loss is anticipated, intraoperative use of the cell saver will be of help. Finally, by appropriate fluid management using crystalloids or colloids in a carefully monitored patient, blood transfusion may be safely avoided even though the hematocrit or hemoglobin levels temporarily fall below usually accepted limits.

References

1. Wilson PD Jr, Amstutz HC, Czerniecki A, et al: Total hip replacement with fixation by acrylic cement: A preliminary study of 100 consecutive McKee-Farrar prosthetic replacements. *J Bone Joint Surg* 1972;54A:207–236.
2. Carlson DC, Robinson HJ Jr: Surgical approaches for primary total hip arthroplasty: A prospective comparison of the Marcy modification of the Gibson and Watson-Jones approaches. *Clin Orthop* 1987;222:161–166.
3. Colville J, Raunio P: Charnley low-friction arthroplasties of the hip in rheumatoid arthritis: A study of the complications and

results of 378 arthroplasties. *J Bone Joint Surg* 1978;60B:498–503.

4. Roberts JM, Fu FH, McClain EJ, et al: A comparison of the posterolateral and anterolateral approaches to total hip arthroplasty. *Clin Orthop* 1984;187:205–210.

5. Robinson RP, Robinson HJ Jr, Salvati EA: A comparison of the transtrochanteric and posterior approaches for total hip replacement. *Clin Orthop* 1980;147:143–147.

6. Bond AG: Conduction anaesthesia, blood pressure and haemorrhage. *Br J Anaesth* 1969;41:942–946.

7. Wiesman HJ Jr, Simon SR, Ewald FC, et al: Total hip replacement with and without osteotomy of the greater trochanter: Clinical and biomechanical comparisons in the same patients. *J Bone Joint Surg* 1978;60A:203–210.

8. Sculco T, Ranawat C: The use of spinal anesthesia for total hip-replacement arthroplasty. *J Bone Joint Surg* 1975;57A:173–177.

9. Weaver JK: Total hip replacement: A comparison between the transtrochanteric and posterior surgical approaches. *Clin Orthop* 1975;112:201–207.

10. Nelson C, Olin F, Lawson N, et al: Hip surgery without transfusion, in *The Hip: Proceedings of the Fifth Open Scientific Meeting of the Hip Society.* St. Louis, CV Mosby, 1977, pp 274–282.

11. Coventry MB, Beckenbaugh RD, Nolan DR, et al: 2,012 total hip arthroplasties: A study of postoperative course and early complications. *J Bone Joint Surg* 1974;56A:273–284.

12. Nelson CL, Bowen WS: Total hip arthroplasty in Jehovah's Witnesses without blood transfusion. *J Bone Joint Surg* 1986;68A:350–353.

13. Aledort LM: Risks associated with homologous blood transfusion. *J Cardiothorac Anesth* 1988;2:2–6.

14. Rosina F, Saracco G, Rizzetto M: Risk of post-transfusion infection with the hepatitis delta virus. *N Engl J Med* 1985;312:1488–1491.

15. Stevens CE, Aach RD, Hollinger FG, et al: Hepatitis B virus antibody in blood donors and the occurrence of non-A, non-B hepatitis in transfusion recipients: An analysis of the transfusion-transmitted viruses study. *Ann Intern Med* 1984;101:733–738.

16. Bailey TE Jr, Mahoney OM: The use of banked autologous blood in patients undergoing surgery for spinal deformity. *J Bone Joint Surg* 1987;69A:329–332.

17. Blood, blood components, and blood substitutes, in *Drug Evaluations,* ed 6. Chicago, American Medical Association, 1986, pp 625–641.

18. Thomson JD, Callaghan JJ, Savory CG, et al: Prior deposition of autologous blood in elective orthopaedic surgery. *J Bone Joint Surg* 1987;69A:320–324.

19. Woolson ST, Marsh JS, Tanner JB: Transfusion of previously deposited autologous blood for patients undergoing hip-replacement surgery. *J Bone Joint Surg* 1987;69A:325–328.

20. Office of Medical Applications of Research, National Institutes of Health: Consensus Conference: Perioperative red blood cell transfusion. *JAMA* 1988;260:2700–2703.

21. Toy PTCY, Strauss RG, Stehling LC, et al: Predeposited autologous blood for elective surgery: A national multicenter study. *N Engl J Med* 1987;316:517–520.

22. Committee on Transfusion and Transplantation: *General Principles of Blood Transfusion.* Chicago, American Medical Association, 1973.

23. Cowell HR, Swickard JW: Autotransfusion in children's orthopaedics. *J Bone Joint Surg* 1974;56A:908–912.

24. Csencsitz TA, Flynn JC: Intraoperative blood salvage in spinal deformity surgery in children. *J Fla Med Assoc* 1979;66:39–41.

25. Flynn JC, Metzger CR, Csencsitz TA: Intraoperative autotransfusion (IAT) in spinal surgery. *Spine* 1982;7:432–435.

26. Young JN, Ecker RR, Moretti RL, et al: Autologous blood retrieval in thoracic, cardiovascular, and orthopedic surgery. *Am J Surg* 1982;144:48–52.

27. Blundell J: Experiments on the transfusion of blood by the syringe. *Med Chir Trans* 1818;9:56.

28. Duncan J: On re-infusion of blood in primary and other amputations. *Br Med J* 1886;1:192.

29. Klebanoff G: Early clinical experience with a disposable unit for the intraoperative salvage and reinfusion of blood loss (intraoperative autotransfusion). *Am J Surg* 1970;120:718–722.

30. Mattox KL: Comparison of techniques of autotransfusion. *Surgery* 1978;84:700–702.

31. Turner RH, Steady HM: Cell washing in orthopaedic surgery, in Haver JM, Thurer RL, Dawson RB (eds): *Autotransfusion Symposium (1st).* New York, Elsevier North Holland, 1981, pp 43–50.

32. Wilson JD, Taswell HF, Utz DC: Autotransfusion: Urologic applications and the development of a modified irrigating fluid. *J Urol* 1971;105:873–877.

Total Shoulder Arthroplasty

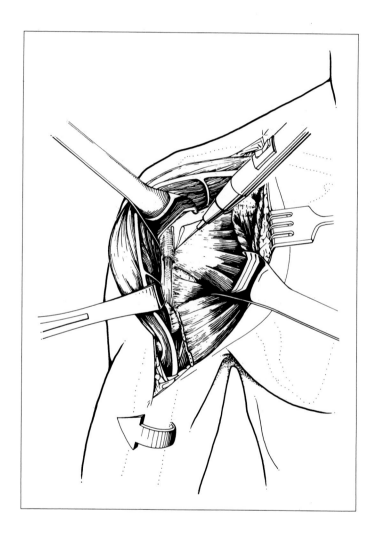

The Technique of Total Shoulder Arthroplasty

Charles A. Rockwood, Jr., MD

General Principles

The technique of total shoulder arthroplasty requires great familiarity with the anatomy of the shoulder. This chapter illustrates the key points of the technique. Critical to the procedure is the realization that the operation can be performed through an extended deltopectoral incision without detaching the origin or insertion of the deltoid muscle. This basic surgical approach can be used for hemiarthroplasty, for total shoulder arthroplasty, or for a variety of other procedures about the proximal humerus, such as open reduction and internal fixation of fractures. For total shoulder arthroplasty, several knowledgeable surgical assistants are required. One assistant stands on the side of the patient opposite the surgeon to retract the pectoralis major and the conjoined tendons. A second assistant stands to one side of the surgeon near the superior aspect of the shoulder to retract the deltoid. A third assistant stands at the other side of the surgeon to support and manipulate the arm. A nurse or scrub technician passes the instruments. One of the three assistants can also control the electric coagulation unit.

It is essential that the patient be positioned at the top and at the side of the operating table, so that the arm of the involved shoulder can easily be extended downward without interference from the table. The table is situated so that the patient is in the beach-chair position, with back and shoulders elevated and hip and knees flexed. The standard headrest portion of the table is removed and is replaced with a Mayfield neurosurgical headrest. This setup leaves the top of the patient's shoulder free and accessible. In addition to the overhead light, I prefer to use the fiberoptic head light so that a bright and intense beam of light is available, permitting better visualization of important anatomic features such as the axillary nerve and facilitating control of bleeding points. Before the sterile preparation begins, I use surgical skin drapes to block off any unwanted anatomy from the surgical wound.

At the time of induction 1 g of cephalosporin is administered intravenously. A second gram of cephalosporin is put into the intravenous fluid bottle. For 24 to 48 hours following surgery 1 g of cephalosporin is given intravenously every six hours. If the patient is sensitive to cephalosporin, intravenous erythromycin is used instead.

An irrigation solution is used throughout the procedure to keep the wound moist and clear of debris.

The irrigation fluid contains a 1-ml ampule of antibiotic per liter of saline. The fluid contains 40 mg of neomycin sulfate and 200,000 units of polymyxin. Only moist lap sponges are used during the procedure. The usual 4-inch-square sponges are not used because they are too small and because it is too easy to leave or lose one of them in the depths of the wound. The prosthetics used in this procedure are the Neer II humeral component and a standard non-metal-backed, high-density polyethylene glenoid prosthesis.

Incision

The incision extends from the origin of the deltoid on the clavicle to the insertion of the deltoid on the mid-humerus. It begins at the clavicle and extends across the coracoid process and down onto the anterior aspect of the arm near the insertion of the deltoid (Figs. 1 and 2). With the arm abducted 20 degrees, the incision is almost a straight line. The incision is carried down through the subcutaneous fat to the fascia that overlies the deltopectoral muscles.

The deltoid is carefully separated from the pectoralis major muscle and the cephalic vein, which is adhered to the deltoid, should be retracted laterally with the deltoid muscle (Fig. 3). The cephalic vein, which lies in the deltopectoral interval, should be carefully identified and protected throughout the procedure. I stress the importance of leaving the cephalic vein intact. Because the origin of the deltoid is significantly retracted, it is important to maintain adequate venous drainage of that muscle. There is no question that the patient whose cephalic vein remains intact at the end of the procedure has an easier postoperative course and far less pain than one in whom the vein has been ligated. Any of the veins that enter the cephalic vein medially from the pectoralis major must be clamped and ligated. Only occasionally, in a patient with rheumatoid arthritis, when the head has migrated superiorly, will it be necessary to mobilize the vein medially.

Deltoid Retraction and Release of Pectoralis Major Tendon

The deltoid is retracted laterally and must be freed completely from its deep surface to expose the coracoid process and conjoined tendons, the anterior surface of

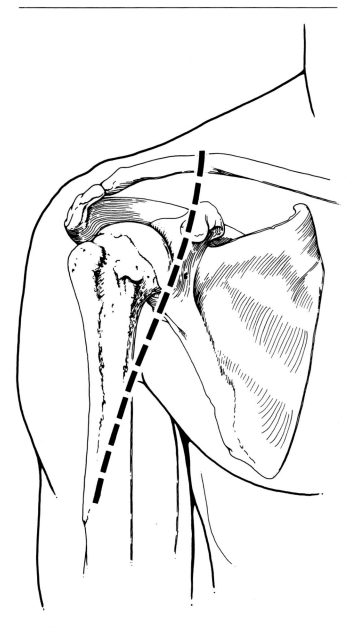

Fig. 1   Extent of skin incision from clavicle over the top of the coracoid down to the insertion of the deltoid.

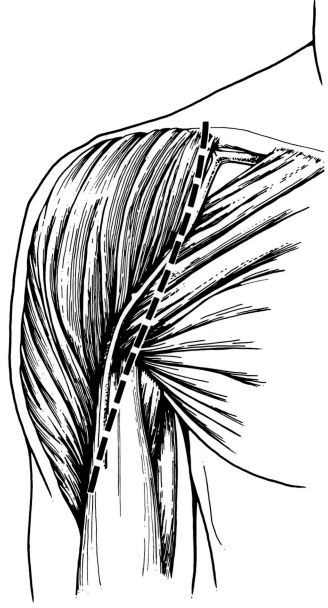

Fig. 2   The incision is basically in the deltopectoral interval.

the humerus, and the insertion of the pectoralis major tendon. It is very important to free the deep surface of the deltoid from the clavicle down to its insertion into the humerus. The deltoid is retracted laterally and held with Richardson retractors. To protect the retracted deltoid muscle and the cephalic vein, I place a moist lap sponge over the medial border of the deltoid and hold it in place with the retractor. The sponge is kept moist throughout the procedure.

The electric cutting knife is then used to release the upper 50% to 80% of the tendinous insertion of the pectoralis major muscle from its insertion into the hu-

merus (Fig. 4, *top*). This is done to allow better visualization of the inferior aspect of the glenohumeral joint and to identify and protect the axillary nerve. If the patient has significant internal rotation contracture (−30 to −40 degrees of external rotation), I do not hesitate to release all of the insertions of the pectoralis major tendons. This is not likely to cause any disability, because the patient has other strong internal rotators of the shoulder, including the teres major, latissimus, and subscapularis muscles.

I do not divide and release the conjoined tendons nor do I perform an osteotomy of the coracoid process.

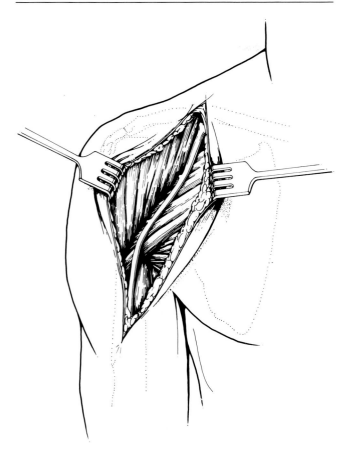

Fig. 3   Cephalic vein is identified in the deltopectoral groove and is carefully preserved, being taken laterally with the deltoid muscle.

I believe it is important to leave the conjoined tendons intact and to retract them medially with a Richardson retractor. The conjoined tendons offer excellent protection for the neurovascular bundle that lies deep and medial to the conjoined tendons. With the conjoined tendon detached, it would be possible for the assistant who is on the opposite side of the table to retract too vigorously and injure the neurovascular bundle. In addition, before retracting the conjoined tendons, it is important to slip a finger under them to locate the exact penetration of the musculocutaneous nerve (Fig. 4, *bottom*).

Only if the head is chronically dislocated anteriorly and is lying posterior to the coracoid process and the conjoined tendon or if there is an associated significant vascular injury have I found it necessary to release the conjoined tendons by performing an osteotomy of the coracoid process.

Subscapularis Release

With the conjoined tendons and the pectoralis major tendons retracted medially and the deltoid retracted

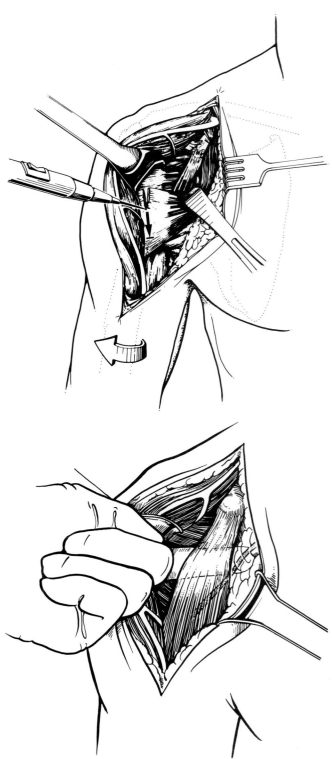

Fig. 4   **Top**, The upper 80% of the pectoralis major tendon is released, allowing better visualization of the inferior aspect of the shoulder joint. If the patient has a severe internal-rotation contracture, the entire pectoralis major tendon can be released. **Bottom**, Palpation of the musculocutaneous nerve into conjoined tendons.

laterally, the subscapularis tendon and the biceps tendon are in clear view. Before the subscapularis tendon is released, I pass my finger down the anterior surface of the subscapularis muscle and hook my finger out anterior and laterally to identify the exact location of the axillary nerve (Fig. 5, *top*). The axillary nerve must be identified and protected throughout the procedure. Before the subscapularis tendon is divided, the anterior humeral circumflex artery and vein, which lie along the inferior aspect of the subscapularis tendon, must be identified and ligated. If the patient has 0 degrees of external rotation or an internal rotational contracture, then the subscapularis tendon must be lengthened by a coronal plane Z-plasty technique (Fig. 5, *center left*). If the patient does not have an internal rotation contracture and easily has 35 to 45 degrees of external rotation, then the subscapularis tendon can be divided in its substance 0.5 inch medial to its insertion. If the patient has a mild internal rotation contracture and can externally rotate only 15 to 20 degrees, I use the electric cutting knife to release the tendon from the lesser tuberosity as close to the bicipital groove as is possible (Fig. 5, *bottom*).

I prefer that the electric knife pass only through the subscapularis tendon, but it sometimes extends down into the capsule attachment. No matter when the capsule is detached from the humerus, it is important that the deep surface of the subscapularis tendon be dissected from the capsule and completely freed. The subscapularis tendon usually adheres to the capsule, creating a tenodesis effect of the tendon down to the glenoid rim. The subscapularis tendon must be freed of all adhesions, particularly from the deep surface of the coracoid process and conjoined tendons and from the capsule, which is attached to the glenoid rim. After it has been dissected off the capsule, the subscapularis tendon must move freely and have a rubbery bounce to it when tugged on (Fig. 5, *bottom right*). During this part of the procedure the axillary nerve must be carefully protected with a Scofield or similar retractor. Three or four 1-mm-thick cottony Dacron sutures are now inserted into the subscapularis tendon. These sutures are later used to reattach the tendon to the neck of the humerus.

Capsule Release and Excision

If the capsule was not detached from the humerus during tenotomy of the subscapularis tendon, it is released now, using the electric cutting knife. The capsular release should begin superiorly, extend anteriorly, and continue inferiorly beyond the 6 o'clock position (Fig. 6). Failure to release the anterior inferior capsule completely will make it more difficult to deliver the head out of the wound for insertion of the humeral prosthesis. I prefer to resect the entire anteroinferior capsule, but, because it is easier, I defer division of the medial capsule from the glenoid until after the head fragment has been removed.

It is essential, as previously described, to position the patient's torso on the edge of the operating-room table so that the arm can be extended and externally rotated, thereby allowing the head of the humerus to be displaced anteriorly out of the wound. A small bone hook placed under the neck of the humerus is used to lift the head out of the glenoid fossa as the arm is extended and externally rotated.

Humeral Head Resection

Once it is established that the head of the humerus can be easily delivered out of the wound, the angles for removal of the head can be planned. Two different planes of removal of the head must be considered: first, the amount of retrotorsion of the head on the shaft, which is normally 30 to 35 degrees; and second, the shaft-neck head angle, which is normally 145 degrees (Fig. 7, *top left*).

The head of the humerus is reduced back into the glenoid and the arm placed in 25 to 30 degrees of abduction. A small Darrach retractor placed along the superior aspect of the head, between the head and the biceps tendon, serves to expose the superior aspect of the articular surface of the head of the humerus. It also protects the biceps tendon and the posterior cuff insertion into the greater tuberosity during removal of the head. The normal amount of humeral head retrotorsion is 30 to 35 degrees (Fig. 7, *top right*). Thus, with the elbow flexed 90 degrees and the arm held in 30 to 35 degrees of external rotation, a saw cut made with the blade perpendicular to the floor will ensure the placement of the humeral prosthesis in the correct degree of retrotorsion (Fig. 7, *bottom*). However, before making the cut, it is necessary to determine the proper varus-valgus orientation. Because the articular surface of the head of the humerus is almost always distorted into a varus position, the surgeon must avoid using the line along the anatomic neck to guide the saw cut. The most reliable way of determining the proper angle of saw cut is to place a humeral prosthesis template, or the stem of the small trial prosthesis, parallel to the long axis of the shaft of the humerus, which is held externally rotated 30 to 35 degrees. The electric cutting Bovie is then used to mark the normal 130-degree angle of the head of the humerus that will be removed. The humeral head is than removed with either the oscillating saw, which I prefer, or the osteotome.

Insertion of Trial Humeral Prosthesis

The resultant flat cancellous bone surface of the proximal humerus is now delivered out of the wound

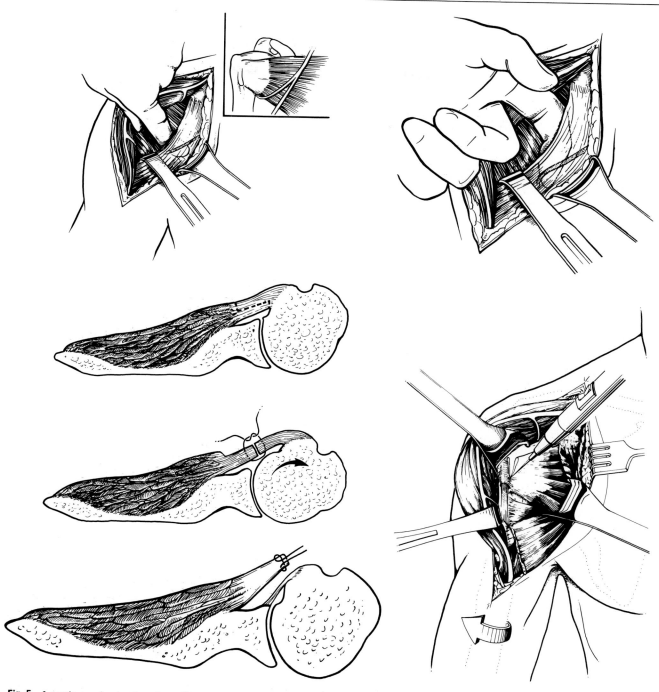

Fig. 5 Locating and palpating the axillary nerve. **Top left,** The index finger is passed along the anterior surface of the subscapularis muscle and under the axillary nerve. **Top right,** The index finger is hooked out laterally, which picks up and identifies the axillary nerve. **Center left,** When the patient has severe loss of external rotation, a Z-plasty lengthening of the subscapularis tendon should be done in the coronal plane. **Bottom right,** Release of the subscapularis tendon from the lesser tuberosity just medial to the biceps tendon. If the patient's arm can be externally rotated 45 degrees, then the subscapularis tendon can be divided in its tendinous portion and not necessarily taken off from its attachment into the tuberosity. **Bottom left,** Three or four 1-mm Dacron sutures are used to tag the end of the subscapularis tendon. Note that the tendon has been separated from the capsule.

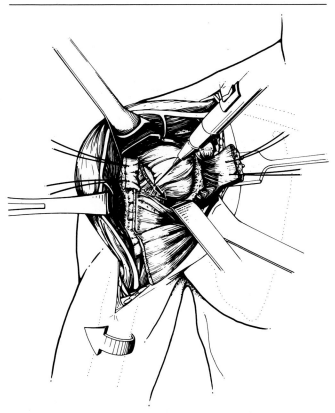

Fig. 6 With the arm in external rotation, the capsule is released from its attachment on the humerus from the top all the way down to the 6 o'clock position. Note that the axillary nerve is being retracted inferiorly out of the way with a Scofield retractor.

for inspection. This is done by means of a bone hook to engage the inferior neck of the proximal humerus. The delivery of the proximal humerus is completed by simultaneously externally rotating the arm and hyperextending the arm down off the side of the table. I do not remove any of the cancellous bone from the proximal neck and upper shaft of the humerus, nor do I use reamers to ream out the medullary canal. Examination of radiographs can help in determining whether the patient will require a small-, medium-, or a large-stem prosthesis, which are 6.3 mm, 9.5 mm, and 12.7 mm in diameter, respectively.

I always first insert the small-stem, thin, 15-mm-head trial prosthesis down through the cancellous bone of the neck of the humerus and gently down into the shaft. The penetration by the stem of the prosthesis should be into the superior surface of the cancellous bone. Remember that once the prosthesis is seated, the head of the prosthesis should be superior to the greater tuberosity of the humerus. Occasionally the lateral fin will run into the cancellous bone adjacent to the greater tuberosity and tend to push the prosthesis too far inferiorly. To remedy this, use the air burr or a small curette and remove just enough of the cancellous bone

to allow the lateral fin to sit adjacent to the cortex of the greater tuberosity. Just before the fins begin to engage the cancellous bone of the proximal humerus, check the rotation of the prosthesis to make sure that the undersurface of the head of the prosthesis is parallel to and will sit perfectly flat on the cut surface of the neck of the humerus. The prosthesis is then seated with the driver and the impactor. The lateral fin of the prosthesis should sit just posterior to the bicipital groove.

With the thin, 15-mm-head trial humeral prosthesis in place, the shoulder should be relocated to determine the relationship of the prosthesis with the glenoid fossae and to make sure the subscapularis tendon is long enough to be reattached to the neck of the humerus. The subscapularis tendon must be long enough to be reattached to the neck of the humerus and still allow 30 to 35 degrees of external rotation. If, with the thick-head prosthesis in place, the tendon is too short to allow 35 to 40 degrees of external rotation, then the thin, 15-mm-head prosthesis should be used. I prefer to use the thick, 22-mm-head prosthesis whenever possible.

Anteroposterior and lateral radiographs can be taken to ensure that the stem is correctly positioned in the medullary canal. A periosteal elevator is then used to pry the small-stem prosthesis gently out of the humerus, with care taken not to alter the four fin cuts made by the prosthesis into the cancellous bone (Fig. 8, *top*). Then the medium-stem trial prosthesis is inserted the same way, with the fins engaged in the same slots in the humerus created by the fins of the small-stem prosthesis. Observe how loose or tight the medium stem is in the canal of the humerus. If by the time the medium stem is two thirds of the way into the canal, it is clearly getting tight, then I know I will be able to use the medium stem. If the medium stem can be seated easily, then I know I will use the large-stem prosthesis.

I prefer to obtain a press-fit of the prosthesis stem into the proximal humerus cancellous bone and down into the medullary canal without using bone cement. I rarely use humeral shaft reamers in routine cases and use them in patients with deficient bone in the proximal humerus only when I have to secure the prosthesis with cement. Cement is used only if the bone in the proximal humerus is deficient; if there are large cysts, as in some patients with rheumatoid arthritis; or if for some reason a stable press-fit cannot be obtained. When the bone in the proximal humerus is deficient, I pack all of the resected humeral head, cut into small pieces, into the proximal humerus and down into the shaft, and use the large-stem prosthesis. I then use an amount of cement only about the size of a Ping-Pong ball, applying it only in the upper flare portion of the humerus to secure fixation of the fins of the prosthesis.

When using cement, I do not use a plug down into the canal. There are two reasons to avoid putting it all the way down the medullary canal to the tip of the

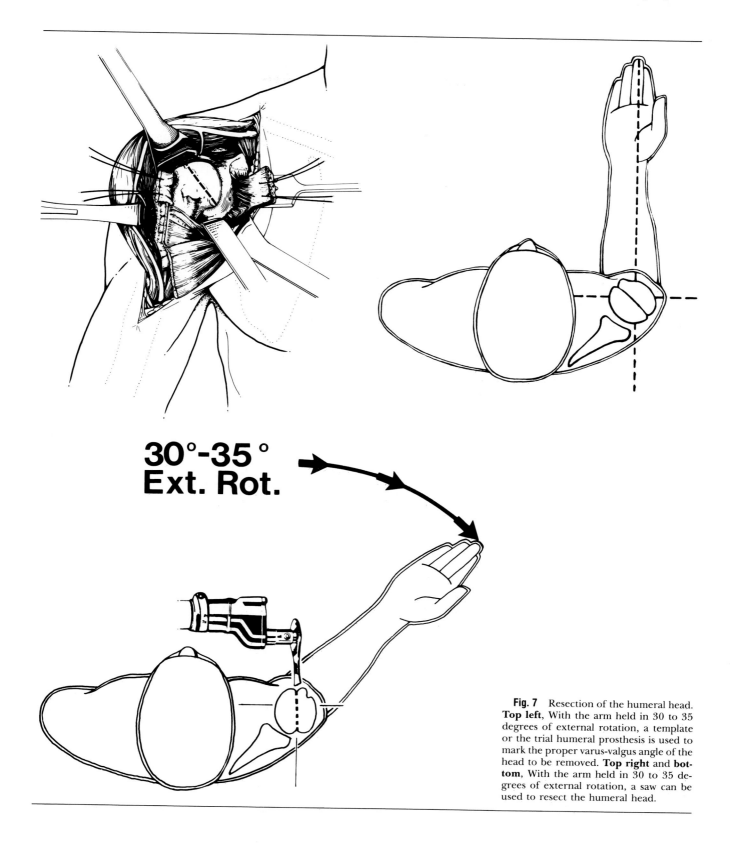

**30°-35°
Ext. Rot.**

Fig. 7 Resection of the humeral head. **Top left**, With the arm held in 30 to 35 degrees of external rotation, a template or the trial humeral prosthesis is used to mark the proper varus-valgus angle of the head to be removed. **Top right** and **bottom**, With the arm held in 30 to 35 degrees of external rotation, a saw can be used to resect the humeral head.

prosthesis. First, that amount of cement is not necessary for fixation. Second, and more importantly, if it is ever necessary to remove the humeral component, I know from previous experience that it is extremely difficult to remove a secure, fully cemented prosthesis. Only in unusual cases, when even the largest stem is

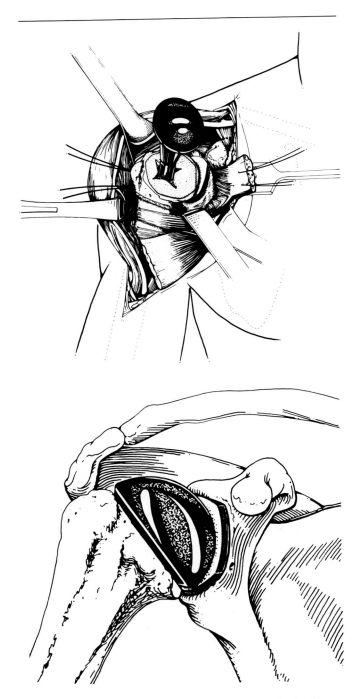

Fig. 8 Press-fit technique of the trial humeral prosthesis with care taken to maintain the fin tracks in the cancellous bone of upper humerus. A press-fit of the humeral prosthesis without cement is ideal.

tom). When the thickness of the humeral head and the proper stem size have been determined, the trial prosthesis should be removed. The humeral head retractor is used to displace the head posteriorly out of the way, exposing the glenoid fossa in preparation for the glenoid prosthesis (Fig. 9, *top*). Any remaining tags of anteroinferior capsule, together with the labrum, should be removed.

Insertion of Trial Glenoid Prosthesis

I prefer to use the football-shaped air burr to create the slot in the glenoid fossa for the prosthesis (Fig. 9). It is important to place a finger along the anterior aspect of the neck of the scapula to get an idea of the slope of the neck of the scapula and hence the slope angle for the trough into the neck of the scapula. The air burr and the curettes are used to enlarge the trough enough to accept the keel of the prosthesis. I do not drill holes into the remaining glenoid face for glenoid fixation, because I prefer not to remove any of the dense cortical bone of the face of the glenoid. However, I do use the burr on a deformed face of the glenoid to insure the proper flush fit of the prosthesis against the face of the glenoid.

The bone trough must be deep enough to allow the trial glenoid prosthesis to sit flat on the glenoid. Thumb pressure all along the glenoid prosthesis should reveal no rocking of the prosthesis. I undermine the bone trough in the neck of the glenoid up into the base of the coracoid and down the lateral border of the scapula to help with cement fixation. The bone trough in the glenoid is carefully irrigated and then packed with a dry sponge while the cement is being mixed. If there is a bleeding point within the bony trough, I coagulate it with the electric coagulation unit or place a small piece of surgical gauze on the bleeding point and hold it in place with pressure by the sponge.

I recommend using only the high-density polyethylene glenoid prosthesis without the metal backing. This is because I am concerned that the forces across and on the superior, inferior, anterior, and posterior borders of the metal-backed glenoid that occur during shoulder motion will be transmitted to the metal keel of the prosthesis and in time loosen the glenoid component.

I use a half package of methylmethacrylate for fixation of the glenoid prosthesis. I do not use the cement in the semiliquid stage, nor do I use a cement gun. The cement is ready for insertion when it is no longer sticks to your gloves. I remove the sponge from the bone trough and divide the cement into three or four equal portions. Each portion is forced sequentially, using heavy thumb pressure, into the bone trough. Between portions I carefully remove any excess cement. I do not put any cement on the back surface of the prosthesis

unstable, will it be necessary to use some cement in the medullary canal to achieve stability.

Once it has been determined whether the thin (15 mm) or the thick (22 mm) humeral head is to be used, the excess bone inferior to the trial prosthesis, which includes the usual inferior head osteophyte, should be removed with an osteotome and rongeur (Fig. 8, *bot-*

or on the face of the glenoid because I do not want it to loosen and float about the joint. The glenoid prosthesis is inserted and held with thumb pressure until the cement has hardened (Fig. 9, *bottom*). All excess cement is carefully removed.

When the glenoid component is secure, the joint is thoroughly irrigated. The bone hook is used again to lift the proximal humerus out of the wound while the arm is extended and externally rotated. If the subscapularis tendon was simply divided, or if it was lengthened, then it is repaired to itself with the previously placed Dacron tape sutures. If the subscapularis tendon has been taken down from its bony insertion, holes are drilled through the lateral upper shaft into the cancellous portion of the neck of the humerus. The 1-mm Dacron sutures that were previously placed in the subscapularis tendon are placed through these drill holes. The loops of the sutures are held inferiorly out of the way in preparation for the insertion of the humeral component. As previously mentioned, I prefer to press-fit the humeral prosthesis, avoiding the use of bone cement. In addition to the press-fit, I usually pack some small pieces of the bone from the resected head of the humerus into the slots in the proximal humerus and down into the upper shaft.

Wound Closure

When the subscapularis is securely reattached, the patient should have 30 to 40 degrees of external rotation without excessive tension on the repair. The wound is thoroughly irrigated with the antibiotic solution. Portable wound evacuation tubes are inserted into the depths of the wound and the wound is closed. The muscles and subcutaneous tissues are infiltrated with 30 ml of 0.25% bupivacaine, which significantly reduces the amount of postoperative pain for six to eight hours. I do not reattach the pectoralis major tendon, and it is not necessary to put any sutures in the deltopectoral muscle interval. I simply reapproximate the subcutaneous tissue. This is done in two layers. The deepest layer is closed with 2-0 Dexon sutures, and the more superficial fatty layer is closed with plain catgut. The skin is closed with a subcutaneous running nylon suture. The final postoperative radiographs are taken, with the arm in neutral rotation, in the operating room or in the recovery room (Fig. 10, *top*). This radiograph is used to demonstrate to the patient and the patient's family the difference between the final result and the preoperative radiograph (Fig. 10, *bottom*).

Postoperative Management

It is essential that the surgeon play an integral part in the rehabilitation program. I agree with Neer that

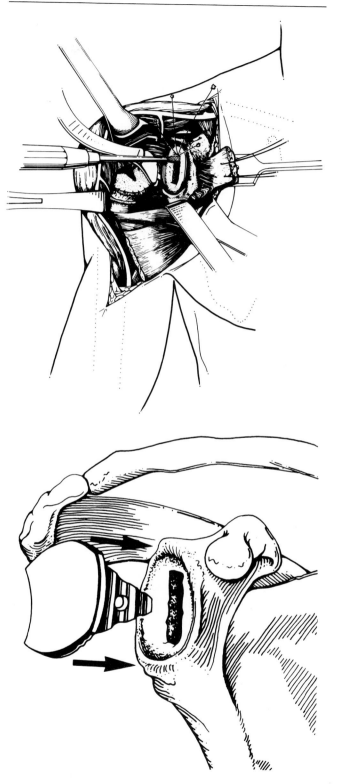

Fig. 9 Using a humeral head retractor, the proximal end of the humerus is retracted posteriorly out of the way. The air burr and curettes are used to create a bone trough into the neck of the glenoid to receive the trial prosthesis. When the trough is deep enough so that the trial glenoid fits flat on the glenoid fossa, bone cement is used to anchor the glenoid prosthesis in place.

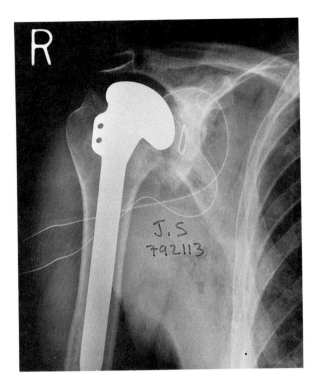

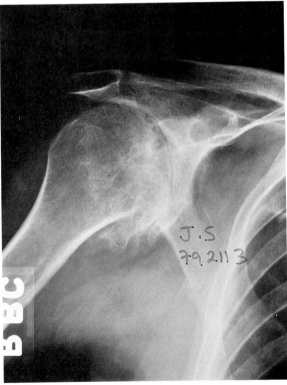

Fig. 10   Top, Following the total shoulder replacement, note that the head of the press-fit humeral prosthesis sits above the top of the greater tuberosity and that the fin fills the medullary canal of the humerus. The small rectangular piece of wire identifies the base of the keel of the glenoid prosthesis. **Bottom,** A preoperative radiograph of the right shoulder in a 79-year-old patient with advanced degenerative arthritis. Note the narrowing of the joint space, sclerosis about the joint, and inferior osteophytes.

postoperative management is as important as the surgery itself. I personally instruct the patient in all exercise programs, which I call "ortho-therapy." I also give patients diagrams of their prescribed exercise program.

I believe that early passive flexion and external rotation is the key to achieving satisfactory functional range of motion. Passive motion of the shoulder—flexion and external rotation—begins the afternoon of the day of surgery. In many instances, after the patient has been moved from the operating room table and is in bed, I connect the arm to a continuous passive movement unit. This unit is used for two to three hours morning and afternoon. Its use is ordinarily discontinued after 24 hours because by then the patient is usually able to use the normal arm to put the treated arm through passive flexion up to 90 degrees and to use a 3-foot stick to obtain passive external rotation. On the first day after surgery, the patient is out of bed in a chair and continues to do the passive flexion exercises. On the second day we encourage the patient to get up and walk to the bathroom and into the halls. On the second day the patient is also taught shoulder pendulum exercises, which are to be done four to six times per day before doing the passive flexion and external rotation while in the supine position. On the second or third day the patient is encouraged to use the arm for gentle everyday living activities. This includes using the arm for eating, brushing teeth, and writing. They are also taught how to use the overhead pulley to increase passive flexion.

The patient usually leaves the hospital on fourth day, and continues to perform pendulum exercises, passive flexion, and external rotation using the normal arm, an overhead pulley, or a 3-foot stick. A sling is worn for one or two weeks, but only when the patient is out in public. Early active use of the arm can and should be encouraged, because the only significant muscle that was completely detached is the subscapularis, and it has been securely reattached to the proximal humerus with the three or four 1-mm Dacron sutures. Because the deltoid is intact, it is not unusual for the patient on the first postoperative day to be able to support the arm actively in 90 degrees of flexion while in the supine position. I have seen patients in the erect position on the third day after surgery actively flex the arm 90 degrees and place the involved hand on top of the head.

The patient continues the "ortho-therapy" program at home four to six times per day, including passive flexion, external rotation, and gentle active use of the arm for activities of daily living. The sutures are removed two weeks after surgery. Between the second and sixth weeks the patient is encouraged to use the arm as much as possible, and to continue with the exercise program, including wall climbing and use of an overhead pulley system. At six weeks the patient begins active resistive exercises to strengthen the rotator cuff and the three parts of the deltoid.

Acknowledgment

The author is indebted to Charles S. Neer II, MD, for his teaching and innovations in the development of the prosthetic component used for the total shoulder arthroplasty procedure.

Carol Mercer (Columbus, Georgia) and Nancy Place (San Antonio, Texas) created the illustrations for this chapter.

Total Shoulder Arthroplasty: Complications and Revision Surgery

Robert H. Cofield, MD

Bradley C. Edgerton, MD

Introduction

In the last 15 years much has been learned about arthritis of the shoulder, its treatment by total shoulder arthroplasty, and the benefits and limitations of this procedure. Numerous articles outlining patient series have given indications, contraindications, and the results to be expected. Complications, including those leading to revision surgery, are uncommon and little has been written about them. This chapter, while it briefly reviews indications, preoperative evaluation, and typical results, concentrates mainly on complications and their surgical treatment. Data will be presented, problems categorized, and solutions suggested. Unfortunately, because of limited experience with revision surgery, the heterogeneity of complications, and the diversity of treatment methods, an analysis of results is not yet available. The goal of revision surgery is to restore normal anatomy insofar as this is possible, essentially the same goal as in caring for patients who have primary prosthetic procedures for glenohumeral arthritis. However, revision surgery is more difficult because of tissue deficiencies and fibrosis.

Indications for Surgery

As the technology for performing total shoulder arthroplasty became available, a number of prostheses were developed to meet treatment needs for a great spectrum of shoulder diseases. Some believed prosthetic arthroplasty might be able to replace rotator-cuff functions and eliminate severe instability in addition to substituting for arthritic joint surfaces. Many types of constrained, ball-in-socket devices were introduced, but complications and revisions occurred too frequently. Currently, most prosthetic components are meant to replace a minimal amount of bone while resurfacing joint surfaces devoid of cartilage, either with or without deformed subchondral bone. Shoulder diseases for which prostheses were applied at our institution are listed in Table 1. In addition to cartilage loss, each disease has specific characteristics.

In osteoarthritis, the humeral head is enlarged and flattened; the glenoid is flat and often has posterior wear. The joint may be subluxated posteriorly. The inferior and posterior aspects of the shoulder capsule may be enlarged and the anterior aspect of the capsule shortened. The manifestations of rheumatoid arthritis vary in degree but not in kind. The bone may be osteopenic or resorbed. The synovium may be active, with hypertrophy, or it may be fibrotic. The rotator cuff may be normal, thin, scarred, or torn. Subluxation

Table 1
Indications by diagnosis for total shoulder arthroplasty

Diagnosis	No. of Shoulders
Osteoarthritis	173
Rheumatoid arthritis	165
Traumatic arthritis	46
Cuff-tear arthropathy	42
Failed surgery	
Total	34
Proximal humeral	21
Fusion	4
Resection	3
Osteonecrosis	15
Old sepsis	5
Other	8

Table 2
Complications of shoulder arthroplasty*

Complications	Unconstrained (%)	Constrained (%)	Hemiarthroplasty (%)
Glenoid loosening	4.7 (0–36)	11.8 (0–25)	0
Humeral loosening	0.4 (0–6.9)	1.0 (0–7.7)	0
Subluxation	0.9 (0–12.5)	0	0
Dislocation	2.7 (0–18.2)	9.4 (6–16.7)	1.7 (2–6.6)
Rotator-cuff tear	2.2 (0.–16.6)	0	2.7 (2–11.5)
Infection	0.5 (0–3.9)	2.9 (0–15.4)	0
Nerve injury	0.5 (0–2)	0	0.4 (0–2)

*Percentages are averages; ranges are in parentheses

Table 3
Component revisions for constrained implants

Authors	No. of Shoulders	Revised (%)
Amstutz et al[1]	10	20
Cofield[13]	12	41.7
Coughlin et al[14]	16	12.5
Kessel and Bayley[21]	18	16.7
Lettin et al[22]	50	34
McElwain and English[23]	13	7.7
Post and Jablon[26]	77	19.5

Table 4
Component revisions for unconstrained implants

Authors	No. of Shoulders	Revised (%)
Amstutz et al[1]	46	10.9
Barrett et al[2]	50	8.0
Cofield[4]	73	4.1
Cruess[15]	26	3.9
Gristina et al[19]	100	5.0
Neer et al[6]	194	3.6
Ranawat et al[7]	29	10.3
Wilde et al[8]	38	5.3
Worland[29]	23	8.7

is usually superior or anterior. In trauma, in addition to scarred, stretched, or occasionally torn soft tissues, the problems are bony—osteonecrosis, malunion, high humeral nonunion, joint impaction, or joint-splitting fractures.

These three diagnoses—osteoarthritis, rheumatoid arthritis, and traumatic arthritis—account for the majority of patients for whom total shoulder arthroplasty is indicated. Three other diagnostic categories include most of the rest: humeral osteonecrosis with associated glenoid arthritis, cuff-tear arthropathy, or other failed reconstructive surgery. Contraindications include recent or active infection, paralysis of the deltoid and rotator cuff, rotator-cuff tearing without arthritis, or instability in the absence of arthritis.

Patient participation in and cooperation with treatment is essential, because soft tissues must be protected during the first months, and early motion exercises must also be done. Persons with neuropathic disease or substance abuse will not do well with prosthetic reconstruction. Neuropathy may be more subtle than one might expect. Alcoholism or other substance abuse may be hidden, denied, or mistakenly described as cured.

Presurgical Assessment

History, physical examination, and plain shoulder radiographs are the essential first steps in preoperative evaluation. Surprisingly, there is seldom a history of injury or, in the absence of rheumatoid arthritis, multiple-joint disease. Pain typically is insidious in onset and progresses over two to ten years. Both shoulders may be involved. Pain occurs with use and, unfortunately, is commonly present at night. Physiotherapy or injections have little effect. Medications for pain are more useful in the daytime than at night.

Range of motion is often restricted to one half or two thirds of normal. Weakness is not a major consideration, because pain prevents strenuous use of the arm and extremity. Standard shoulder-joint radiographic views may fail to demonstrate cartilage loss in the absence of substantial subchondral sclerosis or osteophytes. The axillary view and a well-positioned, 40-degree posterior-oblique view will show cartilage loss and subtle subchondral erosions.

Findings from these basic evaluations may suggest additional study. Other investigations might include general medical examination, rheumatologic consultation, neurologic examination, laboratory or scanning

Table 5
Reoperations on shoulder prostheses

Complications	Hemiarthroplasty	Unconstrained	Constrained	Total
Glenoid loosening	—	13	3	16
Glenoid arthritis	12	—	—	12
Instability	2	7	2	11
Rotator-cuff tear	3	6	—	9
Displaced high-density polyethylene	—	8	—	8
Humeral loosening	1	7	—	8
Infection	4	3	—	7
Unexplained pain	1	—	2	3
Hematoma	—	2	—	2
Fistula	—	—	1	1
Ectopic bone	1	—	—	1
Humeral bone loss	1	—	—	1
Total	25	46	8	79

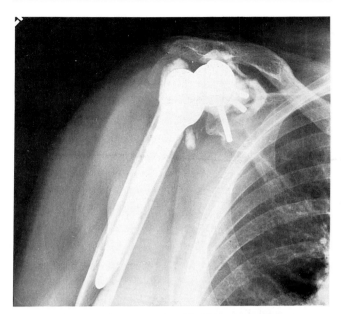

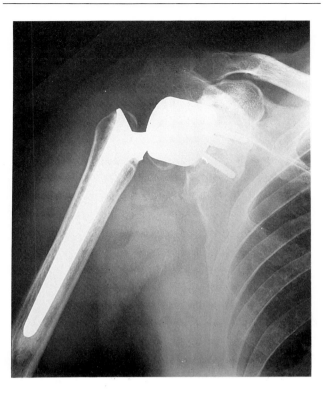

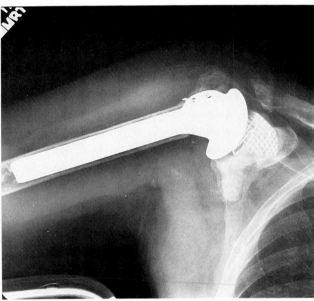

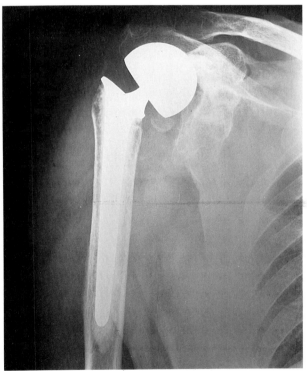

Fig. 1   Top, Loosened glenoid component, Stanmore total shoulder arthroplasty. **Bottom**, The constrained implant was revised to an unconstrained Neer type of implant. There was extensive bone loss within the scapula. This was replaced with methylmethacrylate and wire mesh. Currently, much of this deficiency would be replaced by autogenous iliac crest bone graft.

studies for infection, arthrography with joint aspiration and bacteriologic studies, computed tomography, or magnetic resonance imaging. Some situations call for caution. For example, an elderly patient with long-standing shoulder arthritis and whose treatment included recent cortisone injections suffered a sudden intensification of shoulder pain. This symptom could represent a bacterial infection superimposed on the arthritic condition. Laboratory studies and arthrogra-

Fig. 2   Top, Michael Reese total shoulder arthroplasty with loosened glenoid component and fractured screws. **Bottom**, Bone loss in the scapula precluded placement of a new Michael Reese type of component. Fortunately, the humeral component of the Michael Reese system has a 22-mm head, allowing for placement of a bipolar component in conjunction with glenoid reshaping. Removal of a humeral component that is cemented in place is extremely difficult and may be associated with fracturing and partial destruction of the bone during the process of implant removal.

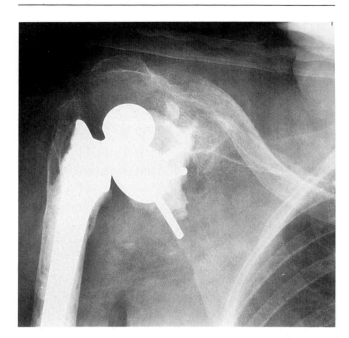

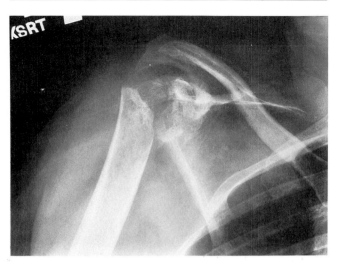

Fig. 3 Dislocated Stanmore total shoulder arthroplasty. Closed reduction was performed and was successful. Unfortunately, the implant again dislocated and revision surgery was required.

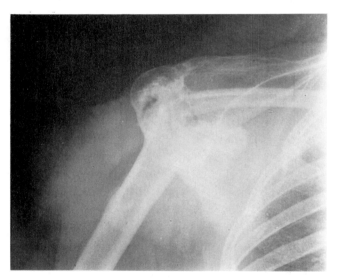

Fig. 4 **Top,** Resection arthroplasty. In addition to the bone deficiencies, the deltoid and rotator cuff have minimal remaining function. Unfortunately, the shoulder was quite painful. **Bottom,** Treatment by shoulder arthrodesis including autogenous iliac crest bone grafts and use of an external fixator.

phy with aspiration and cultures are indicated. In glenohumeral arthritis, and especially in old trauma, the nature and extent of deformities may not be entirely clear despite multiple radiographic views. Computed tomography can aid in determining what osteotomies will be necessary as a part of the surgery.

Expected Results

A number of published series describe results for the relatively unconstrained resurfacing types of total shoulder arthroplasty.[1-8] As with most total joint replacements, pain relief is achieved in approximately 90% to 95% of patients. Return of active movement often depends on the experience of the surgeon and on postoperative management, but motion after surgery as an average approximates two thirds of normal. Major joint replacements in other anatomic areas give similar results. However, return of motion varies more in this operation than in other joint replacements and depends to a great extent on the diagnosis and the degree of soft-tissue or bone deficiencies. In osteoarthritis, return of movement after surgery approximates three quarters or four fifths of normal. The same is true for patients with proximal humeral osteonecrosis and secondary glenoid arthritis. Rheumatoid arthritis affects soft tissues and bone to a greater extent, and this damage is reflected in a return of motion that typ-

ically averages one half to two thirds of normal. In old trauma, extensive fibrosis may further compromise movement after surgery. In such cases, releases can be done, and capsule and tendon can be thinned or lengthened, but often the inflexible tissue cannot be excised for fear of creating joint instability.

Cuff-tear arthropathy with bone, capsule, and rotator-cuff deficiencies is an example of a disease for which surgical goals typically are limited.[6] Here rehabilitation seeks first to maintain stability, with the hope of eventually regaining one third to one half of normal movement.

In the absence of complications, results reported by experienced surgeons are usually quite satisfactory.

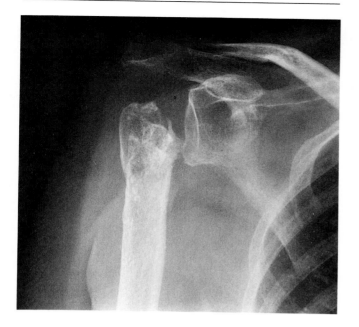

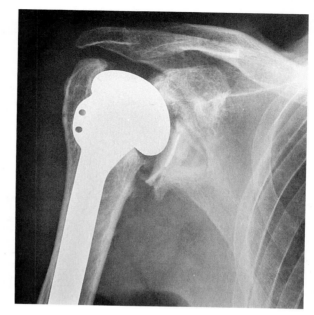

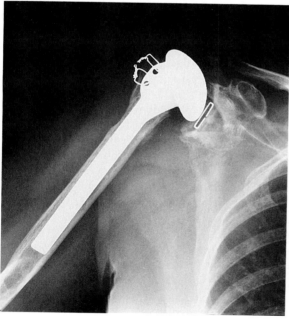

Fig. 5   Top, Resection arthroplasty. The deltoid is intact, and the rotator cuff is present and functioning. Unfortunately, the shoulder was extremely painful. **Bottom**, Placement of unconstrained total shoulder arthroplasty eliminated the pain and allowed moderate return of shoulder function.

Fig. 6   Top, Painful unconstrained total shoulder arthroplasty with loosened glenoid and humeral components. The glenoid component has shifted inferiorly and impacted into the scapula. The humeral component has impacted into the humerus. **Bottom**, At revision surgery, both components were replaced—the glenoid replaced with a slightly larger component and the humeral component positioned slightly more proximal to contour smoothly with the humeral tuberosities.

Should complications occur, either pain relief or postoperative motion and strength may be compromised. If revision surgery is required, it is likely that the absence of bone or the presence of more scar and less flexible capsule or tendon tissues will lead to results inferior to those achieved in primary surgical reconstructions.

Complications and Revision Surgery

Since 1972, 29 studies of shoulder arthroplasty have included sufficient data on complications to make analysis possible.[1-29] For ease of understanding, Table 2

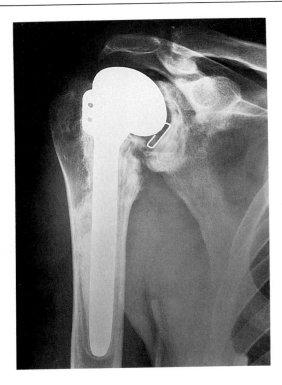

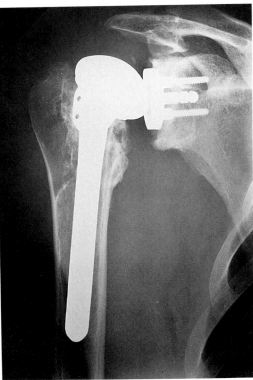

Fig. 7 **Top**, Loosened glenoid component, unconstrained total shoulder arthroplasty. The component has changed position, moving inferiorly, tilting upward, and impacting into the scapula. There was an extensive histiocytic response to the loosened component and fragmented methylmethacrylate. **Bottom**, The shoulder was revised to an unconstrained implant incorporating bone ingrowth characteristics in this patient with sensitivity to polymethylmethacrylate.

groups the studies according to prosthetic type: unconstrained, constrained, or hemiarthroplasty. In order of frequency, major complications for unconstrained implants are glenoid loosening, subluxation or dislocation, and rotator-cuff tearing. Humeral loosening, infection, and nerve injury are less common. Complications are more frequent for constrained prostheses, including those with hooded glenoid components or ball-in-socket designs. Complications for these types of implant, by order of frequency, are glenoid component material failure or loosening of the component, dislocation, and infection.

For a number of patients, these complications led to the need for revision surgery (Tables 3 and 4). In two series of constrained prostheses, no component revisions were reported,[10,25] but the average rate of component revision in a third series was 22%, clearly a much higher rate than in those series reporting revisions of unconstrained prostheses, in which the need for revision surgery averaged 6.6%.

Patient Evaluation

When an individual experiences difficulties after total shoulder arthroplasty, it is necessary first to define the problem. This may not be easy because several minor problems may act together to produce a poor result.

Neer and Kirby[30] suggested a broad approach to evaluating the shoulder arthroplasty with complications or failure. They recommended reviewing general preoperative considerations, surgical considerations (including soft tissues, bone, and prosthesis), and postoperative considerations. This is the only publication that specifically addresses revision surgery for shoulder arthroplasty. In this study, which included 40 humeral head prostheses and total shoulder arthroplasties requiring revision surgery, the causes of failure were often multiple. For failed fixed-fulcrum arthroplasty, the most important of these were loss of the external rotators and mechanical failure. For failed unconstrained arthroplasty, major causes of failure were deltoid scars and detachment, a tight subscapularis, adhesions and impingement of the rotator cuff, a prominent or retracted tuberosity, loss of humeral length, glenoid slope and centralization, and inadequately supervised rehabilitation.

Patient Series

Between 1976 and 1988, our institution handled 79 complications leading to reoperations on shoulder prostheses (Table 5). These complications and the treatments chosen for them are described and illustrated below. Supporting data from the literature are presented when available.

Revision Surgery for Constrained Implants

During this 12-year period, revision surgery was deemed necessary for three implants with glenoid loos-

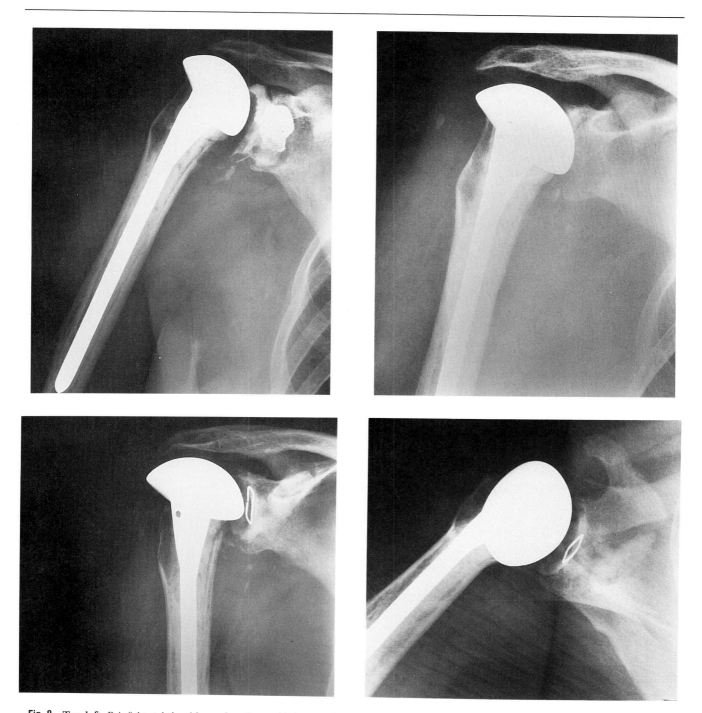

Fig. 8 **Top left**, Painful total shoulder arthroplasty with loosened glenoid component and substantial glenoid bone loss, both centrally and peripherally on the anterior glenoid neck. **Top right**, At surgery, the bone loss was so extensive that a new glenoid component could not be placed. The bone deficiencies were eliminated by bone grafting. **Bottom**, Unfortunately, the patient did not achieve satisfactory pain relief following removal of the loosened glenoid component and bone grafting. Two years later, it was possible to reoperate on the patient and cement a new glenoid component in the presence of adequate scapular bone stock.

ening (Figs. 1 and 2), two with unexplained pain, two with instability (Fig. 3), and one with a synovial fistula. The fistula was excised and closed. In the two patients with pain, although it was thought that the components might be loosened, surgery showed them to be secure. The implants were revised to unconstrained total shoulder arthroplasties, but pain persisted. As a result of this experience, revision surgery on a painful total shoulder

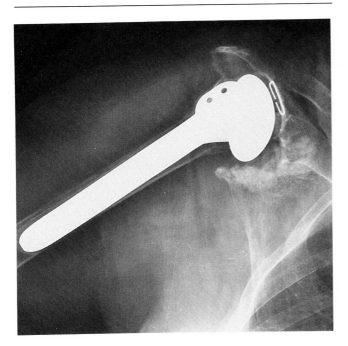

Fig. 9   Unconstrained total shoulder arthroplasty with fractured high density polyethylene glenoid component. The fracture occurred near the junction of the face of the glenoid component with the keel. The keel remains firmly cemented in the scapula. The face of the component has migrated superiorly.

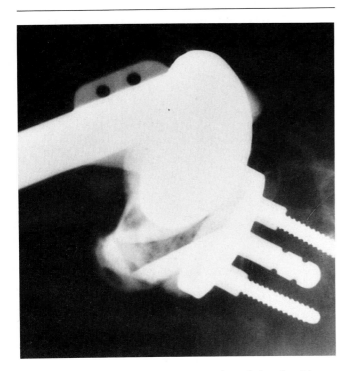

Fig. 10   High-density polyethylene portion of the glenoid component has become displaced from the metal tray of the glenoid implant. This was treated by revision surgery and placement of a one-piece glenoid component.

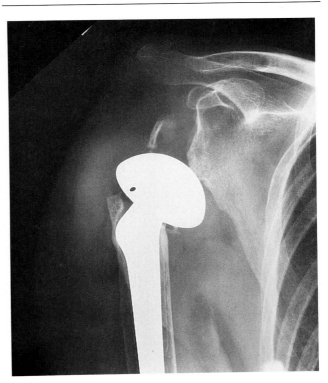

Fig. 11   Inferior dislocation of a proximal humeral prosthesis following surgery for comminuted fracturing of the proximal humerus. Humeral bone loss has occurred, and the implant was positioned to mate with the remaining humeral bone rather than the glenoid surface. Treatment would require replacement of the humeral component, positioning it opposite the glenoid, and eliminating bone deficiencies of the proximal humerus with bone graft.

arthroplasty is not advised unless a definite abnormality can be identified.

The failure of constrained implants often includes glenoid component loosening, material failure, or both. Unfortunately, this is commonly associated with substantial loss of scapular bone stock. Figure 1 illustrates the use of methylmethacrylate and wire mesh to correct these bone deficiencies. However, current techniques include replacing lost bone with an autogenous iliac crest bone graft instead of methylmethacrylate. Lettin and associates[22] suggested excision arthroplasty to treat failed Stanmore total shoulder arthroplasties. In eight of nine patients so treated, the level of pain was reduced, and the return of active abduction and flexion averaged 55 degrees. Subjective evaluation indicated that, compared with their preoperative arthritic condition, three of the patients felt they were better, three felt they were unchanged, and three felt their condition was worse. Unfortunately, resection arthroplasties of the shoulder sometimes fail to achieve satisfactory pain relief. The patient shown in Figure 4 had additional muscle deficiencies that required the use of shoulder fusion to eliminate pain. Figure 5 illustrates a second patient with pain after resection arthroplasty. In this

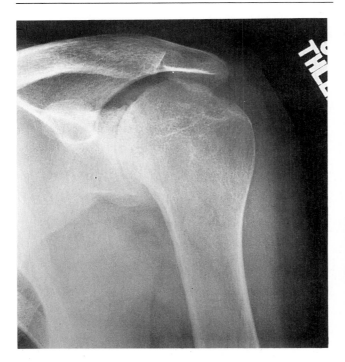

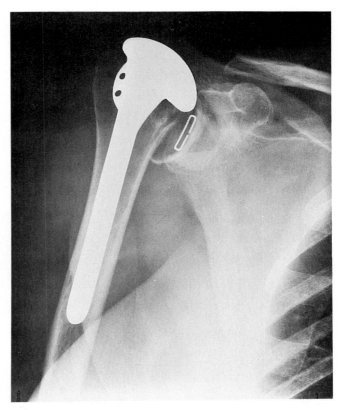

Fig. 13 Superiorly dislocated humeral component of an unconstrained total shoulder arthroplasty. The patient's underlying diagnosis was cuff-tear arthropathy, and at surgery a massive rotator-cuff tear was repaired. The current radiographic findings indicate retearing of the patient's repaired rotator cuff.

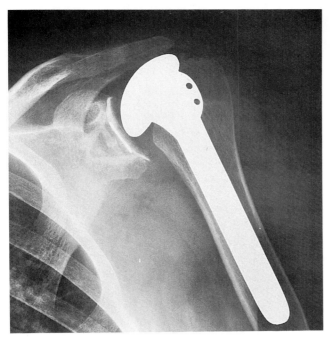

Fig. 12 Top, Rheumatoid arthritis, cartilage loss, osteopenia, and attrition of the rotator cuff with upward subluxation of the humeral head. **Bottom**, Following total shoulder arthroplasty, the proximal humeral prosthesis remains in the slightly upward subluxated position, indicating attrition or thinning of the rotator cuff.

patient, the deltoid and rotator-cuff muscles were functioning, allowing placement of an unconstrained prosthetic system to relieve pain.

Post and Jablon[26] reported eight revisions for bent or broken humeral necks with Series I Michael Reese total shoulder replacements. The broken implants were successfully revised. The design of this implant system was changed to eliminate humeral component fracturing, but unfortunately the point of failure appears to have been transferred to the glenoid component and its fixation (Fig. 2). Orr and associates,[31] using finite-element analysis, found that, compared with less constrained designs, constrained designs resulted in increased forces at the bone-cement interface of the glenoid component.

Revision Surgery for Unconstrained Implants

During the period of review, unconstrained shoulder arthroplasties were revised to correct the following complications: glenoid loosening, a displaced or worn high-density polyethylene component, dislocation, rotator-cuff tearing, infection, hematoma, humeral loosening, and axillary nerve laceration.

There are a number of treatment options for patients with glenoid component loosening. When possible, replacing the loosened component by securely recementing a slightly larger component is preferred (Fig.

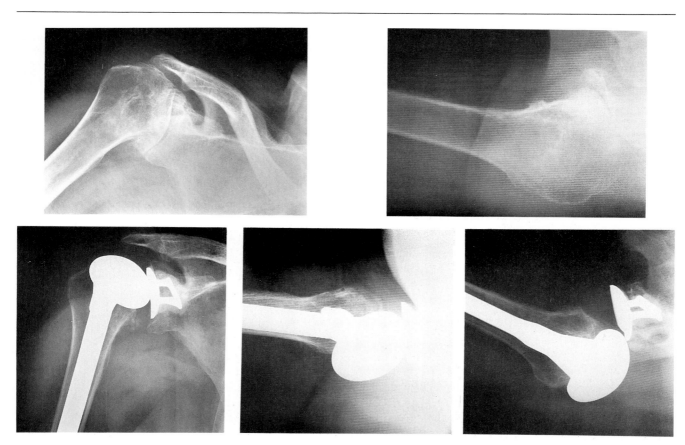

Fig. 14   **Top,** Osteoarthritis of the shoulder with flattening of the humeral head, posterior subluxation of the humerus, and posterior glenoid erosion. **Bottom left** and **bottom center,** Unconstrained total shoulder arthroplasty. The humeral component was positioned in 35 degrees of retrotorsion; the glenoid component was positioned on the glenoid face to mate with the remaining glenoid bone leaving the component facing in a retroverted position. Stability was present at the time of surgery, but the tendency for posterior subluxation remained. **Bottom right,** Sixteen months following surgery, the humeral component dislocated associated with stretching of the posterior structures, lengthening of the subscapularis repair, and erosion of the polyethylene portion of the glenoid component. At revision surgery, it was necessary to revise both components, to tighten the posterior capsular structures, and to rerepair the subscapularis.

6). Alternatively, it is possible to remove the loosened component, the fragmented cement, and histiocytic tissue, and then to graft bone deficiencies and use an ingrowth system like that illustrated in Figure 7. This treatment is appropriate for an individual who had an excessive tissue response to the methacrylate fragmentation associated with loosening.

Unfortunately, it was possible to replace a glenoid component in only four of the 13 shoulders treated for glenoid loosening. The remaining nine shoulders had too little remaining glenoid bone to allow fixation of a component (Fig. 8). This circumstance required removal of the loosened glenoid component, the fragmented methacrylate, and the histiocytic tissue. Autogenous iliac-crest bone graft was used to correct glenoid bone deficiencies, and the total shoulder arthroplasty was essentially converted to a hemiarthroplasty. One patient so treated did not achieve satisfactory pain relief. Two years later it was possible to repeat her shoulder surgery and, with better bone present in

the glenoid, to recement a glenoid component and achieve a satisfactory result.

Compared with other implant materials, high-density polyethylene is relatively weak. It is possible for the polyethylene component of the glenoid implant to fracture at the junction of the component face with a securely fixed keel (Fig. 9). Neer[32] reported two such cases. He now advises the use of a metal-reinforced polyethylene glenoid component, especially in patients who are quite active or who have sloping glenoid surfaces. This treatment involves removal of the fractured glenoid pieces and placement of a new glenoid component, preferably one with metal backing. When the glenoid component has multiple parts, it is possible for the polyethylene portion of the glenoid component to become dislodged from the metal tray (Fig. 10). In this circumstance, it is tempting, at the time of revision surgery, to remove the dislodged polyethylene portion of the glenoid component and replace it with a new polyethylene part. However, the polyethylene compo-

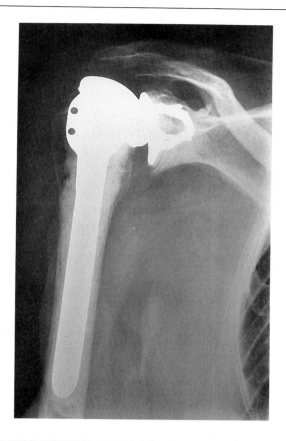

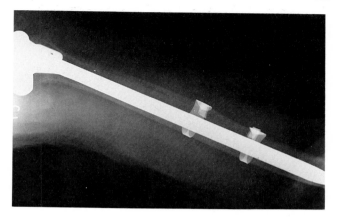

Fig. 16 Patient with rheumatoid arthritis requiring prosthetic shoulder arthroplasty. Bones are quite osteopenic. At surgery, a spiral fracture of the humeral shaft occurred. This was treated by use of a long-stem humeral component and encircling bands. This allowed for stability and uninterrupted progression in postoperative rehabilitation.

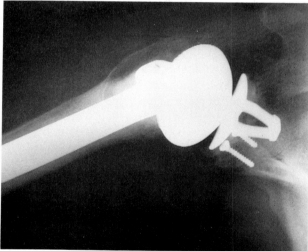

Fig. 15 Osteoarthritic shoulder with pathology similar to that depicted in Figure 14. At initial surgery, the humeral component was positioned in 5 to 10 degrees of retrotorsion, the glenoid bone wear was eliminated by placement of a bone graft, and the glenoid component was cemented in the neutral position relative to version. This eliminated any tendency for residual instability.

nent apparently dislodges only when minor, but often uncorrectable, instability is present in the joint arthroplasty. Replacing the entire multipart glenoid component with a one-piece glenoid component precludes the possibility of polyethylene displacement in the future.

Instability Instability in total shoulder arthroplasty varies in both degree and direction. Subluxations and dislocations have been reported, as have instabilities in superior, inferior, anterior, and posterior directions. Dislocation is more common with constrained implants than with unconstrained designs. Although Lettin and associates[22] successfully treated two dislocated Stanmore prostheses with closed reduction, other designs of constrained implants may not be amenable to closed reduction[7,26] and may require surgical treatment. Of 21 reported dislocations in constrained implants, 16 were treated surgically. Of these, 13 experienced a successful outcome.

Among various types of unconstrained arthroplasties, 28 cases have been reported with a significant instability. The direction of instability was anterior in 11, posterior in nine, inferior in three, and not stated in five. Inferior subluxation that occurs early in the postoperative period may resolve with external support and muscle exercises.[17,24,33] Inferior instability associated with loss of humeral length may not resolve with time, and weakness may persist (Fig. 11).[6]

Some superior subluxation of the humeral component on the glenoid may be expected in patients with rheumatoid arthritis whose rotator cuff and capsular mechanism show attrition but are not torn (Fig. 12). However, in patients without attritional rotator-cuff thinning, significant upward subluxation of the humeral component on the glenoid is almost invariably associated with rotator-cuff tearing (Fig. 13). If this situation occurs soon after surgery, one might consider early rotator-cuff rerepair. If, however, the problem is chronic, treatment should probably parallel that used to treat chronic rotator-cuff tearing when there is no implant. That is, the amount of symptoms, pain, and

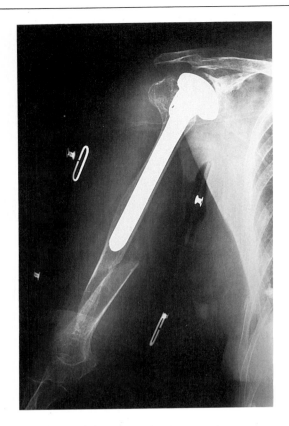

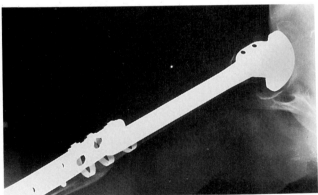

Fig. 17 Top, Humeral shaft fracture as a result of a fall in a patient with a previously performed total shoulder arthroplasty. Satisfactory reduction was achieved. The patient was treated with a coaptation splint and Velpeau dressing support. Unfortunately, no bony callus formed, and nonunion resulted. **Bottom,** Open reduction, internal fixation, and bone grafting of the humeral shaft nonunion. The fracture went on to unite.

lack of function will determine whether or not to undertake surgical rerepair of the rotator cuff.

Of 11 cases of anterior instability reported in the literature, four were treated by closed reduction[8,16,24] and immobilization, and seven were treated by surgery.[8,19,24,29] In this setting, the components may be malpositioned, but certainly the subscapularis repair has

Table 6
Treatment of failed shoulder arthroplasty

Complications	Surgical Treatment Options
Glenoid loosening	Revise component; remove and bone graft
Humeral loosening	Revise component
Glenoid arthritis	Glenoid component
Instability	Soft-tissue repair; revise components
Rotator-cuff tear	Repair
Infection	Implant removal; primary or secondary exchange

become disrupted. The authors found this type of instability extremely difficult to treat successfully.

Posterior instability is seldom mentioned in the literature, which is surprising because posterior translocation of the humeral head on the glenoid and posterior glenoid wear frequently accompany osteoarthritis of the shoulder (Fig. 14). If the components are positioned in osteoarthritis as the bones would suggest they should be, there is the danger that with time the lax posterior structures may stretch further, the subscapularis repair may lengthen, and the polyethylene will deform, resulting in excessive posterior instability and dislocation. When a patient demonstrates this pattern of bone erosion and posterior subluxation, it may be prudent at the initial surgery to decrease the amount of humeral retrotorsion and to consider bone grafting to replace the posteriorly eroded glenoid bone (Fig. 15).[34]

Fractures Intraoperative and postoperative fractures of the glenoid or humerus are rare, but they are more often associated with the use of constrained implants than with unconstrained systems. It would seem sensible to treat intraoperative fractures with rigid internal fixation at the time of prosthetic replacement to facilitate postoperative rehabilitation (Fig. 16). It is suggested that late fractures following surgery can be treated on their own merit. However, many of these fractures occur in patients with rheumatoid arthritis who have softened bones and a lessened tendency for callus formation. Although conservative care is attractive, I have been disappointed in the success of healing following such care and now favor open reduction and internal fixation for fractures that occur in bones adjacent to implanted shoulder prostheses (Fig. 17).

Infection As in other prosthetic arthroplasties, infections may be acute, immediately following surgery, or they may be delayed. Delayed infections represent either a chronic infectious process or a delayed acute infection, metastatic from another site. Infections after total shoulder arthroplasty are not common. Those that occur are usually delayed and are related to hematogenous spread from other infected sites (Fig. 18). *Staphylococcus aureus* is the only bacterial organism recognized in the literature as causing infections in shoulder

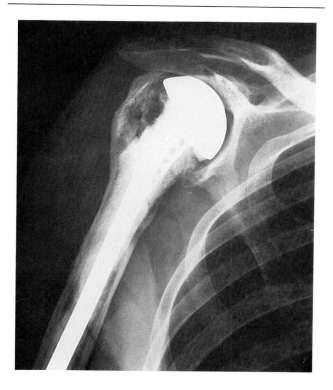

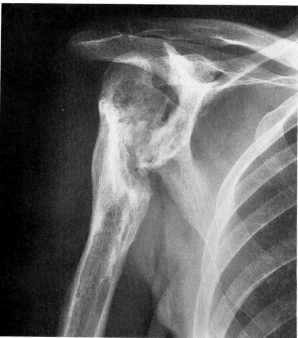

Fig. 18 Top, Patient with multiple-joint osteoarthritis who previously had had a proximal humeral prosthesis placed. Her total knee arthroplasty became infected, and subsequently infection spread to the humeral implant and adjacent bone of the upper humerus. A draining sinus was present in the patient's midarm. **Bottom,** Treatment was by debridement, removal of the prosthesis and adjacent cement, delayed wound closure, use of a suction-irrigation system, and prolonged parenteral antibiotics. The infection resolved; the shoulder became stiffened, but fortunately the patient complained of little pain.

arthroplasties. A *Candida* infection has been reported in an intravenous drug user.[35] There is currently no information in the literature on the use of immediate or delayed reimplantation procedures such as those that have been suggested for septic total hip and total knee arthroplasties. In the literature, with one exception,[1] resection arthroplasty has been necessary for patients with infected shoulder implants.

I have treated two patients who had loosened components but no other indication of the possibility of a septic process. One of these had a painful proximal humeral prosthesis and the second had a painful total shoulder arthroplasty. At surgery, fibrous tissues surrounding the implants were slightly pinker and slightly less firm than usual. Histologic study showed scattered areas of polymorphonuclear leukocytes indicative of a low-grade infectious process. Bacteriologic studies confirmed the presence of infection with *S aureus* in one patient and *Pseudomonas aeruginosa* in the other. Because of the low-grade nature of the infection, these patients underwent debridement and immediate reinsertion of total shoulder components that had either bone ingrowth capabilities or that were fixed with antibiotic-impregnated cement. At two years after surgery, both patients remained pain-free and free of infection. Thus, it would seem, as in other anatomic regions, low-grade infectious processes can be treated with primary or secondary exchange of prosthetic components. However, it must be emphasized that because most patients with infection also have extensive osteomyelitis, resection arthroplasty is the treatment of choice.

Nerve Injuries Despite the close proximity of major nerves to the surgical field, nerve injuries are rarely reported in prosthetic shoulder arthroplasty. In the series considered here, only six nerve injuries occurred.[2,4,9,17,19,28] In every case but one, injury was to the axillary nerve.[17] Three axillary nerve injuries resolved spontaneously. In a fourth, a laceration of the anterior portion of the nerve was not repaired; in the fifth, a laceration to the major portion of the nerve was repaired. Both of these lacerations occurred in heavily scarred surgical fields. The reported injury to the musculocutaneous nerve did not heal. Thus, although nerve injury is not common, it can occur as a part of this procedure. It is fortunate that, in the absence of laceration, contusions or stretch injuries to the nerves almost always recover.

Summary

Fortunately, revision surgery after prosthetic shoulder arthroplasty is rarely required.[36] However, various complications or combinations of complications can lead to the need for revision surgery. For many of these, several treatment options are possible (Table 6). Recognizing all the problems that contributed to failure in an individual patient may be difficult before revision surgery. Understanding the abnormality present at the time of surgery requires considerable experience. For example, glenoid loosening, in addition to being accompanied by scapular bone loss, may be associated with rotator-cuff tearing,[37] instability, or joint contracture. In addition to the component loosening, all of these must also be treated if the revision procedure is to be successful.

When addressing glenoid loosening, it seems to be best to revise the component, if possible. If there is extreme bone loss, one may have to bone graft the deficiencies and not replace the glenoid component. Fortunately, clinically significant humeral loosening is rare. When it occurs, revision of the component is justified and almost always possible. In hemiarthroplasties with pain, conversion to a total shoulder arthroplasty by placing a glenoid component is highly effective. In instability after shoulder arthroplasty, soft-tissue repair does not always create stability. Unfortunately, for most patients, component revision is a necessary part of the revision surgery. When rotator-cuff tearing is acute, repair is indicated; for chronic rotator-cuff tearing, repair depends on the severity of the symptoms. When infection develops after shoulder arthroplasty, implant removal is almost always necessary, but occasionally, in low-grade infections, a primary or secondary exchange procedure may be possible.

References

1. Amstutz HC, Thomas BJ, Kabo JM, et al: The Dana total shoulder arthroplasty. *J Bone Joint Surg* 1988;70A:1174–1182.
2. Barrett WP, Franklin JL, Jackins SE, et al: Total shoulder arthroplasty. *J Bone Joint Surg* 1987;69A:865–872.
3. Bell SN, Gschwend N: Clinical experience with total arthroplasty and hemiarthroplasty of the shoulder using the Neer prosthesis. *Int Orthop* 1986;10:217–222.
4. Cofield RH: Total shoulder arthroplasty with the Neer prosthesis. *J Bone Joint Surg* 1984;66A:899–906.
5. Kelly IG, Foster RS, Fisher WD: Neer total shoulder replacement in rheumatoid arthritis. *J Bone Joint Surg* 1987;69B:723–726.
6. Neer CS II, Watson KC, Stanton FJ: Recent experience in total shoulder replacement. *J Bone Joint Surg* 1982;64A:319–337.
7. Ranawat CS, Warren R, Inglis AE: Total shoulder replacement arthroplasty. *Orthop Clin North Am* 1980;11:367–373.
8. Wilde AH, Borden LS, Brems JJ: Experience with the Neer total shoulder replacement, in Bateman JE, Welsh RP (eds): *Surgery of the Shoulder*. Philadelphia, BC Decker, 1984, pp 224–228.
9. Averill RM: Neer total shoulder arthroplasty. *Orthop Trans* 1980;4:287.
10. Bodey WN, Yeoman PM: Prosthetic arthroplasty of the shoulder. *Acta Orthop Scand* 1983;54:900–903.
11. Brumfield RH Jr, Schilz J, Flinders BW: Total shoulder replacement arthroplasty: A clinical review of 21 cases. *Orthop Trans* 1981;5:398–399.
12. Clayton ML, Ferlic DC, Jeffers PD: Prosthetic arthroplasties of the shoulder. *Clin Orthop* 1982;164:184–191.
13. Cofield RH: The Bickel glenohumeral arthroplasty, in *Joint Replacement in the Upper Limb*. London, The Institution of Mechanical Engineers Conference Publications, 1977, pp 21–25.
14. Coughlin MJ, Morris JM, West WF: The semiconstrained total shoulder arthroplasty. *J Bone Joint Surg* 1979;61A:574–581.
15. Cruess RL: Shoulder resurfacing according to the method of Neer. *J Bone Joint Surg* 1980;62B:116.
16. Figgie HE III, Inglis AE, Goldberg VM, et al: An analysis of factors affecting the long-term results of total shoulder arthroplasty in inflammatory arthritis. *J Arthrop* 1988;3:123–130.
17. Frich LH, Møller BN, Sneppen O: Shoulder arthroplasty with the Neer Mark-II prosthesis. *Arch Orthop Trauma Surg* 1988;107:110–113.
18. Friedman RJ, Ewald FC: Arthroplasty of the ipsilateral shoulder and elbow in patients who have rheumatoid arthritis. *J Bone Joint Surg* 1987;69A:661–666.
19. Gristina AG, Romano RL, Kammire GC, et al: Total shoulder replacement. *Orthop Clin North Am* 1987;18:445–453.
20. Jónsson E, Egund N, Kelly I, et al: Cup arthroplasty of the rheumatoid shoulder. *Acta Orthop Scand* 1986;57:542–546.
21. Kessel L, Bayley I: Prosthetic replacement of shoulder joint: Preliminary communication. *J R Soc Med* 1979;72:748–752.
22. Lettin AW, Copeland SA, Scales JT: The Stanmore total shoulder replacement. *J Bone Joint Surg* 1982;64B:47–51.
23. McElwain JP, English E: The early results of porous-coated total shoulder arthroplasty. *Clin Orthop* 1987;218:217–224.
24. Neer CS: Replacement arthroplasty for glenohumeral osteoarthritis. *J Bone Joint Surg* 1974;56A:1–13.
25. Pahle JA, Kvarnes L: Shoulder replacement arthroplasty. *Ann Chir Gynaecol* 1985;74(suppl 198):85–89.
26. Post M, Jablon M: Constrained total shoulder arthroplasty: Long-term follow-up observations. *Clin Orthop* 1983;173:109–116.
27. Swanson AB: Bipolar implant shoulder arthroplasty, in Bateman JE, Welsh RP (eds): *Surgery of the Shoulder*. Philadelphia, BC Decker, 1984, pp 211–223.
28. Thornhill TS, Karr MJ, Averill RM, et al: Total shoulder arthroplasty: The Brigham experience. *Orthop Trans* 1983;7:497.
29. Worland RL: Shoulder joint replacement. *Va Med* 1985;112:382–383.
30. Neer CS II, Kirby RM: Revision of humeral head and total shoulder arthroplasties. *Clin Orthop* 1982;170:189–195.
31. Orr TE, Carter DR, Schurman DJ: Stress analyses of glenoid component designs. *Clin Orthop* 1988;232:217–224.
32. Neer CS II: Involuntary inferior and multidirectional instability of the shoulder: Etiology, recognition, and treatment, in Stauffer ES (ed): American Academy of Orthopaedic Surgeons *Instructional Course Lectures, XXXIV*. St. Louis, CV Mosby, 1985, pp 232–238.
33. Rao JP, Berkman AR, LaPilusa SJ: A spontaneous relocation of a dislocated Neer prosthesis: Occurs with recovery of brachial plexus lesion. *Orthop Rev* 1986;15:453–456.
34. Neer CS II, Morrison DS: Glenoid bone-grafting in total shoulder arthroplasty. *J Bone Joint Surg* 1988;70A:1154–1162.
35. Lichtman EA: *Candida* infection of a prosthetic shoulder joint. *Skeletal Radiol* 1983;10:176–177.
36. Cofield RH: Total shoulder arthroplasty: Associated disease of the rotator cuff, results, and complications, in Bateman JE, Welsh RP (eds): *Surgery of the Shoulder*. Philadelphia, BC Decker, 1984, pp 229–233.
37. Franklin JL, Barrett WP, Jackins SE, et al: Glenoid loosening in total shoulder arthroplasty: Association with rotator cuff deficiency. *J Arthrop* 1988;3:39–46.

Musculoskeletal Sepsis

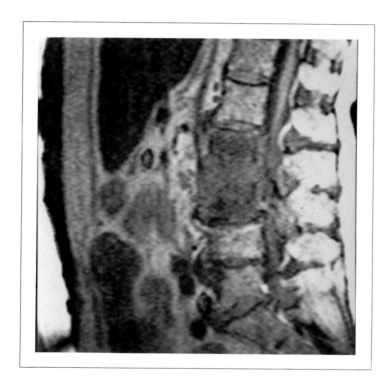

Current Concepts of Antimicrobial Therapy

Robert H. Fitzgerald, Jr., MD

Introduction

The complex surgical procedures used to restore function in the patient with afflictions or traumatic injuries of the spine or the extremities necessitate the optimal use of antimicrobial agents to prevent and treat musculoskeletal sepsis. Ideally, whenever antimicrobial agents are indicated, the surgeon should strive to prescribe the most effective and the safest agent. It is important to avoid the habit of using one or two agents in every situation.

When considering the prophylactic administration of an antimicrobial, it is first necessary to decide whether the indication is appropriate. If it is, then the following variables must be considered: the likely causal organism should an infection complicate the procedure; the ability of the agent to achieve bactericidal concentration at the surgical site; any toxic side effects of the agent under consideration; the patient's history of drug allergies; and whether there is a major cost differential among the potential agents.

When selecting an antimicrobial for therapy, identification of potential causal microorganisms and their susceptibility patterns is critical. When antimicrobials are administered therapeutically, the duration of administration is likely to be prolonged and the potential for toxic side effects becomes greater. Once potential side effects have been identified, methods to monitor for them can be instituted. Finally, the surgeon must decide upon the duration of therapy.

Although many surgeons consider the administration of antimicrobial agents to a patient with an open fracture to be prophylactic in nature, such administration is in reality treatment of an incipient infection.[1-3] In this situation, the surgeon must know what organisms are most apt to contaminate the wound and must prescribe agents specific for each. Timing and duration of administration are also important parameters to consider.

The Prophylactic Administration of Antimicrobial Agents

In the past, the prophylactic administration of antimicrobials was controversial. Several studies have shown the routine administration of prophylactic antimicrobials to be unnecessary or associated with an elevated incidence of sepsis.[4-9] The disastrous consequences of postoperative infections following the surgical implantation of foreign bodies precipitated the many studies that subsequently solidified the opinions of orthopaedists. Fogelberg and associates[10] were among the first proponents of prophylactic antibiotics for surgical procedures of long duration, those with deep dissection, and those associated with hematoma formation. Boyd and associates[11] formally established the efficacy of the prophylactic administration of antimicrobials in adult reconstructive procedures in which a metallic foreign body is implanted. Their findings have been confirmed by Hill and associates,[12] Gustilo and associates,[13,14] and subsequently Patzakis and associates,[2,3] who demonstrated the efficacy of antimicrobial agents in treating traumatic injuries to the musculoskeletal system.

Although the value of prophylactic administration of antimicrobial agents to patients who will have a foreign body implanted, a bone graft procedure, residual deadspace or hematoma following surgery, or a procedure lasting two or more hours is well documented, the routine use of prophylactic antimicrobials in soft-tissue and diagnostic arthroscopic procedures is not so well established. The ideal agents to be administered prophylactically should be active against organisms commonly isolated from infected wounds, for example, *Staphylococcus aureus*, *Staphylococcus epidermidis*, streptococci, anaerobic gram-negative cocci, and anaerobic gram-positive bacilli. Gram-negative bacilli are rarely recovered from postoperative infections complicating elective surgery,[1] but they are commonly encountered in traumatic injuries to the musculoskeletal system. Thus, the antimicrobial agents used for elective procedures often differ from those used for trauma surgery.

Antimicrobial Agents

Two classes of antimicrobial agents offer excellent coverage for elective musculoskeletal procedures. The semisynthetic penicillinase-resistant penicillins, which include methicillin, nafcillin, oxacillin, cloxacillin, and dicloxacillin, are very effective against staphylococci and streptococci, but not against methicillin-resistant staphylococci and enterococci. Methicillin has been associated with nephrotoxicity. It has also been associated with pneumonitis in patients with previous pulmonary damage. Although frequently administered in the past, these complications have led to its replacement by other agents in this class of drugs. Oxacillin and nafcillin are effective agents in this group. Nafcillin can cause local vein toxicity, limiting its therapeutic use. However, this should not be a problem with prophylaxis of short duration.

The cephalosporins are a second class of agents with effective antistaphylococcal and antistreptococcal activity. The cephalosporins are divided into three groups—the first, second, and third generations. The second- and third-generation cephalosporins, which are more active against the gram-negative bacilli, are poor choices for prophylactic agents in elective procedures. The first-generation cephalosporins, in contrast, are primarily antistaphylococcal agents with some gram-negative bacillary coverage. Cephalothin, cephradine, cephapirin, cefazolin, and ceforamide constitute the first-generation cephalosporins. Because cefazolin has a longer half-life, it can be administered every eight hours rather than every four or six hours. Furthermore, it is more competitively produced, reducing its cost without sacrificing activity. Thus, cefazolin is the drug of choice. Since cefazolin has some gram-negative bacillary coverage in addition to its excellent gram-positive activity, it seems superior to oxacillin or nafcillin. It is not active against methicillin-resistant staphylococci or enterococci.

Recently, Kaiser and associates[15] reported that cefamandole with or without gentamicin was statistically superior to cefazolin with or without gentamicin for cardiac surgery. Slama and associates[16] indicated that cefuroxime is statistically superior to cefazolin or cefamandole in patients undergoing coronary artery bypass grafting or cardiac valve replacement surgery. However, the incidence of postoperative infection in these studies was either higher than or just comparable to that considered acceptable following total hip surgery with the prophylactic administration of cefazolin (Table 1). Thus, although these agents have some applicability in cardiac surgery, they do not appear to offer any advantage in elective musculoskeletal surgery.

Timing and Duration of Administration

The timing of administration of prophylactic antimicrobial agents has become fairly standardized. Initially, surgeons administered the agents prophylactically following the surgical procedure. Burke[19] demonstrated that the effective administration of prophylactic agents required their presence when the operative hematoma formed. This, of course, necessitated their administration either before surgery or early during the procedure. It has become common to administer the initial dose of prophylactic agents either as the patient is transported to the operating room or at the time of anesthetic induction.[1,20-23] The administration of an antimicrobial agent one or more days before surgery should be strongly discouraged because it alters the patient's normal bacterial flora, but does not afford any additional protection against sepsis.[1]

The duration of administration of prophylactic antimicrobials remains poorly defined. Some physicians believe that only one or two doses are necessary. Others recommend administering the antimicrobial for a week. Most surgeons continue to administer antimicrobials until the surgical drains are removed, 36 to 72 hours after surgery.[1]

Josefsson and associates[24] have suggested that depot administration of antimicrobials in bone cement may be superior to intravenous administration. However, their study was flawed. Deep sepsis was not documented bacteriologically. In one center included in this multicenter study, the incidence of postoperative sepsis was 6% with the parenteral administration of antimicrobials. Certainly, this is an unacceptably high incidence of sepsis following total hip arthroplasty. Thus, this study did not substantiate the depot administration of antimicrobials for routine prophylaxis. Antibiotic-impregnated bone cement has been used successfully to treat infected total hip arthroplasties and osteomyelitis (see Cierny, Chapter 62).[25]

Table 1
Prophylactic antimicrobials and postoperative sepsis

Investigators	Drugs	Types of Surgery	Incidence of Sepsis (%)
Slama et al[16]	Cefazolin	Cardiac	9
Slama et al[16]	Cefamandole	Cardiac	6
Slama et al[16]	Cefuroxime	Cardiac	5
Kaiser et al[15]	Cefazolin	Cardiac	1.2
Kaiser et al[15]	Cefazolin and gentamicin	Cardiac	2.4
Kaiser et al[15]	Cefamandole	Cardiac	0.8
Kaiser et al[15]	Cefamandole and gentamicin	Cardiac	0
Schutzer and Harris[17]	Cefazolin	Total hip arthroplasty	0.3
Lidwell et al[18]	None	Total hip arthroplasty/ total knee arthroplasty	1.2
Lidwell et al[18]	Cefazolin	Total hip arthroplasty/ total knee arthroplasty	0.3

Open Fractures

The administration of antimicrobial agents to patients with an open fracture or fracture-dislocation is not prophylaxis but is treatment of an incipient infection, because all such wounds are contaminated.[1,2] Because the causal organisms recovered from tissue obtained from these wounds when infection does occur are invariably a mixture of gram-positive and gram-negative bacilli, the antistaphylococcal agents used for elective surgery are inadequate.[3,26] The antimicrobial selected is based on the anticipated microorganism(s) should infection occur and usually combines an antistaphylococcal agent, such as a first-generation cephalosporin, with an agent with considerable activity against gram-negative bacilli, such as an aminoglycoside. One agent, however, provides both of these activities in a single drug and is therefore particularly attractive. This agent is cefamandole, a second-generation cephalosporin. Unfortunately, it is not active against *Pseudomonas aeruginosa*. When an open fracture occurs in association with the use of farm implements or is heavily contaminated by soil, one must consider the possibility of a *Clostridium perfringens* infection, as well as other anaerobic microorganisms. Certainly even the remote possibility of a *C perfringens* infection necessitates the addition of penicillin to the antimicrobial regimen. Because most open fractures are contaminated with soil, many surgeons wish to provide routine coverage against anaerobic microorganisms by adding clindamycin or mitronidazole. In summary, a combination of antimicrobial agents is usually indicated for a patient with an open fracture. Frequently, this combination includes a first-generation cephalosporin (cefazolin), an aminoglycoside (gentamicin), and an agent active against anaerobes (clindamycin). If the injury occurred in the agricultural industry or has been heavily contaminated, penicillin should be added. If the patient is allergic to penicillin, consider metranidazole or chloramphenicol, because nearly all isolates of Clostridia are susceptible to these two drugs. In patients with minimal contamination, a single agent such as cefamandole might suffice.

The Therapeutic Administration of Antimicrobial Agents

Some investigators[27,28] have suggested that the recalcitrant nature of musculoskeletal infections is caused by a blood-bone barrier to antimicrobial penetration similar to that known to exist in the central nervous system (Figs. 1 and 2). Recent steady-state experiments[29-33] have demonstrated that beta-lactam agents, aminoglycosides, and tetracyclines are able to enter the interstitial fluid space of normal and osteomyelitic osseous tissue in concentrations equivalent to the simultaneous serum level (Fig. 3). Thus, no blood-bone barrier exists. Furthermore, these experiments document

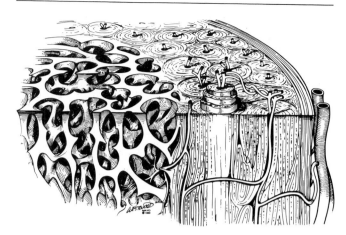

Fig. 1 An artist's rendition of the vascular supply to cortical bone. The periosteal and endosteal vessels supply arterioles that eventually divide into capillaries for each haversian system.

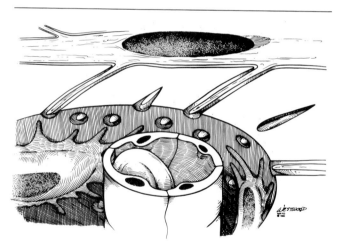

Fig. 2 An artist's rendition of a haversian canal with tight endothelial junctions of the capillary. Antimicrobial agents must cross the endothelial cell to reach the interstitial fluid space of bone. Thus, a blood-bone barrier would be present. Fortunately, physiologic data and ultrastructural studies document rapid transport of solutes from the capillary to the interstitial fluid space of bone.

that one antimicrobial agent is not superior to another in its ability to enter osseous tissue. When an antimicrobial is selected, its ability to enter and achieve bactericidal concentration in osseous tissue need not be a consideration.

The antimicrobial treatment of an established musculoskeletal infection rests upon identification of the causal organism(s) and the susceptibility studies. Once this information is available, selection of the agent of choice necessitates knowledge of the toxicity of each agent under consideration. Only with this information is one able to institute appropriate tests to monitor for early symptoms and signs of toxicity (Table 2).

SERUM AND INTERSTITIAL FLUID CONCENTRATIONS

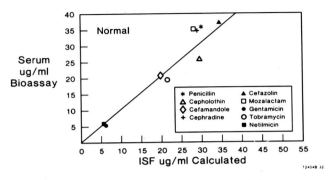

SERUM AND INTERSTITIAL FLUID CONCENTRATIONS

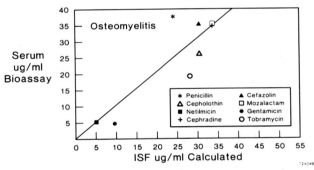

Fig. 3 The relationship of the serum and osseous interstitial fluid concentrations of antimicrobials in a canine model. The serum concentration was measured with bioassay techniques. The interstitial fluid concentration was calculated once the size of the various fluid spaces had been measured with volume of distribution techniques and the osseous and serum concentrations had been measured following the administration of a radioactive antimicrobial. **Top,** The relationship in normal osseous tissue. There is a very close correlation between the two values. **Bottom,** The relationship in osteomyelitic bone. The aminoglycosides appear to be concentrating in bone fluid. Otherwise, the serum and interstitial fluid levels are equivalent.

Three of the newer antimicrobial agents—ciprofloxacin, imipenem, and aztreonam—are particularly suited to treatment of established musculoskeletal infection. Ciprofloxacin is a member of the fluoroquinolone family of drugs, which are all related to nalidixic acid.[34] Its broad spectrum of antibacterial activity includes methicillin-resistant staphylococci and *P aeruginosa*. Ciprofloxacin inhibits bacterial DNA gyrase, an important enzyme in the process of transcription. This unique mechanism of action makes cross-resistance with other agents unlikely. *Bacteroides fragilis, Clostridium difficile, Pseudomonas maltophilia,* and *Pseudomonas cepacia* are resistant. In addition to its broad spectrum, one of the most attractive aspects of ciprofloxacin is the fact that it is an oral agent. Gastrointestinal upsets can compli-

Table 2
Antimicrobial toxicity

Drugs	Side Effects	Monitoring
Gentamicin	Ototoxicity, nephrotoxicity	Weekly audiograms calorics; serum creatinine every other day; serum peak and trough levels
Cephalosporins	Leukopenia, neutropenia	Weekly leukocyte count with differential
Vancomycin	Nephrotoxicity	Serum creatinine
Clindamycin	Colitis	*C difficile* titer
Moxalactam	Superinfection	Repeat culture

cate ciprofloxacin therapy, but this happens only rarely. Even with prolonged therapy required in the treatment of osteomyelitis, ciprofloxacin is a relatively safe drug. Convulsions and central nervous system toxicity may occur with the administration of high doses, especially in the elderly. The drug should not be used in children or pregnant women because it accumulates in and destroys the articular cartilage of developing animals. Clinical use in the treatment of musculoskeletal infections to date has been impressive.

Imipenem, a carbapenem, possesses the broadest spectrum of activity of all antimicrobial agents.[35-37] It is active against penicillin and methicillin-resistant staphylococci, all streptococci except enterococci, Enterobacteriaceae, anaerobic gram-positive and gram-negative bacilli, and most strains of *P aeruginosa*. It is resistant to degradation by bacterial beta-lactamases, which in part explains its extreme potency against such a variety of microorganisms. Nausea and elevation of liver function tests have been observed in a small number of patients treated with imipenem. Seizures have been reported in a small number of patients who received high doses and had histories of seizures, obtundation, or renal insufficiency. When administered with cilastin, its metabolic breakdown by the kidneys is inhibited.

Aztreonam is a monobactam agent that is resistant to beta-lactamases produced by gram-negative bacilli such as *P aeruginosa* and Enterobacteriaceae. It is similar to the aminoglycosides and is not active against gram-positive aerobic or anaerobic microorganisms. It is an ideal agent for treating resistant aerobic gram-negative bacillary infections that previously required aminoglycoside therapy. It is also well suited to the treatment of elderly patients, particularly those with renal insufficiency and hearing loss. The possible side effects—gastrointestinal upset, hypersensitivity reaction, and skin rash—are uncommon.

Specialized Infections of the Musculoskeletal System

Two specialized musculoskeletal infections—puncture wounds of the foot and human-bite injuries—re-

Table 3
Antimicrobial therapy: Dosage and serum peak trough levels

Agent	Usual Dosage	Route	Dosage Interval	Peak Orally	Serum Level (mg/dL)	
					IM	IV
Cefazolin	1 to 2 g	IM, IV	8 hours	—	59	121
Cefamandole	1 to 2 g	IM, IV	4 hours	—	28	32
Cefoperazone	2 g	IM, IV	8 to 12 hours	—	75	133
Cefotaxime	1 to 3 g	IM, IV	4 to 5 hours	—	13	47
Penicillin G	0.125 to 2.5 g	IM, IV	4 hours	—	4.4	16
Oxacillin	1.5 to 2 g	Orally, IM, IV	4 hours	6	16	10
Azlocillin	2 to 4 g	IV	4 hours	—	—	85
Ticarcillin	4 to 5 g	IM, IV	4 to 6 hours	—	27	124
Carbenicillin	5 to 6 g	IM, IV	4 hours	—	24	99
Mezlocillin	2 to 4 g	IM, IV	4 hours	—	15	94
Piperacillin	2 to 4 g	IM, IV	4 hours	—	36	141
Imipenem	0.25 to 0.5 g	IV	4 hours	—	—	22
Ciprofloxacin	0.5 to 0.75 g	Orally	12 hours	1.5	—	—
Gentamicin	1.7 mg/kg	IV	8 to 12 hours	—	—	4–8
Tobramycin	1.7 mg/kg	IV	8 hours	—	—	4–8

quire special types of antimicrobials. When puncture wounds of the foot are complicated by infection, *P aeruginosa* will be isolated from the vast majority of the wounds. *P aeruginosa* has been isolated from the shoes, especially tennis shoes, of injured patients. Thus, therapy must be directed against this microorganism until the results of aerobic and anaerobic incubation of tissue-specimen cultures become available. Therefore, parenteral therapy with an aminoglycoside is usually given, although aztreonam or imipenem are other possibilities. Ciprofloxacin is a very attractive choice because it is an oral agent. Unfortunately, puncture wounds occur most frequently in children, and, as mentioned above, ciprofloxacin should not be administered to individuals with developing cartilage (children or pregnant and lactating women).

Human-bite injuries, usually to the clenched fist, are contaminated with several microorganisms that are part of the normal oral flora. These include *alpha-hemolytic* streptococci, *Eikenella corrodens*, and *S aureus*. Additionally, half of these injuries will be contaminated with anaerobic microorganisms such as *Bacteroides* species and *Fusobacterium nucleatum*. In addition to surgical debridement, antimicrobials should be given, including penicillin and a first generation cephalosporin. The penicillin is active against *E corrodens*, the streptococci, and anaerobes. The cephalosporin is active against *S aureus*.

When using older agents such as the aminoglycosides, carefully monitor the serum peak and trough levels (Table 3). Maintaining serum levels within appropriate ranges can help prevent side effects. This concept basically applies to all antimicrobials administered for therapeutic reasons.

Finally, many orthopaedic surgeons recommend administering antimicrobial agents to patients with total joint implants before they have dental manipulations or other types of invasive examinations.[37,38]

References

1. Fitzgerald RH Jr, Thompson RL: Cephalosporin antibiotics in the prevention and treatment of musculoskeletal sepsis. *J Bone Joint Surg* 1983;65A:1201–1205.
2. Patzakis MJ, Harvey JP, Ivler D: The role of antibiotics in the management of open fractures. *J Bone Joint Surg* 1974;56A:532–541.
3. Patzakis MJ, Ivler D: Antibiotic and bacteriologic considerations in open fractures. *South Med J* 1977;70(suppl 1):46–48.
4. Barnes J, Pace WG, Trump DS, et al: Prophylactic postoperative antibiotics: A controlled study of 1,007 cases. *Arch Surg* 1959;79:190–196.
5. Karl RC, Mertz JJ, Veith FJ, et al: Prophylactic antimicrobial drugs in surgery. *N Engl J Med* 1966;275:305–308.
6. Rocha H: Postoperative wound infection: A controlled study of antibiotic prophylaxis. *Arch Surg* 1962;85:456–459.
7. Sanchez-Ubeda R, Fernand E, Rousselot LM: Complication rate in general surgical cases: The value of penicillin and streptomycin as postoperative prophylaxis. A study of 511 cases. *N Engl J Med* 1958;259;1045–1050.
8. Tachdjian MO, Compere EL: Postoperative wound infections in orthopedic surgery: Evaluation of prophylactic antibiotics. *J Int Coll Surgeons* 1957;28:797–805.
9. Stevens DB: Postoperative orthopaedic infections: A study of etiological mechanisms. *J Bone Joint Surg* 1964;46A:96–102.
10. Fogelberg EV, Zitzmann EK, Stinchfield FE: Prophylactic penicillin in orthopaedic surgery. *J Bone Joint Surg* 1970;52A:95–98.
11. Boyd RJ, Burke JF, Colton T: A double-blind clinical trial of prophylactic antibiotics in hip fractures. *J Bone Joint Surg* 1973;55A:1251–1258.
12. Hill C, Flamant R, Mazas F, et al: Prophylactic cefazolin versus placebo in total hip replacement: Report of a multicentre double-blind randomised trial. *Lancet* 1981;1:795–796.
13. Gustilo RB, Anderson JT: Prevention of infection in the treatment of one thousand and twenty-five open fractures of long

bones: Retrospective and prospective analyses. *J Bone Joint Surg* 1976;58A:453–458.

14. Gustilo RM, Mendoza RM, Williams DN: Problems in the management of type III (severe) open fractures: A new classification of type III open fractures. *J Trauma* 1984;24:742–746.

15. Kaiser AB, Petracek MR, Lea JW IV, et al: Efficacy of cefazolin, cefamandole, and gentamicin as prophylactic agents in cardiac surgery: Results of a prospective, randomized, double-blind trial in 1,030 patients. *Ann Surg* 1987;206:791–797.

16. Slama TG, Sklar SJ, Misinski J, et al: Randomized comparison of cefamandole, cefazolin, and cefuroxime prophylaxis in open-heart surgery. *Antimicrob Agents Chemother* 1986;29:744–747.

17. Schutzer SF, Harris WH: Deep-wound infection after total hip replacement under contemporary aseptic conditions. *J Bone Joint Surg* 1988;70A:724–727.

18. Lidwell OM, Lowbury EJ, Whyte W, et al: Effect of ultraclean air in operating rooms on deep sepsis in the joint after total hip or knee replacement: A randomized study. *Br Med J* 1982;285: 10–14.

19. Burke JF: The effective period of preventive antibiotic action in experimental incisions and dermal lesions. *Surgery* 1961;50:161–168.

20. Henley MB, Jones RE, Wyatt RW, et al: Prophylaxis with cefamandole nafate in elective orthopedic surgery. *Clin Orthop* 1986; 209:249–254.

21. Pollard JP, Hughes SP, Scott JE: Antibiotic prophylaxis in total hip replacement. *Br Med J* 1979;1:707–709.

22. Pavel A, Smith RL, Ballard A, et al: Prophylactic antibiotics in elective orthopedic surgery: A prospective study of 1,591 cases. *South Med J* 1977;70(suppl 1):50–55.

23. Burnett JW, Gustilo RB, Williams DN, et al: Prophylactic antibiotics in hip fractures: A double-blind, prospective study. *J Bone Joint Surg* 1980;62A:457–462.

24. Josefsson G, Lindberg L, Wiklander B: Systemic antibiotics and gentamicin-containing bone cement in the prophylaxis of postoperative infections in total hip arthroplasty. *Clin Orthop* 1981; 159:194–200.

25. Fitzgerald RH Jr: Experimental osteomyelitis: Description of a canine model and the role of depot administration of antibiotics

in the prevention and treatment of sepsis. *J Bone Joint Surg* 1983; 65A:371–380.

26. Bergman BR: Antibiotic prophylaxis in open and closed fractures: A controlled clinical trial. *Acta Orthop Scand* 1982;53:57–62.

27. Verwey WF, Williams HR Jr, Kalsow C: Penetration of chemotherapeutic agents into tissues. *Antimicrob Agents Chemother* 1965; 5:1016–1024.

28. Rosin H, Rosin AM, Kramer J: Determination of antibiotic levels in human bone: I. Gentamicin levels in bone. *Infection* 1974;2: 3–6.

29. Bloom JD, Fitzgerald RH Jr, Washington JA II, et al: The transcapillary passage and interstitial fluid concentration of penicillin in canine bone. *J Bone Joint Surg* 1980;62A:1168–1175.

30. Lunke RJ, Fitzgerald RH Jr, Washington JA II, et al: Pharmacokinetics of cefamandole in osseous tissue. *Antimicrob Agents Chemother* 1981;19:851–858.

31. Hall BB, Fitzgerald RH Jr: The pharmacokinetics of penicillin in osteomyelitic canine bone. *J Bone Joint Surg* 1983;65A:526–532.

32. Quinlan WR, Hall BB, Fitzgerald RH Jr: Fluid spaces in normal and osteomyelitic canine bone. *J Lab Clin Med* 1983;102:78–87.

33. Williams EA, Fitzgerald RH Jr, Kelly PJ: Microcirculation in bone, in Mortillaro NE (ed): *The Physiology and Pharmacology of the Microcirculation.* New York, Academic Press, 1983, vol 2, pp 267–324.

34. Walker RC, Wright AJ: Symposium on antimicrobial agents: The quinolones. *Mayo Clin Proc* 1987;62:1007–1012.

35. Barza M: Imipenem: First of a new class of beta-lactam antibiotics. *Ann Intern Med* 1985;103:552–560.

36. MacGregor RR, Gentry LO: Imipenem/cilastatin in the treatment of osteomyelitis. *Am J Med* 1985;78:100–103.

37. Neu HC, Labthavikul P: Comparative in vitro activity of n-formimidoyl thienamycin against gram-positive and gram-negative aerobic and anaerobic species and its B-lactamase stability. *Antimicrob Agents Chemother* 1982;21:180–187.

38. Lattimer GL, Keblish PA, Dickson TB Jr, et al: Hematogenous infection in total joint replacement: Recommendations for prophylactic antibiotics. *JAMA* 1979;242:2213–2214.

Molecular Mechanisms in Musculoskeletal Sepsis: The Race for the Surface

Anthony G. Gristina, MD

Paul T. Naylor, MD

Lawrence X. Webb, MD

Introduction

Infection complicating the use of biomaterials is resistant, recurrent, frequently catastrophic, and always costly.[1-4] An infected total joint, internal fixation device, or vascular graft will usually require reoperation or amputation and can result in osteomyelitis or death.[1-5] Infected cardiac, abdominal, and extremity vascular prostheses have a 50% combined rate of death or amputation.[4,6-8] Transcutaneous intravenous catheters, as well as peritoneal dialysis and urologic devices, also frequently become infected.[9-16] Vascular grafts become infected in 2% to 6% of cases,[17-20] and intravascular catheters in 25%, depending on length of implantation.[17,21]

Infection rates for orthopaedic implants have diminished because of prophylactic antibiotics, clean air, and improved technique. However, total hip replacements become infected 0.1% to 1% of the time[6,22-25]; total knees, 1% to 4%[26]; and total elbows, 4% to 7%.[27,28]

Even with excellent treatment, the polytrauma patient with multiple closed fractures stabilized by internal fixation may develop a chronic infection based on damaged or dead tissue and retained biomaterials. Septic complications directly contribute to 78% of the late mortality in polytrauma patients.[29]

Interfaces: Tissue Cells, Bacteria, Biomaterials

Progress has been excellent in developing stable, "inert," compatible biomaterials with regard to thrombogenicity, corrosion, and immunogenicity. However, at the molecular level, material surfaces produce an inflammatory interface so that tissue integration, a homeostatic, chemical, cell-to-surface association, is seldom achieved.

Perceptions of foreign-body-centered infection are long-standing, but an understanding of pathogenesis and the molecular mechanisms began only a decade ago. Recent studies[30,31] suggest that tissue integration, which involves the development of normal tissue layers with intact extracellular polysaccharides, may be crucial in preventing bacterial infection.

Bacterial infection about biomaterials and damaged tissues involves adhesion to and colonization of biomaterial surfaces. Tissue integration depends on an even more sensitive adhesion by tissue cells to biomaterials. In fact, tissue integration and bacterial adhesion are chemically parallel, mutually exclusive, and competitive. Surfaces colonized by healthy tissue cells with intact membranes are resistant to infection because of competent extracellular polysaccharides; however, bacterial colonies on surfaces are seldom replaced by tissue cells, and are resistant to treatment and host defense mechanisms.

Microbial Adhesion and Pathogenesis

Implant-associated sepsis is characterized by (1) adhesive bacterial colonization by *Staphylococcus epidermidis*, *Staphylococcus aureus*, and *Pseudomonas aeruginosa* on a biomaterial or damaged-tissue substratum; (2) resistance to host defense mechanisms and antibiotic therapy; (3) specificity; (4) transformation of nonpathogens or opportunistic pathogens into virulent organisms; (5) polymicrobial infection; (6) persistence of the infection until the substratum is removed; and (7) the absence of adequate tissue integration at the biomaterial-tissue interface.

Biomaterials implanted in an animal tissue or organ system provide a preferred substrata for colonization because they provide surfaces that facilitate chemical interactions, allowing increased use of metabolites and directly inhibiting host defense mechanisms.[31-34] A lower inoculum of bacteria can then initiate surviving microcolonies in physiologic environments, regardless of host defense mechanisms.[35] Tissues, especially those traumatized by injury, surgery, and tissue implantation (allografts and organ transplants) also provide ideal substrata for bacterial colonization because they lack optimal cellular or systemic defense mechanisms.

Bacteria may attach to surfaces using specific receptor-ligand or receptor-lectin-ligand chemical interactions, or nonspecifically by charge-related, hydrophobic, and extracellular polysaccharide-based interactions (Fig. 1). The interaction of physical and biologic factors then allows bacterial attachment and adhesion. Proteinaceous adhesins (fimbriae for *Escherichia coli*), polysaccharide polymers (*S epidermidis*), and substances in the milieu then interact to form a "slime" or biofilm. Symbiotic bacterial species may join as a polymicrobial infection. Bacterial adhesion, therefore, is a critical factor in pathogenesis of damaged tissue, osteomyelitis, and biomaterial infections (Fig. 2).[36-39]

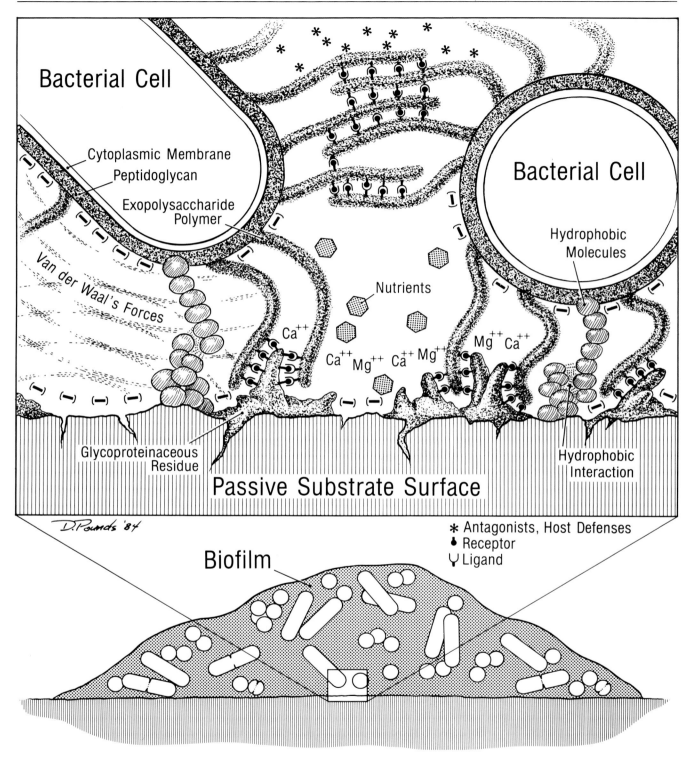

Fig. 1 At specific distances, the initial repelling forces of the negative bacterium and substrate surface charges are overcome by attracting van der Waals forces. There are also hydrophobic interactions between molecules. Under appropriate conditions, an extensive exopolysaccharide polymer develops, facilitating ligand-receptor interactions and bacterial attachment and adhesion to the substrate. (Reprinted with permission from Gristina AG, Oga M, Webb LX, et al: Adherent bacterial colonization in the pathogenesis of osteomyelitis. *Science* 1985;228:990–993.)

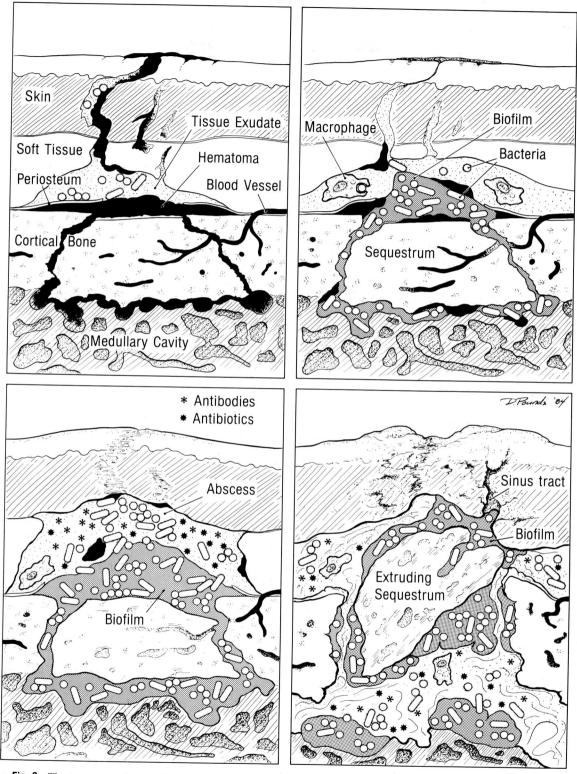

Fig. 2 The sequence of pathogenesis in osteomyelitis: **Top left,** Initial trauma produces soft-tissue destruction and bone fragmentation, as well as contamination by bacteria. In closed wounds, contamination may occur by hematogenous seeding. **Top right,** As the infection progresses, bacterial colonization occurs within a protective exopolysaccharide biofilm. The biofilm is particularly abundant on the devitalized bone fragment, which acts as a passive substratum for colonization. **Bottom left,** Host defenses are mobilized against the infection but cannot penetrate the biofilm and are ineffective. **Bottom right,** Progressive inflammation and abscess formation result in the development of a sinus tract, and in some cases, ultimate extrusion of the sequestrum, which is the focus of the resistant infection. (Reprinted with permission from Gristina AG, et al: Microbial adhesion and biofilm in the pathogenesis of biomaterial-centered infections and osteomyelitis, in Gustilo R, Gruninger R, Peterson P (eds): *Current Concepts in the Management of Musculoskeletal Infections.* Philadelphia, WB Saunders Co., in press.)

The Bacteria

Curiously, a few species seem to dominate biomaterial-centered infections. S epidermidis and S aureus have been most frequently isolated from infected biomaterial surfaces,[37,40,41] but E coli, P aeruginosa, Proteus mirabilis, beta-hemolytic streptococci, and enterococci have also been isolated.[37,41]

S epidermidis, a commensal, human skin saprophyte, commonly infects vascular prostheses, neurosurgical shunts, orthopaedic implants,[7,8,17,40] and implanted polymers such as the total artificial heart, total joints, vascular grafts, catheters, and shunts.[41] When polymers are absent, S epidermidis is less frequently a pathogen, although it may also be a constituent organism in polymicrobial infections of substrata such as metals, compromised bone, and tissue.[41,42]

S aureus is often the major pathogen isolated from metallic, bone-and-joint, and soft-tissue infections; it is the most common pathogen isolated in osteomyelitis when damaged or dead bone acts as a substratum.[5,43,44] The association of S aureus with infection of metallic implants may be directed in part by the tissue environment about the device.

P aeruginosa is the most frequent cause of bacterial keratitis caused by extended-wear contact lenses.[45,46] As the use of polymers increases, P aeruginosa may become the primary pathogen at special sites.[45,47]

Substratum-centered infections are also frequently polymicrobial. Studies have revealed that two thirds of osteomyelitic infections in adults are polymicrobial.[5,42] Among the pathogens that have been isolated are S aureus and S epidermidis, and Pseudomonas, Enterococcus, Streptococcus, Bacillus, and Proteus species.

In vitro and in vivo studies suggest that S epidermidis preferentially colonizes polymers and S aureus preferentially colonizes metals.[17,41,42] The specificity of bacterial species isolated to date may change as sampling techniques and methodology focus on adhesive, biomaterial-centered infections. Infectivity will certainly be strain-related within species.

Extracapsular Polysaccharides (Slime)

Bacterial extracapsular slime may be defined as any polysaccharide-containing moiety outside of but related to the cell wall.[48,49] The polysaccharide slime appears to be virulence-related, and it has been shown to confer resistance to host defense mechanisms such as engulfment by phagocytes,[50] surfactants,[51] and antibodies,[52] as well as resistance to antibiotics.[53] Thus, the formation of adhesive, biofilm-enclosed microcolonies appears to be an inherent protective mode of bacterial growth. This protective mode of growth may allow some bacterial infections to exist in a subtle subclinical state, with intermittent cycling of inflammation or clinical disease, characteristic of S epidermidis infection of total joints and the total artificial heart.

Matrix Substances, Adhesive Proteins, and Conditioning Films

Both bacteria and tissue cells are able to attach directly to clean surfaces in nature or in the laboratory. However, a more natural or physiologic interfacial relationship is achieved via large organic molecules. When implanted, biomaterials or tissues are immediately coated with a glycoproteinaceous film derived from protein and ambient ions, tissue debris, and contaminants. The constituents of this film provide receptor sites for bacterial or possibly tissue adhesion.[17,54] The specific role of each of the macromolecules or constituents of this layer differs for each organism or type of tissue cell involved and possibly will be different on each biomaterial. Fibronectin, collagen, fibrinogen, and laminin are among the more frequently recognized adhesive molecules.

A hypothetical sequence of cell-to-surface adhesion is suggested by extrapolations from colloid physics, microbiology, and biochemistry. For modeling purposes, bacterial particles less than 1 μ in size may be thought to behave as colloids. The following model is derived from suggestions of many researchers and is undoubtedly accurate only in part for each cell and surface.

Bacteria may arrive randomly near the surface of a biomaterial, foreign body, or tissue substrata by direct contamination; by contiguous spread, as occurs from adjacent epithelial cells or by means of transcutaneous drive lines in the total artificial heart; or by hematogenous seeding, as occurs in heart-valve and joint replacements or in osteomyelitis (Fig. 3).[31]

Surface atoms of a biomaterial are not completely bound or satisfied on their open interface, and therefore are available as binding sites for environmental interactions.[55] Most metallic implants have a thin (10 to 20 nm) oxide layer that acts as the true interface for subsequent interactions.[56] Polymer surfaces are dominated by high-energy rearrangements and are also reactive. For both polymers and metals, binding sites are also modified by surface texture, manufacturing processes, trace chemicals, and debris, and by ionic and glycoproteinaceous constituents of the host environment. Surfaces may also act as catalytic stages for molecular and cellular activities.[41,56,57] Detailed profiles of biomaterial surfaces in biologic environments, including electronic state, oxidation layers, contamination level, and sequence of glycoprotein coating have not been created but can be assumed to be specific to the material involved, its environment, and the type of cell attempting adhesion or integration.[17,54,56]

Initial attachment (reversible nonspecific adhesion) depends on the physical characteristics of the bacterium, the fluid interface, and the substratum. Subsequent to this initial attachment, a specific irreversible adhesion occurs. This possibly time-dependent, chemical process depends in part upon specific protein adhesin-receptor interactions, as well as on carbohydrate polymer synthesis.[37,40,58,59] Subsequent to aggregation

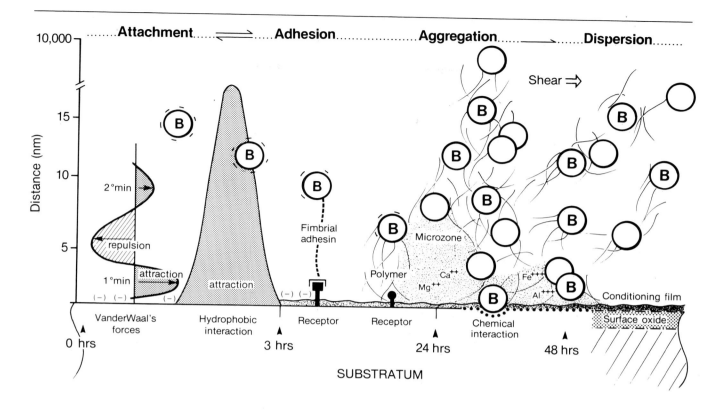

A.G. Gristina — after G.W. Jones/R.M. Pashley

Fig. 3 Molecular sequence in bacterial (B) attachment, adhesion, aggregation, and dispersion at substratum surface. A number of possible interactions may occur depending on the specificities of the bacteria or substratum system (nutrients, contaminants, macromolecules, species, and materials). (Reprinted with permission from Gristina AG: Biomaterial-centered infection: Microbial adhesion versus tissue integration. *Science* 1987;237:1588–1595. Copyright 1987 by AAAS.)

and colony maturation, cells on the periphery of the expanding mass may disaggregate, detach, and disperse. At the cellular and molecular level, disaggregation is a function of growth phase, colony size, nutrient conditions, and hemodynamic or mechanical shear forces. Changes in extracellular polysaccharide polymer production and composition may play an important role in detachment or disaggregation.[60,61] In dynamic environments (hematologic, ocular, intra-articular, and organ systems), when a theoretical maximum surface area is reached, or when aggregational factors decrease, large numbers of bacteria may be detached by shear forces. This sequence may explain the relatively intermittent or short-term phenomena of "bacterial showers" or disseminated bacterial emboli.

Tissue Cell Adhesion (Integration)

The mechanisms of tissue integration are similar to those involved in microbial adhesion. Tissue cells also produce exopolysaccharides (glycocalyces), are highly specialized, and therefore are less adaptive than bac-

teria to environment and substrata. Their ability to interact with substrata depends on a narrow order of chemical and physical interactions based on the nature of the substratum and intervening matrix substances. This specificity explains in part difficulties in compatibility, foreign-body reactions, immunogenicity, and infection of implanted biomaterials and tissue and organ transplants.

Tissue integration implies homeostasis, the lack of an inflammatory response, and a natural proteoglycan or glycoprotein cell-to-surface interface.

The Race for the Surface: Adhesion vs Integration

The fate of a biomaterial surface may be conceptualized as a "race for the surface" by macromolecules and bacteria and tissue cells. If tissue cells arrive first at a biomaterial surface and a secure bond is established, arriving bacteria are confronted by living, integrated cells resistant to bacterial colonization through intact cell membranes, extracapsular polysaccharides, and functioning host defense mechanisms. However, bacteria, being prevalent in biologic environments, may colonize the biomaterial first, producing infection and preventing tissue integration. Tissue cells are generally unable to displace pioneer bacterial colonies, and biomaterials usually do not facilitate tissue integration. Because of this, biomaterial and compromised tissue surfaces are the "eminent domain" primarily of organic and inorganic moieties and of bacteria, not tissue cells. Therefore, infection may be prevented by encouraging colonization (integration) of material surfaces with tissue cells.

Characteristics of Biomaterials and Tissue as Substrata

Biomaterials

Metals and Alloys Metals are composed of regular, repetitive, crystalline lattices. The addition of small amounts of one or more elements to form an alloy may markedly improve tensile and yield strengths, fracture toughness, fatigue properties, and workability. Alloying also improves resistance to corrosion and may be a factor in cell adhesion responses. Metal alloys naturally form, and are treated to form, an oxide layer 20 to 30 nm thick on their surfaces that acts as a passivation layer. Biomolecules interact with this oxide surface layer, the chemical qualities of which may be inconsistent.

When implanted in bone, surgical alloys are surrounded by a thin, fibrous tissue capsule. One exception is titanium and its alloys. Covalent, ionic, or hydrogen bonding may occur at the boundary between the bone tissue and the titanium oxide surface.[56] Titanium alloys have been shown to form a direct bone-(osteocyte)-implant contact (osseointegration) at the ultrastructural level.[62,63] Titanium and titanium alloy surfaces readily and directly colonized by osteoblasts or tissue cells may be protected to a higher degree against colonization by bacterial pathogens.

Ceramics These biomaterials are crystalline structures, used as dental and orthopaedic implants. Bioactive glass ceramics are composed of silicon oxide interspersed with various crystalline substances.[64]

Clean ceramic surfaces or those passivated by appropriate glycoproteins may be suitable substrata for tissue integration. A bioactive glass ceramic-tissue interface is to a degree reactive but is noninflammatory and nonresorbable. Bacterial adhesion to ceramics and glass ceramics has been demonstrated,[65,66] but the clinical significance and microbiologic characteristics should be further studied before any conclusions are drawn.[31,32,67]

Polymers Most medical polymers are amorphous. There are three that are in part crystalline: polytetrafluoroethylene, polyethylene, and polypropylene.[68] Crystalline zones (spherulites) confer structural rigidity and amorphous zones confer resistance to wear. Methylmethacrylate has a noncrystalline, porous structure that, in effect, provides surface area for diffusion and molecular interaction. High-molecular-weight medical polymers in general are thought to be resistant to bacterial deterioration. However, polyvinylchloride, for example, contains low-molecular-weight plasticizers (polypropylene sebacate) that are vulnerable to attack by *P aeruginosa* and *Serratia marcescens*.[68] Our studies indicated a higher rate of bacterial adhesion to polymers than to metals for *S epidermidis*, both in vitro and in vivo.[41,67,69] Interestingly, antibiotic resistance and host defense inhibition may be greater for infections centered on polymers.

Tissue as Substrata

Bone A composite structure composed of calcium hydroxyapatite crystals and a collagen matrix, bone is grossly similar to synthetic composites or to partially crystalline polymers. Calcium phosphate crystals (45 × 29.9 × 3 nm) are formed in plates between collagen fibrils. Proline-rich proteins found in collagen seem to act as ligands for bacterial adhesion.[70] Traumatized bone is devoid of normal periosteum and blood supply, exposing collagen protein matrix and acellular crystal faces to which bacteria may bind.[5]

Cartilage and Intra-articular Surfaces Recent studies indicate that the pathogenesis of intra-articular sepsis depends on the ability of certain strains of staphylococci to bind preferentially to a cartilage matrix.[71] Microscopic examination of infected joints in a rabbit model suggested that bacteria colonize cartilage more readily than synovial surfaces.[71] These findings are consistent with the biochemical identification of collagen receptors on the cell surfaces of certain strains of *S aureus*.[72] Several strains of *S aureus* produce collagenase, which, along with host-originated inflammatory products, is probably the main cause of progressive cartilage destruction.[73,74] The mechanisms involved in bacterial adhesion to collagen epitopes in articular sepsis and osteomyelitis may also operate when collagen is present as a substratum in allografts or on the surface of a biomaterial.[71,75] Binding by collagen receptors can be inhibited by using a synthetic peptide (pro-gly-pro)$_n$ believed to be similar to the collagen epitope.[72]

Allografts Being a traumatized tissue rich in nutrient material, ligands, and lectins, an allograft provides a surface for colonization by bacteria with the appropriate receptors. Avascular bone allografts represent a particularly large mass of dead tissue, bone, and cartilage, and have demonstrated a clinical infection rate of 5% to 14%.[76]

Endothelial Cells These cells are surrounded by a well-developed glycocalyx. When this is traumatized by viruses, toxins, or inflammation, fibronectin and possibly other receptor sites are exposed.[77-79] These sites may then be susceptible to bacterial adhesion and colonization. This may explain infection of aortofemoral vascular grafts by *S epidermidis* and other bacteria. Endothelial damage may also be a factor in site localization of osteomyelitis. Healthy endothelial cell tissue cultured and seeded over vascular graft polymer surfaces might prevent bacterial adhesion or thrombogenic events.[80,81]

Platelets Gram-positive bacteria, the most common causes of bacterial endocarditis, bind to fibronectin, fibrin, or platelets.[82,83] Trauma to natural heart valves or conditioning of plastic valves by fibronectin, fibrin, and platelet vegetations may be the initial and pivotal step in the colonization of heart valves. Platelets binding to other damaged tissue may allow or enhance bacterial colonization.[37,77,78] This is another possible mechanism in trauma-induced osteomyelitis.[37]

Substratum Disruption

Biomaterial surfaces after implantation are disturbed by corrosion, wear, or chemical interactions, resulting in the release of ions or molecules into the peri-implant matrix (Fig. 4). Within closed spaces, ionic disassociations of iron and other heavy metals may not be subject to binding by lactoferrin or transferrin and are available to enhance bacterial virulence and diminish macrophage effectiveness.[31-34,84]

Antibiotic Resistance

Infections centered on biomaterials or damaged tissues are often resistant to antibiotic therapy and require the removal of the substrata to resolve the infection. Resistance persists even when an organism is isolated and appropriate antibiotics are administered. Various local factors, including the biomaterial's surface characteristics and composition, the bacteria's ability to elaborate a protective exopolysaccharide biofilm, and the medium's composition have been reported to affect bacterial sensitivity to antibiotics and host defense systems.[34,85]

In recent studies we compared biomaterial-adherent *S epidermidis* and *S aureus* with standard suspension cultures for sensitivity to nafcillin, vancomycin, gentamicin, and LY146032, and examined antibiotic killing kinetics on surfaces.[85,86] Biomaterials colonized were stainless steel, polymethylmethacrylate (PMMA) and ultra-high-molecular-weight polyethylene (UHMWPE).

The minimum bactericidal concentrations (MBCs) obtained were twofold- to 250-fold higher for bioma-

Substratum Disruption

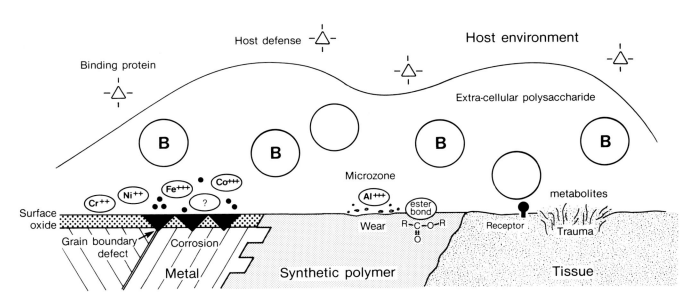

Fig. 4 Surface disruption by wear, corrosion, trauma, or bacterial mechanisms frees metabolites or ions that are then available to bacteria (B) within a biofilm microenvironment. At microzones, metal ions required by pathogenic bacteria are not lost by diffusion and may be shielded from host protein-binding complexes. Bacteria are also protected by biofilms and may metabolize polymer or tissue components. Interactions occur between exposed receptors on bacteria or surfaces. (Reprinted with permission from Gristina AG: Biomaterial-centered infection: Microbial adhesion versus tissue integration. *Science* 1987;237:1588–1595. Copyright 1987 by AAAS.)

terial-adherent bacteria than for bacteria in suspension (Table 1). The MBCs were independent of slime production and specific not only for the organism but also the biomaterial. Bacteria adhering to PMMA were routinely more resistant to antibiotics than organisms adhering to stainless steel. Killing kinetic studies indicated that organisms adherent to PMMA were more difficult to kill even at concentrations above their MBCs when compared with those adhering to stainless steel and UHMWPE.[85,86]

The elevated MBCs were independent of slime production. This observation is somewhat surprising but is also supported by recent studies that indicate that extracapsular polysaccharides may not present a diffusion barrier to antibiotics.[87] This issue requires further resolution.

If biomaterial-adherent organisms have higher MBCs than those determined for suspension cultures, and these sensitivities are organism- and biomaterial-specific, then a sensitivity testing technique will be needed to guide the management of biomaterial-related infections.

Orthopaedic Applications

For orthopaedic applications, methylmethacrylate and polyethylene are quite adhesive for bacteria and stimulate the creation of a fibroinflammatory layer rather than bone or tissue integration. Metal alloys appear to be less adherent than polymers for bacteria, and seem to be more amenable to tissue integration.

The development of stable orthopaedic prostheses with true tissue ingrowth will depend on an understanding of the relationship between osteocytes and bone matrix molecules and metallic or improved biomaterial surfaces. True stable ingrowth will require a chemical bonding of osteocyte and matrix to the prosthetic surface, not gross mechanical interference ingrowth, as is now obtained.

The pathway to perfect compatibility and progress of tissue integration is via a directed sequence of protein macromolecule adsorption specific for tissue adhesion. Bacteria and tissue cells possess multiple binding mechanisms that use covalent and noncovalent (strong and weak) bonds, as well as receptor-ligand interactions. Neutralization or control of all binding forces and receptor interactions is essentially impossible, but with an understanding of each mechanism a degree of direction of substratum effects may be possible.

It is reasonable to hypothesize the development of an almost perfect, fully saturated, low-energy, minimally adhesive surface of inorganic or organic composition for hematologic or special interfaces. It should also be possible to achieve transitional surfaces with programmed and specific adhesive qualities based on weak or strong binding forces and/or lectin-like molecular recognition processes for vascular junction and tissue contact (bone or solid tissue interfaces). Surfaces selectively adsorptive for a particular glycoprotein could be formed that would, in turn, select the next chemical or final receptor interaction with a specific tissue cell type or glycoprotein.

Programmed, proadhesive surfaces would be ideal for certain prosthetic tissue ingrowth devices. During the initial period after implantation, and while awaiting tissue adhesion (when the surface is also susceptible to bacterial colonization), prophylactic antibiotics could be used.

Future Strategies

Prophylactic antibiotics, systemically delivered or in situ in biomaterials, are effective because they act on bacteria in suspension populations (bacteremia) or at surfaces before biofilm-shielded colonization has occurred (Fig. 5).

Effective prevention and treatment strategies should also include improved surgical and sterile techniques in primary surgery, and adequate debridement of in-

Table 1
Antibiotic sensitivity of S hominis SP-2 and S hyicus SE-360 in suspension and biomaterial-adherent in minimum bactericidal concentrations (µg/ml)*

Drug	Suspension	Stainless Steel	Ultra-High-Molecular-Weight Polyethylene	Polymethylmethacrylate
		S hominis SP-2		
Nafcillin	0.5	8	0.5	128
Vancomycin	8	16	8	64
Gentamicin	16	32	32	128
LY146032	1	1	16	16
		S hyicus SE-360		
Nafcillin	0.5	16	6	>256
Vancomycin	16	16	32	128
Gentamicin	2	32	32	64
LY146032	2	16	16	32

*24-hour colonization; 24-hour antibiotic exposure.

Antiobiotic — Analog Strategy

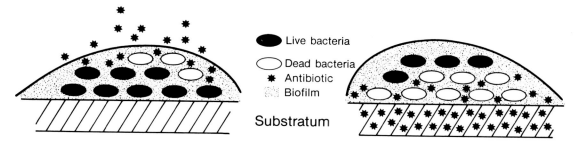

Live bacteria
Dead bacteria
Antibiotic
Biofilm

Substratum

Fig. 5 The polysaccharide biofilm acts as a barrier to antibiotics. (Reproduced with permission from Gristina AG, et al: Microbes, metals, and other nonbiological substrate in man. Substratum and substrate factors in infection, in Gustilo R, Gruninger R, Peterson P (eds): *Current Concepts in the Management of Musculoskeletal Infections.* Philadelphia, WB Saunders Co., in press.)

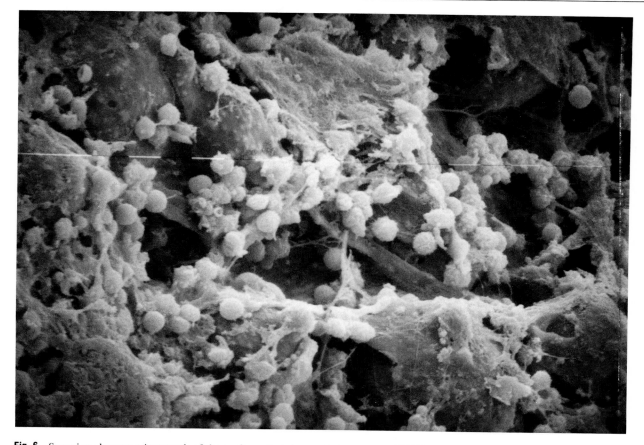

Fig. 6 Scanning electron micrograph of the surface of a tobramycin-impregnated PMMA bead (2.4 g/30 g PMMA) retrieved from a patient with an infected hip wound. Culture of the surface of the bead yielded four bacterial species (*S epidermidis* I, *S epidermidis II*, diphtheroids, and *Streptococcus*).

fected tissue, biomaterials, and bone in revision surgery. Local antibiotic delivery may be appropriate after debridement in specific applications. The use of methylmethacrylate antibiotic beads, combined with adequate surgery to treat osteomyelitis, has advantages and disadvantages. Short-range delivery concentrations are high, but placement is critical because antibiotic levels decay rapidly with time and distance, and the retained beads may act as a substratum (especially in open wounds) for new resistant colonizing bacteria (Fig. 6).

Characterization of biomaterial surfaces and an understanding of interfacial phenomena will be accomplished using advanced instrumentation such as scanning tunneling and atomic force microscopy, Auger electron spectroscopy, and electron spectroscopy for chemical analysis. Surface modification will be one of the keys to controlled biologic response. Surfaces of the future will be modified to diminish adhesion by bacterial cells. Alternatively, adhesive zones may be created for tissue integration or seeding. Heavy ion implantation, chemical vapor deposition, and vacuum evaporation may be used to create a surface that "directs" tissue or desired macromolecular integration in tissue and hemodynamic systems. The biomaterials of the future will no longer be "foreign bodies."

References

1. Gristina AG, Kolkin J: Current concepts review: Total joint replacement and sepsis. *J Bone Joint Surg* 1983;65A:128–134.
2. Gristina AG, Costerton JW: Bacterial adherence to biomaterials: The clinical significance of its role in sepsis. *Soc Biomater '84 Trans* 1984;7:175.
3. Zimmerli W, Waldvogel FA, Vaudaux P, et al: Pathogenesis of foreign body infection: Description and characteristics of an animal model. *J Infect Dis* 1982:146:487–497.
4. Henderson DK: Infections associated with prostheses, shunts, and implants, in Yoshikawa TT, Chow AW, Guze LB (eds): *Infectious Diseases: Diagnosis and Management*. Boston, Houghton Mifflin, 1980, pp 274–285.
5. Gristina AG, Oga M, Webb LX, et al: Adherent bacterial colonization in the pathogenesis of osteomyelitis. *Science* 1985;228:990–993.
6. Dougherty SH, Simmons RL: Infections in bionic man: The pathobiology of infections in prosthetic devices. Part II. *Curr Probl Surg* 1982;19:265–319.
7. Bandyk DF, Berni GA, Thiele BL, et al: Aortofemoral graft infection due to *Staphylococcus epidermidis*. *Arch Surg* 1984;119:102–108.
8. Masur H, Johnson WD Jr: Prosthetic valve endocarditis. *J Thorac Cardiovasc Surg* 1980;80:31–37.
9. Birnbaum DW: Safety of maintaining intravenous sites for longer than 48 H. *J Clin Microbiol* 1981;13:833–835.
10. Peters G, Locci R, Pulverer G: Microbial colonization of prosthetic devices: II. Scanning electron microscopy of naturally infected intravenous catheters. *Zentralbl Bakteriol Mikrobiol Hyg* [B] 1981;173:293–299.
11. Sugarman B, Musher D: Adherence of bacteria to suture materials. *Proc Soc Exp Biol Med* 1981;167:156–160.
12. Sugarman B: In vitro adherence of bacteria to prosthetic vascular grafts. *Infection* 1982;10:9–14.
13. Marrie TJ, Nelligan J, Costerton JW: A scanning and transmission electron microscopic study of an infected endocardial pacemaker lead. *Circulation* 1982;66:1339–1341.
14. Marrie TJ, Costerton JW: A scanning electron microscopic study of urine droppers and urine collecting systems. *Arch Intern Med* 1983;143:1135–1141.
15. Gokal R: Peritonitis in continuous ambulatory peritoneal dialysis. *J Antimicrob Chemother* 1982;9:417–420.
16. Krothapalli R, Duffy WB, Lacke C, et al: *Pseudomonas* peritonitis and continuous ambulatory peritoneal dialysis. *Arch Intern Med* 1982;142:1862–1863.
17. Dankert J, Hogt AH, Feijen J: Biomedical polymers: Bacterial adhesion, colonization, and infection. *CRC Crit Rev Biocompat* 1986;2:219–301.
18. Hepp W, Schulze T: The management of infected grafts in reconstructive vascular surgery. *Thorac Cardiovasc Surg* 1986;34:265–268.
19. Lorentzen JE, Nielsen OM, Arendrup H, et al: Vascular graft infection: An analysis of sixty-two graft infections in 2411 consecutively implanted synthetic vascular grafts. *Surgery* 1985;98:81–86.
20. Jensen LJ, Kimose HH: Prosthetic graft infections: A review of 720 arterial prosthetic reconstructions. *Thorac Cardiovasc Surg* 1985;33:389–391.
21. Sheth NK, Franson TR, Rose HD, et al: Colonization of bacteria on polyvinyl chloride and Teflon intravascular catheters in hospitalized patients. *J Clin Microbiol* 1983;18:1061–1063.
22. Eftekhar NS: Long-term results of cemented total hip arthroplasty. *Clin Orthop* 1987;225:207–217.
23. Eftekhar NS, Nercessian O: Incidence and mechanism of failure of cemented acetabular component in total hip arthroplasty. *Orthop Clin North Am* 1988;19:557–566.
24. Strathy GM, Fitzgerald RH Jr: Total hip arthroplasty in the ankylosed hip: A ten-year follow-up. *J Bone Joint Surg* 1988;70A:963–966.
25. Schutzer SF, Harris WH: Deep-wound infection after total hip replacement under contemporary aseptic conditions. *J Bone Joint Surg* 1988;70A:724–727.
26. Jacobs MA, Hungerford DS, Krackow KA, et al: Revision of septic total knee arthroplasty. *Clin Orthop* 1989;238:159–166.
27. Ross AC, Sneath RS, Scales JT: Endoprosthetic replacement of the humerus and elbow joint. *J Bone Joint Surg* 1987;69B:652–655.
28. Morrey BF, Ryan RS: Revision total elbow arthroplasty. *J Bone Joint Surg* 1987;69A:523–532.
29. Molnar JA, Burke JF: Prevention and management of infection in trauma. *World J Surg* 1983;7:158–163.
30. Albrektsson T: Bone tissue response, in Branemark P-I, Zarb GA, Albrektsson T (eds): *Tissue-integrated Prostheses: Osseointegration in Clinical Dentistry*. Chicago, Quintessence Publishing, 1985, pp 129–143.
31. Gristina AG: Biomaterial-centered infection: Microbial adhesion versus tissue integration. *Science* 1987;237:1588–1595.
32. Gristina AG, Naylor PT, Myrvik Q: The race for the surface: Microbes, tissue cells, and biomaterials, in Switalski L, Hook M, Beachey EH (eds): *Molecular Mechanisms of Microbial Adhesion*. New York, Springer-Verlag, 1989, pp 177–211.
33. Gomer R: Surface diffusion. *Sci Am* 1982;247:98–109.
34. Brown MR, Williams P: The influence of environment on envelope properties affecting survival of bacteria in infections. *Annu Rev Microbiol* 1985;39:527–556.
35. Elek SD, Conen PE: The virulence of *Staphylococcus pyogenes* for man: A study of the problems of wound infection. *Br J Exp Pathol* 1957;38:573–586.
36. Beachey EH (ed): *Bacterial Adherence: Receptors and Recognition, Series B*. London, Chapman & Hall, 1980.
37. Christensen GD, Simpson WA, Beachey EH: Adhesion of bacteria to animal tissues: Complex mechanisms, in Savage DC, Fletcher

M (eds): *Bacterial Adhesion: Mechanisms and Physiologic Significance.* New York, Plenum Press, 1985, pp 279–305.

38. Gibbons RJ, van Houte J: Bacterial adherence and the formation of dental plaques, in Beachey EH (ed): *Bacterial Adherence: Receptors and Recognition, Series B.* London, Chapman & Hall, 1980, vol 6, pp 63–104.

39. Savage DC, Fletcher M (eds): *Bacterial Adhesion: Mechanisms and Physiologic Significance.* New York, Plenum Press, 1985.

40. Sugarman B, Young EJ (eds): *Infections Associated With Prosthetic Devices.* Boca Raton, Florida, CRC Press, 1984.

41. Gristina AG, Hobgood CD, Barth E: Biomaterial specificity, molecular mechanisms and clinical relevance of *S. epidermidis* and *S. aureus* infections in surgery, in Pulverer G, Quie PG, Peters G (eds): *Pathogenesis and Clinical Significance of Coagulase-negative Staphylococci.* Stuttgart, Gustav Fischer Verlag, 1987, pp 143–157.

42. Gristina AG, Webb LX, Barth E: Microbial adhesion, biomaterials, and man, in Coombs R, Fitzgerald R (eds): *Infection in the Orthopedic Patient.* London, Butterworths Press, in press.

43. Cierny G III, Couch L, Mader J: Adjunctive local antibiotics in the management of contaminated orthopaedic wounds. Presented at the 53rd Annual Meeting of the American Academy of Orthopaedic Surgeons, New Orleans, Feb 20–25, 1986.

44. Merritt K, Turner GE: Adherence of bacteria to biomaterials. Presented at the 11th Annual Meeting of the Society for Biomaterials, San Diego, April 25–28, 1985.

45. Slusher MM, Myrvik QN, Lewis JC, et al: Extended-wear lenses, biofilm, and bacterial adhesion. *Arch Ophthalmol* 1987;105:110–115.

46. Wilson LA, Schlitzer RL, Ahearn DG: *Pseudomonas* corneal ulcers associated with soft contact-lens wear. *Am J Ophthalmol* 1981;92:546–554.

47. Gristina AG, Dobbins JJ, Giammara B, et al: Biomaterial-centered sepsis and the total artificial heart: Microbial adhesion vs tissue integration. *JAMA* 1988;259:870–874.

48. Costerton JW, Irvin RT, Cheng KJ: The bacterial glycocalyx in nature and disease. *Annu Rev Microbiol* 1981;35:299–324.

49. Bennett HS: Morphological aspects of extracellular polysaccharides. *J Histochem Cytochem* 1963;11:14–23.

50. Schwarzmann S, Boring JR III: Antiphagocytic effect of slime from a mucoid strain of *Pseudomonas aeruginosa. Infect Immun* 1971;3:762–767.

51. Govan JRW: Mucoid strains of *Pseudomonas aeruginosa:* The influence of culture medium on the stability of mucus production. *J Med Microbiol* 1975;8:513–522.

52. Baltimore RS, Mitchell M: Immunologic investigations of mucoid strains of *Pseudomonas aeruginosa:* Comparison of susceptibility to opsonic antibody in mucoid and nonmucoid strains. *J Infect Dis* 1980;141:238–247.

53. Govan JRW, Fyfe JAM: Mucoid *Pseudomonas aeruginosa* and cystic fibrosis: Resistance of the mucoid form to carbenicillin, flucloxacillin and tobramycin and the isolation of mucoid variants *in vitro. J Antimicrob Chemother* 1978;4:233–240.

54. Baier RE, Meyer AE, Natiella JR, et al: Surface properties determine bioadhesive outcomes: Methods and results. *J Biomed Mater Res* 1984;18:337–355.

55. Tromp RM, Hamers RJ, Demuth JE: Quantum states and atomic structure of silicon surfaces. *Science* 1986;234:304–309.

56. Kasemo B, Lausmaa J: Surface science aspects on inorganic biomaterials. *CRC Crit Rev Biocompat* 1986;2:335–380.

57. Lehninger AL: *Principles of Biochemistry.* New York, Worth Publishers, 1982.

58. Fletcher M: Effect of solid surfaces on the activity of attached bacteria, in Savage DC, Fletcher M (eds): *Bacterial Adhesion: Mechanisms and Physiologic Significance.* New York, Plenum Press, 1985, pp 339–362.

59. Jones GW, Isaacson RE: Proteinaceous bacterial adhesins and their receptors. *CRC Crit Rev Microbiol* 1983;10:229–260.

60. Wrangstadh M, Conway PL, Kjelleberg S: The production and release of an extracellular polysaccharide during starvation of a marine *Pseudomonas* sp. and the effect thereof on adhesion. *Arch Microbiol* 1986;145:220–227.

61. Galleja GB, Atkinston B, Garrod DR, et al: Aggregation: Group report, in Marshall KC (ed): *Microbial Adhesion and Aggregation.* Berlin, Springer-Verlag, 1984, pp 303–321.

62. Albrektsson T: The response of bone to titanium implants. *CRC Crit Rev Biocompat* 1985;1:53–84.

63. Brånemark P-I, Hansson BO, Adell R, et al: Osseointegrated implants in the treatment of the edentulous jaw: Experience from a 10-year period. *Scand J Plast Reconstr Surg* 1977;16(suppl):1–132.

64. Blenckè BA, Brömer H, Deutscher KK: Compatibility and long-term stability of glass-ceramic implants. *J Biomed Mater Res* 1978;12:307–316.

65. Gross U, Strunz V: The interface of various glasses and glass ceramics with a bony implantation bed. *J Biomed Mater Res* 1985;19:251–271.

66. Hench LL, Paschall HA: Direct chemical bond of bioactive glass-ceramic materials to bone and muscle. *J Biomed Mater Res* 1973;7(symposium 4):25–42.

67. Oga M, Sugioka Y, Hobgood CD, et al: Surgical biomaterials and differential colonization by *Staphylococcus epidermidis. Biomaterials* 1988;9:285–289.

68. Mears DC: *Materials and Orthopaedic Surgery.* Baltimore, Wiliams & Wilkins, 1979.

69. Barth E, Myrvik QN, Wagner W, et al: In vitro and in vivo comparative colonization of *Staphylococcus aureus* and *Staphylococcus epidermidis* on orthopedic implants materials. *Biomaterials,* in press.

70. Gibbons RJ, Hay DI: Adsorbed salivary proline-rich proteins as bacterial receptors on apatitic surfaces, in Switalski L, Hook M, Beachey E (eds): *Molecular Mechanisms of Microbial Adhesion.* New York, Springer-Verlag, 1989, pp 143–163.

71. Voytek A, Gristina AG, Barth E, et al: Staphylococcal adhesion to collagen in intra-articular sepsis. *Biomaterials* 1988;9:107–110.

72. Speziale P, Raucci G, Visai L, et al: Binding of collagen to *Staphylococcus aureus* Cowan 1. *J Bacteriol* 1986;167:77–81.

73. McCarty DJ: *Arthritis and Allied Conditions: A Textbook of Rheumatology,* ed 10. Philadelphia, Lea & Febiger, 1985.

74. Smith RL, Schurman DJ: Comparison of cartilage destruction between infectious and adjuvant arthritis. *J Orthop Res* 1983;1:136–143.

75. Gristina AG, Kammire G, Voytek A, et al: Intraarticular sepsis: The shoulder. Molecular mechanisms and pathogenesis, in Rockwood C, Matsen F (eds): *The Shoulder.* Philadelphia, WB Saunders, in press.

76. Burwell RG, Friedlaender GE, Mankin HJ: Current perspectives and future directions: The 1983 Invitational Conference on Osteochondral Allografts. *Clin Orthop* 1985;197:141–157.

77. Ryan US: Metabolic activity of pulmonary endothelium: Modulations of structure and function. *Annu Rev Physiol* 1986;48:263–277.

78. Birinyi LK, Douville EC, Lewis SA, et al: Increased resistance to bacteremic graft infection after endothelial cell seeding. *J Vasc Surg* 1987;5:193–197.

79. Hamill RJ, Vann JM, Proctor RA: Phagocytosis of *Staphylococcus aureus* by cultured bovine aortic endothelial cells: Model for postadherence events in endovascular infections. *Infect Immun* 1986;54:833–836.

80. Rutter PR, Vincent B: Physicochemical interactions of the substratum, microorganisms, and the fluid phase, in Marshall KC (ed): *Microbial Adhesion and Aggregation.* Berlin, Springer-Verlag, 1984, pp 21–38.

81. Webb LX, Myers RT, Cordell AR, et al: Inhibition of bacterial adhesion by antibacterial surface pretreatment of vascular prostheses. *J Vasc Surg* 1986;4:16–21.

82. Christensen GD, Simpson WA, Beachey EH: Microbial adherence in infection, in Mandell GL, Douglas RG Jr, Bennett JE (eds): *Principles and Practice of Infectious Diseases*, ed 2. New York, John Wiley & Sons, 1985, pp 6–23.

83. Baddour LM: Twelve-year review of recurrent native-valve infective endocarditis: A disease of the modern antibiotic era. *Rev Infect Dis* 1988;10:1163–1170.

84. Black J: Does corrosion matter?, editorial. *J Bone Joint Surg* 1988; 70B:517–520.

85. Naylor PT, Jennings R, Webb LX, et al: Antibiotic sensitivity of biomaterial-adherent *Staphylococcus epidermidis*. *Orthop Trans* 1988;12:524–525.

86. Naylor PT, Ruch D, Brownlow C, et al: Fibronectin binding to orthopedic biomaterials and its subsequent role in bacterial adherence. Presented at the 35th Annual Meeting of the Orthopaedic Research Society, Las Vegas, Feb 6–9, 1989.

87. Nichols WW, Dorrington SM, Slack MP, et al: Inhibition of tobramycin diffusion by binding to alginate. *Antimicrob Agents Chemother* 1988;32:518–523.

Management of Soft-Tissue Wounds Associated With Open Fractures

John L. Esterhai, Jr., MD

The importance of the soft-tissue envelope to fracture healing is recognized by all orthopaedic surgeons.[1] This chapter addresses the basic science background associated with wound repair, covers the effects of the patient's nutrition, soft-tissue wound dressings, and soft-tissue transfers, and includes specific recommendations.

Basic Science Background

The phases of wound healing can be approached by emphasizing the timing and morphology of wound repair, repair physiology, or specific cell involvement.

Immediately after injury and in the hours that follow, vessels develop fibrin occlusion and microthrombi. Inflammatory cells accumulate at the wound site. Over the ensuing days, if the wound is superficial and clean, re-epithelialization occurs by a process of migration, mitosis, and ultimately epithelial cell maturation. Wound contracture also contributes to such wound closing. If the wound is deeper, neoangiogenesis, involving endothelial mitosis and recanalization of the thrombotic vessels, must occur (Outline 1).

From a physiologic standpoint, Hunt and associates[2] have documented that deep wound repair begins with damage to the local circulation, and the resultant inflammatory reaction, local hypoxia, and anaerobic metabolism lead to lactate production, stimulation of fibroblasts, and ultimately vascular ingrowth. Macrophage and platelet-derived growth factors have been identified (Fig. 1).

Much of the classic work concerning epidermal healing is now 20 years old. Winter[3] documented that the mitotic rate of regenerating epidermal cells was five to ten times faster in a moist, oxygen-rich environment than in a desiccated wound environment. Epidermal cell movement across a granulating wound bed is energy-dependent. The cells accumulate glycogen before mitosis or migration occur. Aerobic glycolysis releases 17 times the energy released anaerobically. Therefore, supplying oxygen to an epithelializing wound makes sense physiologically. The negative effects of dehydration on wound healing have been documented.[4,5] Human epidermal healing occurs faster under the protection of an intact vesicle than when the wound is allowed to desiccate.[6]

Specific wound chemoattractants have effects on tar-

Outline 1
Phases of wound healing

Hours
  Vessel microthrombi
  Fibrin occlusion
  Inflammatory cell accumulation
Days
  Reepithelialization
    Migration
    Mitosis
    Maturation
  Wound contracture
  Neoangiogenesis
    Endothelial mitosis
    Recanalization
Weeks
  Dermal reconstitution
    Removal
    Synthesis
    Remodeling
    Strengthening

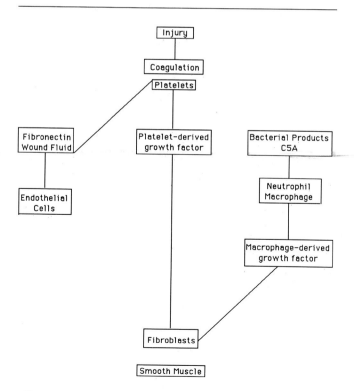

Fig. 1 Schematic emphasizing specific cell involvement in wound-repair physiology.

get cells leading to activation of those cells. Platelet factor IV, elastin peptides, lymphokines, and complement peptides affect the neutrophils and monocytes, leading to phagocytosis and the production of macrophage-derived growth factor. Fibronectin and platelet-derived growth factor affect fibroblasts and smooth muscle cells, leading to matrix production. Fibronectin, laminin, and the monokines affect endothelial cells, leading to vascular system proliferation (Fig. 1 and Table 1).[7]

Specific cells have been shown to respond to platelet-derived growth factor by migration. The migration of fibroblasts has been shown to be enhanced almost 600%, that of smooth muscle cells 400%, and that of endothelial cells, monocytes, and neutrophils 20% to 30%.[8]

The macrophage is believed by many to be the most important cell in wound healing. Its functions include debridement and local killing of bacteria. Proteolytic enzymes assist with debridement. Production of superoxide, hydroxyl radical, and singlet oxygen by the macrophage assists its killing of ingested bacteria. It has been documented[9,10] that the central portion of an experimentally created chronic wound in an animal model is hypoxic, with an oxygen pressure of 0 to 20 torr compared with the normal value of 30 to 60 torr. The pH in a chronic experimental wound is 7.1, and the Pco_2 is 60 to 100 torr.

When macrophages are cultured at oxygen concentrations similar to those found in chronic wounds (2% oxygen, 15 torr), macrophage-derived growth factor is produced. However, macrophages cultured at normal arterial oxygen tension produced no macrophage-derived growth factor. Macrophage-derived growth factor stimulates fibroblast, smooth muscle, and endothelial cell growth in vitro and in vivo and neoangiogenesis in vivo.

Fibroblasts proliferate optimally in hypoxic conditions. The oxygen dose-response curve for dermal fibroblasts shows the greatest fibroblast proliferation at 5% oxygen (Balduini and associates, unpublished data).

Table 1
Wound repair chemoattractants

Chemoattractants	Target Cells	Functions of Target Cells
Platelet factor 4, elastin peptides, lymphokines, monokines complement peptides	Neutrophils, monocytes	Phagocytosis, macrophage-derived growth factor
Fibronectin	Fibroblasts, smooth muscle cells	Matrix production
Fibronectin laminin monokines	Endothelial cells	Vascular system

Increased oxygen tension adversely affects vessel ingrowth in the chronic wound.[10] In summary, biochemical signals translate mechanical injury into messages that cells can recognize. The magnitude and duration of the body's wound-healing response are determined by the extent of injury, host status, and the method of wound closure; however, more research is necessary to define precisely what starts the wound-healing process and what ultimately stops it.

Nutrition and Wound Healing

Half of metropolitan medical/surgical patients have overt or subclinical protein and calorie malnutrition.[11] Protein malnutrition is responsible for increased mortality and morbidity.[12] Two laboratory parameters—serum albumin and total lymphocyte count—can be used to evaluate a patient's nutritional status rapidly.[12] A serum albumin value of less than 3.5 mg/dl or a total lymphocyte count of less than 1,500 cells/ml is considered to be significant. Hypoalbuminemia has an adverse effect on intravascular oncotic pressure; amino acid, zinc, and fatty acid transport; and amino acid availability for metabolism. The importance of the lymphocyte count is related to the documented loss of immunocompetence in patients with a low lymphocyte count. The lymphocyte count returns to normal after nutritional recovery.

The patient with multiple trauma and open fracture has increased nutritional demands.[13,14] To produce adequate nutritional support, basal energy expenditure requirements, which are normally affected by the patient's age, height, weight, and sex, must be adjusted upward either by multiplying by a stress factor to obtain calculated energy expenditure, or by monitoring the patient's actual energy expenditure after trauma to provide adequate nutritional support.[15]

Soft-Tissue Wound Dressings

The eight performance characteristics to be considered in choosing a soft-tissue wound dressing are effect on the rate and quality of wound healing, effectiveness as a bacterial barrier, capacity to absorb exudate, occlusivity, biocompatibility, hypoallergenicity, wound contact and release characteristics, and thermal insulation. Desiccation and suboptimal wound oxygen concentrations are counterproductive. From the patient's viewpoint, desirable dressing performance characteristics include improved comfort and convenience, control of wound odor, and reduction of pain. Dressings should minimize nursing time and optimize treatment costs. The human body is magnificently able to overcome hardships, some of which, when it comes to our dressing techniques, might be iatrogenic.

Four types of newer wound dressings include semipermeable films, hydrogels, occlusive hydrocolloids, and synthetic skin substitutes. Semipermeable films and semiocclusive hydrogels are permeable to water vapor and oxygen, but are impermeable to liquids and bacteria. The occlusive hydrocolloids are impermeable even to water vapor and oxygen (Outline 2).

Several semipermeable films are available on the market (OpSite, Tegaderm, and Bio-occlusive). Their permeability to water vapor is 2,500 g/m²/24 hr: their permeability to oxygen is 4,000 to 10,000 cc/m²/24 hr. Single-polymer hydrogels are three-dimensional networks of hydrophilic polymer that are more oxygen-permeable than the film dressings. Vigilion is a gelatinous sheet of insoluble cross-linked polyethylene oxide copolymer and polyethylene film. Impermeable or occlusive hydrocolloids have a permeability to water vapor and oxgen of 30 g/m²/24 hr and 150 cc/m²/24 hr, respectively. Duoderm is an example of impermeable hydrocolloid. It has an outer impermeable polyurethane foam and an inner adherent surface. In contrast to the hydrocolloids, Epigard, a synthetic skin substitute, is a two-layer, nontextile, open-matrix polyurethane, backed by a microporous polytetrafluoroethylene film. Wound exudate is absorbed by the hydrocolloids and skin-substitute matrices, and newly developing microcirculation grows into the matrix interstices of the Epigard mesh foam sheet.

The relative disadvantages of these synthetic wound dressings are cost and the potential for accumulation of exudate, hematoma, or seroma. Although application of the synthetic dressings is facilitated by the presence of a healthy soft-tissue border about the wound, such a border is not mandatory. Alvarez and associates[16] compared the rates of wound healing beneath occlusive dressings to that seen with exposure. Re-epithelialization occurred most rapidly under hydrocolloid wound dressing, followed, in descending order of rapidity, by polyurethane film, desiccation by air exposure, and wet-to-dry dressing changes. Collagen synthesis was equal in the hydrocolloid and polyurethane dressed wounds and was greater than that seen in wounds that were exposed to air. The evolution of dressings for the open traumatic wound has progressed from the age of passive absorbent plugs and covers to interactive dressings establishing a controlled microenvironment. The next stage will be the delivery of active substances (macrophage-derived growth factor or platelet-derived growth factor) impregnated into the dressing to speed wound repair.

Soft-Tissue Transfers

Soft-tissue transfers include simple skin grafts, local skin flaps, cross-leg flaps, jump flaps, and muscle and musculocutaneous pedicle flaps. The local pedicled muscle and myocutaneous flaps that are available in the lower extremity include the sartorius, fascia lata, vastus medialis, vastus lateralis, and gracilis in the thigh; the gastrocnemius, sartorius, and gracilis about the knee; the gastrocsoleus in the proximal one third of the lower leg; and the gastrocsoleus, tibialis anterior, or flexor digitorum in the middle aspect of the lower leg. In the distal one third of the leg the options, which are limited, include the soleus, extensor digitorum longus, extensor hallucis longus, and peroneus brevis. Obviously, transferring these muscles at this level runs the risk of failure as well as functional compromise.

The initial work on microvascular free-tissue transfers was performed by Goldwyn and associates[17] over 25 years ago. The first human cutaneous transfer was reported in 1973 by Taylor and Daniel.[18] The indications for a free vascularized flap include extensive soft-tissue loss, osteomyelitis, infected prostheses, poor vascularization, and defects in the distal one third of the tibia.

There are five different vascular pedicle types. The tensor fascia lata has one vascular pedicle. The gracilis has several dominant pedicles. The gluteus maximus has two, the sartorius has segmental pedicles, and the latissimus has one dominant and several secondary vascular pedicles. Available cutaneous flaps include scapular, iliofemoral vessel-based groin flap, dorsalis pedius-based flaps, deltopectoral, and axillary flaps. The free muscle and myocutaneous flaps include latissimus, gracilis, tensor fascia lata, pectoralis major, gastrocnemius, and rectus abdominis.

The question of when to perform the transfer in the acute setting has not been defined. Work published by Godina[19] emphasized early microvascular transfer. In analyzing his early work it became apparent that the percentage of flap failures, infection rate, time to bone healing, and number of procedures required depended on whether the patient's free muscle transfer was accomplished within 72 hours of the injury. When the microvascular transfer was performed within 72 hours, Godina had only a 0.75% flap failure rate and a 1.5% infection rate. The average time to bone healing was 6.8 months, and the average of surgeries per patient was 1.3. Patients who were treated in a delayed fashion, with microvascular transfer between 72 hours and three

Outline 2
Permeability of types of wound dressings

Semipermeable films
  Permeable to water vapor and oxygen
  Impermeable to water and bacteria
Semiocclusive hydrogels
  Permeable to water vapor and oxygen
  Impermeable to water and bacteria
Occlusive hydrocolloids
  Impermeable to water vapor and oxygen

months, had a 12% flap failure rate, 17% infection rate, 12 months for bone healing, and an average of 4.1 surgeries per patient. When the procedure was delayed beyond three months, the flap failure rate was 9.5%, the infection rate was 6%, and the time to healing extended to more than two years, with an average of 7.8 surgeries per patient. There are no comparable United States series. Just as our management of long-bone fractures in trauma patients has become more aggressive in the recent past, I believe that we will develop the teamwork and expertise required to be able to do extensive soft-tissue reconstruction procedures safely within the first several days after a patient's injury. With dedicated operating room time and appropriate assistance, such transfers could be accomplished at the time of second-look surgical debridements for appropriate grade III open fractures.

Specific Recommendations

Authors from Ger[20] in 1970 to Gustilo[21] and Patzakis[22] have defined and reiterated the need for appropriate wound grading, intravenous antibiotics, meticulous debridement, and the mechanics of stabilization and reconstruction. My specific recommendations for management of the soft-tissue wound associated with grade III long-bone fractures include aggressive rapid debridement, removal of all foreign material and necrotic bone, and the application of an external fixator. I believe that the new soft-tissue wound dressings are superior to povidone-iodine- or saline-soaked gauze dressings in most applications, because they minimize wound desiccation and subsequent soft-tissue necrosis. By eliminating the need for dressing changes by personnel outside of the operating-room environment, they decrease the risk of contamination with hospital-based organisms and minimize the patient's discomfort. The patient's nutritional status must be determined and optimized as rapidly as possible. Subsequent redebridement of the wound at approximately 48 hours and delay of wound closure until the surgeon is convinced that all compromised tissue has been removed is in order.

References

1. Wray JB: Factors in the pathogenesis of non-union. *J Bone Joint Surg* 1965;47A:168–173.

2. Hunt TK, Conolly WB, Aronson SB, et al: Anaerobic metabolism and wound healing: An hypothesis for the initiation and cessation of collagen synthesis in wounds. *Am J Surg* 1978;135:328–332.

3. Winter GD: Epidermal regeneration studied in the domestic pig, in Maibach HI, Rovee DT (eds): *Epidermal Wound Healing*. Chicago, Yearbook Medical Publishers, 1972, pp 71–112.

4. Winter GD: Formation of the scab and the rate of epithelization of superficial wounds in the skin of the young domestic pig. *Nature* 1962;193:293–294.

5. Hinman CD, Maibach H: Effect of air exposure and occlusion on experimental human skin wounds. *Nature* 1963;200:377–378.

6. Odland GF: The fine structure of the interrelationship of cells in the human epidermis. *J Biophys Biochem Cytol* 1958;4:529–538.

7. Glaser BM, D'Amore PA, Seppa H, et al: Adult tissues contain chemoattractants for vascular endothelial cells. *Nature* 1980;288:483–484.

8. Grotendorst GR, Pencev D, Martin GR, et al: Molecular mediators of tissue repair, in Hunt TK, Heppenstall RB, Pines E, et al (eds): *Soft and Hard Tissue Repair*. New York, Praeger Press, 1984, pp 20–40.

9. Knighton DR, Silver IA, Hunt TK: Regulation of wound-healing angiogenesis-effect of oxygen gradients and inspired oxygen concentration. *Surgery* 1981;90:262–270.

10. Thakral KK, Goodson WH III, Hunt TK: Stimulation of wound blood vessel growth by wound macrophages. *J Surg Res* 1979;26:430–436.

11. Jensen JE, Jensen TG, Smith TK, et al: Nutrition in orthopaedic surgery. *J Bone Joint Surg* 1982;64A:1263–1272.

12. Seltzer MH, Fletcher HS, Slocum BA, et al: Instant nutritional assessment in the intensive care unit. *JPEN* 1981;5:70–72.

13. Smith TK: Prevention of complications in orthopedic surgery secondary to nutritional depletion. *Clin Orthop* 1987;222:91–97.

14. Kay SP, Moreland JR, Schmitter E: Nutritional status and wound healing in lower extremity amputations. *Clin Orthop* 1987;217:253–256.

15. Cortes V, Nelson LD: Errors in estimating energy expenditure in critically ill surgical patients. *Arch Surg* 1989;124:287–290.

16. Alvarez OM, Hefton JM, Eaglestein WH: Healing wounds: Occlusion or exposure. *Infect Surg* 1984;173–181.

17. Goldwyn RM, Lamb DL, White WL: An experimental study of large island flaps in dogs. *Plast Reconstr Surg* 1963;31:528–536.

18. Taylor GI, Daniel RK: The free flap: Composite tissue transfer by vascular anastamosis. *Aust NZ J Surg* 1973;43:1–3.

19. Godina M: Early microsurgical reconstruction of complex trauma of the extremities. *Clin Plast Surg* 1986;13:619–620.

20. Ger R: The management of open fractures of the tibia with skin loss. *J Trauma* 1970;10:112–121.

21. Gustilo RB: Current concepts in the management of open fractures, in Griffin PP (ed): American Academy of Orthopaedic Surgeons *Instructional Course Lectures, XXXVI*. Park Ridge, Illinois, American Academy of Orthopaedic Surgeons, 1984, pp 359–366.

22. Patzakis MJ: Management of open fracture wounds, in Griffin PP (ed): American Academy of Orthopaedic Surgeons *Instructional Course Lectures, XXXVI*. Park Ridge, Illinois, American Academy of Orthopaedic Surgeons, 1987, pp 367–369.

Antibiotic Management of Open Fractures

Dean T. Tsukayama, MD

Ramon B. Gustilo, MD

Introduction

Prevention of wound sepsis is a major goal in the treatment of open fractures. Loss of life, amputation, or nonunion can result from infection. The surgical aspects of management—including immediate, meticulous, and repeated debridement; fracture stabilization; and appropriate wound coverage—are of paramount importance. The benefit of empiric antibiotic therapy, although not universally accepted in the past as necessary,[1,2] is well documented in the literature.[3,4] In a prospective, double-blind, randomized study, Patzakis and associates[3] reported an infection rate of 13.9% in the placebo group, compared with 2.3% in the group treated with cephalothin. Experimental studies have also demonstrated the efficacy of antibiotics in preventing infections when administered just before, or shortly after, bacterial contamination.[5,6] The basic principles guiding the use of antibiotics in the early management of open fractures have evolved from key observations made in investigations over the past 20 years. It has been shown that the majority of open fractures are contaminated with bacteria at the time of injury, that both facultative gram-negative bacilli and aerobic gram-positive cocci are major pathogens in fracture-associated infections, and that the risk of infection in open fractures depends on the degree of severity of the associated soft-tissue injury.

Selection of an Appropriate Antibiotic Regimen

Soft-tissue injuries associated with open fractures can be classified into three major types as follows: A type I fracture has a wound that is clean and less than 1 cm long. A type II fracture has a laceration more than 1 cm long without extensive soft-tissue damage, flaps, or avulsions. A type III fracture is an open fracture with extensive soft-tissue damage. This type includes open segmental fractures, farm injuries, arterial injuries, high-velocity gunshot injuries, shotgun injuries, and untreated injuries more than eight hours old. Type III fractures can be further classified into three subtypes. In type IIIA there is adequate soft-tissue coverage of a fractured bone despite extensive laceration or flaps, or high-energy trauma irrespective of the size of the wound. Type IIIB has extensive soft-tissue injury with periosteal stripping and bony exposure. Type IIIC in-

volves an open fracture associated with arterial injury requiring repair.

The incidence of infection in open fractures correlates directly with the extent of soft-tissue damage (Table 1). Infection rates in type I and type II open fractures are low; from 1976 to 1984 we experienced a 0% infection rate in 190 type I open fractures and a 3.1% infection rate in 158 type II open fractures. However, the infection rate in 162 type III open fractures during the same time period was 19% (Table 2). The increased incidence of infection in type III, and especially type IIIB, open fractures has been demonstrated in many studies.[7-9]

Of open fractures, 60% to 70% are contaminated with bacteria before any surgical or antibiotic therapy.[3,4,10] The majority of the bacteria cultured are normal skin flora (*Staphylococcus epidermidis, Propionibacterium acnes, Corynebacterium* species, *Micrococcus*) or environmental contaminants (*Bacillus* species, *Clostridium* species), which infrequently cause infection.[10] However, when more virulent pathogens, especially gram-negative bacilli, are cultured initially, the risk of infections with these bacteria appears to be higher.[3,10] Specific pathogens are also associated with certain types of environmental exposure. Gas gangrene caused by *Clostridium perfringens* can follow farm-related injuries.[7] Exposure to fresh water is associated with infections by *Pseudomonas aeruginosa* and *Aeromonas hydrophila*.[11,12] Saltwater contamination is associated with infection by *Aeromonas, Vibrios,* and *Erysipelothrix*.[13-15] Therefore the early institution of antibiotics is indicated as therapy (as opposed to prophylaxis) of wounds that are already contaminated and have a high likelihood of becoming clinically infected. Penicillin is added to our antibiotic regimen for farm-related trauma.

Case 1

A 29-year-old man driving in a rural area was thrown from his pick-up truck and suffered a type IIIB open tibial fracture. He lay in a pasture for five hours before assistance arrived. Immediate debridement was performed and an external fixator applied. Cultures obtained at the second debridement four days after admission grew *C perfringens, Enterobacter agglomerans,* and *Bacillus coagulans*. The patient was started on cefazolin and gentamicin and, later, because of concern about gas gangrene, clindamycin and penicillin were added. The patient was transferred to our facility eight days after admission. Despite numerous debridements, hy-

Table 1
Relationship of infection rate to severity of open fracture

Study	No. of Patients	Fracture Type			Antibiotic Regimen
		I*	II*	III*	
Patzakis, et al[18]	109	1.9	2.3	20.0	Cefamandole plus tobramycin
Gustilo, et al[7]	303	0	2.5	13.7	Cefazolin plus tobramycin
Dellinger, et al[17]	248	4.0	6.0	23.0	Cefonicid or cefamandole

*Numbers are infection rates per 100.

Table 2
Fracture-site infections of type III open fractures (Hennepin County Medical Center, 1961–1988)

Study Period	No. of Cases	Antibiotic Regimen	Infection Rate
1961 to 1968	36	Penicillin plus chloramphenicol or ampicillin	44.0%
1969 to 1975	98	Oxacillin plus ampicillin	10.2%
1976 to 1979	82	Cefazolin	24.2%
1980 to 1984	80	Cefazolin alone or cefazolin plus aminoglycoside*	13.7%
1985 to 1988	63	Cefazolin or cefamandole plus aminoglycoside	12.9%

*Not all cases received both drugs.

Table 3
Antimicrobial activity* of selected new broad-spectrum antibiotics

Drug	Coagulase-Positive Staphylococcus	Enteroccocus	Enteric Gram-Negative Bacilli	*Pseudomonas aeruginosa*	Anaerobes
Ceftriaxone	3	0	4	1	2
Ceftizoxime	3	0	4	1	3
Ceftazidime	2	0	4	4	1
Ampicillin-sulbactam	4	4	4	0	4
Ticarcilin-clavulanate	4	2	4	3	4
Imipenem	4	3	4	4	4
Ciprofloxacin	3	1	4	4	1

*Activity is as follows: 0 = none, 1 = poor, 2 = moderate, 3 = good, and 4 = excellent.

perbaric oxygen therapy, and antibiotics, including tobramycin, clindamycin, and penicillin, the infection could not be controlled, and the patient underwent below-knee amputation six days later.

Comment This case illustrates the pathogenic role of bacteria that contaminate the fracture site at the time of injury. It also demonstrates the importance of *C perfringens* as a pathogen in the rural setting. The long interval between injury and initiation of medical care probably also contributed to the fulminant course of his infection.

Fracture-related infections can also occur as a result of nosocomial pathogens.[16] The frequent recovery of *P aeruginosa* and *S aureus* from infected patients contrasts with the infrequent recovery of these pathogens from initial wound cultures,[7,10,17] implying that these bacteria colonize wounds after hospital admission. The role of hospital-acquired bacteria in the pathogenesis of infection at the fracture site underscores the im-

portance of early wound coverage in the management of open fractures.[8] It also suggests that despite optimal antibiotic therapy, a certain number of infections, especially those involving resistant pathogens, may be inevitable. On the other hand, the duration of initial therapy may be limited to minimize wound colonization by resistant nosocomial pathogens.

Case 2

A 48-year-old man sustained a type IIIB open tibial fracture following an assault. He underwent immediate debridement and external fixator placement on the day of admission, and was started on cefazolin and tobramycin. Initial wound cultures were negative. He underwent repeated debridement on day 2 and day 4 after admission. Despite the continuation of antibiotics throughout his hospital course, the wound became infected one week after admission and enterococcus was cultured at the time of surgical debridement on day seven.

Table 4
Organisms recovered from open fracture wounds prior to treatment

Organisms	Incidence
Gram-positive	
Coagulase-negative staphylococci	9
Bacillus	5
Diphtheroids	4
Viridans streptococcus	1
Gram-negative	
Pseudomonas maltophilia	1
Acinetobacter	1
Serratia	1
Escherichia coli	1
Enterobacter cloacae	1
Enterobacter agglomerans	1
Anaerobes	
Micrococcus	1
Peptostreptococcus	1
Propionibacterium	1
Lactobacillus	1
Fungi	
Rhodoturula	1
Curvularia	1
Alternaria	1

Table 5
Infecting bacterial pathogens in type III open fractures

Pathogen	No. of cases
Gram-positive	
Coagulase-positive staphylococci	3
Enterococcus	2
Coagulase-negative staphylococci*	1
Diphtheroids	1
Gram-negative	
Pseudomonas aeruginosa	3
Serratia	1
*Enterobacter**	2
Klebsiella	1
Pseudomonas maltophilia	1
Anaerobes	
Clostridia	2

*Organisms isolated in original pretreatment culture.

The antibiotic was changed to vancomycin and the wound infection was controlled. However the patient subsequently developed osteomyelitis with the same organism, which required further surgery for debridement and fracture nonunion and additional courses of antibiotic therapy were required.

Comment In this case, wound cultures taken before treatment were negative. The patient developed a wound infection one week after hospitalization with bacteria resistant to the antibiotics he was receiving. Enterococcus is rarely recovered from initial cultures of trauma-related wounds but is a frequent nosocomial pathogen. The prolonged course of antibiotic therapy did not help and may have selected the resistant organisms that colonized and later infected the wound.

S aureus and facultative gram-negative bacilli are the most common pathogens causing infections after open fractures.[4,7,17,18] The emergence of gram-negative bacilli as significant pathogens has led to a modification of antibiotic regimens originally recommended when gram-positive cocci were the predominant pathogen.[18,19] First-generation cephalosporins have been supplanted by second-generation cephalosporins or a combination of a cephalosporin and an aminoglycoside. In a randomized prospective study of type III open fractures, Gustilo and associates[7] reported an infection rate of 29.1% using a cephalosporin alone in contrast to 8.8% with a cephalosporin plus aminoglycoside. A number of recently introduced antibiotics may be useful in the early management of open fractures (Table 3). Several of these agents, characterized by broad-spectrum activity (including excellent gram-negative coverage) and a low incidence of adverse reactions, might be used as monotherapy but at present published clinical experience using these agents is lacking.

The optimal duration of early antibiotic therapy has been the subject of recent reports.[9,17] Although therapy must be continued long enough to prevent clinical infection, an unnecessarily prolonged course is associated with greater cost, increased risk of adverse drug reactions, and colonization with resistant organisms. In a double-blind prospective study of 248 patients, Dellinger and associates[17] concluded there was no difference between a one-day course and a five-day course of a second-generation cephalosporin in the prevention of fracture-site infections. One-day therapy with combination antibiotic therapy has not been evaluated. We prefer to administer three days of a cephalosporin plus aminoglycoside initially, with brief courses of antibiotics restarted for such major surgical procedures as wound coverage, hardware implantation, and skin closure.

Type III Open Fractures at Hennepin County Medical Center, 1985–1988

For 63 type III open fractures treated at our facility between 1985 and 1988, surgical management was conventional, but all patients received a cephalosporin and aminoglycoside as part of their initial management. Cultures were obtained from 29 patients before surgical debridement or antibiotics. Organisms were recovered from 68.9% (Table 4). However, only two of 32 organisms initially isolated (7%) were implicated in later infections. Overall there were eight fracture-site infections within three months of injury, an infection rate of 12.9%. Bacteria cultured from these infections are listed in Table 5.

From 1980 to 1988, our incidence of fracture-site infections in type III open fractures has been less than 15%. We believe this is due largely to improved gram-negative coverage in our antibiotic regimen. In 1987 and 1988, cefamandole replaced cefazolin as the cephalosporin in our antibiotic combination, but this change did not appear to improve the clinical outcome.

Summary and Recommendations

Optimal antibiotic management of open fractures includes initiating therapy as soon as possible after injury, choosing agents that are active against gram-negative bacilli and gram-positive cocci, and limiting the duration of therapy in the absence of clinical infection. Our recommendations for therapy are cefazolin for type I fractures, and cefazolin plus aminoglycoside for type II and III fractures. On the basis of experience, we continue antibiotic therapy for three days although recent data suggest that a shorter duration may be adequate. As discussed above, monotherapy with a newer broad-spectrum agent may prove to be as effective as our current regimen and has the potential advantages of lower cost and less toxicity.

References

1. Copeland CX Jr, Enneking WF: Incidence of osteomyelitis in compound fractures. *Am Surg* 1965;31:156–158.
2. Epps CH Jr, Adams JP: Wound management in open fractures. *Am Surg* 1961;27:766–769.
3. Patzakis MJ, Harvey JP Jr, Ivler D: The role of antibiotics in the management of open fractures. *J Bone Joint Surg* 1974;56A:532–541.
4. Gustilo RB, Anderson JT: Prevention of infection in the treatment of one thousand and twenty-five open fractures of long bones: Retrospective and prospective analyses. *J Bone Joint Surg* 1976;58A:453–458.
5. Bowers WH, Wilson FC, Greene WB: Antibiotic prophylaxis in experimental bone infections. *J Bone Joint Surg* 1973;55A:795–807.
6. Worlock P, Slack R, Harvey L, et al: The prevention of infection in open fractures: An experimental study of the effect of antibiotic therapy. *J Bone Joint Surg* 1988;70A:1341–1347.
7. Gustilo RB, Gruninger RP, Davis T: Classification of type III (severe) open fractures relative to treatment and results. *Orthopedics* 1987;10:1781–1788.
8. Caudle RJ, Stern PJ: Severe open fractures of the tibia. *J Bone Joint Surg* 1987;69A:801–807.
9. Dellinger EP, Miller SD, Wertz MJ, et al: Risk of infection after open fracture of the arm or leg. *Arch Surg* 1988;123:1320–1327.
10. Lawrence RM, Hoeprich PD, Huston AC, et al: Quantitative microbiology of traumatic orthopedic wounds. *J Clin Microbiol* 1978;8:673–675.
11. Pollack M: *Pseudomonas aeruginosa*, in Douglas RG, Bennett JE (eds): *Principles and Practice of Infectious Diseases*, ed 2. New York, Wiley, 1985, pp 1236–1247.
12. Hanson PG, Standridge J, Jarrett R, et al: Fresh water wound infection due to *Aeromonas hydrophilia*. *JAMA* 1977;238:1053–1054.
13. Joseph SW, Daily OP, Hunt WS, et al: *Aeromonas* primary wound infection of a diver in polluted waters. *J Clin Microbiol* 1979;10:46–49.
14. Bonner JR, Coker AS, Berryman CR, et al: Spectrum of *Vibrio* infections in a gulf coast community. *Ann Intern Med* 1983;99:464–469.
15. Poretz DM: *Erysipelothrix rhusiopathiae*, in Mandell GL, Douglas RF, Bennett JE (eds): *Principles and Practice of Infectious Diseases*, ed 2. New York, John Wiley & Sons, 1985, pp 1185–1186.
16. Roth AI, Fry DE, Polk HC Jr: Infectious morbidity in extremity fractures. *J Trauma* 1986;26:757–761.
17. Dellinger EP, Caplan ES, Weaver LD, et al: Duration of preventive antibiotic administration for open extremity fractures. *Arch Surg* 1988;123:333–339.
18. Patzakis MJ, Wilkins J, Moore TM: Considerations in reducing the infection rate in open tibial fractures. *Clin Orthop* 1983;178:36–41.
19. Gustilo RB, Mendoza RM, Williams DN: Problems in the management of type III (severe) open fractures: A new classification of type III open fractures. *J Trauma* 1984;24:742–746.

Clostridial Myonecrosis

Michael J. Patzakis, MD

Clostridial myonecrosis, or gas gangrene, is an infection that is associated with a high morbidity and mortality. This disease can occur very rapidly and is characterized by necrosis of muscle and soft tissue and by the production of gas and toxins. It is imperative that the orthopaedic surgeon take all measures to prevent this catastrophe when dealing with traumatic wounds.

Clostridial myonecrosis requires ideal conditions that include ischemia with low or absent oxygen tension, necrotic tissue, and clostridial organisms. Clostridial organisms are gram-positive, spore-forming bacilli that produce lethal exotoxins. *Clostridium welchii*, renamed *C perfringens* in 1897, is responsible for the majority of clostridial myonecrosis cases.[1-3] Other species of *Clostridia* that can cause gas gangrene include *C septicum* and *C novyi*.

Although the production of gas is generally present in classic clostridial myonecrosis, I have seen several cases of gas gangrene without gas production. In addition, certain gram-negative organisms, such as the paracolons, can produce gas in certain types of infections, specifically in patients with diabetes mellitus.

Etiology and Incidence

Hitchcock and associates[4] have estimated that from 900 to 1,000 cases of clostridial myonecrosis occur in the United States each year. Although the majority of cases occur following such injuries as open fractures, traumatic wounds, and burns, clostridial myonecrosis has also been reported in cases of clean surgery. Parker[5] reported 56 cases of gas gangrene in clean surgical cases in 55 British Hospitals over a two-year period. I have treated a patient who developed clostridial myonecrosis following an injection given to him in Mexico. Therefore, gas gangrene can occur after any type of trauma in both contaminated and clean surgical environments.

Brown and Kinman[2] reported 27 cases of gas gangrene over a ten-year period in the Miami, Florida, metropolitan area. Seventeen of these cases occurred in association with open fractures and ten with injuries received in a single plane crash. All 27 cases had inadequate debridement as well as primary closure of their wounds, and all of them cultured *C welchii* (*perfringens*).

Altemeier and Furste[1] reviewed 187,937 open fractures. They found an incidence of clostridial myonecrosis ranging from 0.03% to 5.2% depending on the treatment given.

The United States Army incidence of gas gangrene in wounds during wartime has been reported as 1.8% for World War I, 0.5% for World War II, 0.2% for Korea, and 0.16% for the Vietnam War.[2]

At my facility an estimated 7,600 open fractures were treated between 1970 and 1989. There were two cases of gas gangrene, and both of these patients received no antibiotics and primary wound closure. Both cases were treated and have been reported elsewhere.[6]

Contributing Factors

Factors that increase the risk of clostridial myonecrosis in contaminated wounds include primary wound closure, inadequate debridement, and inadequate antibiotic therapy. Experimentally, Patzakis and associates[7] reported on the effect of antibiotic therapy and wound closure on *Clostridia*-contaminated, open-fracture wounds in rats. The lowest mortality, 4%, was in animals that received penicillin at the time of wounding and whose open fracture wounds were left open. Animals that received no antibiotics and had primary closure of their wounds had the highest incidence (44%). Administering cephalothin at the time of wounding reduced the mortality to 4%, but when cephalothin was not given until three hours after wounding, the mortality increased to 28%.

Treatment of Open Fractures

In treating open fractures, it is paramount to minimize the risk of gas gangrene. The three cardinal principles in prevention are immediate effective antibiotic therapy, thorough surgical debridement and irrigation of the wound, and leaving the original fracture wound open. I recommend the immediate administration of wide-spectrum antibiotics effective against both gram-positive and gram-negative organisms,[8] for example, a first- or second-generation cephalosporin combined with an aminoglycoside. Penicillin is added for farm, stable, crush, vascular, and compartment injuries, which are more likely to develop gas gangrene.

Thorough debridement and irrigation of the wound is advocated for all open fracture wounds, regardless

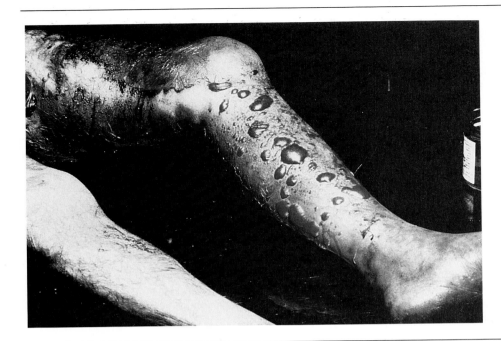

Fig. 1 Note the swollen gangrenous extremity with large bullae.

of type. For type I and type II wounds I do partial closures as described by Patzakis and associates.[7] In this procedure, the initial wound is left open, but the wound that is extended to facilitate debridement is closed. If there is a wound over a bone, this part of the wound is closed and the part that has been extended is left open. All type III wounds are left open, and secondary wound closure or muscle-flap tissue coverage is done within the first seven days. Virtually all open fracture wounds are left open initially.

Clinical Findings

Signs and symptoms indicative of clostridial myonecrosis include disproportionate pain, edema, clinical signs of toxicity, fever, shock, skin gangrenous changes, and the production of gas. Gram staining should be done on any wound suspected of clostridial myonecrosis, because the Gram stain often clarifies diagnosis by demonstrating dumbbell-shaped gram-positive rods.

Figure 1 shows a 57-year-old man who had been given an injection, thought to be an antibiotic, in Mexico. He subsequently developed gas gangrene and was brought to my facility. At the time of admission, the skin was gangrenous (Fig. 2), radiographs demonstrated gas production (Fig. 3), and a Gram stain showed gram-positive rods (Fig. 4). In addition, the patient was in renal failure, and myoglobinuria from muscle breakdown was present. This patient died within one hour after admission.

Treatment of Clostridial Myonecrosis

Treatment of clostridial myonecrosis includes the use of as much as 20 to 25 million units of intravenous penicillin per day. Sodium penicillin is given rather than potassium penicillin, because these patients are in renal

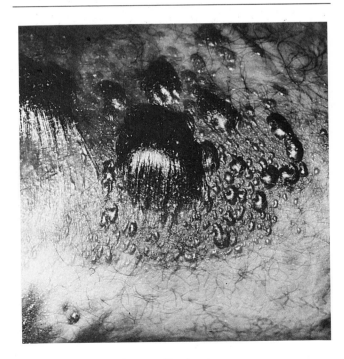

Fig. 2 Gangrenous bullous skin changes.

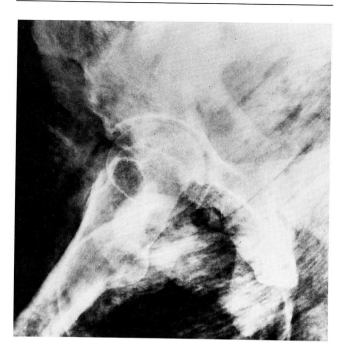

Fig. 3 Radiograph of the hip showing the presence of air in the soft tissues.

failure and the cellular breakdown from the exotoxins causes release of more potassium. Otherwise, the resultant hyperkalemia could cause cardiac arrhythmias. Clindamycin and an aminoglycoside are often added, because other anaerobic and polymicrobial organisms may also be present. Debridement is essential and amputation may be necessary. The use of hyperbaric oxygen has been advocated by a number of investigators[9] and personal experience has proven it to be of value. In addition, supportive therapy, including intravenous fluid hydration and other medical management, is indicated. The use of antitoxin has proven ineffective and is not recommended.

Hart and associates,[8] who reported on 139 cases of clostridial myonecrosis, advocate the use of hyperbaric oxygen for treating gas gangrene. They also found that a delay in treatment adversely affected survival. Patients treated within the first 12 hours had the highest survival rate. Patients who died had a mean lag treatment period of approximately 32 hours. In addition, they reported that the presence of shock and a compromised host were associated with a poor prognosis.

Summary

The best treatment for gas gangrene is prevention by following the principles of thorough debridement, immediate effective parenteral antibiotic therapy, and delayed closure of open fractures.

References

1. Altemeier WA, Furste WL: Collective review: Gas gangrene, abstract. *Surg Gynec Obst* 1947;84:507–523.
2. Brown PW, Kinman PB: Gas gangrene in a metropolitan community. *J Bone Joint Surg* 1974;56A:1445–1451.
3. MacLennan JD: The histotoxic clostridial infections of man. *Bacteriol Rev* 1962;26:177–276.
4. Hitchcock CR, Demello FJ, Haglin JJ: Gangrene infection: New approaches to an old disease. *Surg Clin North Am* 1975;55:1403–1410.
5. Parker MT: Postoperative clostridial infections in Britain. *Br Med J* 1969;3:671–676.
6. Patzakis MJ, Harvey JP Jr, Ivler D: The role of antibiotics in the management of open fractures. *J Bone Joint Surg* 1974;56A:532–541.
7. Patzakis MJ, Dorr LD, Hammond W, et al: The effect of antibiotics, primary and secondary closure on clostridial contaminated open fracture wounds in rats. *J Trauma* 1978;18:34–37.
8. Patzakis MJ, Wilkins J, Moore TM: Considerations in reducing the infection rate in open tibial fractures. *Clin Orthop* 1983;178:36–41.
9. Hart GB, Lamb RC, Strauss MB: Gas gangrene: I. A collective review. II. A 15-year experience with hyperbaric oxygen. *J Trauma* 1983;23:991–1000.

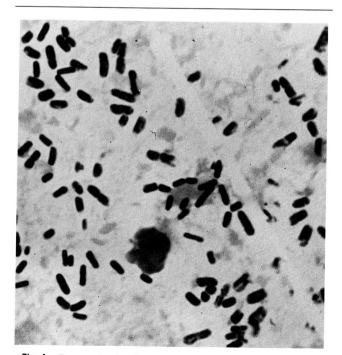

Fig. 4 Gram stain showing gram-positive bacilli. Note the dumbbell appearance of the rods.

Chronic Osteomyelitis: Results of Treatment

George Cierny III, MD

The management of patients with chronic osteomyelitis requires consideration of physiologic, anatomic, psychosocial, and institutional variables. The interplay of these factors determines the goal of therapy: simple or complex, curative or palliative, limb-sparing or ablative. The patient's medical history, the options for osseous stabilization, and the experience of each clinical team affect the process of selecting patients and the methods used to manage debridement defects.

The first step in treatment is debridement to viable and well perfused tissue margins. Secondly, the host's immune and metabolic capacity must be operational and effective throughout therapy. With viable tissue, cells from the immune system can attack the remaining bacteria. At that time, antibiotics can also be effective in helping to remove all bacteria.

Host factors that adversely affect wound healing and, thus, the prognosis include both local and systemic factors. Local factors are chronic lymphedema, venous stasis, major vessel disease, arteritis, extensive scarring, and radiation fibrosis. Systemic factors are malnutrition, immune deficiency, chronic hypoxia, malignancy, diabetes mellitus, old age, renal or liver failure, and tobacco abuse. Local conditions limit perfusion and systemic factors affect the immunologic, hemopoietic, and/or metabolic capabilities of the host.

A series of 538 patients was prospectively staged according to the Cierny-Mader classification.[1] In this system, the local extent of the disease (the nidus) is designated by one of four anatomic types (Fig. 1). In type I (medullary osteomyelitis) the nidus is endosteal. In type II or superficial osteomyelitis, an outer surface of bone is infected because of a refractory defect in the soft-tissue envelope. Localized osteomyelitis (type III) is a well-marginated sequestration of cortical bone that often combines the features of types I and II; the entire lesion can, however, be completely excised without causing segmental instability. In type IV lesions, the process is permeative, involves an entire segment of bone, and often has characteristics of types I, II, and III. These later lesions (diffuse osteomyelitis) are biomechanically unstable both before and after debridement.

The host is stratified with regard to physiologic capacity to withstand infection, treatment, and the morbidity of the disease. A-hosts are normal, healthy patients; the B-host has either a local (B^L), systemic (B^S), or a combined local and systemic (B$^{L/S}$) compromise.

ANATOMIC CLASSIFICATION OF ADULT OSTEOMYELITIS

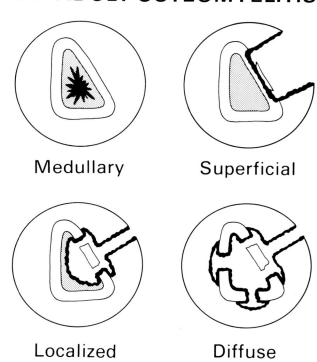

Medullary

Superficial

Localized

Diffuse

Fig. 1 Medullary and superficial lesions are limited to the inner and outer surfaces of the bone respectively. When full-thickness sequestra are present, treatment and prognosis depend on the stability (localized) or instability (diffuse) of the skeletal segment.

The C-host is one who, for whatever reason, is not a treatment candidate. In this category, the disability is either minimal or the potential morbidity of therapy is too great to warrant curative measures (Fig. 2).

The physiologic stratification of this series of 538 patients was as follows: for type I, 12 patients were A-hosts and 19 were B-hosts; for type II, 21 were A-hosts and 43 were B-hosts; for type III, 74 were A-hosts and 24 were B-hosts; and for type IV, 167 were A-hosts and 178 were B-hosts. Note that 50% of the patients seen from 1981 through 1988 had wound-healing deficiencies (B-hosts) and were at risk for treatment failure regardless of the etiology, the anatomic site, or the type and number of bacteria present.

The clinical staging of osteomyelitis in the preoper-

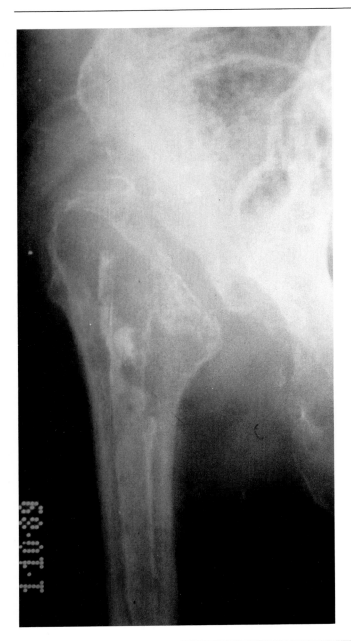

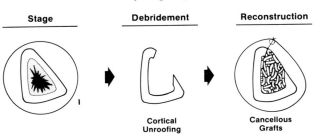

Fig. 2 **Left,** A 72-year-old woman with a painless resection arthroplasty of the hip following removal for sepsis. Polymethylmethacrylate was not removed from the canal. **Right,** Drainage has persisted for three years with the wound limited in size and the discharge controllable with one gauze pad daily. This patient is not a treatment candidate (C-host).

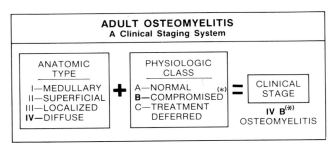

Fig. 3 The anatomic type is matched with a physiologic class to designate one of 12 possible clinical stages of osteomyelitis.

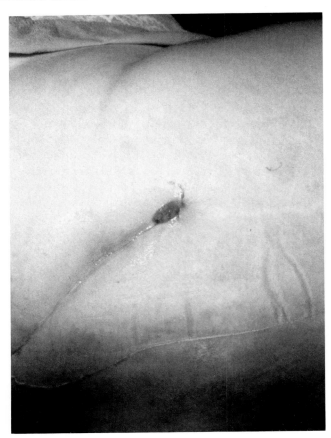

Fig. 4 In many instances of medullary osteomyelitis, it is not necessary to graft the deadspace, for example, after reaming for an infected intramedullary nail.

Superficial Osteomyelitis
(Stage II)

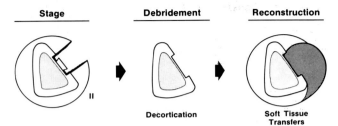

Stage — Debridement — Reconstruction

Decortication — Soft Tissue Transfers

Fig. 5 Stage II osteomyelitis is primarily a soft-tissue problem in patients with local compromise of healing.

Localized Osteomyelitis
(Stage III)

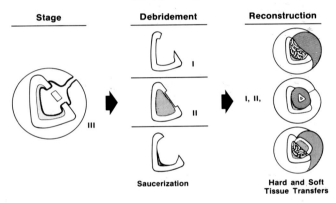

Stage — Debridement — Reconstruction

Saucerization — Hard and Soft Tissue Transfers

Fig. 6 The treatment of type III lesions combines the techniques used for types I and II with simple methods of stabilization and rather complicated bony reconstructions.

Diffuse Osteomyelitis
(Stage IV)

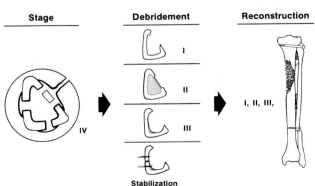

Stage — Debridement — Reconstruction

Stabilization

Fig. 7 Stages IVA and IVB osteomyelitis are basically infected non-unions requiring complex stabilizations, reconstructions, and rehabilitation.

Table 1
Adult osteomyelitis (arrest rates at 2+ years)*

Stage	Host Type	Percent	(No. of Patients)
I	A	100%	11
I	B	89%	9
II	A	100%	9
II	B	79%	19
III	A	98%	43
III	B	92%	13
IV	A	98%	66
IV	B	80%	75

*Overall figures equal 91% (245 patients)

Table 2
Deadspace management

Authors	No.	Success (%)
Closed/Irrigation Systems		
1973 Clawson et al	97	74%
1970 Kelly et al	44	71%
1987 Perry et al	21	72%
Papineau Grafts		
1988 Cabanela	25	72% (100%)*
1973 Burri et al	21	? (90%)*
1988 Cierny	20	80% (90%)*
1983 Green and Dlabal	15	? (87%)*
Myoplasty		
1988 Nahai and Cierny	74	95%
1985 Fitzgerald et al	42	93%
1983 Mathes and Nahai	21	86%
1977 Ger	17	82%
Free (Soft) Flaps		
1988 Nahai and Cierny	57	91%
1985 May	53	98%
1986 Irons and Wood	33	66%
1984 Weiland et al	23	70%
Free Bone Flaps		
1985 Wood et al	20	60%
1984 Wood et al	11	91%
1984 Weiland et al	11	55%
1988 Nahai and Cierny	10	80%

*Initial success rate (eventual success rate).

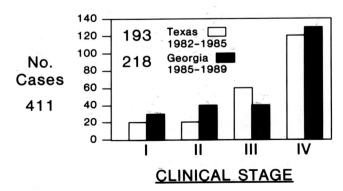

Fig. 8 The spectrum of adult osteomyelitis has not changed over the years in either type or stage (see text).

Biologic Dead Space Management

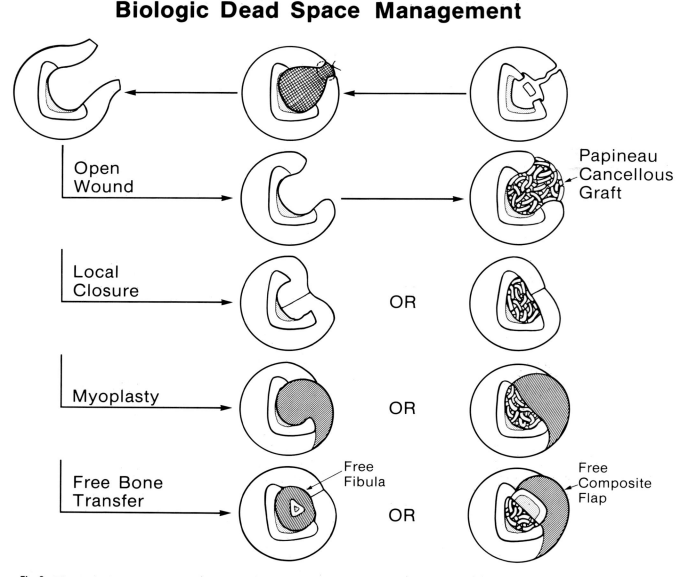

Fig. 9 The methods used to manage deadspace following debridement range from complex to simple depending on the requirements for each individual site.

ative assessment helps determine the treatment and is a prognostic indicator (Figs. 3 to 7; Table 1): stage I = simple deadspace and simple closures; stage II = no deadspace and complex closures; stage III = simple stabilizations with complex deadspaces and complex closures; stage IV = complex stabilizations, deadspaces, and closures. Figure 8 compares the types of infections seen in two geographic regions of the USA: Galveston, Texas (1983–1985) and Atlanta, Georgia (1985–1988). The anatomic distribution was similar in both regions. The C-host category, in Atlanta, plateaued at 8% and the primary amputation rate at 10%. Thus, 82% of patients evaluated in these clinics are offered limb salvage.

Deadspace Management

When managing infected, contaminated wounds, the methods and materials for deadspace management are limited; wounds heal by second intention healing, local approximations, or closures with distant tissues (Figs. 9 and 10). Reconstruction may require bone grafts to restore form and/or function. The requirements for each wound differ according to the anatomic site of infection, host variables, and institutional resources.

There are no recent publications supporting protocols advocating second intention healing alone. The series of Shannon and associates[2] is, however, instructive:

freshly debrided surfaces were skin grafted for a long-term success rate of 60% to 70%. Immediate skin grafts prevent the accumulation of dense scar tissue on the bony surface. This method does not, however, address the need for surface revascularization, nor does it help eliminate the contamination present after each debridement. Unless new tissue, with its own perfusion, is brought to the surface, bacteria may persist in the exposed interstitial lamellae and small fissures. The same problems exist if these defects are closed without deadspace obliteration over closed irrigation systems.[3-5] The same 70% success rates occur because scar and granulation tissue accumulate on the surface, where they temporarily entrap the organisms in an ischemic cocoon. Washing this space with high doses of antibiotics, detergents, or astringents has not changed the prognosis (Table 2).

The open cancellous grafting technique popularized by Papineau is the simplest method used to obliterate defects of both hard and soft tissue.[6,7] The debridement

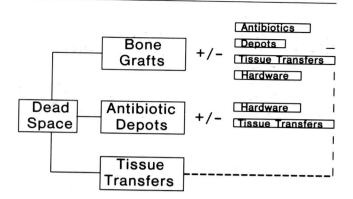

Fig. 10 Defects are filled with grafts, antibiotic depots, or soft tissue. The timing for each method depends on several factors, including the sterility of the wound, the condition of the host, institutional resources, and anatomic limitations.

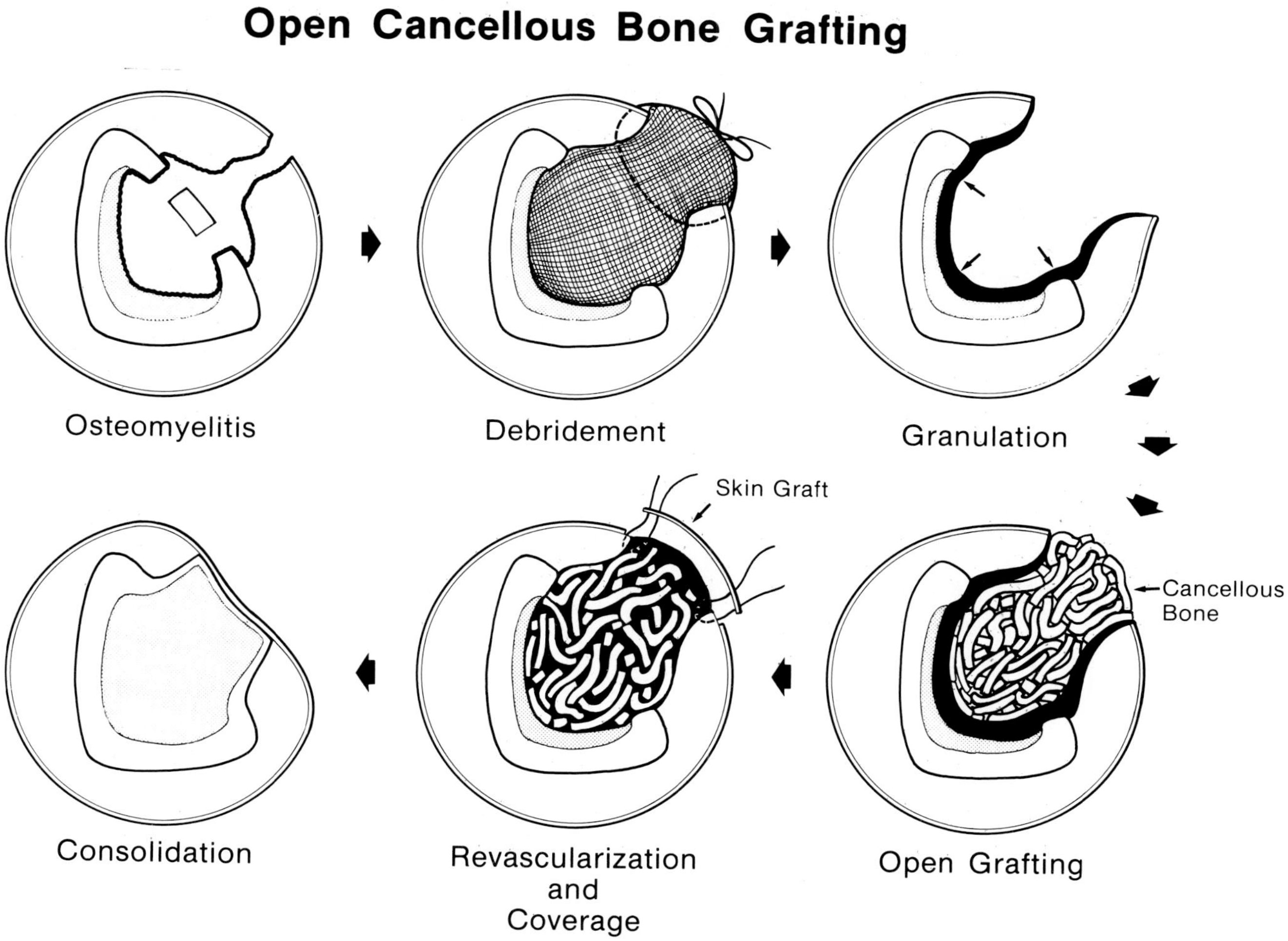

Open Cancellous Bone Grafting

Osteomyelitis

Debridement

Granulation

Consolidation

Skin Graft

Revascularization and Coverage

Open Grafting

Cancellous Bone

Fig. 11 The coverage gained in this technique is either a spontaneous epithelialization or split-thickness skin graft.

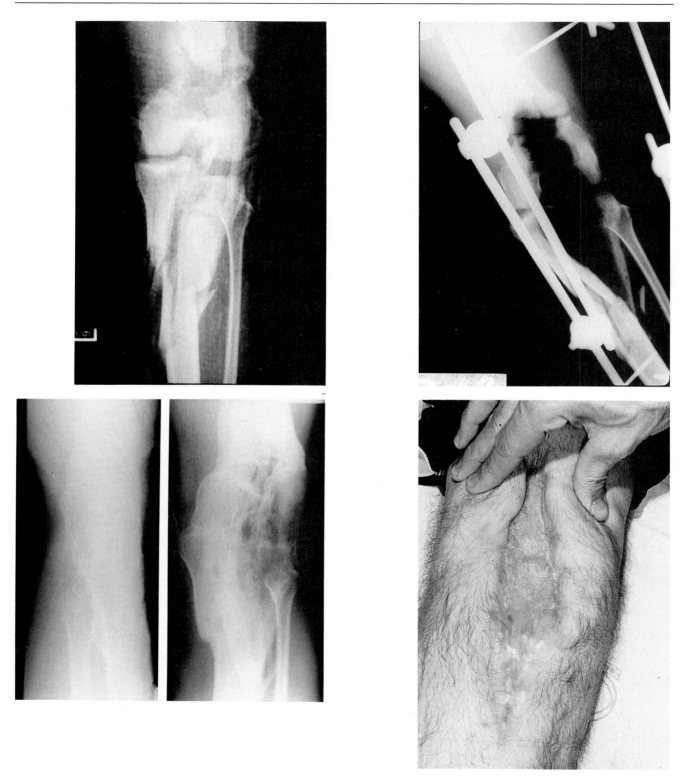

Fig. 12 **Top left**, An infected fracture of the distal femur, knee, and proximal tibia. **Top right**, The debridement defect. **Bottom left**, Open cancellous grafting (two serial grafts) was used to gain a solid knee fusion. **Bottom right**, Coverage is adequate but adherent, vulnerable to trauma, and cosmetically displeasing.

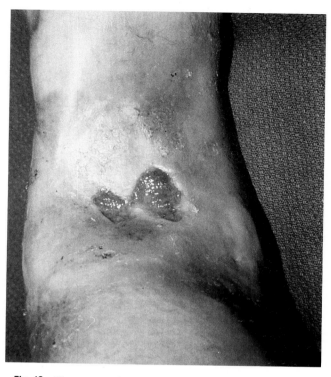

Fig. 13 Three years after a successful ankle fusion using the Papineau technique, this patient is functional but is troubled by a recurrent cellulitis, pain, swelling, and drainage from this persistent ulcer.

Table 3

The amount of antibiotic (weight) that can be mixed with the acrylic powder is volumetrically determined.*

Drugs	Antibiotic Bead Cocktails (g)†
Cephalosporins	
Cefazolin	6.0
Moxalactam	6.0
Cefotaxime	10.0
Tobramycin	9.6
Vancomycin	5.0
Ticarcillin	12.0

*Theoretically, any powdered antibiotic can be used. (Wt = vol [24 ml] antibiotic/pk [120 ml] cement)
†Mix/40 g pk Simplex-P

Table 4

Risk factors pertaining to complications encountered during treatment using the Ilizarov methodology

Authors	Tibial Nonunion		
	No. of Patients	Union (%)	Risk (%)
Paley and Catagni	25	100	36
Morandi and Zembo	42	95	38
Biasibetti and Gallinaro	62	74	28

Table 5

Deadspace management (Method/Failure Associations)*

Technique	Failure (%)		No. of Cases
	1st Treatment	2nd Treatment	
Papineau graft	20%	10%	20
Immediate graft	7%	5%	86
Beads/graft	14%	8%	114
Free flap	12%	9%	57
Myoplasty	11%	5%	74
Free bone	30%	20%	10

*The results achieved in 361 cases treated prospectively by the same team of physicians (Galveston and Atlanta). Overall case results were improved by re-treatment or adjunctive measures.

Outline 1

Comparing the results when treating A-hosts and B-hosts with type I, II, III vs type IV lesions

Adult Osteomyelitis (2+ year follow-up)		
Stable (Types I, II, and III lesions)		
Normal (A-host)	98%	
		> 93% (104)
Compromised (B-host)	85%	
Unstable (Type IV lesions)		
Normal (A-host)	98%	
		> 89% (141)
Compromised (B-host)	80%	

is followed by a brief waiting period (ten to 14 days). When the wound surfaces develop a flush mat of 1/8 inch of healthy granulation tissue (Fig. 11), fresh, autogenous, cancellous grafts are gently compressed into the defect and slightly above the bony surface, because some graft is lost with dressing changes. The wound must be saucerized; overhanging soft tissues are marsupialized to the bone edges to prevent "lipping" and the accumulation of fluids. Once the implants are revascularized, split-thickness skin is applied if the spontaneous reepithelialization is insufficient to seal the wound. The result of this type of "open" management differs from others: the cancellous grafts induce a permanent revascularization of the defect; eventually, the remodeled structure has a cortex, endosteum, and marrow. However, the patient should be an A-host, the bone subcutaneous, and the wound adequately contoured to contain the grafts during mobilization. Furthermore, there must be a reserve of autogenous cancellous grafts to fill the defect. Serial graftings will be necessary to contour and fill large defects, because each layer should be limited to a thickness no greater than 2 cm. This latter detail will prevent central graft necrosis. B-hosts are not candidates for this technique; they cannot support the metabolic requirement of revascularization, graft incorporation, and wound consolidation in the face of persistent bacterial contamination. A case example using this method is seen in Figure 12.

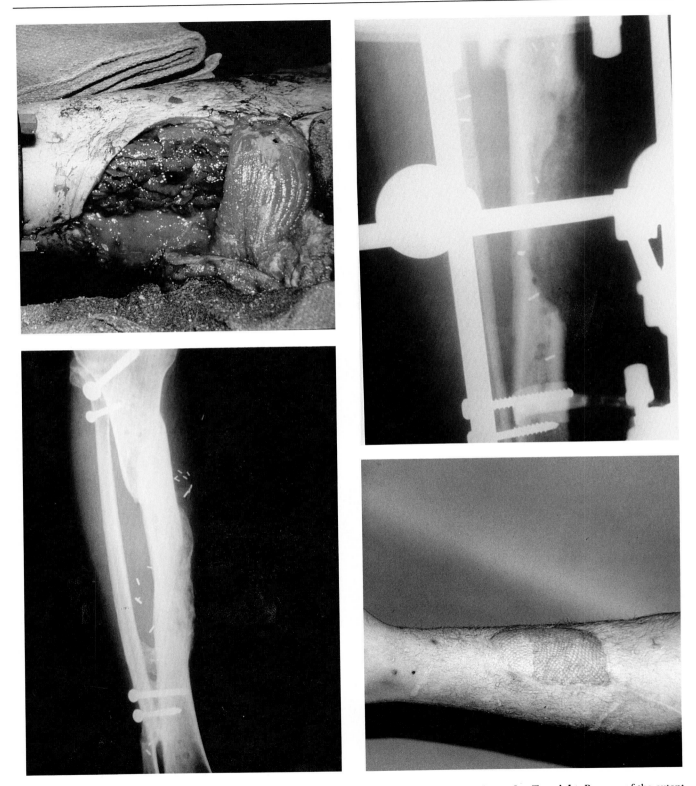

Fig. 14 **Top left**, A massive cancellous graft was performed at the time of a free latissimus dorsi transfer. **Top right**, Because of the extent of bone lost at debridement, an ipsilateral fibular transfer was used to augment the cancellous grafts. **Bottom left**, Ten months later the patient is walking brace-free without drainage. **Bottom right**, The latissimus has atrophied leaving a well-contoured extremity.

Staged Dead Space Management
(Antibiotic Beads)

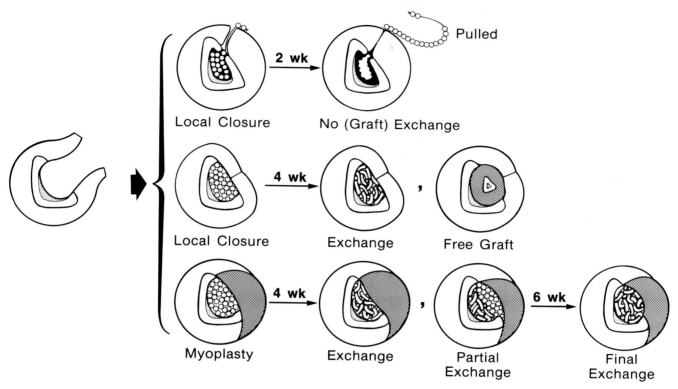

Fig. 15 In most instances, the beads precede a biologic repair. Exceptions to this include small type I or type III lesions.

The most common problem encountered with the open graft technique is persistent drainage and/or breakdown of coverage rather than a failure to consolidate the grafts (Fig. 13). Superficial ulcerations occur and persist until more sophisticated techniques of coverage are used. The method itself is successful in 70% to 80% of cases (Table 2). Ten percent to 20% of the patients must later be managed with some other technique. Overall, the cases do quite well; 90% to 96% of the patients treated eventually have a successful result[6-8] (M.E. Cabanela, personal communication, February 1989). At times, the choice of a Papineau graft over another method may be a circumstantial or simply a matter of resource availability.

Closed-Wound Techniques

The disadvantages of open-wound protocols are (1) patient selection is limited to A-hosts; (2) the defects treated should be small or flat; (3) they require wound care and patient cooperation; and (4) the success rates are moderate. When the debridement defect can be obliterated with live tissues, these problems are over-

come. The best results come from techniques wherein muscle[9] is used as either a transposition or a free flap to completely obliterate the deadspace. The overall success rates of these two methods (Table 2) are comparable and quite excellent.[9-14] However, the perfusion of transferred tissue with a microvascular reanastomosis is often superior to a local transposition, because it is harvested and perfused from outside the zone of injury. Furthermore, a free flap may be used anywhere in the body, but transpositions are limited to their anatomic arc.[15] Each microsurgical anastomosis is, however, a complex undertaking. Success depends on the skill and experience of the surgeon, the condition of the wound, and the physiologic status of the patient.

When To Bone Graft

As a rule, most infected nonunions require a bone graft. Indeed, in my series of 78 such lesions, patients averaged 1.6 grafts per site. However, the indication for a structural (osseous) augmentation is a 30% to 50% loss of volume.[16,17] Treatment options, in the order of

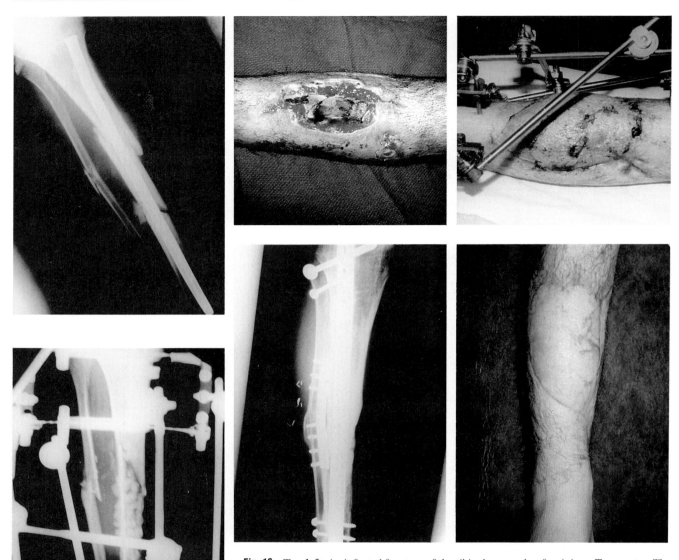

Fig. 16 **Top left**, An infected fracture of the tibia three weeks after injury. **Top center**, The initial and surgical trauma caused extensive hard- and soft-tissue loss. **Top right**, The soft tissues were replaced by a free latissimus transfer. **Bottom left**, Beneath the free flap, the deadspace was maintained with antibiotic beads while the wound matured. Length and alignment were maintained with a simple external frame. **Bottom center**, The final reconstruction reverted to medullary fixation, augmenting the repair with cancellous grafts, and an ipsilateral fibular transfer. **Bottom right**, At three years the patient is ambulating without restrictions, drainage, or pain.

technical difficulty, include the Papineau technique, closed cancellous grafts,[18] pedicled osseous transfers, bone distraction-transport systems, and free bone flaps.

In a series of patients seen from 1983 through 1988, 86 patients received cancellous bone grafts at the time of delayed primary closure, five to seven days after the debridement. The success rate for these grafts was 93% (Fig. 14). The long-term success of these cases was 95%, with augmentative techniques used to gain union, reconstitute bone, and restore function. In contrast, 114 grafts, placed an average of 34 days after an implant of antibiotic beads,[18-21] had an initial success rate of 86% and an overall rate of 92%. I do not have experience with a management protocol wherein the space is first filled with muscle and then later bone grafted[10]; the overall success rate of delayed vs immediate grafts has not been statistically different. The presence of bacteria did not influence the prognosis in my series,[20] as the bacterial counts were low, the hosts primed, and systemic antibiotics tailored to the wound pathogens. I have always added powdered, pathogen-specific antibiotic to the grafts at the time of insertion. Immediate

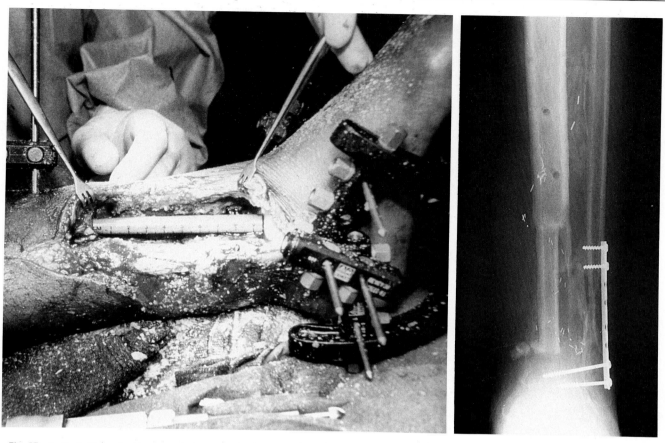

Fig. 17 **Left**, A 12-cm hard- and soft-tissue defect following debridement of this distal tibia and talus. **Right**, Coverage was gained with a free latissimus flap while bony continuity was restored using a free and ipsilateral fibular construct.

grafting, however, is only offered to A-hosts with well-perfused tissue beds in logistically feasible sites.

Antibiotic Bead Implantation

When immediate reconstruction cannot be performed, a staged deadspace management is recommended. Since 1983, this method was used in the 114 cases mentioned above. Following debridement, wound coverage was secured, but the deadspace was maintained with customized antibiotic beads (Fig. 15). The antibiotics (Table 3) were tailored to the sensitivities of the bacteria present in the wound. The overall success rate in these cases was 92%, indicating that the delayed technique is a reasonable alternative to immediate management (95%). The indications for using beads—compromised hosts, staging grafts longer than 50 cc, internal fixation, and complex wound closures—address issues affecting the technical aspects of coverage and the physiologic status of the host (Fig. 16).[22] In my experience, B-hosts are at risk for graft resorption and failure if grafted primarily. These wounds are first covered and sterilized with beads; the patients are brought back at a later date when the infection is arrested, their immune system recovered, and their wound-healing capacity restored.

Free Bone Flaps

These procedures[12,23,24] are technically difficult, because the vascular pedicles are short, the fixation techniques are typically complex, and the reconstructions are often performed within the primary zone of injury. Furthermore, the bones available for transfer, such as the fibula, rib, iliac crest, and scapula, are usually inferior in size and structure to the missing skeletal segment (Fig. 17). As a result of these problems, the procedures have met with fewer successes. Wound complications are frequent, because most of the patients are compromised (type B) hosts. The stabilization methods are limited; two unions are required; and stress fractures are common. Furthermore, a late salvage is difficult because an onlay, Phemister bone graft[25,26] for delayed union may totally devascularize the

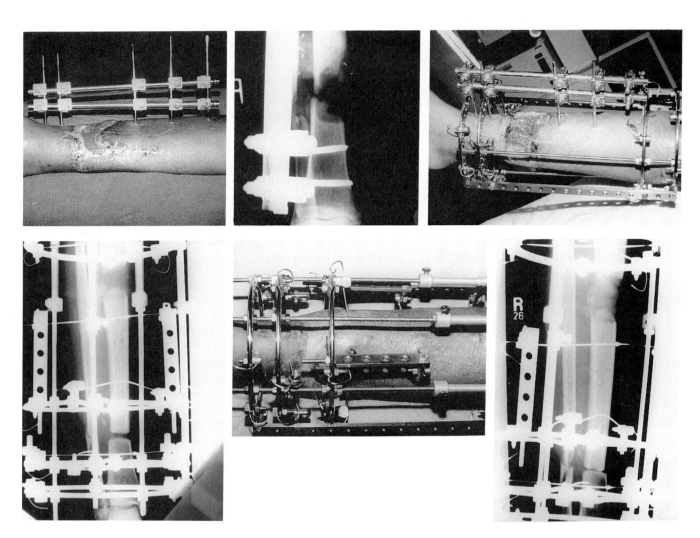

Fig. 18 **Top left**, A 54-year-old woman suffering a IIIC open fracture of the tibia and the loss of three free-tissue transfers at another institution to attempt coverage and fracture union. **Top center**, Alignment had been maintained with a unilateral frame. **Top right**, Following debridement, a 4-cm hard- and soft-tissue defect existed. An Ilizarov construct was applied with the unilateral frame in place. **Bottom left**, Following a proximal corticotomy, a central segment of diaphysis was mobilized at the rate of 1 mm per day on the transport ring. **Bottom center**, Closure of the soft-tissue defect took place spontaneously without skin grafts and flaps. **Bottom right**, Radiograph documenting the completed transportation, excellent alignment, and early distraction osteogenesis at the corticotomy site.

transferred segment as a result of subperiosteal stripping. The method must be perfect from every standpoint right from the start. However, considering that they are being performed in situations in which the bone gaps are larger than 4 cm, such rates are admirable (Table 2).

Bone Transportation

Bone transport mechanisms,[27,28] using in situ regenerate "grafts" provide an attractive alternative to free bone flaps (Fig. 18). The indications, quite interestingly, do not exclude B-hosts; distraction osteogenesis is reportedly quite successful even in the face of these factors. Furthermore, the method is suitable for many patients unable to participate in conventional protocols because they lack autogenous graft reserves, suitable vessels, or adequate length or because of a shortage of microvascular surgeons. Furthermore, shortened extremities can be simultaneously lengthened with the technique.

The method of Ilizarov is not without its problems. The techniques are complicated, many outpatient adjustments are required, and the internal transports and lengthenings are painful. The operations are, however, relatively bloodless, limited to the extremity, usually percutaneous, and can be done by one surgeon. The results of treatment are difficult to assess. Table 4 lists the experience of other authors attempting to heal non-unions by the Ilizarov methods.[29-31] Union can be achieved in 74% to 100% of the cases. Various problems, including deformities at joints, iatrogenic neuropathies, dystrophies, nonunion, and pin-tract infections, occur in 28% to 38% of cases. However, the overall complication rates I experienced when using conventional methods to treat my patients with infected nonunions was 33%. For normal patients the rate was 25%, and for compromised patients it was 62%. Thus, the Ilizarov methodology compares favorably.

Summary

As stated previously, approximately 8% of the patients evaluated do not require curative treatment and palliative treatment with suppressive therapy may be successful (Fig. 2). For the most part, these are C-hosts for whom the morbidity of treatment is greater than the morbidity of disease or exceeds the expected gain. The overall spectrum of treatment in 411 of my patients (1983–1988) is seen in Table 5. Of the 411 patients, 228 (55%) required a bone graft; of these, 42% were primary grafts. Soft-tissue reconstructions were required in 37% of the entire patient population and in 59% of the type IV lesions. The overall amputation rate was 9%. There were no statistical differences in success rates between stable and unstable lesions, nor when cases were stratified for the type or number of bacteria present. However, compromised patients had a statistically inferior prognosis compared with patients who had normal physiologic profiles (Outline 1).

Conclusions

The prognosis in adult osteomyelitis is host-dependent. Irrigation systems and second intention healing are to be avoided for anything other than small defects. Papineau grafts and free bone flaps are acceptable alternatives when indications are closely scrutinized. Deadspace obliteration with well perfused soft tissue offers the best chance for cure following a debridement to viable margins, host rescue, and the administration of pathogen-specific antibiotics. Distraction osteogenesis coupled with bone transport appears promising in the management of segmental hard- and soft-tissue defects.

References

1. Cierny G, Mader JT, Penninck JJ: A clinical staging for adult osteomyelitis. *Cont Orthop* 1985;10:5.

2. Shannon JG, Woolhouse FM, Eisinger PJ: The treatment of chronic osteomyelitis by saucerization and immediate skin grafting. *Clin Orthop* 1973;96:98–107.

3. Clawson DK, Davis FJ, Hansen ST Jr: Treatment of chronic osteomyelitis with emphasis on closed suction-irrigation technic. *Clin Orthop* 1973;96:88–97.

4. Kelly PJ, Martin WJ, Coventry MB: Chronic osteomelitis: II. Treatment with closed irrigation and suction. *JAMA* 1970;213:1843–1848.

5. Perry CR, Davenport K, Vossen MK: Local delivery of antibiotics via an implantable pump in the treatment of osteomyelitis. *Clin Orthop* 1988;226:222–230.

6. Cabanela ME: Open cancellous bone grafting of infected bone defects. *Orthop Clin North Am* 1984;15:427–440.

7. Green SA, Dlabal TA: The open bone graft for septic nonunion. *Clin Orthop* 1983;180:117–124.

8. Burri C, Passler HH, Henkemeyer H: Treatment of posttraumatic osteomyelitis with bone, soft tissue, and skin defects. *J Trauma* 1973;13:799–810.

9. Mathes SJ, Alpert BS, Chang N: Use of the muscle flap in chronic osteomyelitis: Experimental and clinical correlation. *Plast Reconstr Surg* 1982;69:815–829.

10. Fitzgerald RH Jr, Ruttle PE, Arnold PG, et al: Local muscle flaps in the treatment of chronic osteomyelitis. *J Bone Joint Surg* 1985;67A:175–185.

11. Ger R: Muscle transposition for treatment and prevention of chronic post-traumatic osteomyelitis of the tibia. *J Bone Joint Surg* 1977;59A:784–791.

12. May JW: Symposium: The use of muscle flaps in the treatment of osteomyelitis in the lower extremity. *Contemp Orthop* 1985;10:127.

13. Weiland AJ, Moore JR, Daniel RK: The efficacy of free tissue transfer in the treatment of osteomyelitis. *J Bone Joint Surg* 1984;66A:181–193.

14. Irons GB Jr, Wood MB: Soft-tissue coverage for the treatment of osteomyelitis of the lower part of the leg. *Mayo Clin Proc* 1986;61:382–387.

15. Mathes SJ, Nahai F: *Clinical Applications of Muscle and Musculocutaneous Flaps.* CV Mosby, St. Louis, 1982.

16. Beals RK, Lawton GD, Snell WE: Prophylactic internal fixation of the femur in metastatic breast cancer. *Cancer* 1971;28:1350–1354.

17. Harrington KD, Johnston JO, Turner RH, et al: The use of methylmethacrylate as an adjunct in the internal fixation of malignant neoplastic fractures. *J Bone Joint Surg* 1972;54A:1665–1676.

18. Cierny G: The classification and treatment of adult osteomyelitis, in Evarts CM (ed): *Surgery of the Musculoskeletal System,* ed 2. Churchill Livingstone, 1989.

19. Klem K: *Die Behandlung chronischer knochen Infektionen mit Gentamicin-PMMA-ketten and Kygelin in gentamicin-PMMA-kette Symposium,* muchen Contzen H (ed). Erlanger Verlag surlehrmittel, Wissenschaft und Forschung, 1976, pp 20–25.

20. Cierny G, Mader JT, Couch L: Adjunctive local antibiotics in the management of contaminated orthopaedic wounds. *Orthop Trans* 1986;10:465.

21. Nahai F, Cierny G: Soft tissue reconstruction of the lower leg. *Perspect Plast Surg* 1987;1:1–32.

22. Campanacci M, Zanoli S: Double tibiofibular synostosis (*fibula pro tibia*) for non-union and delayed union of the tibia: End result review of one hundred seventy-one cases. *J Bone Joint Surg* 1966;48A:44–56.

23. Wood MB, Cooney WP III, Irons GB Jr: Skeletal reconstruction by vascularized bone transfer: Indications and results. *Mayo Clin Proc* 1985;60:729–734.

24. Wood MB, Cooney WP, Irons GB: Lower extremity salvage and reconstruction by free-tissue transfer: Analysis of results. *Clin Orthop* 1985;201:151–161.

25. Phemister DB: Treatment of ununited fractures by onlay bone grafts without screw or tie fixation and without breaking down of the fibrous union. *J Bone Joint Surg* 1947;29:946–960.

26. Rokkanen P, Slätis P: Subcortical cancellous bone grafting in the treatment of delayed union of tibial shaft fractures. *J Trauma* 1972;12:1075–1082.

27. Ilizarov GA: The tension-stress effect on the genesis and growth of tissues: Part I. The influence of stability of fixation and soft-tissue preservation. *Clin Orthop* 1989;238:249–281.

28. Ilizarov GA: The tension-stress effect on the genesis and growth of tissues: Part II. The influence of the rate and frequency of distraction. *Clin Orthop* 1989;239:263–285.

29. Paley D, Catagni MA, Argnani F, et al: Ilizarov treatment of tibial nonunions with bone loss. *Clin Orthop* 1989;241:146–165.

30. Morandi M, Zembo M: Management of tibial nonunions with or without bone defect, soft tissue defect or osteomyelitis. Presented at the symposium on Ilizarov techniques, Washington, DC, May 16–18, 1988.

31. Biasibetti A, Gallinaro P: Nonunions and bone defects: A comprehensive approach. Presented at the symposium on Ilizarov techniques, Washington, DC, May 16–18, 1988.

The Use of Septopal (Polymethylmethacrylate Beads With Gentamicin) in the Treatment of Chronic Osteomyelitis

J. David Blaha, MD

Carl L. Nelson, MD

Larry F. Frevert, MD

Stephen L. Henry, MD

David Seligson, MD

John L. Esterhai, Jr., MD

R. Bruce Heppenstal, MD

Jason Calhoun, MD

Jose Cobos, MD

Jon Mader, MD

Introduction

The treatment of osteomyelitis is expensive and time-consuming for both patient and medical staff. A treatment that would decrease expense and inconvenience would be distinctly advantageous. From the time of Hippocrates to Paré and Orr, debridement has been the most important part of therapy for osteomyelitis, but even from the time of the Smith papyrus (circa 4000 BC), the local application of substances to the wound has been used to augment therapy.[1]

The current standard treatment for osteomyelitis combines debridement, adequate coverage of the defect with soft tissue, and administration of antibiotics. This chapter reports on the treatment of osteomyelitis with a new drug, Septopal, developed by Klaus Klemm, a German physician. Extending the work of Jenny and associates,[2] who packed methylmethacrylate into osteomyelitic cavities, and Buchholz and associates,[3] who added gentamicin to bone cement, Klemm experimented with placing antibiotic-containing cement in osteomyelitic cavities. Initial failures were attributed to lack of drainage, inability of the granulation tissue to grow into the cavity, and difficulty of removing the cement. Klemm then tried rolling the cement into spheres, which not only overcame the problems of using the cement in bulk form, but also increased the surface area of the cement, allowing a greater elution of antibiotic.[4] This treatment has proven quite successful in the hands of Klemm and another European surgeon.[5]

Study Protocol

A randomized, multicenter, controlled study to compare the use of polymethylmethacrylate antibiotic beads (without long-term intravenous antibiotics) with conventional intravenous antibiotic therapy was set up according to FDA guidelines. The protocol, by controlling for surgical and wound treatment, makes the variable either systemic antibiotics given in an optimized fashion with the consultation of infectious diseases specialists or the local application of Septopal chains. Osteomyelitic cavities are debrided to the extent that the surgeon believes closure of the wound is possible—no open treatment of the wound is allowed under the protocol. Soft-tissue coverage is provided by local or free flaps or skin substitution. Patients are randomly assigned to either the conventional group or the Septopal group. Use of systemic antibiotics in the Septopal group is limited to a five-day maximum course just after surgery to treat the soft-tissue component of infection or for other infections, such as a urinary-tract infection or pneumonia, that might develop.

One "second-look" debridement is allowed during the first 14 days after the index debridement. If more than one debridement is necessary because clinical indicators of infection—local warmth, redness, pain, swelling, and loss of function—are present, the treatment is termed a failure. If additional antibiotic is administered for signs and symptoms related to the original bone infection, the treatment is also termed a failure. Once a case is termed a failure, it remains a failure despite response to subsequent treatment. The study is, then, a "single-treatment" study of surgery plus antibiotics. In comparing this study with others in the literature, be aware that most other reported results represent multiple-treatment (that is, multiple debridements and multiple antibiotics) therapy.

Five of eight participating centers have contributed to this preliminary report. A review of all cases at all centers will be necessary before a comprehensive report can be issued. For this reason, the data have not been collated into a single report but are presented as separate reports detailing the experience at each center.

Reports From Participating Centers

University of Arkansas

Twenty-two patients were entered into the study, 11 into the Septopal group (four hips, five tibias, and one infected knee) and 11 into the conventional treatment group (six hips, four femurs, and one tibia). Patients in the Septopal study group received gentamicin-polymethylmethacrylate beads after surgical debridement and closure of the wound over gravity drainage. Patients in the control group received intravenous antibiotics for a period of four to six weeks following debridement and closure over suction irrigation drains. Following the intravenous drug therapy, several patients received prolonged oral antibiotics. A few patients in both groups required a graft or muscle flap for coverage at the time of closure.

The patients were classified according to the Cierny-Mader clinical osteomyelitis stages (Table 1),[6] and all cases were classified as either III-A, III-B, IV-A, or IV-B. Causative organisms included *Staphylococcus aureus*, *Aerobacter cloacae*, *Staphylococcus epidermidis*, *Pseudomonas aeruginosa*, *Diphtheroid*, *Citrobacter*, *Escherichia coli*, and *Serratia*.

In the Septopal group, nine of the 11 patients (82%) were successful after an average follow-up of 30 months. The nine successful cases included four total hip arthroplasties, one total knee arthroplasty, one hip fusion, one femoral fracture, and two open tibias. The two failures were both open tibial fractures infected with *S aureus*.

In the control group, nine of 11 (82%) patients had no clinical evidence of infection after an average follow-up of 34 months. Infection sites for the nine successful cases included two total hips, one total knee, five femoral fractures, and one osteonecrosis of the femoral head. The two failures were hips infected with *S aureus*, one with a previous endoprosthesis and the other a total hip arthroplasty.

Table 1
Cierny-Mader staging system for adult osteomyelitis

Stages	Description
Anatomic type	
Type I	Medullary osteomyelitis
Type II	Superficial osteomyelitis
Type III	Localized osteomyelitis
Type IV	Diffuse osteomyelitis
Physiologic class	
A-host	Good immune system and delivery
B-host	Compromised locally (B^L) or systemically (B^S)
C-host	Requires suppressive or no treatment; minimal disability; treatment worse than disease; not a surgical candidate
Clinical stage	Type plus class

There were no known side effects with Septopal, although one complication occurred during removal of the beads. This patient had been treated with Septopal for an infection of the midfemoral fracture with *A cloacae*. When beads were removed three weeks later, *S aureus* was cultured from the wound. The patient was lost to follow-up until approximately four months later, when he returned with clinical symptoms of infection. The wound was packed open after being irrigated and debrided. The patient was treated with intravenous antibiotics for five days and then switched to oral antibiotics. His wound healed spontaneously by second intention. He has continued to do well over the past two years and is considered a success with the complication of reinfection at the time of bead removal. The average number of hospital days for the Septopal group was 15.3 days (range, seven to 37 days) vs 26.7 days (range, seven to 70 days) for patients given intravenous therapy.

In this center, the effectiveness of Septopal was comparable to that of traditional intravenous antibiotics. In addition, the patients who received the beads were pleased with the treatment and had no problem adapting to the therapy.

The University of Louisville

Forty-five patients with chronic osteomyelitis were randomly assigned under the Septopal investigational protocol; 22 patients were treated with Septopal and 23 patients were treated with conventional intravenous antibiotic therapy. There were 40 men and five women with a mean age of 41 years (range, 18 to 78 years) in the study. In 33 of 45 patients (73%), the tibia was the site of osteomyelitis; in six (13%), it was the femur, and in three (7%), the acetabulum. Osteomyelitis had been present an average of 6.4 years (range, one month to 45.3 years) before the initiation of therapy. Patients in the Septopal group had a longer duration of osteomyelitis (8.1 years vs 4.7 years) than the antibiotic group because of the randomization of several World War II veterans to the bead group.

Chronic osteomyelitis followed an open fracture in 30 patients, a postoperative infection in 13 patients, and was the result of hematogenous seeding in two patients. Fifty-six organisms were obtained from the exudates and deep surgical specimens of bone and soft tissue. *S aureus* was the organism most commonly isolated (18 patients). Twenty-six (46.4%) of the organisms isolated were gram-negative. Of these, *Pseudomonas*, *Serratia*, and *Proteus* were the most frequently isolated agents. Of interest was the frequency of cultures positive for *S epidermidis*. This organism was the sole isolate in five patients and cultured in mixed flora in five additional patients. In nine patients (20%) with positive Gram stains and with clinical and radiographic signs of chronic osteomyelitis no organisms were cultured. Twenty-three patients demonstrated one organism on culture, and 12 patients demonstrated multiple organisms.

Eighteen (82%) of the patients treated with Septopal antibiotic beads were in clinical remission, and 16 (70%) of the patients treated with intravenous antibiotics were successful. The mean follow-up period for Septopal was 45.6 weeks (range, six to 144 weeks); for conventional treatment it was 47.2 weeks (range, six to 148 weeks).

In this series, elderly and compromised patients who were not candidates for free-tissue transfer were managed successfully with an initial sequestrectomy and saucerization. Beads were then placed in the bone defect and, when clinically indicated, into the intramedullary canal. In most of these patients, marginal soft-tissue coverage was accomplished without the use of flap coverage. Once healed, removal of the beads created a greater soft-tissue risk to the patient than leaving the beads in situ. Ten patients with marginal soft-tissue coverage have retained chains of implanted beads and remain in clinical remission at a mean of 13.2 months after surgery (range, four to 32 months).

Adverse Experiences Complications were reported in two patients receiving systemic intravenous antibiotics. These two patients experienced rapid elevation of serum creatinine levels while receiving aminoglycoside antibiotics. With adjustment of the antimicrobial therapy, the patients' creatinine levels returned to normal and no permanent sequelae were reported. No complications were experienced in patients treated with the Septopal beads.

Costs Septopal patients averaged 27% fewer days of total hospitalization (mean, 30.4 days; range, three to 55 days) than did patients treated with intravenous antibiotics (mean 41.6 days; range, six to 87 days). Calculation of total medical expenses for each patient's therapeutic regime revealed that the average medical expense for patients treated with Septopal beads was $19,880 (range, $1,824 to $36,240). The medical expense for patients treated conventionally was 24% higher (average, $25,671.28; range, $10,152 to $59,157).

University of Pennsylvania

Thirty-seven patients, ten women and 27 men, were entered into the Septopal randomized investigation beginning in October 1985. Average age for the study population was 37 years. The most commonly involved bone was the tibia (23 patients, 62%), followed by the femur (ten patients, 27%), the humerus (three patients, 8%) and the metatarsal (one patient, 3%) The most frequently cultured organism was *S aureus*, followed by β-hemolytic *Streptococcus* and *Streptococcus fecalis*. Of the 37 patients, 27 have more than one year of follow-up: 14 in the Septopal group and 13 in the conventional antibiotic group. In this group, nine of 14 patients (64%) treated with Septopal have no signs or symptoms

of osteomyelitis and ten of 13 (77%) cases in the conventional group are quiescent.

Nine cases from the study have been considered failures. Four required more extensive debridement after entry into the study. We believe that treatment in these patients failed because of inadequate initial debridement. (Three of these patients were in the Septopal group, and one was in the conventional antibiotic group.) Two patients elected to have amputations as definitive treatment for recurrent signs and symptoms of osteomyelitis rather than undergo more extensive debridement. One was an above-knee amputation and one a below-knee. Both of these patients had been randomly assigned to conventional treatment. One patient whose symptoms recurred after reinjury proved to be an intravenous drug user with severe nutritional deficiency. This patient had been randomly assigned to the Septopal treatment group. One patient in whom treatment failed proved to be positive for the human immunodeficiency virus. Treatment failed in another despite repeated surgical attempts to gain soft-tissue coverage.

We believe these failures can be explained as resulting from inadequate debridement, preexisting disease that limited the host response to infection, inadequate soft-tissue cover, and loss of microvascular soft-tissue transfer. Success rates for patients randomly assigned to Septopal and conventional therapy were essentially the same.

Adverse Reactions Only one of the patients in this series had an adverse reaction to antimicrobial therapy. A patient randomly assigned to the conventional group had significant pruritus and diarrhea while being treated with nafcillin. There were no adverse reactions in the Septopal group.

Costs Hospitalization time was shorter for patients treated with Septopal, even though many patients in the conventional treatment group received part of their intravenous antibiotics at home. For the Septopal group, hospital days averaged 12.5 (range, three to 46 days). For the conventional antibiotic group, the average stay was 22 days (range, 11 to 52 days).

The University of Texas at Galveston

Seventy-eight patients were entered into the Septopal study beginning in April 1987. Control patients (39) were treated with debridement therapy and intravenous antibiotics for four to six weeks. The other 39 patients were treated with debridement, intravenous perioperative antibiotics, and Septopal.

Most of the patients (77%) were men; ages ranged from 22 to 87 years. Etiology was typically posttraumatic (58%) or postoperative (35%), and three cases each were paraplegic and hematogenous. The most common sites of infection were the tibia (53%) and the femur (30%). Four cases involved the ischium, three the fibula, two the radius, one the ulna, and one the humerus. Host compromise was common (53%) and most infections were nonunions or infected joints (stage IV) that are difficult to treat.

Microbiologic findings were similar to those in previous reports of chronic osteomyelitis.[7] Polymicrobial cultures were frequent (68%), and gram-positive bacteria were more common than gram-negative bacteria (89% vs 46%). *S epidermidis* was cultured most frequently (53%), followed by *S aureus* (32%) and *P aeruginosa* (24%). One fourth of the *S aureus* cultures were resistant to methicillin. Anaerobic cultures were positive in one fourth of the patients. Serum and seroma levels of gentamicin were measured in all Septopal patients. Serum levels were less than 1 to 2 μg. Seroma levels, between 110 and 200 μg initially, remained bacteriostatic for up to six weeks.

Thirty-seven patients have been followed up for longer than one year. The success rate was 79% for 19 Septopal patients and 67% for the 18 control patients. Patients followed up for less than one year had success rates of 86% for Septopal and 90% for conventional therapy. There was no statistical difference between the groups.

Failures occurred more frequently in stage IV osteomyelitis and in compromised patients. This is consistent with data published by Cierny and Mader.[8] Seven of the eight failures in this series have been successfully re-treated. Two of the other failures required amputation.

A number of the failures had early indications of problems with therapy. Eleven Septopal patients required more than five days of antibiotics for wound cellulitis, postoperative drainage, or muscle-flap problems. Seven of these patients went on to clinical failure. Further treatment of early failures with antibiotics or surgery may have led to a higher success rate.

Adverse Reactions and Costs No complications occurred. Patients benefited from not requiring long-term intravenous catheters or antibiotics and from lower medical costs.

West Virginia University

Twenty-four patients were enrolled in the Septopal randomized investigations beginning in June 1985. The most common problem (62%) was posttraumatic osteomyelitis of the tibia (58%). Other sites involved were the femur (22%), and one case each (4%) of the pelvis, humerus, knee, and ankle. Thirteen patients were randomly assigned to the control group and 11 patients to Septopal therapy. Most conventionally treated patients had oral therapy for a variable time after the four to six weeks of intravenous therapy.

Classification of patients using the Cierny-Mader clinical osteomyelitis stages showed that 19 of 24 patients (79.2%) fell into stages III and IV and that seven patients (29.2%) were classified as compromised hosts. The distribution of patients according to the osteomyelitis stage was approximately equal between the conventional and Septopal groups.

Infection with more than one organism was frequent (63%), with 22 of 24 patients having gram-positive organisms and 13 of 24 having gram-negative organisms. *S aureus* was present in 25% of the isolates, *S fecalis* in 14%, other *Streptococcus* species in 12%, *Pseudomonas* in 9%, and *Aspergillus* in 2% (one case).

Of the 11 patients in the Septopal group, three were treated with free vascularized tissue transfer and two patients were treated with conventional antibiotics in addition to the Septopal therapy for diagnoses not related to the original osteomyelitis (one for urinary-tract infection, one for pin-tract infection). Five patients had additional antibiotics for problems possibly related to the original osteomyelitis (two for positive culture at second reconstructive surgery, two for redness or swelling at the osteomyelitis site without drainage, and one to treat a significant anaerobic infection). Treatment failed in six patients according to the strict definitions of the protocol.

The first patient could not tolerate gradual extraction of Septopal chains, as recommended by Klemm,[4] and had to have the chains totally removed at day 7 after surgery. The wound spontaneously drained 14 days after surgery and the patient was treated with six weeks of intravenous antibiotics without further debridement. He is without evidence of ostoeomyelitis at 43 months after initial debridement.

The second patient had a positive culture for *S aureus*, presumably the same as the initial organism, at the time of major joint reconstruction six months after initial debridement. This patient was treated with six weeks of intravenous antibiotics following the second surgery because of the extent of reconstruction (total hip-femur-knee) and the potential consequences of infection.

The third patient, although without evidence of active infection at five days, had grown a significant number of anaerobes (*Fusobacterium* and *Bacteroides*) and was treated with parenteral ampicillin and clindamycin for six weeks. The Septopal chains were removed after eight days and the patient remains symptom-free at 26 months after debridement.

The fourth patient had a segmental fracture associated with significant soft-tissue and vascular injury. An attempt was made to preserve bone for future reconstruction and, in retrospect, it was apparent that inadequate debridement had been done. This patient had spontaneous drainage at 26 weeks after the initial surgery with culture positive for *S aureus* and *Serratia*—the same as the initial organisms.

The fifth patient had poor soft-tissue cover over a debrided tibia. Because of a positive culture when the beads were removed, this patient was treated for 2.5

weeks with oral antibiotics. At nine months after debridement, the osteomyelitis site drained with culture positive for *S aureus*, one of the organisms originally cultured from the site. Redebridement and free vascularized tissue transfer was apparently successful, and the patient remained symptom-free 14 months after the second debridement.

The sixth patient was symptom-free for 13 months following debridement of an infected tibial pin tract that was positive for *S aureus*. Because of intermittent symptoms of redness and pain, this patient had three courses of oral antibiotics, at 13 months, 24 months, and 37 months after initial debridement surgery. Aspiration of the site revealed no fluid or positive culture. Finally, because of increasing symptoms, redebridement was done at the site of infection. Cultures taken at the second debridement grew only *S epidermidis*.

Of the 13 patients in the conventional antibiotic group, four were treated with free vascularized tissue transfer. Follow-up in this group ranged from one to 190 weeks. All patients in the conventional group have been successful according to the criteria of this study. One patient died of preexisting carcinoma.

These results indicate 100% success wih the conventional treatment and 45% success with Septopal. If, as has been done in other studies, we considered the reappearance of drainage or the requirement for redebridement as indicators of failure, our Septopal success rate would be eight of 11 (73%). At our institution, we have probably overtreated positive cultures and have possibly treated symptoms not necessarily related to osteomyelitis with antibiotics for fear of undertreating an infection. All patients in the Septopal group in whom treatment failed are now symptom-free, with three having required a second debridement for signs and symptoms of infection.

Adverse Experiences At our site, there were 19 adverse experiences related to the use of parenteral antibiotics (six liver-function abnormalities, five cases of leukopenia, three renal-function abnormalities, two cases of pruritus and rash, two gastrointestinal upsets, and one auditory abnormality). There were no permanent sequelae to these problems, many of which were considered to be usual problems encountered with modern antibiotics. Only one adverse experience was related to the use of Septopal chains, in the patient who could not tolerate gradual extraction.

Cost For patients in the conventional group, the average cost of treatment (including inpatient and outpatient treatment) was $37,394.00 with a hospitalization time of 23 days. For patients who had both Septopal and parenteral antibiotics, the treatment cost was $39,307.20 with 25 days of hospitalization. For patients who completed the Septopal treatment without requiring additional antibiotics, the average cost was $24,536.00 with 16 days of hospitalization.

General Discussion

The Septopal study is an ongoing study that compares single-treatment, conventional intravenous antibiotic therapy to single treatment with Septopal beads. On the basis of preliminary data, the results in the two groups are equivalent. Failures have been related to the extent of infection, inadequate debridement, and host factors. Most failures responded to further treatment. Permanent implantation of Septopal beads remains controversial among the Septopal investigators. In those patients with extended placement of beads, no side effects or complications have been reported.

There are significant potential advantages to Septopal over conventional antibiotics. A primary advantage of beads is the release of high levels of antibiotics into the local wound environment. This action is independent of vascular supply or soft-tissue compromise. Implanted beads treatment is less dependent on patient compliance than is conventional intravenous therapy. On the basis of the adverse experience reports, we are encouraged that the Septopal chains will prove safer than parenteral antibiotics. However, use of the Septopal beads may be limited by the sensitivity of the microorganisms to gentamicin. In addition, the patient should also be advised that bead removal can be painful and may require an additional hospitalization and surgical procedure.

Septopal is presently not available for sale in the United States. A number of reports in the literature and at various meetings have dealt with "homemade" antibiotic beads containing various antibiotics. It is not within the scope of this presentation to comment on the results of the use of homemade beads or to make recommendations in that regard. When enough patients have been followed up in this randomized study, overall recommendations about the local use of Septopal and, perhaps by inference, antibiotic-impregnated polymethylmethacrylate beads in general can be made.

General Conclusion

Septopal antibiotic beads are a therapeutic alternative in the management of chronic osteomyelitis. Continued monitoring of the preliminary results of the Septopal protocol will be necessary to determine the clinical significance of Septopal antibiotic beads with longer periods of follow-up.

In the new world of medicine, where cost-effectiveness of new treatments will be of considerable importance, Septopal may show its most significant benefit in reducing the cost and number of hospital days for the treatment of osteomyelitis.

References

1. Pickett JC: A short historical sketch of osteomyelitis. *Ann Med Hist NS* 1935;7:183.
2. Jenny G, Kempf J, Jaeger JH, et al: Utilisation de billes de ciment acrylique a la gentamycine dans le traitement de l'infection osseuse. *Rev Chir Orthop* 1977;63:491.
3. Buchholz HW, Elson RA, Engelbrecht E, et al: Management of deep infection of total hip replacement. *J Bone Joint Surg* 1981; 63B:342–353.
4. Klemm K: Clinical experience with Septopal chains in West Germany, in Smith TWD (ed): *Treatment of Chronic Bone Infections With Septopal.* Proceedings of a Symposium. Ed: BDH Pharmaceuticals Ltd., Lenten House, Alton Hants, p 21.
5. Walenkamp GHIM: *Gentamicin-PMMA Beads.* Darmstadt, E Merck, 1983.
6. Cierny G III, Mader HT, Panninck JJ: A clinical staffing system for adult osteomyelitis. *Contemp Orthop* 1985;10:17–37.
7. Fitzgerald RH Jr, Hughes SPF (eds): *Musculoskeletal Infections.* Chicago, Year Book Medical Publishers, 1986.
8. Cierny G III, Mader JT: Management of adult osteomyelitis. Surgery of the musculoskeletal system. *Orthop Clin North Am* 1983; 10:15–35.

Spinal Infections

Thomas W. McNeill, MD

Pyogenic Osteomyelitis of the Spine

History and Epidemiology

Although some aspects of the natural history of spinal infection have been known since antiquity, the modern era began in the 19th century. In 1879, Lannelongue first distinguished pyogenic osteomyelitis of the spine from tuberculosis.[1] A year later, Pasteur described the bacterial etiology of pyogenic osteomyelitis.[2] It was not until 1933 that Smith[3] described the benign nature of childhood diskitis.

The natural history of pyogenic osteomyelitis of the spine has changed during the present century. In 1929, Steindler described the disease as one primarily of children, but now the disease more often affects adults.[4] In Kulowski's[5] series of 102 cases, published in 1936, most of the patients were adults with an average age of 31 years; however, the largest cluster of patients were those in their second decade. The majority of the spine infections came from superficial skin lesions or from pneumonia. Then, as now, the infection involved the vertebral bodies, was more common in the lumbar vertebrae than in the thoracic or cervical spine, and had a male-to-female ratio of two to one.

In 1971, Griffiths and Jones[6] presented a series of 28 patients, of whom 15 were more than 50 years of age. Where it could be determined, the source in more than half (six of 11) was from the genitourinary system. Now, in adults, this has become a disease of older men[7,8] and the trend continues that the infection is often secondary to genitourinary manipulation or sepsis, and intravenous drug use.[9] Many of the patients today are diabetic. Digby and Kersley[10] estimated that their cases "represented an approximate annual incidence of one in 250,000 of the population."

In the past, there was a high mortality rate from pyogenic osteomyelitis of the spine (25% in Kulowski's[5] series), and when the infection involved the central nervous system it exceeded 50%. Ten percent of Griffiths and Jones'[6] patients died. The mortality rate continues to fall because of improved antibiotic therapy. Before the antibiotic era (approximately 1944), reported cases of pyogenic osteomyelitis were often those of an acute fulminant disease with the subacute and chronic varieties being less commonly reported. In recent years the subacute variety seems to have become more common,[11] with early healing often being observed at the time of diagnosis. The subacute variety of the disease

may be confused with tuberculosis even though the offending organism is actually *Staphylococcus*.

Hematogenous pyogenic osteomyelitis in children is usually a disease of long bones,[2,12,13] but when it does occur in the spine of children, it remains a very serious disease.[14] After the first year of age, osteomyelitis of the spine is usually caused by *Staphylococcus aureus*. In neonates the offending organism more often is group B β-hemolytic streptococci introduced during delivery.[15] Streptococci continue to be the dominant organisms up to 1 year of age.

Pathophysiology and Pathology

Bacteria enter the bone in both adult and childhood osteomyelitis through the nutrient artery.[16] Batson's[17] venous plexus has been shown to be a route for the spread of prostate carcinoma to the vertebrae. This route has been assumed to be the source of spinal infection related to the genitourinary tract; however, because the pressure gradient in the venous blood is greater in the vertebrae than in the venous system, Batson's plexus is not the probable route of spread of pelvic infection to the vertebrae. Furthermore, experimental production of vertebral infection by the venous route has not been achieved.[18]

The vertebral body appears to be the primary site in the vast majority of cases of pyogenic vertebral osteomyelitis.[5,6,8,19] Kemp and associates[20] argued that the disk may be the primary site of seeding in pyogenic vertebral osteomyelitis. This is probably not the case except in children, or when pathologic neovascularization has occurred.[2,10,21] Coventry and associates[22] confirmed earlier findings that the blood supply to the intervertebral disk is gradually obliterated during childhood and is absent by the third decade. The initial site of seeding is probably the capillary end loop of vessels in the bone adjacent to the end plate,[23] and the disks are involved only secondarily.[4] In staphylococcal osteomyelitis, the disk space narrowing results in bacterial enzyme action, causing chondrolysis of the disk. A few cases associated with an epidural abscess have involved the posterior elements, the facet joints, and an area of spondylolysis.[24,25] Pyogenic osteomyelitis has also been reported as a complication of a closed compression fracture[26] and as a complication of spinal tumors.[27]

Bacteriology

S aureus remains the organism most commonly found in adult patients. This organism accounts for approximately 50% of the cases in Digby and Kersley's[10] patients and about 60% in those reported by Waldvogel and Papageorgiou.[13] Following *S aureus* in incidence is *Escherichia coli, Proteus, Streptococcus,* and *Pseudomonas,*[28] with occasional cases of *Salmonella,*[29] *Aspergilla, Haemophilus,*[30] and *Brucella.*[31] Intravenous drug users have *Pseudomonas* more often than other patient groups.[7]

Clinical Features

Kulowski[5] described three types of clinical presentations for pyogenic vertebral osteomyelitis: acute, subacute, and chronic. In the acute form, the disease can be fulminant and has a sudden onset, with fever, chills, and signs of septicemia. More often, however, the disease is subacute.[4,6,10,11] In the subacute form, the onset is insidious. There may have been a febrile episode as a prodromal event. Back pain that is not relieved by rest is a constant feature of pyogenic osteomyelitis of the spine. The back pain may be so severe that any activity causes severe spasm and increased pain; more often, the pain is moderate, but it rarely abates completely. Digby and Kersley[10] did not describe local tenderness in their patients. It has been my experience that local tenderness and spasm are universally present. Radicular findings and deformity are more often late features of the disease. Kyphosis is the typical deformity,[32] but scoliosis may also be present.

Investigations

Acutely the patient may have a high fever; later in the disease, fever may be absent or low grade. The leukocyte count is often normal or slightly elevated; however, the erythrocyte sedimentation rate is consistently elevated.[11] Blood cultures may be positive early in the illness. Mid-stream urine cultures may yield the offending organism. Digby and Kersley[10] had difficulty with needle biopsy and obtained a positive culture in only one of the four cases attempted. My associates have attempted needle biopsy or open biopsy in every case in which blood cultures were negative. In 1985 my colleagues and I reported our first 16 cases of presumed diskitis.[33] In these cases, cultures were positive in 13 patients and sterile in three. More recent, but untabulated, experience in our institution leads me to believe that the correct percentage of positive cultures in patients with radiographic and clinical findings of diskitis is closer to 50%. Kirkaldy-Willis and Thomas[34] recommended an anterior approach for diagnosis and treatment of all cases of spinal infection. Their argument was that other infections could mimic tuberculosis and that adequate treatment could not be designed without cultures and sensitivities. This principle still applies in many instances.

Various imaging techniques provide valuable information in treating patients with vertebral osteomyelitis. Because the yield from an attempted culture may be 50% or less, it may be necessary to provide treatment empirically, based on a radiographic and clinical diagnosis.

Plain radiographs demonstrate changes approximately ten days after the onset of the illness. Roentgenograms of spinal infections are not comparable to those of osteomyelitis in other bones. Disk-space narrowing, which may resemble degenerative disk disease,[10] will be the first sign (Fig. 1). Following this stage, radiographs demonstrate destruction of the bone adjacent to the disk. This can range from minimal to severe destruction and significant deformity (Fig. 2). Swelling of the adjacent soft tissues is often an associated feature (Fig. 3). Later changes include osteopenia of adjacent bone, new bone formation, and even fusion. In the diagnosis of vertebral osteomyelitis, radiographs have an accuracy of about 73%, with a sensitivity of 82% and a specificity of 57%.[35] Computed tomography is also capable of demonstrating the changes of infection and may help differentiate an infectious process from similar radiographic changes seen with tumors (Fig. 4).[36] Radiographic changes that have been confused with those of osteomyelitis or diskitis include tumor,[37] Char-

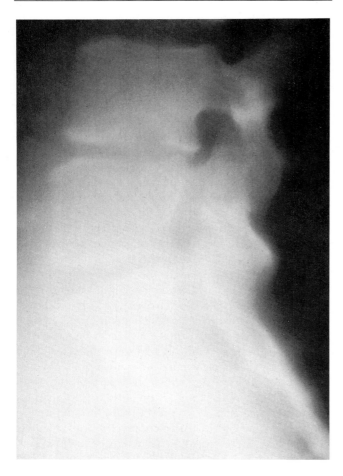

Fig. 1 Vertebral pyogenic osteomyelitis. Lateral tomographic views showing early disk narrowing and defect in the vertebral bodies on either side of the disk.

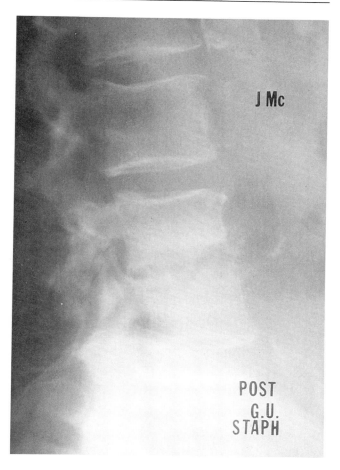

Fig. 2 Vertebral pyogenic osteomyelitis. Plain radiographic views showing moderately severe destruction of two vertebral bodies and the adjacent disk. Organism was *S aureus* and was secondary to genitourinary manipulation in an 80-year-old man.

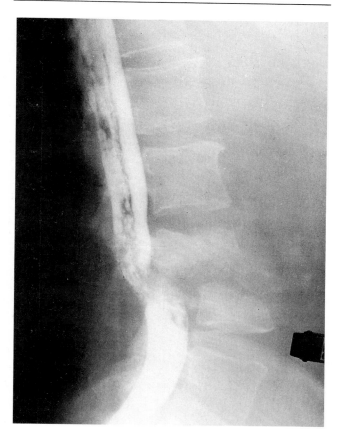

Fig. 3 Vertebral pyogenic osteomyelitis. Myelogram in patient with severe deformity and cauda equina syndrome.

cot spine, and spinal pseudarthrosis.[38] Gout[39] and pseudogout[40] may also bear a superficial resemblance to infectious diseases of the vertebra.

Radioisotope scanning of the spine is valuable in the diagnosis and follow-up assessment of vertebral osteomyelitis. Technetium phosphate bone scans are more sensitive and more accurate than plain radiographs in the early diagnosis of a spinal infection. The accuracy of technetium bone scans in the diagnosis of spinal infection was estimated by Tom and Power[35] to be 86% vs 73% for plain radiographs. Furthermore, technetium bone scans are more sensitive than plain radiographs (90% vs 82%) in arriving at the initial diagnosis of spinal infection. Combined gallium and technetium bone scan improves the accuracy to 94%. Ouzounian and associates[41] stated that indium-111 leukocyte imaging is quite specific for musculoskeletal sepsis with false-positive results seen only in rheumatoid arthritis and fractures and in the immediate postoperative period. My experience with this technique is limited.

Although magnetic resonance imaging has a reported accuracy of 94% in vertebral osteomyelitis,[35] this level of accuracy has not been maintained in my experience. In pyogenic vertebral osteomyelitis, T_1-weighted images (Fig. 5) should show a decreased signal from the vertebral body on either side of the disk and loss of the signal from the disk. The T_2-weighted images should demonstrate a bright signal from the vertebral bodies with the intervening disk being distorted and showing an abnormal signal.[35]

Treatment

The treatment of vertebral pyogenic osteomyelitis has five general categories: initial biopsy for precise bacterial diagnosis, emergency surgery for epidural abscess when present, bed rest and antibiotics, surgery for drainage of other abscesses, and surgical treatment of late spinal deformity.

The biopsy technique depends on the location. The preferred method in the lumbar spine uses a Craig needle (trephine biopsy) with associated needle aspiration. In the thoracic spine, thoracotomy or costotransversectomy are direct and effective methods. In a few instances, I have been able to perform a thoracic

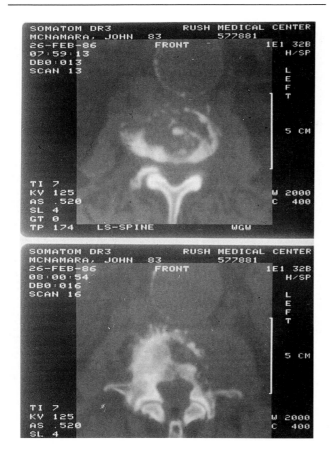

Fig. 4 Vertebral pyogenic osteomyelitis. Computed tomography demonstrating severe destruction of bone and disk in same case shown in Figure 2.

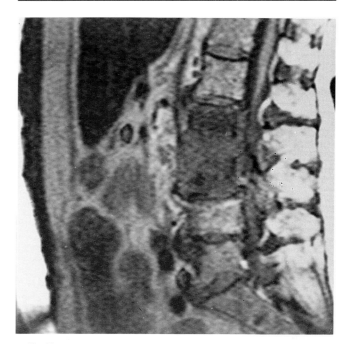

Fig. 5 Vertebral pyogenic osteomyelitis. Magnetic resonance imaging T_1-weighted image showing loss of signal from the vertebral bodies and intervening disk.

biopsy using a transpedicular approach. In the cervical spine, an anterior approach either with a needle or formal open biopsy is simple and direct.

An epidural abscess, as a complication of vertebral osteomyelitis, constitutes a surgical emergency[42] because permanent neurologic injury will result if it is neglected. This most often appears to be related to involvement of the posterior elements.[24,25]

The mainstay of treatment remains bed rest until the acute pain subsides and intensive antibiotic therapy for four to six weeks. Treatment need not require prolonged hospitalization. A Hickman catheter provides an easy means of delivering antibiotic therapy at home,[43] and a custom-molded spinal orthosis can provide adequate support after the acutely painful period has passed. I continue brace treatment for six months or until fusion has taken place. Late treatment of deformity or painful instability may become necessary in a small minority of cases of pyogenic osteomyelitis.[32,42]

Diskitis

Since the first description of diskitis in childhood, researchers[44,45] have debated whether or not this disease is of bacterial origin. Hensinger argued that diskitis of childhood is caused by bacterial infection because, with the exception of inoculation, it only occurs at ages when vessels enter the disk.[46] Fraser and associates,[47] by injecting a very few viable *Staphylococcus epidermidis* organisms, demonstrated an experimental diskitis that is identical to the clinical disease. In this experiment, viable organisms could not be recovered after three months. Furthermore, the syndrome is clinically typical of infection, both direct cultures and blood cultures[48] have been obtained from patients with diskitis, and paravertebral abscesses have occurred in patients with diskitis.

The clinical features of diskitis of childhood are somewhat age-dependent. The younger child may refuse to stand, walk, or sit. In the older child,[45,49] nonspecific complaints and clinical findings may also be a problem. Hip pain and abdominal pain with or without back pain may be present. Constitutional symptoms, such as fever, restlessness, nausea, and vomiting, are less common. In most series, boys slightly outnumber girls. The mean age is about 7.5 years with the range from toddlers to teenagers.[48]

In adults, diskitis is usually secondary to direct inoculation during disk surgery or other invasive procedures into or adjacent to the disk.[47,50-53] In Lindholm and Pylkkänen's[52] series, the incidence of diskitis following surgery was 0.75%, approximately the same as that for surgical infection in general. In Pilgaard's[54] series, the rate was 2.8%. However, the incidence following chemonucleolysis can be as high as 3.2%.[47] Although Fraser and associates[47] classified many episodes as chemical diskitis, a bacterial etiology has generally been accepted since that time.

In Lindholm and Pylkkänen's[52] surgical patients, the onset of the disease was 35 days with a range from one day to one year. In Pilgaard's[54] series, all patients had symptoms beginning two to 28 days after surgery. The typical history includes initial relief of the preoperative sciatica, followed by recurrence within one month after surgery of low back pain and sciatica. Because the pain is severe and out of proportion to the findings, the patients are often thought to be hysterical.[54] Adults may also complain of pelvic pain.[52] The diagnosis of diskitis in adults, whether it is primary or secondary, is often difficult because the symptoms may be nonspecific and the onset insidious. Diagnostic delay is the rule rather than the exception and averaged 14 weeks in one series.[55]

A *de novo* diskitis may occur in adults, but this is uncommon and probably occurs when neovascularization is present secondary to injury or degenerative changes. McCain and associates[55] presented convincing evidence of primary disk-space infection in 12 of 15 patients with a variety of medical and preexisting spinal diseases. I have seen only one such case, which was caused by *Candida albicans* in an immunocompromised host. Holmes and associates[56] described two cases of *Aspergillus* diskitis in immunocompromised adult hosts, but on review I believe that these patients had osteomyelitis rather than diskitis.

Investigations

Positive identification of the bacterial agent is difficult in both adults and children. When positive cultures have been obtained in postdiskectomy diskitis, *S aureus* was the organism most often found. In the majority of my recent patients, suspected diskitis followed diskography or chemonucleolysis. Despite concerted efforts to obtain direct cultures, the yield has been less than 50%. Where an organism was found, it was often one of low-grade pathogenicity, such as *S epidermidis* or *Propionibacterium acne*. In children the erythrocyte sedimentation rate is consistently elevated.[48] In adults an elevated erythrocyte sedimentation rate is routinely present initially, but the percentage of abnormal results for this test decreases with time.[53]

Following laminectomy, most patients with diskitis will have fever[54] and an elevated leukocyte count.[53] In both adults and children the *sine qua non* of diskitis remains the radiographic changes of disk-space narrowing with end-plate erosions. These changes are best seen on tomography of either the standard or computed type (Fig. 6).

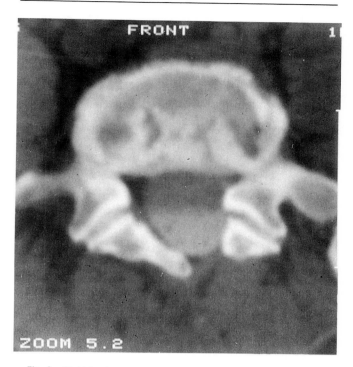

Fig. 6   Diskitis. Computed tomography showing typical end-plate erosions.

Technetium

Technetium bone scanning is almost always positive in children[48,57] and may give the diagnosis even before the radiographs show diagnostic changes, but in adult patients the bone scan may not be diagnostic.[58]

Magnetic resonance imaging as a diagnostic tool in diskitis has been studied in a rabbit model.[59] Magnetic resonance imaging was found to be more sensitive than bone scanning or radiographs in the diagnosis of experimental diskitis. Both false-negative and false-positive results occurred but were unusual. The imaging changes demonstrated a decreased signal from the disk and an increased signal from the adjacent end plate (Fig. 7). Schmorl[60] subscribed to the idea that the diskitis may start in the end plate and extend from there to the disk. Gabriel and Crawford[61] present a case of "diskitis" in a child in whom they detected imaging changes more like those of vertebral osteomyelitis. This case led them to the conclusion that "the results of this scan substantially support the opinion that diskitis in a child is vertebral osteomyelitis with involvement of a disk." This may be correct, but I would recommend caution in any attempt to extrapolate from one case to general principles relating to all cases, especially with an entirely new technology such as magnetic resonance imaging. Furthermore, vertebral osteomyelitis and diskitis should be considered distinct clinical entities from the point of view of care and prognosis (Fig. 8).[44,62]

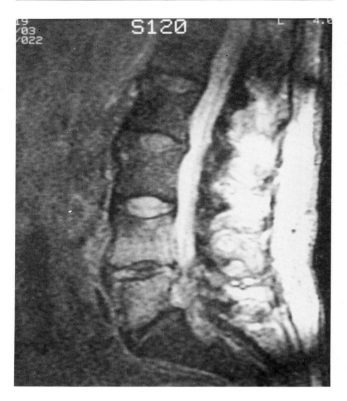

Fig. 7 Diskitis. Magnetic resonance imaging T$_2$-weighted image showing some increased signal from adjacent vertebral bodies and loss of signal from involved disk.

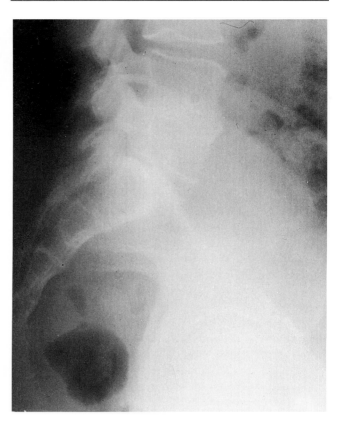

Fig. 8 Diskitis. Fusion following diskitis. (Reproduced with permission from Andersson GBJ, McNeill TW, in *Lumbar Spine Syndromes: Evaluation and Treatment*. New York, Springer-Verlag, 1989.)

Treatment

Before the antibiotic era, children with diskitis were treated with bed rest, Bradford frame, or double hip spica with successful resolution of the symptoms in most instances. Some authors[44,49] have suggested that this treatment is still appropriate in most instances. Except when there were positive cultures, Spiegel and associates[45] found no difference in the resolution of the acute symptoms between those treated with antibiotics and those who were not. Wegner and associates[48] recommended the use of antibiotics in these patients, and the use of a brace if the symptoms warrant.

In adult, postlaminectomy diskitis, Fernand and Lee[53] recommended bed rest followed by an ambulatory body jacket with the addition of antibiotics only if there was a positive culture or if the course was clearly septic. I have been more aggressive recently and have given six weeks of antibiotics in all cases in which there was clinical and radiographic evidence of diskitis, even in the absence of bacterial confirmation of continuing infection. The added value of this aggressive posture is as yet unproven.

In some instances the loss of disk height may be sufficient to result in symptomatic neuroforamenal stenosis, which may require surgical decompression (Fig. 9). Surgical fusion is also required in a minority of cases for persistent mechanical pain.

Granulomatous Infection of the Spine

Tuberculosis

On Jan 3, 1988, the *New York Times* reported a "substantial increase in tuberculosis in the United States for 1986," an increase due, at least in part, to acquired immune deficiency syndrome (AIDS). This was the first increase in three decades except for 1980 when a large number of infected refugees arrived from Southeast Asia. Until the recent reversal, the incidence of spinal tuberculosis had been decreasing in western Europe and the United States during the entire past century.[63] Infection with *Mycobacterium tuberculosis* is usually an infection of the lung (90%), but the second most common site of involvement is the spine. By contrast, atypical mycobacterial infections of the bones and joints seldom involve the spine.[64] Any level of the spine may be involved, but the greatest number of cases are clustered in the lower thoracic spine and upper lumbar

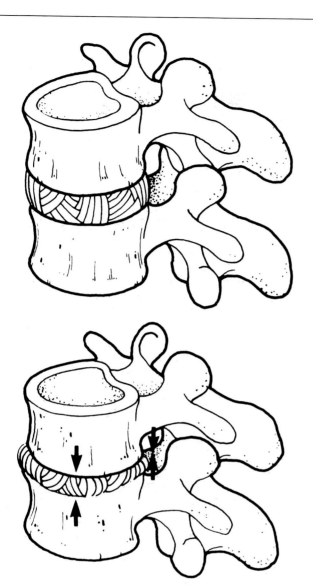

Fig. 9   Diskitis. Loss of disk height resulting in secondary stenosis of the neuroforamen. (Reproduced with permission from Andersson GBJ, McNeill TW, in *Lumbar Spine Syndromes: Evaluation and Treatment.* New York, Springer-Verlag, 1989.)

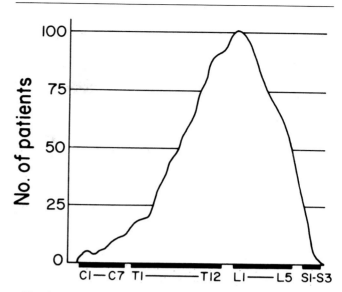

Fig. 10   Tuberculosis of the spine. Graph illustrating the incidence of vertebral tuberculosis by level. (Reproduced with permission form Andersson GBJ, McNeill TW, in *Lumbar Spine Syndromes: Evaluation and Treatment.* New York, Springer-Verlag, 1989.)

spine (Fig. 10). The vertebral body is typically affected,[60] while the posterior elements rarely are involved. Postacchini and Montanaro[65] reported one case of a tuberculous granuloma simulating a herniated intervertebral disk. In Hong Kong, the age distribution of spinal tuberculosis is skewed toward childhood and adolescence.[66] In the United States and Great Britain, the average age is above 35 years.[63]

Clinical findings that should lead one to suspect tuberculosis are weight loss, night sweats, painful spinal deformity, swelling in the groin, thigh, or flank, pain, family history of tuberculosis, AIDS-related complex, and origin from endemic regions.

Investigations

Tuberculosis of the spine develops slowly and can resemble other diseases. The diagnosis may be difficult because the disease is rare in western Europe and the United States and because screening tests may be negative. A skin test may be normal in 14% of cases, a bone scan is negative in 35%, a gallium scan is normal in 70%, and patients with normal radiographs may nonetheless have neurologic changes.[63,67] Radiographic changes observed with spinal tuberculosis include destruction of the vertebrae on either side of the disk (the disease most often begins adjacent to the end plate), central destruction of the vertebral body, anterior scalloping, paravertebral abscess, osteopenia, and kyphosis.[60] Late findings include block vertebra, elongated vertebra, and fixed kyphosis, which may appear to be congenital. Computed tomography and magnetic resonance imaging will accurately demonstrate the extent of the bony loss and the paravertebral abscess.[68] Magnetic resonance imaging also shows involvement of the spinal canal and neural elements (Fig. 11).

Blastomycosis

Blastomyces dermatitidis has been called "Chicago disease," because the early studies and reports came from Cook County Hospital and Rush Medical College[69]; however, the disease occurs in many parts of the world.[64] The primary source of the infection is soil, and most infected persons have worked as gardeners or farmers.

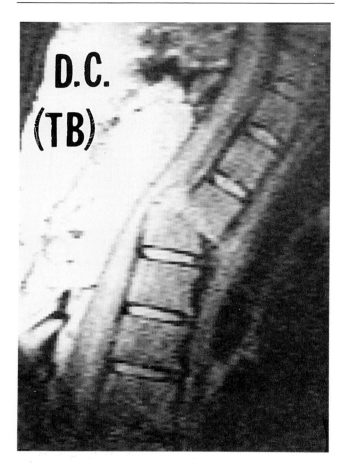

Fig. 11 Tuberculosis of the spine. Magnetic resonance imaging demonstrating the involvement of the spinal cord by tuberculous abscess with significant bony destruction and early kyphosis.

Like tuberculosis, blastomycosis is usually a pulmonary disease; however, the bones and joints may be involved, and, as in tuberculosis, the vertebrae are the bones most commonly involved. The radiographic appearance of the vertebral involvement resembles that in tuberculosis except when the ribs are also involved, a situation that is rare in tuberculosis.[69]

Cryptococcosis

Cryptococcus neoformans infection is most often a complication of another disease, such as sarcoidosis, leukemia, steroid treatment, and Hodgkin's disease.[70,71] The lung and central nervous system are most frequently involved. When the skeleton is involved, there is often a long delay in diagnosis. The patients usually are not febrile. In most cases, the only complaint is local pain and swelling. About 45% of the skeletal cases involve the vertebrae. The lesions produce lytic changes, with some surrounding sclerosis. A bone scan may be negative.

Coccidioidomycosis

Infection with *Coccidioides immitis* is endemic in the southwestern United States, Mexico, and South America.[72] The disease, when it involves the spine, has a striking resemblance to tuberculosis both clinically and radiographically. Blacks and immunocompromised hosts have an increased susceptibility.[73]

Other Granulomatous Diseases

Actinomyces israelii, Arachnia propionica, Sporothrix schenckii, Brucella abortus, and *Candida albicans* may all produce chronic granulomatous infection of the musculoskeletal system.[56,62,64] Infection with any of these agents may result in a clinical course and radiographic appearance resembling tuberculosis.

Treatment of Granulomatous Spinal Infection

The treatment of granulomatous infection of the spine follows the same general plan outlined for vertebral osteomyelitis. The Medical Research Council[74,75] recommends surgical debridement "when appropriate facilities and enough hospital beds are available, together with experienced spinal surgeons. . . ." Kirkaldy-Willis and Thomas[34] rightly pointed out that biopsy for diagnosis is essential, whether treatment is to be surgical or with chemotherapy alone. There do not appear to be any important differences between the treatment of fungal infections and tuberculosis except for the choice of the appropriate antibiotic. Surgical debridement, anterior grafting, and correction of late deformity are equally effective whatever the organism.

References

1. Steindler A: *Diseases and Deformities of the Spine and Thorax.* St. Louis, CV Mosby, 1929.
2. Gillespie WJ, Nade S: *Musculoskeletal Infections.* Melbourne, Blackwell Scientific Publications, 1987, pp 1–28, 213–247.
3. Smith AD: A benign form of osteomyelitis of the spine. *JAMA* 1933;101:335–337.
4. Stauffer RN: Pyogenic vertebral osteomyelitis. *Orthop Clin North Am* 1975;6:1015–1027.
5. Kulowski J: Pyogenic osteomyelitis of the spine: An analysis and discussion of 102 cases. *J Bone Joint Surg* 1936;18:343–364.
6. Griffiths HED, Jones DM: Pyogenic infection of the spine: A review of twenty-eight cases. *J Bone Joint Surg* 1971;53B:383–391.
7. Sapico FL, Montgomerie JZ: Pyogenic vertebral osteomyelitis: Report of nine cases and review of the literature. *Rev Infect Dis* 1979;1:754–776.
8. Garcia A Jr, Grantham SA: Hematogenous pyogenic vertebral osteomyelitis. *J Bone Joint Surg* 1960;42A:429–436.
9. Chan KM, Leung PC, Lee SY, et al: Pyogenic osteomyelitis of the spine: A review of 16 consecutive cases. *J Spinal Disorders* 1988;1:224–231.
10. Digby JM, Kersley JB: Pyogenic non-tuberculous spinal infection: An analysis of thirty cases. *J Bone Joint Surg* 1979;61B:47–55.

11. Harris NH, Kirkaldy-Willis WH: Primary subacute pyogenic osteomyelitis. *J Bone Joint Surg* 1965;47B:526–532.

12. Waldvogel FA, Medoff G, Swartz MN: Osteomyelitis: A review of clinical features, therapeutic considerations and unusual aspects [three parts]. *N Engl J Med* 1970;282:198–206,260–266,316–322.

13. Waldvogel FA, Papageorgiou PS: Osteomyelitis: The past decade. *N Engl J Med* 1980;303:360–370.

14. Eismont FJ, Bohlman HH, Soni PL, et al: Pyogenic and fungal vertebral osteomyelitis with paralysis. *J Bone Joint Surg* 1983;65A:19–29.

15. Baxter MP, Finnegan MA: Skeletal infection by group B beta-haemolytic streptococci in neonates: A case report and review of the literature. *J Bone Joint Surg* 1988;70B:812–814.

16. Trueta J: The three types of acute haematogenous osteomyelitis: A clinical and vascular study. *J Bone Joint Surg* 1959;41B:671–680.

17. Batson OV: The function of the vertebral veins and their role in the spread of metastases. *Ann Surg* 1940;112:138–149.

18. Wiley AM, Trueta J: The vascular anatomy of the spine and its relationship to pyogenic vertebral osteomyelitis. *J Bone Joint Surg* 1959;41B:796–809.

19. Puig Guri J: Pyogenic osteomyelitis of the spine: Differential diagnosis through clinical and roentgenographic observations. *J Bone Joint Surg* 1946;28:29–39.

20. Kemp HBS, Jackson JW, Jeremiah JD, et al: Pyogenic infections occurring primarily in intervertebral discs. *J Bone Joint Surg* 1973;55B:698–714.

21. Ratcliffe JF: Anatomic basis for the pathogenesis and radiologic features of vertebral osteomyelitis and its differentiation from childhood discitis: A microarteriographic investigation. *Acta Radiol [Diagn]* 1985;26:137–143.

22. Coventry MB, Ghormley RK, Kernohan JW: The intervertebral disc: Its microscopic anatomy and pathology. Part I. Anatomy, development, and physiology. *J Bone Joint Surg* 1945;27:105–112.

23. Crock HV: *Practice of Spinal Surgery*. Vienna, Springer-Verlag, 1983, pp 223–241.

24. Roberts WA: Pyogenic vertebral osteomyelitis of a lumbar facet joint with associated epidural abscess: A case report with review of the literature. *Spine* 1988;13:948–952.

25. Yu L, Emans JB: Epidural abscess associated with spondylolysis: A case report. *J Bone Joint Surg* 1988;70A:444–447.

26. Fellmeth BD, Da Silva RM, Spengler DM: Hematogenous osteomyelitis complicating a closed compression fracture of the spine. *J Spinal Disorders* 1988;1:168–171.

27. Eismont FJ, Green BA, Brown MD, et al: Coexistent infection and tumor of the spine: A report of three cases. *J Bone Joint Surg* 1987;69A:452–458.

28. Yang EC, Neuwirth MG: *Pseudomonas aeruginosa* as a causative agent of cervical osteomyelitis: Case report and review of the literature. *Clin Orthop* 1988;231:229–233.

29. Ingram R, Redding P: *Salmonella virchow* osteomyelitis: A case report. *J Bone Joint Surg* 1988;70B:440–442.

30. Oill PA,, Chow AW, Flood TP, et al: Adult *Haemophilus influenzae* type B vertebral osteomyelitis: A case report and review of the literature. *Clin Orthop* 1978;136:253–256.

31. Samra Y, Hertz M, Shaked Y, et al: Brucellosis of the spine: A report of 3 cases. *J Bone Joint Surg* 1982;64B:429–431.

32. O'Brien JP: Kyphosis secondary to infectious disease. *Clin Orthop* 1977;128:56–64.

33. Lafer L, McNeill TW, Andersson GBA, et al: Post invasive diskitis: Characterization of clinical syndrome. *Arthritis Rheum* 1986;29:389.

34. Kirkaldy-Willis WH, Thomas TG: Anterior approaches in the diagnosis and treatment of infections of the vertebral bodies. *J Bone Joint Surg* 1965;47A:87–110.

35. Tom BM, Power TC: Diagnosis of spinal column infections. *Spine: State Art Rev* 1988;2:395–406.

36. Rothman SLG, Glenn WV: *Multiplanar CT of the Spine*. Baltimore, University Park Press, 1985, pp 319–322.

37. Greenfield GB: *Radiology of Bone Diseases*, ed 4. Philadelphia, JB Lippincott, 1986, pp 460–491.

38. Fang D, Leong JCY, Ho EKW, et al: Spinal pseudarthrosis in ankylosing spondylitis: Clinicopathological correlation and the results of anterior spinal fusion. *J Bone Joint Surg* 1988;70B:443–447.

39. Das De S: Intervertebral disc involvement in gout: Brief report. *J Bone Joint Surg* 1988;70B:671.

40. Berghausen EJ, Balogh K, Landis WJ, et al: Cervical myelopathy attributable to pseudogout: Case report with radiologic, histologic, and crystallographic observations. *Clin Orthop* 1987;214:217–221.

41. Ouzounian TJ, Thompson L, Grogan TJ, et al: Evaluation of musculoskeletal sepsis with indium-111 white blood cell imaging. *Clin Orthop* 1987;221:304–311.

42. Abramovitz JN, Batson RA, Yablon JS: Vertebral osteomyelitis: The surgical management of neurologic complications. *Spine* 1986;11:418–420.

43. Couch L, Cierny G, Mader JT: Inpatient and outpatient use of the Hickman catheter for adults with osteomyelitis. *Clin Orthop* 1987;219:226–235.

44. Boston HC Jr, Bianco AJ Jr, Rhodes KH: Disk space infections in children. *Orthop Clin North Am* 1975;6:953–964.

45. Spiegel PG, Kengla KW, Isaacson AS, et al: Intervertebral disc-space inflammation in children. *J Bone Joint Surg* 1972;54A:284–296.

46. Andersson GBJ, McNeill TW: *Lumbar Spine Syndromes*. Vienna, Springer-Verlag, 1988.

47. Fraser RD, Osti OL, Vernon-Roberts B: Discitis following chemonucleolysis: An experimental study. *Spine* 1986;11:679–687.

48. Wegner DR, Bobechko WP, Gilday DL: The spectrum of intervertebral disc-space infection in children. *J Bone Joint Surg* 1978;60A:100–108.

49. Smith RF, Taylor TKF: Inflammatory lesions of intervertebral discs in children. *J Bone Joint Surg* 1967;49A:1508–1520.

50. Thibodeau AA: Closed space infection following removal of lumbar intervertebral disc. *Clin Neurosurg* 1966;14:337–360.

51. El-Gindi S, Aref S, Salama M, et al: Infection of intervertebral discs after operation. *J Bone Joint Surg* 1976;58B:114–116.

52. Lindholm TS, Pylkkänen P: Discitis following removal of intervertebral disc. *Spine* 1982;7:618–622.

53. Fernand R, Lee CK: Postlaminectomy disc space infection: A review of the literature and a report of three cases. *Clin Orthop* 1986;209:215–218.

54. Pilgaard S: Discitis (closed space infection) following removal of lumbar intervertebral disc. *J Bone Joint Surg* 1969;51A:713–716.

55. McCain GA, Harth M, Bell DA, et al: Septic discitis. *J Rheumatol* 1981;8:100–109.

56. Holmes PF, Osterman DW, Tullos HS: *Aspergillus* discitis: Report of two cases and review of the literature. *Clin Orthop* 1988;226:240–246.

57. Ailsby RL, Staheli LT: Pyogenic infections of the sacroiliac joint in children: Radioisotope bone scanning as a diagnostic tool. *Clin Orthop* 1974;100:96–100.

58. Merkel KD, Fitzgerald RH Jr, Brown ML: Scintigraphic evaluation in musculoskeletal sepsis. *Orthop Clin North Am* 1984;15:401–416.

59. Szypryt EP, Hardy JG, Hinton CE, et al: A comparison between magnetic resonance imaging and scintigraphic bone imaging in the diagnosis of disc space infection in an animal model. *Spine* 1988;13:1042–1048.

60. Schmorl G: *The Human Spine in Health and Disease*, ed 2 (Beseman EF, trans-ed). New York, Grune & Stratton, 1971.

61. Gabriel KR, Crawford AH: Magnetic resonance imaging in a child who had clinical signs of discitis: Report of a case. *J Bone Joint Surg* 1988;70A:938–941.

62. Eismont FJ, Bolhman HH, Soni PL, et al: Vertebral osteomyelitis in infants. *J Bone Joint Surg* 1982;64B:32–35.

63. Hughes SPF, Fitzgerald RH Jr: *Musculoskeletal Infections.* Chicago, Year Book Medical Publishers, 1986.

64. Pritchard DJ: Granulomatous infections of bones and joints. *Orthop Clin North Am* 1975;6:1029–1047.

65. Postacchini F, Montanaro A: Tuberculous epidural granuloma simulating a herniated lumbar disk: A report of a case. *Clin Orthop* 1980;148:182–185.

66. Hodgson AR, Stock FE: Anterior spine fusion for the treatment of tuberculosis of the spine: The operative findings and results of treatment in the first one hundred cases. *J Bone Joint Surg* 1960;42A:295–310.

67. Lifeso RM, Weaver P, Harder EH: Tuberculous spondylitis in adults. *J Bone Joint Surg* 1985;67A:1405–1413.

68. Ramsey RG: *Neuroradiology,* ed 2. Philadelphia, WB Saunders, 1987, pp 702–703.

69. Riegler HF, Goldstein LA, Betts RF: Blastomycosis osteomyelitis. *Clin Orthop* 1974;100:225–231.

70. Matsushita T, Suzuki K: Spastic paraparesis due to cryptococcal osteomyelitis: A case report. *Clin Orthop* 1985;196:279–284.

71. Chleboun J, Nade S: Skeletal cryptococcosis. *J Bone Joint Surg* 1977;59A:509–514.

72. Winter WG Jr, Larson RK, Zettas JP, et al: Coccidioidal spondylitis. *J Bone Joint Surg* 1978;60A:240–244.

73. Bried JM, Galgiani JN: *Coccidioides immitis* infections in bones and joints. *Clin Orthop* 1986;211:235–243.

74. Medical Research Council Working Party on Tuberculosis of the Spine: Five-year assessments of controlled trials of ambulatory treatment, debridement and anterior spinal fusion in the management of tuberculosis of the spine: Studies in Bulawayo (Rhodesia) and in Hong Kong. *J Bone Joint Surg* 1978;60B:163–177.

75. Medical Research Council Working Party on Tuberculosis of the Spine: A 10-year assessment of a controlled trial comparing debridement and anterior spinal fusion in the management of tuberculosis of the spine in patients on standard chemotherapy in Hong Kong. *J Bone Joint Surg* 1982;64B:393–398.

Infections of the Hand

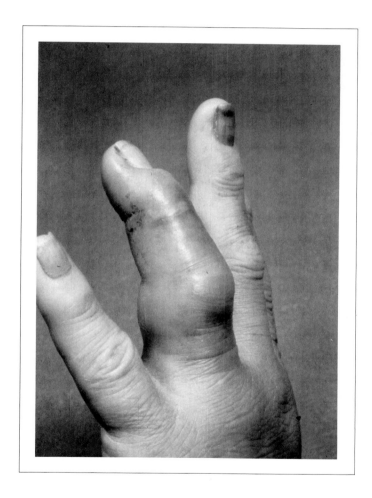

Introduction and Overview

Stephen F. Gunther, MD

The overall spectrum of hand infections has changed over the past 50 years, largely because of the introduction and continuing development of antibiotics. Although the diabetic hand is still a serious problem, rampant necrotizing fasciitis, Meleney's ulcers, and neglected synovial infections with necrotic tendons are uncommon. Septicemia from ascending lymphangitis can now be controlled, and advanced tuberculosis in the hand is nearly gone. Nevertheless, the potential for these problems remains, and there are numerous severe infections of other types (Fig. 1).

Figure 2 shows how different factors are involved in hand infections. In a general way, this schema applies to any infection or disease. To make a correct and timely diagnosis, the physician must be familiar with each of these factors and with their interaction in the production and spread of infection.

Almost any organism can be involved. Some are predictable from the clinical presentation, but most are not. With rare exceptions, it is imperative that the offending organisms be identified by culture and drug-sensitivity characteristics, even if empiric antibiotic treatment has already been started. The complex anatomy of the hand determines to a large extent the patterns of spread of infections. The treating physician must be familiar with the various tissues, synovial sheaths, and potential spaces to which organisms have access by inoculation or by hematogenous seeding. The level of the patient's immunologic competence is also important. A number of conditions can increase a patient's susceptibility to infections, and these have a bearing on the type of infection as well as the severity.

Not shown in the schema is the physician, the final variable in determining outcome. What the physician does or fails to do, and when, are tremendously important factors in the course of the disease and its eventual resolution.

The Organism

In general, the hand can be infected by almost any organism that infects wounds or peripheral tissues elsewhere. Sometimes, the organism can be predicted with reasonable accuracy from the type of clinical presentation. Examples are *Pasteurella* species in dog and cat bites and atypical mycobacteria in chronic synovial proliferation following skin puncture. In some cases, two common and very different organisms can produce a remarkably similar picture at initial presentation. An example is the felon, which can be caused by a bacterium, such as *Staphylococcus*, or by herpes simplex, a virus. At other times, the organisms are less predictable but are known as strong possibilities. A typical example is *Eikenella corrodens*, found in many human-bite infections.

Table 1 matches some clinical infections and the organisms commonly associated with them. The list includes far fewer than half of the infections that are seen, and the surgeon should understand that it is not possible to guess the organism with adequate reliability. The surgeon should strive for proof by culture in every case. Nevertheless, most infections demand the early

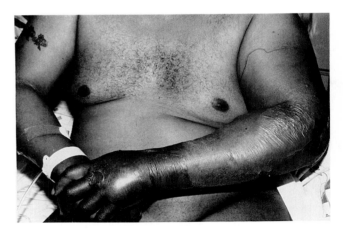

Fig. 1 This massive infection developed from a dime-sized abrasion on the dorsum of the long finger in this previously healthy 38-year-old man. He had a fever of 104.6 F and went on to renal shutdown despite intravenous antibiotics for β streptococcus and *Staphylococcus aureus*. He made an immediate turnaround within 12 hours of a surgical incision from the long finger to midbrachium. There was no infection beneath the muscle fascia.

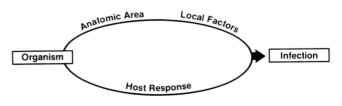

Fig. 2 Factors causing and affecting hand infections.

Table 1
Clinical situations in which the organisms can usually be predicted

Clinical Situations	Organisms
Home and workplace injuries	Gram-positive, *Staphylococcus aureus*
Farm, lawn, soil	Gram-negative
Dog and cat bites	*Pasteurella*
Human bites	*Eikenella corrodens*
Lymphangitis	*Streptococcus*
Felon	*S aureus*, herpesvirus
Chronic paronychia	Fungus
Chronic synovial or skin infections	Atypical mycobacteria

administration of antibiotics, and the decision to use a certain drug or drugs should be based on experience and on knowledge gained from the literature.

In my experience, *Pasteurella* species have been responsible for every dog- and cat-bite infection requiring hospitalization, whether cellulitis, abscess, synovitis, or osteomyelitis. These organisms are sensitive to both penicillin and the cephalosporins.

E corrodens, a gram-negative rod found in the human mouth, is responsible for the rapid tissue and bone necrosis seen in some hand infections caused by punching teeth or being bitten.[1] This vicious organism prefers an anaerobic environment, and it not uncommonly leads to joint resection or even ray amputation (Fig. 3).

Ascending lymphangitis occasionally emanates from small infections that look innocuous in themselves. These infections are marked by chills and fever, red streaks up the arm, and positive blood cultures. Streptococci are usually responsible, but resistant staphylococci must be sought if penicillin does not bring a rapid response.

Felons are difficult problems early on because there are no hallmarks to distinguish bacterial from viral felons before enough time has passed for the viral ones to form typical vesicles on the skin. The surgeon cannot wait on a staphylococcal felon, but must surgically drain pus and administer antibiotics, although neither of these treatments will help a herpetic infection.

Paronychias can also be confusing. Most acute ones are bacterial, but chronic paronychias are frequently fungal. The treatments are very different. The former require drainage and appropriate antibiotics. The latter will not be helped by either of these but will respond to drops of a simple drying agent such as 3% thymol in ether.

Diagnosis of atypical mycobacterial and fungal infections requires considerable suspicion on the part of the physician. Tissue biopsy and culture is imperative, but treatment must sometimes be rendered despite the fact that the organisms are not seen on smear or grown on culture.[2]

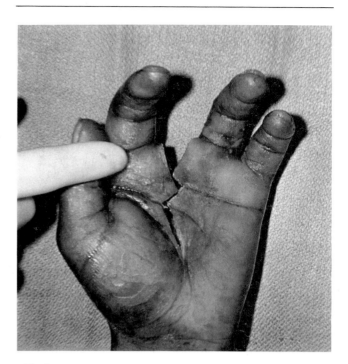

Fig. 3 Ray amputation was necessary ten days after this 60-year-old man punched his 30-year-old son in the mouth. The patient had osteomyelitis, tendon-sheath infection, and a thenar space infection with *Eikenella corrodens*.

Anatomy

Many infections are named according to the anatomic area involved. Paronychias and eponychias are infections adjacent to and above the nail fold. Felons are infections of the pulp, a specialized fibrofatty tissue that does not easily allow spread. Subungual osteomyelitis results from infection under the nail bed. Tenosynovitis obviously refers to infections within the synovial sheaths, and deep-space infections are yet another example of occurrence and spread within a specific anatomic area. It is only through knowledge of hand anatomy that the surgeon can look for, and therefore appreciate, the full extent of certain infections (Fig. 4). The urgency and techniques of surgical drainage differ for these different areas.

Local Factors

Two local conditions that often predispose to infection are ischemia and the presence of foreign bodies. Ischemia can be acute after trauma, or it can be the result of vasculitis and really be a local expression of a systemic disease. The latter is usually worse because it will not improve over time, whereas ischemia from trauma usually will. Foreign bodies are generally introduced as acute contaminants of trauma and can remain

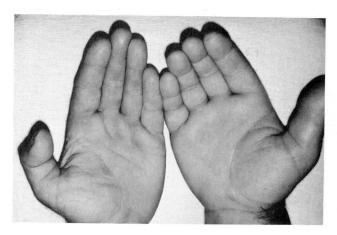

Fig. 4 Within three days of an injection into the synovial sheath to treat trigger thumb, this healthy 52-year-old man developed a "horseshoe abscess" as the infection spread along the radial bursa to the wrist and back out the ulnar bursa to the little finger. Five incisions were necessary to drain this. The organism was *Acinetobacter*.

as chronic indwelling irritants. Chronic drainage through a small festering sinus long after a laceration should raise the physician's suspicion of glass or vegetable foreign bodies, most of which are invisible on radiographs.

The Host

As is true anywhere in the body, some apparently healthy patients seem to handle hand infections less well than others. There are measurable parameters of immune defense, such as leukocyte and lymphocyte function and the humoral defense system, but there are no practical tests for common usage in these patients who are otherwise healthy. Certain groups of patients are more susceptible to infection than others. The worst are diabetics, patients immunosuppressed by steroid medication, and those with acquired immune deficiency syndrome (AIDS). Others include alcoholics, the malnourished, patients with hypogammaglobulinemia, and those with any chronic illness.

Every surgeon is aware of the diabetic foot as a special situation, but many do not realize that the diabetic hand can be just as bad. We do not see it as often as the foot, but it certainly exists. At present, the patients most likely to have a combination of gangrene and infection in the hand are severe diabetics who are receiving chronic hemodialysis for renal failure.[3] These are patients who did not survive 20 and 30 years ago. Amputations of fingers, rays, or even whole hands are frequently necessary (Fig. 5). As with the foot, seemingly small problems should be taken quite seriously in the diabetic hand.

Patients on long-term steroid medication are liable

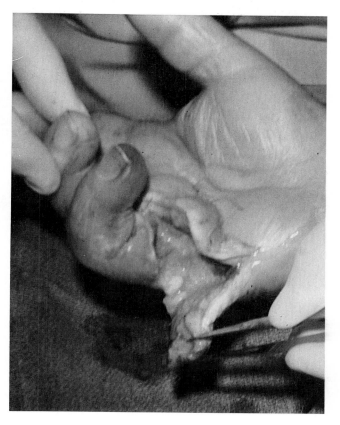

Fig. 5 This 62-year-old man with diabetes lacerated his little finger on a crab claw. The hand is seen here with massive infection and gangrene after partial amputation. This patient died of an arrhythmia three days later.

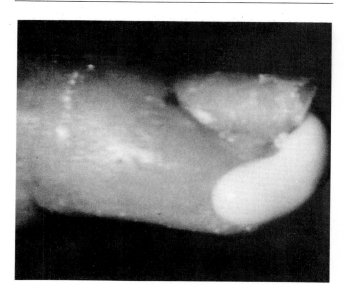

Fig. 6 This elderly woman, who had been taking high doses of prednisone for years to treat lupus erythematosus, came for treatment of a six-month-old felon that had never been drained. A small incision released the pus seen here. The distal two thirds of the phalanx was necrotic inside. The finger was amputated through the middle phalanx.

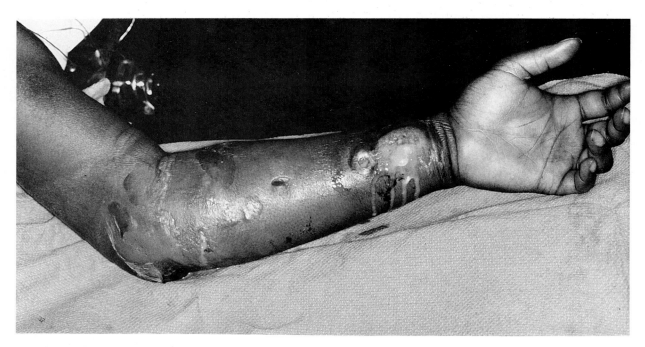

Fig. 7 This 30-year-old woman (a transsexual) came for treatment of abscesses, myositis, and tenosynovitis related to heroin injections. She did not know that she was positive for human immunodeficiency virus until it was proven during this admission. An incision from the midpalm to above the elbow was necessary. Because a tourniquet cannot be used in such cases, the surgical team is at increased risk.

to infections that can smolder for a long time before becoming obvious (Fig. 6). In the absence of steroid medications, rheumatoid patients do not seem to be significantly more disposed to infection than others. However, Felty's syndrome, an uncommon form of arthritis accompanied by hypersplenism and decreased white cell function, predisposes patients to postoperative infections. Other rheumatic conditions, such as systemic lupus erythematosus, mixed connective tissue disease, and the CREST variation of scleroderma, can manifest severe vasculitis and digital ischemia, which predispose to infections or necrotic ulcerations (Fig. 6). Superimposed steroid medications exacerbate this situation. I have not found that digital artery sympathectomy brings sufficient improvement to alter the course of amputation in these patients.

The alcoholic is a special case. There may be immunosuppression from chronic malnutrition and organ malfunction, and there is the added problem that these patients often delay seeking treatment for infections that, diagnosed sooner, could have been treated successfully. Interestingly, alcoholics do not pose as great as problem in our area as do diabetics.

We are still learning about AIDS and hand infections. Any of the common infections can occur in these patients, and they can even be the presenting clinical manifestation of the illness (Fig. 7).[4]

Treatment

Appropriate treatment includes surgical debridement and the administration of antibiotics in most cases. Timing is important, because surgery should be performed early, and antibiotics usually should be started before culture results are known. Felons and paronychias can be treated in the emergency room if the surgeon uses a tourniquet, insists on having proper instruments and help, and can anesthetize the digit successfully with local anesthesia. More extensive infections should generally be treated in the operating room, where all infected areas are decompressed or unroofed. This is particularly true with human-bite injuries to the metacarpophalangeal joints.

When all infections are considered, *Staphylococcus aureus* and streptococci are the most common organisms.[5] These are easily cultured by swabbing infected tissue or pus. For this reason a cephalosporin can be used as empiric treatment for most infections,[6] keeping in mind the situations listed in Table 1. One must be aware of the fact that wound infections following injury in soil or grass are a special situation. Such wounds are frequently colonized with any of a wide assortment of gram-negative organisms that are resistant to the cephalosporins.[7] Established infections must be treated with wider-spectrum antibiotics. For prophylaxis of fresh wounds involving soil or grass, it may be best to omit

antibiotics to avoid promoting the growth of resistant organisms. Good surgical debridement is more important than antibiotic administration in the care of fresh wounds, especially wounds of this type.

Conclusion

The variety of infections and their clinical presentations are almost limitless. These chapters cannot cover all situations, although they do cover the major groups. I cannot overstress the importance of the basic principles of diagnosis and treatment that apply to all infections anywhere in the body. The correct techniques of tissue culture in both routine and special situations will be discussed in another chapter. These include early recognition, accurate identification of organisms, and early appropriate treatment with intravenous antibiotics and surgical drainage.

References

1. Goldstein EJ, Barones MF, Mille TA: *Eikenella corrodens* in hand infections. *J Hand Surg* 1983;8:563–567.
2. Gunther SF: Nontuberculous mycobacterial infections of the hand, in Flynn JE (ed): *Hand Surgery*, ed 3. Baltimore, Williams & Wilkins, 1982, pp 730–739.
3. Lagaard SW, McElfresh EC, Premer RF: Gangrene of the upper extremity in diabetic patients. *J Bone Joint Surg* 1989;71A:257–264.
4. Glickel SZ: Hand infections in patients with acquired immunodeficiency syndrome. *J Hand Surg* 1988;13A:770–775.
5. Stern PJ, Staneck JL, McDonough JJ, et al: Established hand infections: A controlled, prospective study. *J Hand Surg* 1983;8:553–559.
6. Robson MC, Schmidt D, Heggers JP: Cefamandole therapy in hand infections. *J Hand Surg* 1983;8:560–562.
7. Fitzgerald RH Jr, Cooney WP III, Washington JA II, et al: Bacterial colonization of mutilating hand injuries and its treatment. *J Hand Surg* 1977;2:85–89.

Treating Infections of the Hand: Identifying the Organism and Choosing the Antibiotic

Charles S. Levy, MD

Introduction

This chapter offers a guide to the steps in identifying infecting organisms and selecting appropriate drug treatment. A number of new antibiotics and some combinations of familiar drugs are replacing more traditional therapy. These are described along with older treatments. Depending on their experience with infections, orthopaedic surgeons may be familiar with much or little of this material. Part of it is presented in chart form (Table 1), not to serve as a cookbook for antibiotic treatment, but for ease of access. The three authors of this section on infections are in agreement that a specialist in infectious diseases should be part of the treating team for potentially grave hand infections.

Diagnosis

Hand infections can be caused by bacteria, fungi, and viruses. Although empiric antibiotic therapy is usually a practical initial approach, it is important that the infected material be obtained for special stains and culture before instituting a definitive antibiotic regimen. Maximal treatment benefit and minimal toxicity are afforded by drugs specific to a particular organism, and specific treatment requires that all organisms be identified.

Special Stains

Useful information can be obtained quickly and easily through microscopic examination of pus and tissue. This procedure should be performed on all clinical specimens to allow evaluation of the types and proportions of different microorganisms as well as the cellular elements present. The Gram stain is the best for identifying bacteria. This stain dyes cellular elements pink and bacteria either dark blue (gram-positive) or red (gram-negative). When fungi are present, they are gram-positive as well. Artifacts may closely resemble bacteria and can mislead the inexperienced observer. If no pathologist is available, the treating physician can look at the Gram stain, but a pathologist should always be asked to confirm the Gram stain identification.

The Ziehl-Neelsen stain is used for *Mycobacteria* and *Nocardia* species. *Mycobacteria* are small and sparse in most infections, making them difficult to find even with the Ziehl-Neelsen stain. Fluorescent staining has made identification easier, but it is still possible to miss seeing *Mycobacteria*, although they will eventually grow out in culture. Therefore, acid-fast staining is reliable when it is positive but is suspect when negative.

Microscopic examination for fungi is done with specimens prepared with potassium hydroxide, Giemsa, or one of the silver stains. The fungal hyphae, spores, and mycelia are much easier to see than the *Mycobacteria*. Some species may be reasonably identified from the smear alone, but this is not reliable because morphologic features may be distorted. The physician must keep in mind the fact that fungi seen in the chronic wound may be insignificant contaminants in that infection.

Cultures

Special stains are used to establish the fact that organisms are present and to define their general characteristics, but only cultures of infected tissues can provide precise species identification and antibiotic sensitivities. Organisms can be recovered from unopened abscesses if the pus has been properly collected and transported to the laboratory. A sterile specimen, one from which nothing grows, may simply be the result of inadequate collection and processing. When possible, pus should be taken with a sterile syringe and needle rather than a swab. Cultures of abscesses that have previously been opened surgically may yield a variety of microorganisms, which can make it difficult to identify the primary pathogen. Mycobacterial infections are most often caused by *Mycobacterium marinum*, an organism that frequently will not survive and grow at body temperature, 37 C, and should be cultured at 25 to 30 C. *Myobacterium fortuitum-chelonei* usually grows out in seven days, hence the name "rapid growers." *Mycobacterium tuberculosis* usually takes four weeks to grow.

Table 2 summarizes the special stain reagents and usual culture media for the groups of organisms commonly seen. Table 3 matches clinical situations, both acute and chronic, with organisms that commonly cause them and lists current treatments. The material contained in these tables is somewhat general. Empiric therapy can be started right away if the physician is aware of the organisms most likely to be present in a given situation. Appropriate stains and cultures are

Table 1
Drugs, indications, contraindications, and side effects

Drug	Activity	Use With Penicillin Allergy	Dose	Reduce Dosage With Renal Dysfunction	Side Effects
Nafcillin	Group A β-hemolytic streptococci Methicillin-sensitive *S aureus*	No	2 g q 6 hr IV	No	Neutropenia
Cefazolin	Group A β-hemolytic streptococci Methicillin-sensitive *S aureus*	No	1 g q 8 hr IV	Yes	—
Vancomycin	Methicillin-sensitive and -resistant *S aureus*; gram-positive cocci	Yes	500 mg q 6 hr IV	Yes	"Red man syndrome"
Ceftriaxone	Penicillin-sensitive and -resistant gonorrhea; aerobic gram-negative rods	No	1 g q 12 hr IV	Yes	—
Aztreonam	Penicillin-sensitive and -resistant gonorrhea; aerobic gram-negative rods	Yes	2 g q 8 hr IV	Yes	—
Ampicillin-sulbactam (Unasyn)	*Pasteurella, Eikenella* aerobic gram-positive cocci, anaerobes, *S aureus*	No	3 g q 6 hr IV	Yes	—
Amoxicillin-clavulanic (Augmentin)	Same as above	No	500 mg q 8 hrs po	Yes	Diarrhea
Penicillin	Group A β-hemolytic streptococci *Eikenella, Pasteurella*	No	—	No	—
Erythromycin	Group A β-hemolytic streptococci	Yes	500 mg q 6 hr	No	—
Tetracycline	*Pasteurella, Eikenella*	Yes	500 mg q 6 hr	Yes	—

then used to confirm or correct the original diagnosis. Drug therapy and sometimes surgical therapy must be readjusted as the data change.

Animal Bites

The therapy for animal bites must include antibiotics to cover *Pasteurella*. Other common isolates include aerobic gram-positive cocci, anaerobes, and, less commonly, aerobic gram-negative rods. Until recently, two-drug therapy with penicillin plus a cephalosporin has been common, but ampicillin-sulbactam (Unasyn) and amoxicillin-clavulanic acid (Augmentin) provide excellent single drug therapy for animal bites.[1,2] These drugs are safe but cannot be used in an individual with penicillin allergy.

If *Pasteurella* alone is isolated, intravenous penicillin at a dosage of 2 million units every four hours should be adequate. Oral therapy with 500 mg of penicillin every six hours should be satisfactory for mild infection or to complete a course of parenteral therapy. Tetracycline is the choice in the penicillin-allergic individual.

The risk of tetanus from animal bites requires tetanus toxoid and tetanus immune globulin for at-risk individuals. For previously unimmunized individuals or those who have received only one dose of toxoid, tetanus immune globulin and the full series of tetanus toxoid should be given. The previously immunized individual who has not had toxoid in the past ten years should receive a single dose of tetanus toxoid.

Rabies is a potential risk from animal bites. Skunks, bats, foxes, and raccoons are among the animals most likely to spread the disease. Domestic animals in the United States rarely spread rabies. Rodents, birds, and reptiles do not carry the virus. Following exposure, hu-

Table 2
Stain reagents and culture media for commonly encountered organisms

Organism	Stain	Culture	Special Remarks
Bacteria	Gram stain	Aerobic Anaerobic	Anaerobes will not grow well from swab
Fungus	Methenamine silver	Sabouraud's brain-heart infusion (BHI)	—
Mycobacteria	Acid-fast smear, Ziehl-Neelsen fluorochrome	Lowenstein-Jenson, 7H-11	Culture at 25 C for *M marinum*
Viral	Tzanck	Herpes culture	—

Table 3
Clinical situations, causative organisms, and therapies

Situation	Organism	Therapy
	Acute	
Animal bite	*Pasteurella*, streptococcal species	Ampicillin-sulbactam or amoxicillin-clavulanic acid
Human bite	*Eikenella*, streptococcal species, anaerobes, *S aureus*	Ampicillin-sulbactam or amoxicillin-clavulanic acid
Parenteral drug user	Methicillin-resistant *S aureus* Group A β-hemolytic streptococci	Vancomycin
Tenosynovitis	Penicillin-resistant gonococcus	Ceftriaxone
Whitlow	Herpes simplex types 1 or 2	Acyclovir
	Chronic	
Granuloma	*Mycobacterium marinum*	Doxycycline or ethambutol and rifampin
	Mycobacterium kansasii	Isoniazid, ethambutol, and rifampin
	Mycobacterium avium-intracellularae	Clofazamine, ansimycin, ciprofloxacin, and ethambutol
	Mycobacteria fortuitum-chelonei	Cefoxitin, amikacin, doxycycline, and erythromycin (Check sensitivity. Use two drugs.)
	Mycobacterium tuberculosis	Isoniazid, ethambutol, and rifampin

man rabies immune globulin and the series of five injections of human diploid cell rabies vaccine should be given over a four-week period.

Human Bites

In human bites, a two-drug therapy has been necessary to cover *Eikenella*, aerobic gram-positive cocci, *Staphylococcus aureus*, and anaerobes. As with animal bites, ampicillin-sulbactam is a good parenteral therapy and amoxicillin-clavulanic acid a good oral therapy.

If *Eikenella* alone is isolated, intravenous penicillin at a dosage of 2 million units every four hours should be adequate. Oral therapy with 500 mg of penicillin every six hours should be satisfactory for mild infection or to complete a course of parenteral therapy. Tetracycline is therapy for the penicillin-allergic patient.

Ampicillin-sulbactam is a parenteral drug combination that produces the efficacy of ampicillin with enhanced activity against *S aureus*, anaerobes, and gram-negative rods. Amoxicillin-clavulanic acid is an oral drug combination with the same activity. The usual dose of ampicillin-sulbactam is 3 g every six hours, given intravenously, and for amoxicillin-clavulanic acid the dosage is 500 mg every eight hours, given orally.

Drug Addicts

In the parenteral drug user with soft-tissue infection, *S aureus* is the likely cause. Because methicillin-resistant *S aureus* has become prevalent in a number of American cities, vancomycin is now the treatment of choice. Vancomycin, a parenteral drug, has been available for 20 years. The most common reaction is "the red man syndrome," a flushed appearance associated with too rapid an infusion of the drug. This reaction is not a contraindication to subsequent vancomycin. Vancomyin is given in a dosage of 500 mg intravenously every six hours in individuals with normal renal function. If lower doses are used because of impaired renal function, serum vancomycin levels should be monitored. In a patient with methicillin-sensitive *S aureus*, a semisynthetic penicillin such as nafcillin or a first-generation cephalosporin such as cefazolin is indicated. Nafcillin and cefazolin cannot be used in patients with penicillin allergy. Occasionally a patient receiving high-dose nafcillin for several weeks will suffer neutropenia, but this quickly resolves when the drug is stopped. Nafcillin, given intravenously at the rate of 2 g every six hours, does not need to be adjusted with renal dysfunction. Cefazolin, given intravenously at the rate of 1 g every eight hours, must be adjusted with renal impairment.

Group A β-hemolytic streptococci are another common cause of soft-tissue infection in these individuals. With the use of nafcillin, cefazolin, or vancomycin, concomitant penicillin should not be necessary, but if Group A streptococci are the only pathogens isolated, parenteral penicillin alone should be adequate.

Tenosynovitis

Tenosynovitis should be approached as possible disseminated gonorrhea. Although parenteral penicillin was the approach to this problem for more than 40 years, the gonococcal isolates in many American cities are now penicillin-resistant.[3] Even the isolates responsible for disseminated infection, which in the past were exquisitely sensitive to penicillin, can no longer be considered sensitive. An initial approach would be parenteral ceftriaxone at the rate of 1 g every 12 hours.[4] This third-generation cephalosporin is safe and has a long life. A concomitant course of a tetracycline, such as doxycycline, should be given because of the strong association of gonococcal infection with chlamydia.

Ceftriaxone would be contraindicated in an individual with penicillin allergy. Aztreonam, a monobactam, is a parenteral drug with excellent activity against aerobic gram-negative rods. It is also active against both penicillin-sensitive and -resistant gonococcus and can be used in individuals with serious penicillin allergies. The quinolones, such as ciprofloxacin, offer an oral approach.

While aztreonam and ciprofloxacin have efficacy in this situation, the Centers for Disease Control do not endorse these therapies.

Herpes Simplex

Herpetic whitlow usually resolves without treatment. Parenteral or oral acyclovir can speed healing, particularly in an immunocompromised individual.[5] Acyclovir is also useful as prophylaxis to prevent recurrence.

Mycobacteria

In the patient with a chronic infection, a granulomatous reaction secondary to mycobacterium or fungus is likely. An initial approach would be 300 mg of isoniazid, 15 mg/kg of ethambutol, and 600 mg of rifampin administered daily if granulomas are seen but special stains fail to reveal fungus. This will cover *M marinum*, *M kansasii*, and typical tuberculosis. *M kansasii* and *M marinum* may be suspected if tuberculosis stains reveal broad-banded organisms.

Extrapulmonary tuberculosis should be as easy to cure as pulmonary tuberculosis. Experience in Arkansas has demonstrated that two months of isoniazid, ethambutol, and rifampin followed by seven months of isoniazid and rifampin is excellent therapy for both pulmonary and extrapulmonary tuberculosis. Occasional isolates may be resistant, requiring substitution of streptomycin and pyrazinamide.

Therapy with isoniazid, ethambutol, and rifampin is satisfactory for *M kansasii*, although it is not as sensitive to isoniazid as is typical tuberculosis. Because short-course therapy has not been studied, treatment should be continued for at least a year following negative cultures.

M marinum has been treated successfully with trimethoprim, sulfamethoxazole, and with tetracycline alone. Rifampin and ethambutol are also effective. Combination therapy with these two drugs provides excellent results. While long-term therapy for 18 months has been given, shorter treatment should be adequate.

Mycobacterium avium-intracellulare is an extremely resistant organism that may respond to multiple-drug therapy including clofazamine, ansimycin, ciprofloxacin, and ethambutol.

The rapid growers, *M fortuitum* and *M chelonei*, are frequently sensitive to doxycycline, erythromycin, cefoxitin, and amikacin. The sensitivity of these drugs should be tested by disk to determine the isolate sensitivity. *M fortuitum* and *M chelonei* will usually respond to two-drug therapy.[6,7]

Fungus

Fungal causes of hand infection are uncommon. Tissue biopsy is critical for establishing a firm diagnosis. These infections are rare, with cultures and biopsy difficult to interpret. The therapies, including parenteral amphotericin, oral ketoconazole, and new antifungal therapies, such as fluconazole, make an infectious disease consultation advisable.

Sporotrichosis is a fungal cause of lymphocutaneous disease. Often there is a history of contact with thorny plants. The diagnosis is established by culture of infected tissue. Therapy is begun with a saturated solution of potassium iodide at a dose of 5 drops three times a day. Dosage is increased by 3 to 5 drops a day until a total of 120 drops a day is reached. Toxicity requires stopping therapy and then reinstituting it at a lower dose.

References

1. Goldstein EJ, Reinhardt JF, Murray PM, et al: Outpatient therapy of bite wounds: Demographic data, bacteriology, and a prospective, randomized trial of amoxicillin/clavulanic acid versus penicillin ± dicloxacillin. *Int J Dermatol* 1987;26:123–127.
2. Goldstein EJ, Citron DM: Comparative activities of cefuroxime,

amoxicillin-clavulanic acid, ciprofloxacin, enoxacin, and ofloxacin against aerobic and anaerobic bacteria isolated from bite wounds. *Antimicrob Agents Chemother* 1988;32:1143–1148.

3. Hook EW III, Holmes KK: Gonococcal infections. *Ann Intern Med* 1985;102:229–243.

4. Judson J: Management of antibiotic resistant neisseria gonorrhea. *Ann Intern Med* 1989;110:5–7.

5. Schwandt NW, Mjos DP, Lubow RM: Acyclovir and the treatment of herpetic whitlow. *Oral Surg Oral Med Oral Pathol* 1987;64:255–258.

6. Woods GL, Washington JA II: Myobacteria other than mycobacterium tuberculosis: Review of microbiologic and clinical aspects. *Rev Infect Dis* 1987;9:275–294.

7. Wolinsky E: Nontuberculous mycobacteria and associated diseases. *Am Rev Respir Dis* 1979;119:107–159.

Selected Acute Infections

Peter J. Stern, MD

Pulp-Space Infection (Felon)

A felon is an abscess of the digital pulp, usually caused by a penetrating injury. The pulp consists of fatty tissue separated by 15 to 20 fibrous septa that run from the periosteum of the distal phalanx to the skin. If a felon is untreated, it either spreads inward to the terminal phalanx, laterally through the rest of the pulp, or palmarly through the skin.[1]

Felons usually follow a puncture wound and are most frequent in the index finger or thumb. The most common causative organism is *Staphylococcus aureus*. The abscess usually begins centrally and spreads centrifugally, making the entire pulp tense. Radiographs initially demonstrate soft-tissue swelling. If the finger is left untreated, acute osteomyelitis, as evidenced by tuft rarefaction and resorption, can develop within two or three weeks. Occasionally, the acute osteomyelitis progresses to chronic draining osteomyelitis with sinus tracts and sequestrum formation.

On initial examination there is a minor wound with slight swelling and tenderness. The terminal pulp is normally fluctuant, but if the felon is untreated for five to seven days it becomes indurated, red, and exquisitely tender to pressure. It is rare for swelling to extend proximal to the terminal flexor crease (Fig. 1).

Treatment depends on the stage of infection. If the patient is seen early, an antibiotic, such as a cephalosporin, may be effective. The vast majority of felons involve a purulent collection that requires surgical drainage. Assuming there is no proximal lymphangitis or cellulitis, anesthesia can be accomplished with either a digital or a wrist block.

Two incisions are acceptable. The classic incision, a dorsal midaxial hockey stick, is developed directly to periosteum followed by blunt division of the vertical septae from their periosteal attachments to allow drainage of all of the septal compartments (Fig. 2). The incision is placed on the noncontact side of the digit (radial side of the thumb and ulnar side of fingers), should not be through and through, and should not extend around the tip of the finger. After drainage and cultures, the wound is irrigated and loosely packed open. The packing is removed after 48 to 72 hours, and the wound is allowed to close secondarily. Conolly and Kilgore[2] have described drainage through a central longitudinal incision extending from the distal flexion crease to the fingertip (Fig. 3). This incision avoids the

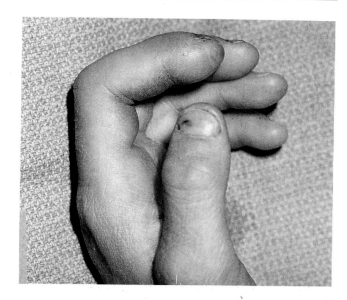

Fig. 1   Felon. Note tense pulp in the index finger.

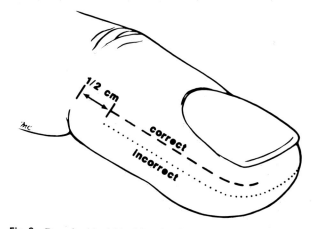

Fig. 2   Dorsal midaxial incision for drainage of a felon. The more volar (incorrect) incision can damage the neurovascular bundle.

neurovascular bundles, heals well, and rarely results in a hypersensitive or painful pulp.

Complications include osteomyelitis, loss of overlying apical pulp tissue, and dorsal spread resulting in a paronychia. Rarely, there is proximal spread into the flexor tendon sheath or distal interphalangeal joint.

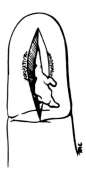

Fig. 3   Alternative volar longitudinal incision of the pulp.

With early treatment and appropriate antibiotic coverage, complications are less frequent.

Herpetic Infections

Herpetic digital infections are self-limited. They most commonly occur after exposure to oropharyngeal secretions and are often seen in nurses who work in intensive-care units, respiratory therapists, and dentists (Fig. 4). These infections usually occur in adults but have also been reported in children[3] and in immunodeficient patients.[4] Less frequently, they follow self-inoculation by gingivostomatitis (herpes simplex virus, type I) or genital (herpes simplex virus 2) herpetic infection.

The incubation period is two to 20 days. Early symptoms are tingling and pain, which may become intense, followed by erythema and vesicle formation on one or more digits. The vesicles may coalesce or enlarge to form bullae.[5] Drainage next occurs and the fluid is either clear or turbid, but never purulent. Confirmation can be made by culture of the fluid or by the Tzanch smear.[6] This is done by unroofing the vesicle, scraping the base onto a glass slide, air drying, and staining by the Giemsa, Wright, or hematoxylin-eosin method. The presence of multinucleated giant cells supports the diagnosis.

Herpetic infection, being self-limited, should be managed conservatively and symptomatically. Surgical drainage is contraindicated. When located adjacent to the nailfold, a herpetic infection can be misdiagnosed as a paronychia, inappropriately surgically drained, and can become superinfected with bacteria. Treatment with topical antiviral agents (adenine-arabinoside or acyclovir) has not proven effective.[5,7]

Tendon-Sheath Infections

The flexor tendons to the digits and thumbs are surrounded by a closed synovium-lined sheath. The thumb

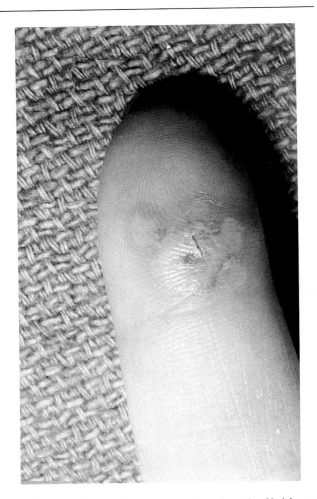

Fig. 4   Herpetic infection in a respiratory therapist. Vesicles are coalescing.

and small finger sheaths often extend proximally through the carpal canal to the radial and ulnar bursa, respectively (Fig. 5). The ulnar bursa surrounds the superficial and deep flexor tendons and the radial bursa surrounds the flexor pollicis longus. In 80% of individuals these bursae communicate,[8] and through this connection an infection arising in one border digit can spread to the opposite border digit to form a horseshoe abscess.

The infection usually reaches the sheath by direct penetration or occasionally by extension from an adjacent abscess. Rarely, the sheath becomes infected secondary to hematogenous spread (as in gonorrhea). When the inoculation results from a puncture wound, it is often at a flexor crease, where the sheath is superficial.

The diagnosis is made when Kanavel's[9] four cardinal signs are present (Fig. 6). These are (1) symmetric swelling over the volar aspect of the entire digit, (2) pain on passive extension, (3) tenderness over the course of the tendon sheath, and (4) flexed posture of the finger.

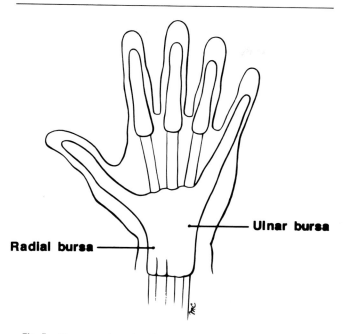

Fig. 5 Flexor tendon sheaths, radial and ulnar bursae.

A subcutaneous abscess can be confused with a tendon-sheath infection. However, passive mobility of the uninvolved segments is painless, and tenderness does not extend over the entire course of the sheath.

Established flexor tendon-sheath infections require surgical drainage. A technique similar to that described by Carter and associates[10] and more recently by Neviaser[11] is recommended. Drainage is accomplished under tourniquet control in the operating room. The sheath is entered just proximal to the first annular pulley at the distal palmar crease through a limited zigzag or transverse incision (Fig. 7). Appropriate cultures are taken. A second drainage incision is made in the distal flexor crease or in the midaxial line of the distal portion of the middle phalanx.

A drainage catheter (No. 5 pediatric feeding tube) is then threaded into the sheath for irrigation with normal saline solution. Sometimes, to facilitate drainage, a third incision is placed over the proximal interphalangeal joint crease. Antibiotics are not added to the irrigating solution because they can produce a chemical synovitis. The hand is elevated in a bulky dressing and the sheath is irrigated every two hours with 25 mL of saline. The irrigations may be painful, and a analgesic may be necessary. At 48 to 72 hours, the dressing is removed, the wounds inspected, and, if there is resolution of the infection, a program of intensive physiotherapy is initiated.

For severe infections with loculations, decompression through a midaxial incision is preferred. This provides excellent drainage and also maintains coverage of the tendon sheath. Drainage of infections through a

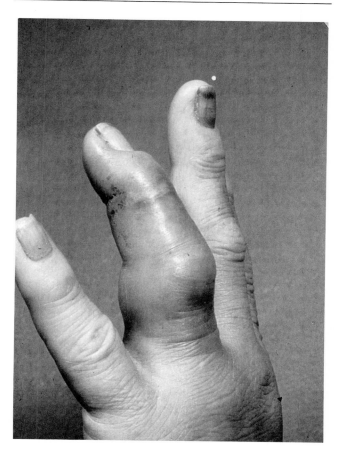

Fig. 6 Tenosynovitis of ring finger.

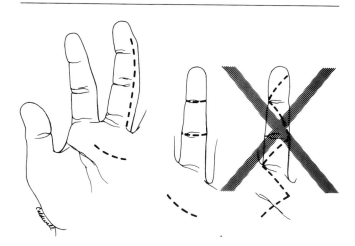

Fig. 7 Midaxial or transverse incisions for flexor-tendon sheath drainage. Zigzag incision contraindicated.

volar zigzag incision is contraindicated, because it leaves the sheath exposed and risks desiccation of the flexor tendons.

The most common complication after flexor tendon-sheath infection is stiffness. This may be secondary to flexor tendon adhesions (or, occasionally, disruption), capsular stiffness of the digital joints, destruction of the sheath (iatrogenic or infectious) causing bowstringing and impaired tendon excursion, or poor patient compliance with the postoperative physiotherapy program. Less commonly, there is loss of volar skin necessitating local or regional flaps, and rarely there can be digital loss, particularly in a diabetic patient. Osteomyelitis, septic arthritis, and suppurative thrombophlebitis have also been noted.

Human-Bite Infections

Human-bite infections, particularly in the pre-antibiotic era, often had a devastating outcome. In 1936, Welch[12] reported amputations in six of 18 patients with clenched-fist injuries. The three factors determining the prognosis are the presence of infection within the joint, the type of infecting organism, and the length of time before surgery (Outline 1).

Bites of the upper extremity involve the hand or fingers 55% of the time.[13] Most morbidity-producing hand bites result from clenched-fist injuries to the dorsum of the middle- and ring-finger metacarpal heads.[14]

Anatomic location of human bites plays a significant role in the ultimate outcome. Most bites proximal to the wrist produce injury to the skin and subcutaneous tissue, and deeper structures are spared. Bites distal to the wrist are more likely to become infected, because such superficial spaces as the dorsal subaponeurotic space, joints, or flexor tendon sheath are at risk for inoculation by saliva.

Many patients with human bites are reluctant or embarrassed to discuss the mechanism of injury. A puncture wound over a metacarpal head should be considered a clenched-fist injury unless proven otherwise. After the mechanism of injury has been established, the physician must determine whether active infection is present as evidenced by cellulitis, lymphangitis, swelling, tenderness, restriction of joint motion, or purulent drainage. The older the wound, the greater the likelihood of an established infection.[15]

Radiographs are taken to assess presence of fractures, such as a metacarpal neck fracture; a foreign body; gas; or osteomyelitis. Aerobic and anaerobic cultures and a Gram stain are mandatory. Culture specimens should be obtained from deep within the wound. Although *S aureus* is the most common organism, gram-negative organisms, such as *Eikenella corrodens*,[16] and anaerobes[17] occur frequently.

Initial selection of a parenteral antibiotic is empiric. There are often multiple pathogens.[17,18] Treatment with a cephalosporin alone,[15,17] a penicillinase-resistant penicillin (or cephalosporin) and penicillin G[16] (for *E corrodens*), and penicillinase-resistant penicillin and an aminoglycoside[19,20] have all been recommended. As soon as culture and sensitivities are available, appropriate modifications can be made.

Surgical Management

Outpatient If the injury is seen in the first 12 hours and it has been determined that active infection is not present, treatment can be carried out in the emergency room with follow-up in 24 to 48 hours as an outpatient. Puncture wounds should be extended proximally and distally. The wound is then explored, debrided, thoroughly irrigated with normal saline or Ringer's lactate solution, and primary wound closure is done. Repair of damaged deep structures, such as tendon, bone, and joint, is contraindicated. A silicone drain is inserted, and the hand is placed in a bulky dressing. Tetanus prophylaxis is administered when indicated. While the wound is being debrided, an intravenous first-generation cephalosporin is usually administered. The patient is then discharged with instructions to return in follow-up in 24 to 48 hours, and a three- to five-day course of oral cephalosporin is indicated.

Inpatient If the injury is not seen until after 12 hours, or if there is an established infection, drainage in the operating room is the mainstay of treatment. Regional anesthesia is permissible, but the anesthetic agent should not be introduced through an area of lymphangitis, cellulitis, or adenopathy because of the risk of bacteremia if there is an intravascular injection. A bloodless field is established through tourniquet control, but to avoid exsanguination with an elastic bandage, the extremity is instead elevated for 60 seconds before tourniquet inflation.

Specific management depends on the area infected.

Outline 1
Management of human-bite infections

Presence of infection
  History and physical examination
  Radiographs
  Tetanus
  Cultures (aerobic/anaerobic)
In emergency room (outpatient)
  Irrigate and debride
  Leave wound open
  No sutures
  Oral antibiotic
  Close follow-up
In operating room (inpatient)
  Irrigate/debride/tissue cultures
  Leave wound open
  Bulky dressing
  Parenteral antibiotics
  "Second look" at 48 to 72 hours
  Wound closure
  Aggressive physiotherapy

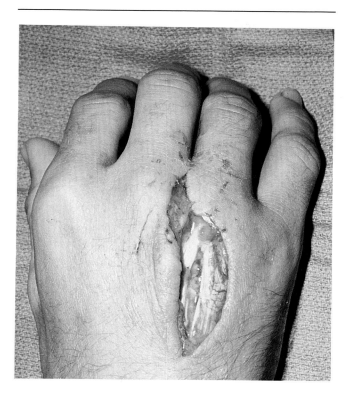

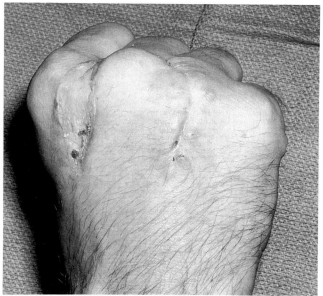

Fig. 8 **Top,** Exposed tendons after drainage of a clenched-fist infection. **Bottom,** Transposition flap for coverage. Donor site covered with a split-thickness skin graft.

Regardless of location, wide drainage and thorough debridement must be accomplished. Injured structures, such as bone, tendon, or nerve, are repaired secondarily. Wounds are never closed and sutures are to be avoided.

Patzakis and associates[21] described 191 patients with

Outline 2
Sources of soft-tissue gas*

Bacterial
   Clostridia
    Bacteroides
   Anaerobic streptococci
   Aerobic aerogenic
     Coliforms
     Mixed
Hemolytic staphylococci
Hemolytic streptococci
Nonbacterial
   Mechanical effect of trauma
   Hydrogen peroxide
   Air-hose injection
   Self injection
   Dysbarism
   Postoperative

*Modified from Altemeier and Fullen.[23]

clenched-fist injuries and noted a 75% incidence of tendon, bone, joint, or cartilage injury. They concluded that all such injuries should be treated with debridement and exploration of deep structures, including the joint.

At 48 to 72 hours, a second look is indicated. If the wound is surgically clean, injured deep structures may be repaired and closure can be considered. I prefer to let wounds heal by secondary intention unless there is exposed tendon or joint, in which case coverage with a local flap may be indicated (Fig. 8). If the wound remains infected, further debridement and careful review of culture data are indicated.

Complications frequently follow human-bite infections. After clenched-fist injuries, stiffness at the metacarpophalangeal and proximal interphalangeal joint frequently occurs. The mobility loss is caused by various factors, including tendon adhesions, loss of articular incongruity, and capsular tightness. To minimize stiffness, a supervised program of active physiotherapy must be initiated once the active infection is under control. Chronic osteomyelitis may necessitate ray amputation. Chronic pain syndromes and reflex sympathetic dystrophy have also been reported.

Gas-Forming Infections

Gas-forming infections are among the most serious treated by the orthopaedic surgeon and are often fatal. To avoid the wrong diagnosis, it is important to remember that trauma may not be the infection's cause,[22] that organisms other than *Clostridia* can produce gas gangrene,[23] that soft-tissue gas may be of nonbacterial origin and does not necessarily indicate infection, and that gas may not be present, particularly in the early stages of infection (Outline 2).

In a literature survey[22], gas gangrene arose from

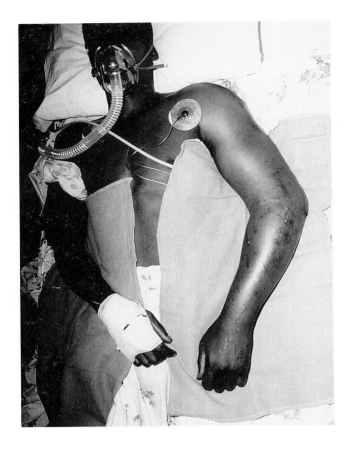

Fig. 9   An intravenous drug abuser with clostridial myonecrosis of the upper extremity. Note needle tracks and swelling of the right upper extremity.

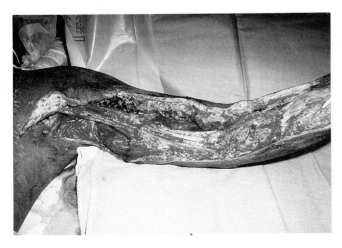

Fig. 10   Appearance after extensive fasciotomy and wound debridement. Infection persisted and necessitated a forequarter amputation. The patient survived.

three sources: trauma (49%), postoperative (35%), and spontaneous (16%). Traumatic causes include open fractures, burns, gastrointestinal trauma, and drug injections. Most postoperative infections occurred after gastrointestinal surgery. The primary diagnoses in spontaneous cases included colon cancer, diabetes, burns, and arteriosclerotic peripheral vascular disease.

Of the many clostridial species capable of causing gas gangrene, *Clostridia perfringens* is the most common. Clostridia are gram-positive, anaerobic, encapsulated bacilli that can be isolated from the soil, the gastrointestinal tract, and the operating-room floor. Clostridial myonecrosis occurs in an environment of low oxygen tension, as in wounds with necrotic muscle and marginal blood supply. The organisms produce histotoxins, such as lecithinase and collagenase, that destroy cell walls. This results in cellular death, thereby perpetuating an environment for clostridial proliferation. *Clostridia* can also cause a crepitant cellulitis that does not produce myonecrosis and that spreads along fascial planes. This infection is less virulent, has a gradual onset, and results in abundant gas production.

Most aerobic aerogenic infections are produced by coliforms such as *Escherichia coli*, *Proteus*, and enterococci. They are often polymicrobial, they are less systemically toxic than clostridial myonecrosis, and they usually occur after pelvic or abdominal surgery.

Streptococcal myositis is an uncommon anaerobic infection capable of producing myonecrosis that is usually less severe than that produced by *Clostridia*. There is extensive cutaneous erythema. This infection is distinguished from clostridial infections on the basis of the Gram stain and subsequent cultures.

Clostridial myonecrosis is the most common of the clostridial infections that the orthopaedic surgeon faces after open fractures. These infections can usually be prevented by meticulous debridement and by avoiding tight casts, tight packing, and prolonged tourniquet time, and by closing of grade III open fractures.

Pain, the outstanding symptom, is commonly out of proportion to the appearance of the wound. The incubation period is less than three days after injury. Swelling of an advancing nature with a purplish or bronze discoloration of the skin (Fig. 9) and hemorrhagic skin blebs are commonplace. There is a thin, brown discharge from the wound with a characteristic odor.

There is a tachycardia early on, but the temperature is minimally elevated. Later, the temperature can be elevated to 41.1 C (106 F). If untreated, a state of shock develops with oliguria and hypotension. Mental changes include apathy and indifference followed by convulsions and coma.

Gas may not be seen on early radiographs. The amount of gas varies depending on the clostridial organism causing the infection (*Clostridia novyi* produces virtually no gas). A feathery pattern suggests a fasciitis;

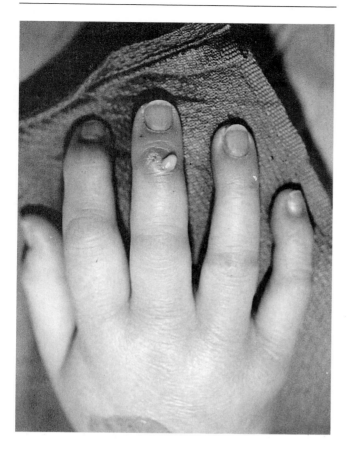

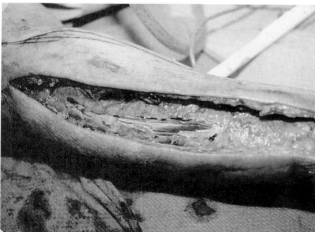

Fig. 11 **Top,** Necrotizing fasciitis. Abrasion of middle finger leading to extensive forearm cellulitis in an alcoholic. **Bottom,** Dorsal longitudinal fasciotomies were performed. Skin with necrotic subcutaneous fat was excised. Muscle was not involved. Split-thickness skin grafts were used for coverage.

bubbles are more commonly associated with myonecrosis.

In confirming the diagnosis, one must have a higher index of suspicion. A Gram stain of the wound drainage showing gram-positive bacilli should be considered an indication of gas gangrene until proven otherwise.[23]

The cornerstone of treatment is prompt surgical debridement (Fig. 10).[24] Mortality in most series is 20%. It is adversely affected by an incubation period longer than 30 hours, shock, and intercurrent disease, such as diabetes and malignancy.[25] When there is extensive myonecrosis, one should not hesitate to perform an open guillotine amputation. At the same time, fluid and electrolyte imbalance is corrected. Intravenous penicillin, 3 million units every three hours, is administered; however, it is not a substitute for surgery. If a concomitant gram-negative infection is suspected, aminoglycosides can be added to the therapeutic regimen. The effectiveness of serum antitoxin has not been proven, and the allergic-reaction side effects preclude its use.[22] Hyperbaric oxygen, if available, is reasonable as an adjunctive treatment. Complications such as central nervous and lung toxicity, barotrauma, and decompression sickness are uncommon.

Necrotizing Fasciitis

Hemolytic streptococcal gangrene was first described by Meleney[26] in 1924. Wilson,[27] in 1952, described the same clinical entity and introduced the term necrotizing fasciitis. Although group A *Streptococcus* is the most common organism, other bacteria, both aerobic and anaerobic, can be isolated.[28]

This disease in the upper extremity is seen in indigent patients with a history of alcoholism and drug abuse (Fig. 11). It begins as an extensive cellulitis after a substance injection, an abrasion, or a surgical procedure. Compression of cutaneous nerves is an early finding and may help with the diagnosis. The infection does not respond to antibiotics, heat, and elevation, and, if left surgically untreated, the skin becomes violaceous or necrotic, bullae form, and the temperature usually reaches as high as 38.9 C (102 F). Laboratory findings consistently reveal leukocytosis.

The primary treatment is surgical. Drainage is accomplished through generous longitudinal incisions. The subcutaneous fat is grayish, hemorrhagic, or necrotic. Vessels within the fat are frequently thrombosed. There are rarely localized purulent collections and muscle is usually not involved. I recommend excision of undermined skin (even if viable) and subcutaneous tissue. The wound is left open and delayed coverage is usually possible through skin grafting.

References

1. Mann RJ: *Infections of the Hand.* Philadelphia, Lea & Febiger, 1988, pp 21–29.
2. Conolly WB, Kilgore ES Jr: *Hand Injuries and Infections: An Illustrated Guide.* London, Edward Arnold, 1979, pp 138–145.

3. Behr JT, Daluga DJ, Light TR, et al: Herpetic infections in the fingers of infants: Report of five cases. *J Bone Joint Surg* 1987; 69A:137–139.

4. Glickel SZ: Hand infections in patients with acquired immunodeficiency syndrome. *J Hand Surg* 1988;13A:770–775.

5. Louis DS, Silva J Jr: Herpetic whitlow: Herpetic infections of the digits. *J Hand Surg* 1979;4:90–94.

6. Blank H, Burgoon CF, Bladridge GD, et al: Cytologic smears in diagnosis of herpes simplex, herpes zoster, and varicella. *JAMA* 1951;146:1410–1412.

7. Levitz R, Ehrenkranz N: Herpetic whitlow: A misunderstood syndrome. *Infect Surg* 1984;832–836.

8. Flynn JE: The grave infections of the hand, in Flynn JE (ed): *Hand Surgery*, ed 3. Baltimore, Williams & Wilkins, 1982, pp 688–706.

9. Kanavel AB: *Infections of the Hand: A Guide to the Surgical Treatment of Acute and Chronic Suppurative Processes in the Fingers, Hand and Forearm*, ed 7. Philadelphia, Lea & Febiger, 1939, pp 241–242.

10. Carter SJ, Burman SO, Mersheimer WL: Treatment of digital tenosynovitis by irrigation with peroxide and oxytetracycline: Review of nine cases. *Ann Surg* 1966;163:645–650.

11. Neviaser RJ: Closed tendon sheath irrigation for pyogenic flexor tenosynovitis. *J Hand Surg* 1978;3:462–466.

12. Welch CE: Human bite infections of the hand. *N Engl J Med* 1936;215:901–908.

13. McDonough JJ, Stern PJ: Human bite infections. *Problems in General Surgery* 1984;1:508–521.

14. Peeples E, Boswick JA Jr, Scott FA: Wounds of the hand contaminated by human or animal saliva. *J Trauma* 1980;20:383–389.

15. Chuinard RG, D'Ambrosia RD: Human bite infections of the hand. *J Bone Joint Surg* 1977;59A:416–418.

16. Goldstein EJC, Barones MF, Miller TA: *Eikenella corrodens* in hand infections. *J Hand Surg* 1983;8:563–567.

17. Stern PJ, Staneck JL, McDonough JJ, et al: Established hand infections: A controlled, prospective study. *J Hand Surg* 1983; 8:553–559.

18. Glass KD: Factors related to the resolution of treated hand infections. *J Hand Surg* 1982;7:388–394.

19. Shields C, Patzakis MJ, Meyers MH, et al: Hand infections secondary to human bites. *J Trauma* 1975;15:235–236.

20. Mann RJ, Hoffeld TA, Farmer CB: Human bites of the hand: Twenty years of experience. *J Hand Surg* 1977;2:97–104.

21. Patzakis MJ, Wilkins J, Bassett RL: Surgical findings in clenched-fist injuries. *Clin Orthop* 1987;220:237–240.

22. Hart GB, Lamb RC, Strauss MB: Gas gangrene: I. A collective review. *J Trauma* 1983;23:991–995.

23. Altemeier WA, Fullen WD: Prevention and treatment of gas gangrene. *JAMA* 1971;217:806–813.

24. DeHaven KE, Evarts CM: The continuing problem of gas gangrene: A review and report of illustrative cases. *J Trauma* 1971; 11:983–991.

25. Hart GB, Lamb RC, Strauss MB: Gas gangrene: II. A 15-year experience with hyperbaric oxygen. *J Trauma* 1983;23:995–1000.

26. Meleney FL: Hemolytic streptococcus gangrene. *Arch Surg* 1924; 9:317–364.

27. Wilson B: Necrotizing fasciitis. *Am Surg* 1952;18:416–431.

28. Schecter W, Meyer A, Schecter G, et al: Necrotizing fasciitis of the upper extremity. *J Hand Surg* 1982;7:15–20.

Chronic Infections

Stephen F. Gunther, MD

Introduction

Forty years ago, a discussion of chronic infections in the upper extremity would have been about tuberculosis. This disease was still a significant killer in this country, and the treatment of skeletal tuberculosis was a significant part of orthopaedic surgical practice. Tuberculous arthritis of the wrist and elbow,[1,2] tenosynovitis of the wrist and hand,[3,4] and dactylitis[5,6] were frequent manifestations of extrapulmonary disease. The principal treatments were rest and surgery.

Fortunately, tuberculosis has now been controlled in most progressive countries. Today, American surgeons rarely encounter it in the upper extremity, but the world in general is still in a 400-year epidemic,[7] which continues to devastate many areas. The diagnosis and treatment are the same as for the atypical mycobacteria, and I will not dwell further on tuberculosis.

At present, the vast majority of chronic infections in the hand are from atypical mycobacteria, and most of the remainder are from fungi.

Atypical Mycobacterial Infections

The Organisms

Atypical, or nontuberculous, mycobacteria have been recognized increasingly over the past 30 years as primary pathogens in the hand and in the body in general.[8,9] At first, they were thought to be harmless saprophytes. Then, they were labeled opportunistic pathogens because it was thought that they infected only patients with compromised immune systems. Although they are still opportunistic in many clinical situations, we know that they infect healthy people as well. A list of the atypical mycobacteria that have been cultured in human hand infections includes at least seven different species. By far the most common is *Mycobacterium marinum*. *M kansasii* is the next most common, and *M avium-intracellulare* is probably next. Some of these, such as *M kansasii* and *M avium-intracellulare* cause pneumonia and can be disseminated throughout the body. On the other hand, *M marinum* cannot survive at body core temperature and has been described only in the skin, the hands and feet, and the bursae of the elbow and knees. All are found in soil, but some have other favorite habitats. An example is *M marinum*, which is prevalent in warm saltwater environments, in certain swimming pools, in fish tanks, and in soil.

Pathogenesis

Most hand infections follow direct inoculation by puncture wounds. This is always true of *M marinum*. However, others can be spread hematogenously from a primary focus, and the most common of these are *M kansasii* and *M avium-intracellulare*.[10] From local foci, the organisms tend to penetrate tendon sheaths, and occasionally they gain entrance into joints as well. Their reproduction is slow, and the associated inflammatory reaction is not dramatic. It is quite common for patients with mycobacterial infections either to have forgotten the inoculating injury or to remember it as a trivial laceration or abrasion followed by a few weeks of redness.

Clinical Presentation

By far the most common presentation is dermatitis from *M marinum*.[11] Chronic ulcerations (Fig. 1) follow scrapes on the underside of boats, punctures by crab claws and fish fins, or any abrasion in contaminated water or soil. These lesions are usually referred to dermatologists for care.

The most common form of deep infection is flexor tenosynovitis (Fig. 2).[10] This can be present either in the wrist or in individual fingers. The flexor synovium becomes distended, and the wrist or finger develops stiffness. Swelling of the digit may be fusiform. There rarely is any pain, and the patient may not be able to say when the swelling started. Motion is usually restricted by the bulk of the synovium. Joint infections are uncommon, but they do occur. The interphalangeal joints are most often involved (Fig. 3), and such infections can be seen with or without tenosynovitis.

Diagnosis

A surgeon familiar with these infections will think of the diagnosis right away when confronted with a chronic tenosynovitis in the hand. Only a short time ago, however, these infections were almost always misdiagnosed and inappropriately treated with cortisone injections, antibiotics, and the like (Fig. 4). Education has changed this, and a high index of suspicion on the part of the treating physician is the key to early recognition.

The diagnosis is made by biopsy and culture. Rice bodies are usually evident in the synovium (Fig. 2, *top right*). Pus is uncommon. Positive proof is visualization of the acid-fast organisms on special smears or growth

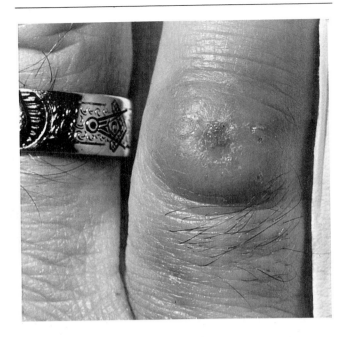

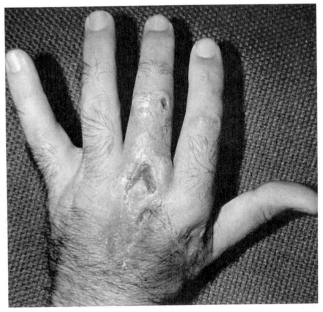

Fig. 1 *M marinum* skin infections. **Top,** This small lesion was photographed twelve weeks after abrasion on barnacles beneath a boat in Florida waters. The ulceration healed in ten months with no treatment other than heat lamps. **Bottom,** These lesions also originated with a scrape on barnacles in Atlantic waters, but this photograph was taken two years after onset and after various unhelpful treatments. Antituberculous medications brought about cure in approximately six months from the time of this photograph. (Reproduced with permission from Gunther S: Nontuberculous mycobacterial infections of the hand, in Flynn JE (ed): *Hand Surgery*, ed 3. Baltimore, Williams & Wilkins, 1982, p 733.)

on special culture media. However, both of these can be negative, despite open biopsy, and the diagnosis then depends on the histologic appearance and a process of

exclusion. The histologic hallmark is granuloma formation (Fig. 2, *bottom*), which is never normal in the synovium or other structures in the hand. In our opinion, a typical clinical presentation combined with granuloma formation seen on histologic sections and negative fungal smears indicates atypical mycobacterial infection. The diagnosis is strengthened by the absence of foreign-body crystals, which are sought under polarized light. It is essential that the surgeon, in addition to looking at the slides, alerts the pathologist to the clinical suspicion of atypical mycobacterium.

Unfortunately, there may not be any granuloma formation early in the course of the illness, and diagnosis may be impossible when the cultures and smears are negative. Only time or a response to a therapeutic trial with antituberculous medication will make the diagnosis in such cases.

Treatment

As has been mentioned, most skin infections from atypical mycobacteria involve *M marinum*. The diagnosis is often made by simple punch biopsy and culture, and the treatment is medicinal. Most dermatologists prefer to use minocycline,[12,13] a form of tetracycline that is highly concentrated in the skin. It is not commonly used for other diseases because it rapidly crosses the blood brain barrier and frequently causes dizziness. The usual dosage is 100 mg twice a day, but this can be cut to 50 mg four times a day if the dizziness is a problem. A response should be seen within two or three months, and it is reasonable to continue the medicine for at least a month after clinical resolution.

As a general rule, the treatment of deep infections is both surgical and medicinal.[10] Although infections with *M kansasii* and even *M marinum* have been cured by antibiotics or surgery alone, it is far safer to employ both. I prefer a nearly complete surgical synovectomy and early institution of antituberculous drugs. When dealing with the flexor tendon apparatus, the surgeon must be careful not to remove the important annular pulleys, even when they obviously are involved in the infection (Fig. 5). These pulleys are essential to tendon function, and the medicines will eradicate any small amount of disease left on them. Because it is common for wounds to break down and drain early in the postoperative period if the anti-tuberculous drugs are not employed,[14] I believe that they should be instituted at the time of surgery without waiting for positive proof of infection in most cases. The usual drugs employed are isoniazid (300 mg per day) and rifampin (600 mg per day). These can be taken as single doses in the morning. It is now standard tuberculosis treatment to add 1200 mg per day of ethambutol hydrochloride to this regimen for two or three months to prevent the emergence of resistant strains. I continue to use ethambutol hydrochyloride in the treatment of atypical mycobacteria in the upper extremity, although others have

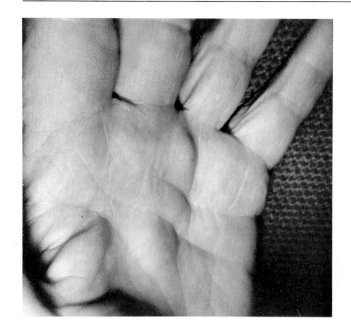
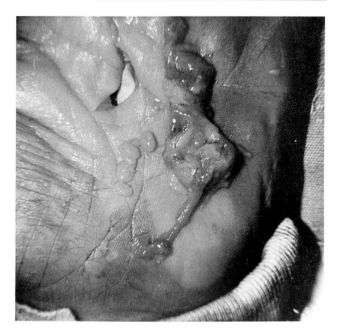

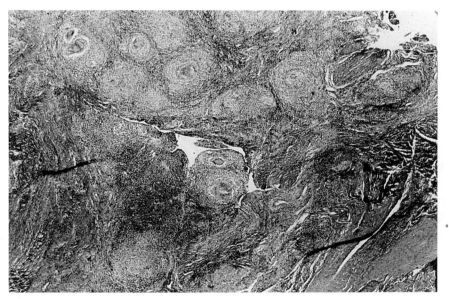

Fig. 2 *M kansasii* tenosynovitis. **Top left**, This hand of a 61-year-old dentist was photographed four years after the onset of synovial swelling. **Top right**, The patient permitted only limited biopsy and synovectomy under local anesthesia. The excised synovium and rice bodies are seen on the hand. The hand returned to normal within eight months of the surgical biopsy and institution of treatment with isoniazid, ethambutol, and rifampin. **Bottom**, The granulomatous nature of this synovium is seen. In our experience, such well formed granulomas with central giant cells are seen in very chronic cases but are not often seen when biopsy is done within six to twelve months of onset. It may take a pathologist to recognize granuloma formation in such cases.

reported good results without it. As mentioned already, the criteria for the institution of these drugs are a chronic infection that is clinically typical of mycobacteriosis, a granulomatous synovitis proven on histologic sections, and negative fungal smears. I do not insist on seeing the acid-fast organisms on special stains, nor do I wait for the cultures, which may take six to eight weeks to grow out. Clinical resolution may take six months or longer. I prefer to continue the drugs for at least three months after the disappearance of any clinical signs of infection when the infection is in the synovium or joints.

It should be noted that some authors describe the successful use of minocycline in the treatment of deep

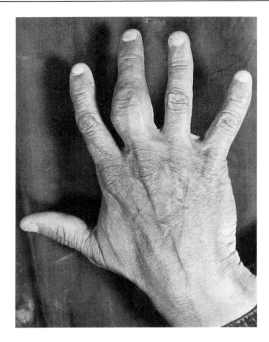

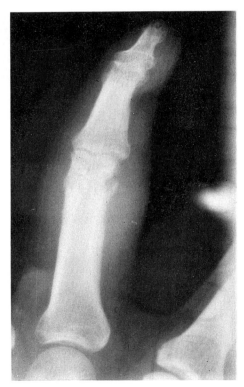

Fig. 3 *M kansasii* in a proximal interphalangeal joint. **Top,** The finger of this 31-year-old airplane mechanic is seen five years after onset of finger swelling and after three surgical synovectomies of the flexor tendon compartment. **Bottom,** The joint space is narrowed and there is bone erosion under the radial collateral ligament. (Reproduced with permission from Gunther S: Nontuberculous mycobacterial infections of the hand, in Flynn JE (ed): *Hand Surgery*, ed 3. Baltimore, Williams & Wilkins, 1982, p 735.)

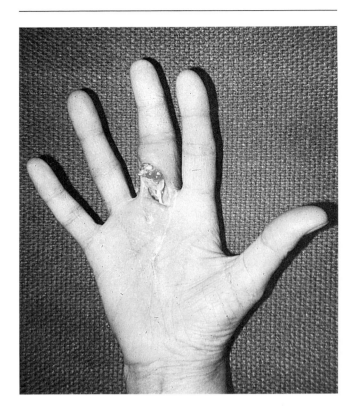

Fig. 4 *M avium-intracellulare* infection seen as ruptured flexor tendons in an open ulcer. Multiple cortisone injections into the flexor sheath over an 18-month period probably contributed to this rare situation. This 54-year-old woman had also been taking prednisone for 20 years as treatment for her chronic asthma.

infections.[12] I have no experience with this. The dosage is the same as for skin infections.

Fungal Infections

Fungi are far more likely to infect the skin and periungual tissues than the deep structures of the hand. This is just the reverse of the pattern of mycobacteria, with the exception of *M marinum*. There are too many cutaneous mycoses to discuss here. Mycoses are most often seen and treated by the dermatologist, who is best equipped to make an accurate diagnosis while ruling out psoriasis, contact dermatitis, intradermal reactions, and the many other conditions that can be confused with fungal infections. The list of fungi that have been documented in the deep structures of the hand and wrist is long. Most of these appear in case reports and are extremely rare. They include species of the following: *Sporothrix, Actinomyces, Aspergillus, Blastomyces, Cryptococcus, Histoplasma, Candida, Nocardia,* and *Coccidioides.*[15-26] These fungi are more likely to cause soft-tissue abscesses called mycetomas, whereas mycobac-

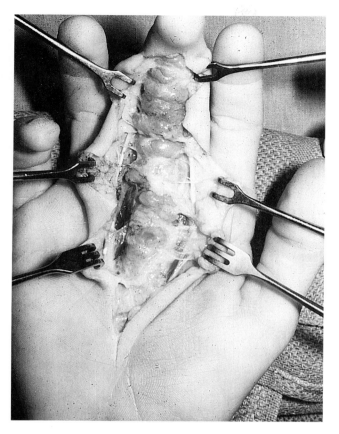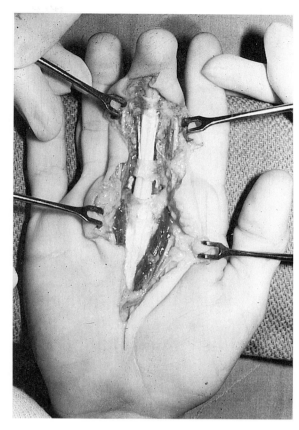

Fig. 5 Surgical synovectomy for *M marinum* flexor tenosynovitis in a 17-year-old boy. **Left**, Intraoperative photograph. The flexor retinaculum is not recognizable. **Right**, After synovectomy. Portions of the A-1, A-2 and A-4 pulleys have been retained even though some infected tissue remains on them.

teria infect synovium. This is only a generalization, however, and both histologic and culture search for fungi should be included any time a mycobacterium is suspected. The medicines used for either one are ineffective against the other, and they carry a significant rate of side effects. They should not be used inappropriately.

Although compromised hosts are more likely to be infected, many infections have been reported in perfectly healthy patients. As is the case with the mycobacteria, the presentation is frequently nonspecific. There may be soft tissue, tendon sheath, or joint swelling. Although the fungi are more likely to present with draining sinuses, this is not always the case. There rarely is fever, although the sedimentation rate is usually elevated. The principles of diagnosis and treatment are the same for the various fungi as for other infections. Most fungi are easily seen on special smears with potassium hydroxide, Giemsa stain, or one of the silver stains. The diagnosis demands histologic examination and culture of surgically obtained material. It is unlikely that any hand surgeon would begin drug therapy for a fungal infection without the guidance of a specialist in infectious diseases, because the recommended drugs change with time and are often dangerous.

Onychomycosis

Clinical

Fungal and yeast infections of the nails and the periungual tissues are more common than most physicians realize. Most are chronic, but painful acute infections can occur as well. Candida species are the most common organisms (Fig. 6).[27] Chronic infections may wax and wane for six months or more before the patient seeks attention, and then the complaint may be the appearance of the nail itself rather than the inflammation that caused it. Because fungal nails have a typical appearance, experience is more helpful than anything else in recognizing the condition. These infections, although persistent, can be treated fairly simply.

Diagnosis

By expressing some discharge or by scraping the nail under inflamed eponychial or paronychial tissues and

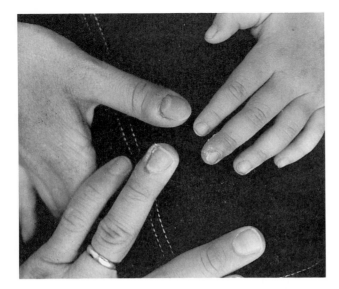

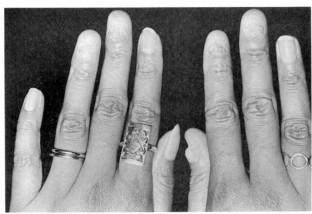

Fig. 6 *Candida* nail infections. **Top,** A child and each parent have acute *Candida* infections of one finger, apparently from a severe diaper rash on the child. The mother's thumb was acutely painful and swollen and had prompted surgical incisions by a general surgeon who assumed that this was bacterial. All three fingers healed with ether drop therapy. In addition, ketoconazole was given to the mother for one week. **Bottom,** Onychomycosis is present in some fingers and not in others.

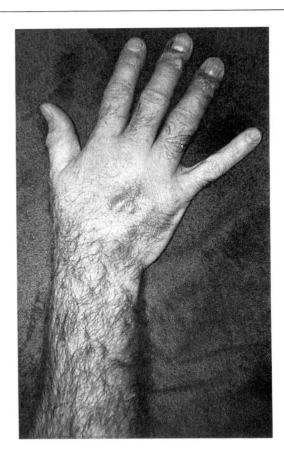

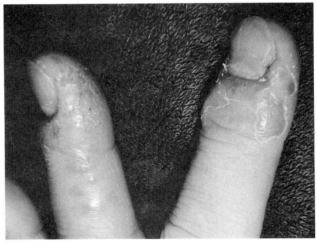

Fig. 7 Sporotrichosis. This man contracted his disease while working in soil. The lesion on the dorsum of the hand was not at all diagnostic, but when combined with the paronychial lesions and others in an ascending pattern up the forearm, it suggested sporotrichosis. **Top,** The whole hand. **Bottom,** The long and ring fingers.

plating the scrapings in 10% potassium hydroxide, an experienced examiner can usually see the budding yeast, branching hyphae, or mycelia. For culture, material should be plated on Sabouraud's or other appropriate medium. Because therapy is not specific to any particular fungus or yeast, this step is frequently bypassed in chronic cases, but in acute cases the physician must be careful to differentiate bacterial from fungal infection.

Treatment

Superficial fungi depend upon a moist environment, and an effective and harmless treatment is the frequent application of a drying agent. After gently unfolding

overlying tissues at the edge of the nail and performing mechanical debridement of loose desquamation, a few drops of 3% thymol in ether are applied. Although not commonly available, this medication can be prepared by any pharmacist. This is done four times a day, and some response is usually seen within five days. Resolution may take as long as a month, and drying therapy should be continued for at least ten days after apparent cure because relapses may occur. Removal of the nail is rarely indicated. Ointments and creams should be avoided because they entrap moisture and do not reach the infected tissues anyway.

Sporotrichosis

Clinical

Sporotrichosis is infection caused by *Sporothrix schenkii*, a fungus incurred from thorn pricks as well as from penetration by infected wood, sphagnum moss,[24] and other such matter. Typical sporotrichosis is seen in the hand as multiple red sores on the involved digit or digits and on the hand and arm in an ascending pattern corresponding to the lymphatic drainage through which the infection spreads. The lesions, which occur on the dorsum of the fingers and hand (Fig. 7), often become raw and may drain spontaneously. Although immunosuppressed people are more likely than others to become infected, anyone can contract it.

Considerably less common are sporotrichal arthritis and tenosynovitis.[15] These usually occur in older men who work in soil. Because the primary focus is in the lung with hematogenous seeding, often there are no skin lesions to suggest a diagnosis. The interphalangeal joints and the wrist follow the knee in rates of occurrence, and there are no telltale signs other than joint swelling and perhaps an elevated sedimentation rate.

Diagnosis

Because the clinical picture is not strongly suggestive unless there are skin lesions that the physician is able to recognize, the suspicious surgeon makes the diagnosis by following the general principles for diagnosing any chronic infection. Infected tissue must be examined histologically, and appropriate fungal cultures must be performed. The hyphae and spores are easily identified on smear in most cases, and the general histologic picture will be a granulomatous synovitis. The organism is readily grown on culture.

Treatment

Potassium iodide administered by mouth is relatively simple and successful in most cases of cutaneous infection. Deep infections in tendon sheaths or joints demand surgical synovectomy, debridement of infected tissues, and frequently require more toxic antifungal drugs. Joint function in the hand and wrist can usually be maintained by such an approach, although failure is common in larger joints.

Summary

The surgeon is rarely the first physician to examine the hand with a chronic infection. In most cases, simple treatment has been tried and has failed. The surgeon must think of atypical mycobacteria and fungi and then systematically make a diagnosis by biopsy and culture and by excluding other diseases and conditions. Because these infections can be very damaging to the hand or wrist, treatment should be rendered promptly and adequately. These general principles are no different from those followed in treating acute hand infections or actually for any disease.

Acknowledgment

Photograph in Figure 6 (bottom) is used courtesy of David Lichtman, MD.

References

1. Berney S, Goldstein M, Bishko F: Clinical and diagnostic features of tuberculous arthritis. *Am J Med* 1972;53:36–42.
2. Robins RHC: Tuberculosis of the wrist and hand. *Br J Surg* 1967; 54:211–218.
3. Adams R, Jones G, Marble H: Tuberculous tenosynovitis. *N Engl J Med* 1940;233:706–708.
4. Fellander M: Tuberculous tenosynovitis of the hand treated by combined surgery and chemotherapy. *Acta Chir Scand* 1956;11: 142–150.
5. Herzfeld G, Tod M: Tuberculous dactylitis in infancy. *Arch Dis Child* 1926;1:295–301.
6. Umansky A, Schlesinger P, Greenberg B: Tuberculous dactylitis in the adult. *Arch Surg* 1947;54:67–78.
7. Youmans GP: *Tuberculosis.* Philadelphia, WB Saunders, 1979.
8. Selkon JB: "Atypical" mycobacteria: A review. *Tubercle* 1969; 50(suppl):70–78.
9. Wolinsky E: Nontuberculous mycobacteria and associated diseases. *Am Rev Respir Dis* 1979;119:107–159.
10. Gunther SF: Nontuberculous mycobacterial infections of the hand, in Flynn JE (ed): *Hand Surgery,* ed 3. Baltimore, Williams & Wilkins, 1982, pp 730–739.
11. Linell F, Norden A: *Mycobacterium balnei:* A new acid fast bacillus occurring in swimming pools and capable of producing skin lesions in humans. *Acta Tuberc Scand* 1954;33(suppl):1–11.
12. Hurst LC, Amadio PC, Badalamente MA, et al: *Mycobacterium marinum* infections of the hand. *J Hand Surg* 1987;12A:428–435.
13. Loria PR: Minocycline hydrochloride treatment for atypical acid-fast infection. *Arch Dermatol* 1976;112:517–519.
14. Gunther SF, Elliott RC: *Mycobacterium kansasii* infection in the deep structures of the hand: Report of two cases. *J Bone Joint Surg* 1976;58A:140–142.
15. Dehaven KE, Wilde AH, O'Duffy JD: Sporotrichosis arthritis and tenosynovitis: Report of a case cured by synovectomy and amphotericin B. *J Bone Joint Surg* 1972;54A:874–877.
16. Iverson RE, Vistnes LM: Coccidioidomycosis tenosynovitis in the hand. *J Bone Joint Surg* 1973;55A:413–417.
17. Linscheid RL, Dobyns JH: Common and uncommon infections of the hand. *Orthop Clin North Am* 1975;6:1063–1104.
18. Brown H: Fungus infections of the hand, in Flynn JE (ed): *Hand Surgery,* ed 3. Baltimore, Williams & Wilkins, 1982, pp 739–756.

19. Hay EL, Collawn SS, Middleton FG: *Sporothrix schenckii* tenosynovitis: A case report. *J Hand Surg* 1986;11A:431–434.

20. Yuan RT, Cohen MJ: *Candida albicans* tenosynovitis of the hand. *J Hand Surg* 1985;10A:719–722.

21. Jones NF, Conklin WT, Albo VC: Primary invasive *aspergillosis* of the hand. *J Hand Surg* 1986;11A:425–428.

22. Duran RJ, Coventry MB, Weed LA, et al: Sporotrichosis: A report of twenty-three cases in the upper extremity. *J Bone Joint Surg* 1957;39A:1330–1342.

23. Monroe PW, Floyd WE Jr: Chromohyphomycosis of the hand due to *Exophiala jeanselmei* (Phialophora jeanselmei, Phialophora gougerotii): Case report and review. *J Hand Surg* 1981;6:370–373.

24. Powell KE, Taylor A, Phillips BJ, et al: Cutaneous sporotrichosis in forestry workers: Epidemic due to contaminated sphagnum moss. *JAMA* 1978;240:232–235.

25. Atdjian M, Granda JL, Ingberg HO, et al: Systemic sporotrichosis polytenosynovitis with median and ulnar nerve entrapment. *JAMA* 1980;243:1841–1842.

26. Lichtman DM, Johnson DC, Mack GR, et al: Maduromycosis (*Allescheria boydii*) infection of the hand: A case report. *J Bone Joint Surg* 1978;60A:546–548.

27. Barlow AJE, Chattaway FW, Holgate MC, et al: Chronic paronychia. *Br J Dermatol* 1970;82:448–453.

The Multiply Injured Patient

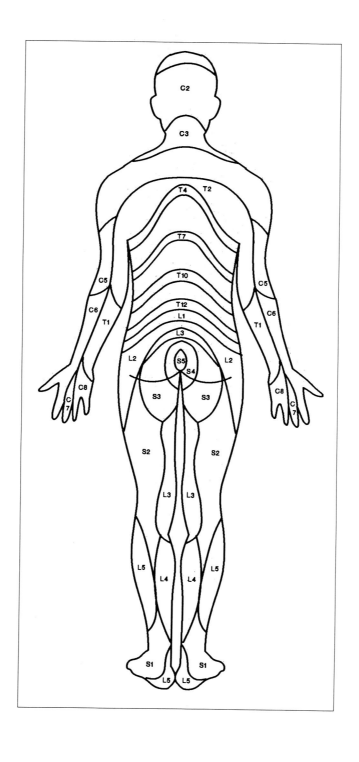

Initial Management of the Patient With Multiple Injuries

Lawrence B. Bone, MD

Michael W. Chapman, MD

Each year, motor-vehicle accidents and sports injuries are responsible for a significant number of severe multiple-system injuries.[1] Patients with these injuries are a challenge to hospitals, their medical staffs, and to society as a whole. The prolonged disability and loss of productivity associated with these injuries are major contributors to the increasing cost of our medical and social programs.

Injuries are the most serious preventable major health problem in the United States. It is estimated that the direct and indirect cost to society is between $75 billion and $100 billion, far exceeding the cost of any other disease.[2] More than 7 million potential years of life are lost annually as the result of injuries, exceeding the combined total for heart disease, cancer, and stroke.[2] Fifty million injuries occur annually in the United States, 10 million of which are disabling.[1] Trauma has become the leading cause of death in persons between 1 and 45 years of age. In 1980, more than 164,000 persons died from traumatic injuries.[2] Injuries are the leading cause of death in children and are responsible for six times as many deaths as cancer, the second leading cause of death in children. Although we have been able to reduce the death rate from cancer in young people, the death rate associated with trauma in persons between the ages of 15 and 24 years increased by 13% from 1960 to 1978.[2]

Better management of shock and fluid loss and the introduction of arterial blood gas determinations, volume cycle ventilator, and nutritional support in the late 1960s are significant advances in management of the trauma victim. The organization and training of emergency medical technicians, the introduction and establishment of regional trauma centers, and the institution of advanced trauma life-support systems during the 1970s have further reduced unnecessary deaths from trauma.

Because of the tremendous improvement in emergency care at the scene of the accident and rapid transport of the patient to the hospital, patients who would have died 15 years ago are surviving. For orthopaedic surgeons, particularly those practicing in smaller community or rural hospitals, these patients often present a complex array of difficult problems that necessitate transferring the patient to a major trauma center.

Field Triage

The responsibility of the emergency medical technician (EMT) is to assess quickly the severity of injury, stabilize the patient from further injury, extract the patient if necessary, and transport the injured patient to the appropriate medical facility. The EMT with advanced training may institute venous access for fluid resuscitation and perform endotracheal intubation when necessary. Unlike the cardiac patient, in whom drug therapy and defibrillation in the field can be life-saving, little can be done in the field to save the life of a dying trauma patient. This person typically has serious hemorrhage or an intracranial expanding lesion and requires emergency surgical management in order to survive. It therefore becomes the responsibility of the EMT to transport the trauma victim as rapidly as possible to the appropriate institution.

Triage systems have been introduced to determine which patients will benefit the most from treatment at a trauma center. Several guides are currently in use to help with triage. Kane and associates[3] use a checklist (Outline 1) of 12 items. If any of these 12 is present, the patient should be taken to the trauma center. West and associates[4] (Outline 2) advocate physiologic parameters as well as location, extent, and mechanism of injury to refine the triage process. Other methods, such as the CRAMS[5] scale and the Trauma Score, use a numerical system based on physiologic and neurologic parameters. These scales have been very helpful in improving the sensitivity of triage, but specificity may be decreased, which means that some patients who do not

Outline 1
Revised triage checklist*†

1. No spontaneous eye opening
2. Abnormal capillary refill
3. Penetrating cranial injuries
4. Penetrating neck injuries
5. Penetrating chest injuries
6. Penetrating abdominal injuries
7. Blunt thoracic trauma with systolic blood pressure under 90 mm Hg
8. Involvement in motor vehicle vs pedestrian accidents (patient is a pedestrian) and sustaining blunt abdominal trauma
9. Flail chest
10. Involvement in motorcycle accident (as a motorcyclist) and sustaining blunt abdominal trauma
11. Fall from a height greater than 15 feet
12. Age less than 5 or greater than 65 years

*A patient with any of the listed conditions would be taken to a trauma center.

†Adapted from Kane G: Empirical Development and Evaluation of Prehospital Trauma Triage Instruments. *J Trauma* 1985;25:484.

Outline 2
Triage list: For automatic triage to a trauma center*

1. Blood pressure below 90 mm Hg
2. Pulse faster than 120 beats/min
3. Respirations faster than 120 or slower than 30/min
4. Penetrating head or torso trauma
5. Unconscious or deteriorating level of consciousness or lateralizing neurologic signs
6. Traumatic amputation above wrist or ankle
7. Flail chest
8. Two or more proximal long-bone fractures

*Adapted from West JG, Murdock MA, Baldwin LC, et al: A method for evaluating field triage criteria. *J Trauma* 1986;26:659.

require it are sent to a trauma center. Although only approximately 5% of trauma patients require the expertise of a trauma center, some overtriage is preferable because the death rate is reduced when trauma centers are utilized.

The pneumatic antishock garment (PASG) is commonly used to help maintain blood pressure in the field. In recent double-blind studies the benefit of the PASG has been questioned.[6] Prolonged use with pressures greater than 30 mm Hg is contraindicated,[7] and the PASG is not recommended in patients with lower-extremity fractures or major soft-tissue injury because of the risk of compartment syndrome. Although originally believed to effect autotransfusion, it actually produces increased cardiac afterload by reducing perfusion to the lower half of the body. The PASG is still considered appropriate for initial stabilization of pelvic fractures to help tamponade pelvic hemorrhage[8] and reduce the pelvis.

Trauma Centers

In two studies from the 1970s, preventable deaths from motor-vehicle accidents (excluding deaths from injuries involving the central nervous system) were found to be 73% and 71%.[9] After regional trauma centers were established, only 9% of deaths were judged to be preventable. In another study, concurrent assessments of trauma care were performed in San Diego County, California, before and after implementation of a trauma system.[10] The care of the multiple-trauma victim was considered suboptimal in 32% of patients before regionalization compared with 4.2% after regionalization. Delays in evaluation and disposition were decreased from 41% to 10% and 53% to 7%, respectively. Suboptimal assessment decreased from 22% to 1%, and the overall mortality was reduced from 26.4% to 8.2% after implementing the trauma system. More importantly, the preventable death rate as determined by autopsy was reduced from 13.6% to 2.7%.

Emergency Management: Initial Assessment and Resuscitation

The Committee on Trauma of the American College of Surgeons has developed an Advanced Trauma Life Support System and course curriculum to improve emergency management of the trauma patient. Each patient should be assessed in an orderly sequence that progresses in a prioritized fashion. Patient management requires rapid primary evaluation, resuscitation of vital functions, a more detailed secondary assessment, and, finally, definitive care.

Primary Survey: Airway, Breathing, Circulation (The "ABCs")

During the primary survey, life-threatening conditions are identified and management is begun. The order of priority is (1) airway, (2) breathing, and (3) circulation.

Airway Establishment of an airway has the first priority. A patient's upper airway must be inspected and cleared of any obstruction such as blood, vomitus, loose teeth, or foreign objects. In a patient who is awake and who complains of pain or tenderness of the cervical spine, in any patient with injuries above the clavicles, and in an unconscious or disoriented patient, the cervical spine must be controlled and protected until a significant cervical spine injury has been ruled out with a cross-table lateral radiograph visualizing all seven cervical vertebrae. In an unconscious patient whose cervical spine is protected, the mandible should be pulled forward, opening the upper airway for improved breathing. Early assessment of oxygenation is determined by obtaining arterial blood gases, and supplemental oxygen may be delivered through a mask with the help of a nasal airway. Arterial blood gas determinations should be repeated quickly after instituting supplemental oxygen to help assess gas exchange.

Breathing The patient's chest should be exposed to assess ventilation and air exchange. Airway patency does not assure adequate ventilation, and oxygenation is determined through arterial blood gases. If the arterial sample contains dark blood, supplemental oxygen should be given. This may be followed by endotracheal intubation after the cervical spine is evaluated. When intubation is necessary before evaluation of the cervical spine can be completed, nasotracheal intubation or endotracheal intubation with proper longitudinal traction on the cervical spine should be used. The cause of inadequate oxygenation must then be found; the first step is inspecting the thoracic cage for evidence of flail segments and open chest wounds. Rapid palpation for tenderness or crepitus caused by rib fractures should be followed by auscultation to determine if there are decreased breath sounds, as occurs in a pneumothorax. It may be necessary to place bilateral chest tubes to decompress potential hemopneumothoraces. Endotracheal intubation is also indicated in patients who are unconscious or have unstable injuries and in patients with inadequate or labored ventilation, flail chest, facial fractures that compromise the airway, or deteriorating blood oxygenation. If possible, endotracheal intubation should be performed by the most experienced member of the trauma team, usually the anesthesiologist. Temporary oxygenation with nasal airway and bag ventilation is preferable to intubation by an inexperienced person. Cricothyroidotomy is rarely indicated and if needed to obtain an airway in children under the age of 12 years, the procedure should be performed with a needle.

Circulation Hypotension in the trauma patient is assumed to be caused by hypovolemia unless another cause can be found. Shock is defined as the decreased delivery of oxygen to the tissues. It is assessed through blood pressure monitoring, pulse rate and quality, and capillary refill. In general, if the radial pulse is palpable, the systolic pressure will be above 80 mm Hg. If the femoral or carotid pulses are palpable, their systolic pressures will be above 70 mm Hg and 60 mm Hg, respectively.[1] Delayed capillary refill with blanching of the nailbed lasting longer than two seconds suggests hypotension. Fluid resuscitation is best monitored by measuring urine output, and determining the pH and bicarbonate levels of arterial blood.

Hemorrhagic shock requires rapid fluid resuscitation, which requires venous access using large-bore catheters usually placed in the upper extremities; they can also be placed through cutdowns in the lower extremities. Hypovolemic shock is reversed through restoration of adequate perfusion of oxygenated blood. This requires adequate ventilation, proper oxygenation, adequate volume replacement, and oxygen-carrying erythrocytes. Vasopressors are contraindicated in the management of hypotension in trauma patients.

Hemorrhage is the acute loss of circulating blood. Normal blood volume is approximately 7% of body weight or 5 L in a 70-kg person. The physiologic response to hemorrhage can be graded on the basis of the degree of acute blood loss. There are four classes of hemorrhage:

In class I, there is loss of 15% or less of blood volume. This amount of blood loss elicits minimal physiologic response, with only minor tachycardia. The movement of interstitial fluid into the intravascular space, as well as vasoconstriction and decreased urine output, maintains adequate blood volume. However, in the presence of other fluid changes, this amount of blood loss can produce clinical symptoms. Replacement with crystalloid fluid will correct the circulatory deficit.

In class II, blood loss is 15% to 30% or approximately 800 to 1,500 ml of blood. The clinical response is generally tachycardia at a rate of approximately 100 beats/min, a decrease in the pulse pressure, and a positive capillary blanch test. Urine output may be only minimally affected with hourly output of between 20 to 30 ml. Management consists of fluid replacement with Ringer's lactate to maintain an adequate urine output of more than 30 ml/h.

In class III, 30% to 40% of blood volume is lost, which represents approximately 2,000 ml in an adult and causes a major physiologic change. Tachycardia, hypotension, tachypnea, and changes in mental status result, which are managed with initial intravenous infusion of Ringer's lactate, usually at three to four times the blood volume lost. If bleeding continues, transfusion with packed red cells is required.

In class IV, more than 40% of the blood volume is lost. Symptoms include marked tachycardia, a significant depression in systolic blood pressure, a very narrow pulse pressure, and negligible urine output. These patients require immediate blood volume replacement in addition to crystalloid replacement. If vital signs are not restored rapidly with blood and crystalloid replacement, surgery to eliminate the source of hemorrhage must be performed. In patients with class IV hemorrhage, it is usually necessary to use Rh-type, ABO-specific blood, because there is not enough time to do a full crossmatch. O negative blood can be given if type-specific blood is not available. When massive transfusion is anticipated, all fluids should be warmed, platelets and fibrin-split products should be monitored, and fresh-frozen platelets should be administered when indicated.

While hypovolemic shock is the most common cause of hypotension in the trauma patient, other causes may exist. Myocardial dysfunction may occur from direct cardiac injury, cardiac tamponade, or, rarely, from myocardial infarction. A history of direct blow to the sternum from deceleration injury would suggest a myocardial contusion. The presence of distended neck veins, decreased arterial pressure, and muffled heart sounds (Beck's triad) suggests cardiac tamponade. An electrocardiogram should be performed to identify myocardial damage or an arrhythmia.

When the clinical situation suggests myocardial dysfunction with elevation of venous pressure, a central venous pressure line should be inserted after establishment of appropriate peripheral venous access. Any clinical evidence of myocardial dysfunction from cardiac tamponade requires immediate pericardiocentesis by insertion of a spinal needle into the pericardial sac. Aspiration of unclotted blood is both diagnostic and therapeutic for cardiac tamponade. Because this condition is immediately life-threatening, pericardiocentesis should be performed before tube thoracostomy to rule out other sources of impaired venous return, such as tension pneumothorax. Arrhythmia secondary to myocardial infarction or myocardial contusion is managed with antiarrhythmic drugs. In a patient with myocardial contusion diagnosed through an elevated creatinine-phosphokinase-MB fraction, close monitoring with Swan-Ganz catheter and proper oxygenation and fluid management can permit safe emergency surgery.

The adequacy of resuscitation should be monitored through hourly urine outputs and arterial blood gas, pH, and bicarbonate levels. The patient with metabolic acidosis and decreased serum bicarbonate is underresuscitated even in the presence of adequate blood pressure. These patients should be treated with increased intravenous fluids. Intravenous sodium bicarbonate is not indicated unless the pH is less than 7.2.

With adequate venous access and initiation of fluid resuscitation, a central venous line may then be inserted to provide a relative gauge to the adequacy of fluid resuscitation. Do not use the central venous line as a primary intravenous fluid resuscitation route. When central lines are placed in a patient who is hypovolemic, iatrogenic injuries to neurovascular structures and the lung frequently occur. Remember that the goal of therapy is the restoration of organ perfusion as signified by appropriate urine output, central nervous system function, good skin color, and return of normal pulse and blood pressure. When the patient fails to respond to adequate therapy, ventilatory problems, unrecognized fluid loss, acute gastric distention, cardiac tamponade, myocardial dysfunction, diabetic acidosis, hypoadrenalism, and neurogenic shock should be considered. Constant reevaluation of the patient is the key to avoiding potential problems. Prolonged shock is a contributing factor to late complications such as adult respiratory distress syndrome, hepatic dysfunction, renal failure, gut-origin septic states, and multisystem organ failure.

Neurologic Assessment

The patient's level of consciousness should be assessed with the Glasgow Coma Scale,[11] an easy to use and reproducible numerical scale of the best response to requests for eye opening, motor activity, and verbal command (Outline 3). Sequential determinations of the Glasgow Coma Scale are useful for defining change in mental status. In any patient with intracranial problems, adequate oxygen transport, reversal of shock, and production of hypocapnia through hyperventilation are necessary resuscitative measures. In the conscious patient, a rapid assessment of extremity function and sensation should also be undertaken at this time.

Secondary Survey

Once the patient's cardiopulmonary resuscitation has begun, perform a secondary survey. Starting with the head, a more thorough physical examination and neu-

Outline 3
Glasgow Coma Scale

Eye opening	
Spontaneous	4
To voice	3
To pain	2
None	1
Verbal response	
Oriented	5
Confused	4
Inappropriate words	3
Incomprehensible sounds	2
None	1
Motor response	
Obeys commands	6
Purposeful movement	5
Withdraw to pain	4
Flexion to pain	3
Extension to pain	2
None	1
Range: 3 to 15	

rologic examination should be performed. The head and scalp should be examined, and any lacerations palpated with a sterilely gloved finger for the presence of a depressed skull fracture. Ecchymoses posterior to the ears (Battle sign), blood in the ears, or fluid draining from the nose may indicate a basilar skull fracture. The face should be palpated for the presence of tenderness or movement suggestive of facial fractures. Examination of the palate and palpation of the mid-face for potential ethmoid plate fractures are important to prevent nasogastric tube misplacement into the cranium. Palpate the cervical spine for swelling, crepitus, tenderness, and misalignment. When major trauma of the head or neck is evident, cervical spine injury should be suspected. The cervical spine should be stabilized with lateral supports and a Philadelphia collar in any patient with a suspected injury.

Head injury is the major cause of mortality from motor-vehicle accidents, accounting for 40% to 60% of deaths.[12] Patients with acute subdural hematoma are more likely to survive if they are taken directly to a trauma center where decompression can be performed within the first four hours.[13,14] The key to diagnosis is close supervision and repeated examinations for such signs of increased intracranial pressure as hypertension, bradycardia, altered consciousness, and pupillary reflex changes. In patients with a history of loss of consciousness, computed tomographic examination of the head is usually indicated. Intracranial lesions caused by hemorrhage may be subdural, usually venous in origin, and are often manifested by loss of consciousness and pupillary changes suggestive of a focal lesion. Diagnosis is made by computed tomography. The treatment is immediate decompression and evacuation of the clot. An epidural lesion is usually arterial in origin and is commonly associated with a fracture about the middle meningeal artery. A history of loss of consciousness followed by a lucid interval and then rapid coma is suggestive of an epidural lesion. Rapid decompression is also necessary. Diffuse cerebral edema is managed with correction of hypoxia, reversal of hypotension, reduction of Pco_2, restriction of fluid, osmotic diuretics, and, when indicated, intracranial pressure monitoring.

Thoracoabdominal Assessment

Chest injuries are present in 50% to 75% of all fatalities caused by blunt trauma and are the second leading cause of death in trauma patients. However, only 15% of chest injuries require surgical intervention.[15] Rib fractures are the most common injury of the thoracic cage. Fractures of the first or second rib, particularly with associated fracture of the clavicle, may be accompanied by injury to the aortic arch or brachial plexus. Radiographic contrast study of the aortic arch is often indicated. Fractures of the lower ribs may indicate injury to the spleen on the left and the liver on the right. Multiple rib fractures are often associated with a pulmonary contusion. Sternal tenderness with or without fracture suggests direct blow to the sternum, and injuries to the underlying structures, such as pulmonary contusion, cardiac contusion, or aortic rupture, must be considered.

Fifteen percent of patients with aortic arch ruptures will survive the first hour.[1] Diagnostic clues to an aortic rupture, as seen on chest radiographs, are widening of the mediastinum, blurred aortic knob or arch, depression of the left mainstem bronchus, and deviation of the esophagus or trachea, as well as major fractures of the upper ribs or clavicle. These, however, are nonspecific signs, and anyone with a history of significant deceleration injury should have an arch aortogram to rule out this injury.

Indications for a thoracotomy are few. They include persistent hemorrhage of more than 100 ml/h over six hours, penetrating injury to the mediastinum, evidence of tracheal, bronchial, or esophageal rupture, and failed pericardiocentesis or failed resuscitation, in which case it may be necessary to cross-clamp the aorta.[1]

Abdominal Trauma

The abdomen is the most common site of undetected hemorrhage in the trauma patient. Liver, spleen, kidney, pancreas, and bowel are the most common organs injured. Care must be taken in evaluating the patient with suspected abdominal trauma in that as many as 25% of patients with hemiperitoneum may not have peritoneal signs.[16] A nasogastric tube and Foley catheter should be placed for decompression of the stomach and bladder. The abdomen should be examined for evidence of contusions, and palpation for lower rib fractures, pelvic instability, or signs of peritoneal irritation should be performed, along with auscultation for bowel sounds. A peritoneal lavage is the diagnostic procedure of choice in patients with suspected injuries indicated by the examination or persistent clinical evidence of hemorrhage. In addition, the patient who has altered consciousness caused by a head injury, or drugs or alcohol, and in whom the diagnostic findings are unreliable should undergo peritoneal lavage. Finally, any patient with multiple trauma who will be lost to continued monitoring, such as those undergoing general anesthesia for associated injuries, should undergo peritoneal lavage. Contraindications to peritoneal lavage are a history of multiple abdominal operations and the presence of an obvious cause for exploratory laparotomy, such as pneumoperitoneum, penetrating trauma, or the presence of peritonitis. A positive peritoneal lavage would include any of the following: aspiration of fluid containing more than 100,000 erythrocytes/ml[3] or more than 500 leukocytes/ml[3], a hematocrit level greater than 2%, or the presence of bile, bacteria, or fecal material.[1]

Computed tomography of the abdomen is now increasingly performed to help rule out intra-abdominal injuries. It has not replaced peritoneal lavage but may be of value in those patients with a negative lavage who have persistent signs or symptoms or in those patients who are symptomatic and stable but who will be lost to continued monitoring.[17]

Genitourinary Injuries

Fifteen percent of abdominal trauma results in genitourinary injuries, and 15% of pelvic fractures result in genitourinary injuries.[18] An early rectal examination should be performed to evaluate the status of the prostate. The meatus of the penis should be examined for the presence of blood. A high-riding or floating prostate or the presence of blood at the end of the meatus generally contraindicates catheterization until a voiding urethrogram or retrograde urethrogram is performed to rule out a urethral injury. The presence of hematuria, whether it is gross or microscopic, is an indication for an intravenous pyelogram and a cystogram. In the presence of a pelvic fracture with hematuria, a cystogram is essential to rule out a bladder rupture. Radiographs, including lateral views with the bladder full and then with the bladder evacuated, should be taken to avoid missing a posterior tear of the bladder. If a kidney cannot be visualized on an intravenous pyelogram, then an arteriogram is indicated to rule out a vascular renal injury. Computed tomography is very helpful in the diagnosis of renal injuries.

In the patient with massive pelvic hemorrhage in association with an unstable pelvis, the temporary use of a PASG or the emergency placement of an external fixator on the pelvis is indicated.[8] The majority of these injuries can be stabilized, which will reduce further hemorrhage.

Extremity Injuries

The extremities should be examined for evidence of swelling, crepitus, and inappropriate motion, as well as neurovascular impairment. Extremities with suspected fractures should be stabilized to avoid further injury. Open fractures should be splinted as they lie, although recent evidence suggests that mild traction, even with an open fracture, is indicated to help reduce motion at the fracture site, reduce further soft-tissue damage, and to help tamponade bleeding.[19] Dislocations should be reduced on an emergency basis with hip and knee reductions performed urgently. Arteriography should be performed in any patient with major skeletal trauma who has altered distal circulation in that extremity compared with the opposite extremity. The vast majority of patients with dislocated knees should have arteriography. Compartment syndrome should be suspected, and compartment pressure should be monitored when clinically indicated, particularly in unconscious patients. Fasciotomies should be performed early when indicated.

Management of Pulmonary Failure, Sepsis, and Multiple-System Organ Failure: Role of Early Fracture Fixation

The adult respiratory distress syndrome (ARDS) is the result of complex sequelae of shock, systemic sepsis, trauma, and other insults. It is both common and lethal, affecting approximately 150,000 persons annually with a mortality rate of 50%.[20] Clinically, ARDS is characterized by declining arterial oxygen tension, decreased pulmonary compliance, increased pulmonary vascular resistance and pulmonary artery pressure, increase in the intrapulmonary shunt, and the appearance of bilateral diffuse alveolar infiltrates on chest radiographs. There is no specific therapy for ARDS. Treatment consists primarily of supportive mechanical ventilation that includes positive end-expiratory pressure.

The systemic septic response frequently seen in the patient with blunt multiple trauma has its beginning with delays in shock management resulting in prolonged tissue anoxia. If the patient has less than adequate debridement and does not undergo early total surgical care, including fracture stabilization, the risk of sepsis is enhanced. This occurs because of the forced supine position, the development of atelectasis through elevation of the diaphragm, and retained secretions. With the patient intubated, oral intake is lacking and the gut mucosa atrophies, thereby enhancing release of endotoxins from the intestines through the gut mucosa. These endotoxins stimulate liver macrophages, which then release their tissue-destructive agents that damage the lung and produce further pulmonary failure.[21] With the patient in the enforced supine position, capillary hydrostatic pressure in the posterior dependent lung is both maximal and fixed, so that the lung is already at risk for interstitial pulmonary edema and a ventilatory-perfusion mismatch.[21] All these factors together contribute to the failure of pulmonary oxygen transport and to pulmonary tissue damage. The damaged pulmonary tissue and the embolic products of fat, activated aggregates of leukocytes, platelets, and debris from blood transfusion together cause activation of the pulmonary alveolar macrophages. These then release their own tissue-destructive immunosuppressive products. If the systemic septic response is allowed to go unchecked, the patient will develop multiple-system organ failure, which represents the late metabolic sequelae of the systemic inflammatory response and carries a high mortality rate.[21] It is characterized by progressive liver failure.

There appears to be a continuum from ARDS through the systemic septic response to multisystem organ failure and death in the trauma patient. Prevention of ARDS is the best management. Early stabilization of the musculoskeletal injury has been shown to reduce the incidence and severity of ARDS.[22,23] In a prospective randomized study of early vs delayed stabilization of femur fractures in the multiply injured patient (Injury Severity Score above 18), there was a 38% incidence of major pulmonary complications in patients with persistently unstable fractures of the femur for 48 hours or more vs a 2% incidence when the femoral fracture was stabilized immediately.[22] This study supports other studies showing that pulmonary failure is reduced in the multiply injured patient when long-bone fractures are stabilized within the first 24 hours.[23-25] By avoiding ARDS, the patients are extubated and fed earlier, with subsequent reduction in the septic state originating in the gut and subsequent liver failure.

The key to salvage of the multiply injured patient is rapid resuscitation with return of oxygen delivery; rapid definitive hemostasis; performance of definitive surgery with debridement of devitalized tissue; stabilization of long-bone fractures within the first 24 hours; and nutritional support through the enteral route to help feed the gut mucosa. These measures minimize the metabolic response to the injury, making recovery more certain and rapid.

Nutrition

The patient with multiple injuries has early nutritional needs that are often not appreciated. The multiply injured patient may require up to 10,000 calories per day. The small stores of carbohydrates present in the body are depleted rapidly. As most patients with multiple injuries are unable to eat in the first few days after injury, nutritional needs demand early attention. Major organ systems demand glucose for energy, and this usually requires the breakdown of amino acids by gluconeogenesis. Despite metabolism of muscle and visceral proteins, hypoproteinemia leads to weakening of vital organ systems and impairment of immune mechanisms. This can lead to such life-threatening complications as multiple-system organ failure and the usual accompanying sepsis.

Nutrition through the alimentary tract protects the endothelium of the gut and provides the best source of nutrients. If patients are unable to eat, supplementary calories and protein can be provided by a feeding tube. In many cases, hyperalimentation by intravenous feeding becomes necessary. This usually requires a nutrition consultation team. Hospitals that are not capable of intravenous hyperalimentation should consider early transfer of polytraumatized patients.

References

1. Committee on Trauma, American College of Surgeons: *Advanced Trauma Life Support Course.* Chicago, American College of Surgeons, 1985.
2. Baker SP: Injuries: The neglected epidemic. Stone Lecture, 1985 American Trauma Society meeting. *J Trauma* 1987;27:343–348.
3. Kane G, Engelhardt R, Celentano J, et al: Empirical development and evaluation of prehospital trauma triage instruments. *J Trauma* 1985;25:482–489.
4. West JG, Murdock MA, Baldwin LC, et al: A method for evaluating field triage criteria. *J Trauma* 1986;26:655–659.
5. Clemmer TP, Orme JF Jr, Thomas F, et al: Prospective evaluation of the CRAMS scale for triaging major trauma. *J Trauma* 1985;25:188–191.
6. Mattox KL, Bickell WH, Pepe PE, et al: Prospective randomized evaluation of antishock MAST in post-traumatic hypotension. *J Trauma* 1986;26:779–786.
7. Christensen KS: Pneumatic antishock garments (PASG): Do they precipitate lower-extremity compartment syndromes? *J Trauma* 1986;26:1102–1105.
8. Moreno C, Moore EE, Rosenberger A, et al: Hemorrhage associated with major pelvic fracture: A multispecialty challenge. *J Trauma* 1986;26:987–994.
9. West JG, Cales RH, Gazzaniga AB: Impact of regionalization: The Orange County experience. *Arch Surg* 1983;118:740–744.
10. Shackford SR, Hollingworth-Fridlund P, Cooper GF, et al: The effect of regionalization upon the quality of trauma care as assessed by concurrent audit before and after institution of a trauma system: A preliminary report. *J Trauma* 1986;26:812–820.
11. Jennit B, Teasdale G, Braakman R, et al: Predicting outcome in individual patients after severe head injury. *Lancet* 1976;1:1031–1034.
12. Becker DP, Miller JD, Ward JD, et al: The outcome from severe head injury with early diagnosis and intensive management. *J Neurosurg* 1977;47:491–502.
13. Seelig JM, Becker DP, Miller JD, et al: Traumatic acute subdural hematoma: Major mortality reduction in comatose patients treated within four hours. *N Engl J Med* 1981;304:1511–1518.
14. Stone JL, Lowe RJ, Jonasson O, et al: Acute subdural hematoma: Direct admission to a trauma center yields improved results. *J Trauma* 1986;26:445–450.
15. Lewis FR: Thoracic trauma. *Surg Clin North Am* 1982;62:97–104.
16. Meyer AA, Crass RA: Abdominal trauma. *Surg Clin North Am* 1982;62:105–111.
17. Peitzman AB, Makaroun MS, Slasky BS, et al: Prospective study of computed tomography in initial management of blunt abdominal trauma. *J Trauma* 1986;26:585–592.
18. Peters PC: Urologic assessment of multiple injured patient, in Meyers MH (ed): *The Multiply Injured Patient with Complex Fractures.* Philadelphia, Lea & Febiger, 1984, pp 55–66.
19. Tscherne H: The management of open fractures, in Tscherne H, Gatzen L (eds): *Fractures with Soft-Tissue Injuries.* Berlin, Springer-Verlag, 1984, p 11.
20. Rinaldo JE, Rogers RM: Adult respiratory-distress syndrome: Changing concepts of lung injury and repair. *N Engl J Med* 1982;306:900–909.
21. Border JR, Hassett J, LaDuca J, et al: The gut origin septic states in blunt multiple trauma (ISS-40) in the ICU. *Ann Surg* 1987;206:427–448.
22. Bone L, Johnson J, Weigelt J, et al: Early versus delayed femoral fracture stabilization: A prospective randomized study. *J Bone Joint Surg* 1989;71A:336–340.
23. Johnson KD, Cadambi A, Seibert, GB: Incidence of adult respiratory distress syndrome in patients with multiple musculoskeletal injuries: Effect of early operative stabilization of fractures. *J Trauma* 1985;25:375–384.
24. Riska EB, Myllynen P: Fat embolism in patients with multiple injuries. *J Trauma* 1982;22:891–894.
25. Seibel R, LaDuca J, Hassett JM, et al: Blunt multiple trauma (ISS 36), femur traction, and the pulmonary failure-septic state. *Ann Surg* 1985;202:283–295.

Management of Fractures of the Femur, Tibia, and Upper Extremity in the Multiply Injured Patient

Kenneth D. Johnson, MD

This chapter discusses victims of falls, airplane crashes, and motor-vehicle, motorcycle, and auto-pedestrian accidents, who have sustained blunt trauma and have multiple injuries. These patients have absorbed a large amount of energy in their torso, resulting in multiple soft-tissue torso injuries, as well as long bone and axial skeletal fractures. The orthopaedic surgeon attending an emergency room must be prepared to deal with these patients. For the purposes of our discussion, major skeletal trauma includes fractures of the femur, pelvis (including the acetabulum), spine, and tibia. Major dislocations are common. Upper-extremity fractures can also have significant impact on patient care, either because of their severity or because they may make it impossible for an individual to use crutches or a walker.

Complications in a multiply injured patient with major skeletal trauma occur early and late. For patients that survive, early complications include respiratory failure, sepsis, and multiple organ-system failure. Persistent instability of major fractures may cause increased soft-tissue injury, excessive blood loss, and excessive pain that can result in multiple transfusions and a need for narcotic pain medication, which can compound these problems. Most late complications in these patients are caused by infection or loss of musculoskeletal function that can result from inadequate early fracture management. Seibel and associates[1] have shown that the majority of acute complications occurring in these patients are in significant part attributable to the forced supine position required for skeletal traction. This position, which contributes to adult respiratory distress syndrome, multiple organ system failure, and sepsis, can lead to death in these patients. Most chronic complications or loss of long-term musculoskeletal function relate to orthopaedic care compromised because appropriate treatment was not accomplished before the patient became too sick to undergo surgery.

The severity of multiple injuries can be quantified by an injury severity scoring system. This system allows a comparison of mortality and morbidity between institutions. Injury severity scoring (ISS) is a generic term. Scoring systems available include the hospital trauma index (ISS-HTI), the abbreviated injury scale (AIS), and the comprehensive research injury scale (CRIS).[2,3] The HTI grades six organ systems—respiratory, cardiovascular, nervous, abdominal, extremities, and skin and subcutaneous tissue—by five levels of injuries.[4] These range from no injuries, scoring 0, to critical or risk of death from injury, scoring 5. The ISS is calculated by totaling the squares of the three highest scores. The maximum possible score is 75. A maximum score of 5 in the respiratory category would be given for a lacerated diaphragm, in the cardiovascular category for a 45% loss of blood volume with an absent blood pressure, and in the extremity category for an open femoral fracture and an unstable pelvis. If all these injuries occurred in one patient, that would represent a maximum score of 75. In our studies, my colleagues and I defined the multiply injured patient as a patient with an injury severity score of 18 to 20 or more.[4,5] We thought that this was significant because it involved either two major injuries, that is $3^2 + 3^2 = 18$; or one severe injury plus one moderate injury, that is $4^2 + 2^2 = 20$. A score of 40 or more means that these patients have at least one critical injury or two severe injuries and are at significant risk of death from their injuries.

A study was undertaken to determine how the timing of fracture stabilization in the multiply injured patient affected the incidence of adult respiratory distress syndrome, systemic infection, and mortality. Patients were divided into two groups. In one group, fractures were stabilized within the initial 24 hours; in the other, fracture stabilization of major long-bone fractures was delayed for 48 hours or longer. A retrospective review was performed of 132 patients from 1982 to 1984.[5] The patients had an average injury severity score of 38, with a range from 18 to 75. The only major difference between the two groups—the timing of fracture stabilization—resulted from the different philosophy of treatment by attending orthopaedic and trauma surgeons taking call. Resuscitation in the emergency room followed a standard protocol dictated by the general surgical trauma service. Patients included in the study were 12 years of age or older, had two long-bone fractures or a long-bone fracture plus a spine or pelvic fracture, had one other associated injury, survived at least 24 hours, and had an injury severity score of 18 or higher. In the 132 patients, there were 511 fractures, averaging 3.9 fractures per patient. Thirty percent of the fractures were open. More than half the patients had ipsilateral tibial and femoral fractures, the floating-knee lesion. Thirty-two patients had three or more major fractures of one extremity. This study showed a statistically significant difference in the incidence of adult respiratory distress syndrome, mortality, systemic sepsis, and hospital cost between those fixed early and

Table 1
Early vs delayed stabilization of fractures in the multiply injured patient

Clinical Data	Early Stabilization		
	Yes	No	Total
No. of patients	83	49*	132
Mean age (yrs)	30.7	30.6	30.6
Mean injury severity scale	38.2	38.0	38.1
Adult respiratory distress syndrome	6	19	25
Major systemic infection	4	12	16
Major orthopaedic infection	17	4	21
Mortality (patients)	2	6	8
Mean intensive care time (days)	4.9	11.1	7.2

*Includes seven patients treated conservatively with no surgical stabilization of major fracture. Adapted from Johnson KD, Cadambi A, Seibert GB: Incidence of adult respiratory distress syndrome in patients with multiple musculoskeletal injuries: Effect of early operative stabilization of fractures. *J Trauma* 1985;25:375–384.

Table 2
Data from prospective study of early vs late stabilization of femoral shaft fractures in patients with an injury severity scale (ISS) greater than 18*

Clinical Data	Fracture Stabilization	
	Early (Within 24 hrs)	Late (After 24 hrs)
Total	30	28
Sex		
Male	25	19
Female	5	9
Age (yrs)	25.6	29.0
Injury severity scale	31.6	32.5
Days in hospital	19.1	28.8
Days in intensive care	3.1	10.5
Days on ventilator	2.7	8.7
Hospital cost	$19,854	$32,915

*Adapted from Johnson KD, Cadambi A, Seibert GB: Incidence of adult respiratory distress syndrome in patients with multiple musculoskeletal injuries: Effect of early operative stabilization of fractures. *J Trauma* 1985;25:375–384.

Table 3
Incidence of respiratory complication in early vs delayed stabilization of femoral shaft fractures*†

Clinical Data	Patient Groups*			
	EI	EM	LI	LM
Total	42	46	53	37
Adult respiratory distress syndrome	—	1	—	6
Pulmonary dysfunction	—	—	—	2
Fat emboli	—	—	—	2
Abnormal blood gases	4	15	12	33
Pulmonary embolism	1	—	2	1
Pneumonia	—	1	—	6
Total patients	4	16	12	32
Total complications	5	17	14	50

*Adapted from Johnson KD, Cadambi A, Seibert GB: Incidence of adult respiratory distress syndrome in patients with multiple musculoskeletal injuries: Effect of early operative stabilization of fractures. *J Trauma* 1985;25:375–384.
†EI = early stabilization, isolated femoral fracture (ISS < 18); EM = early stabilization, multiple injuries (ISS > 18); LI = late stabilization, isolated femoral fracture (ISS < 18); LM = late stabilization, multiple injuries (ISS > 18).

those fixed late. All of these variables were significantly higher in the delayed fracture stabilization group than in the early fracture stabilization group (Table 1).

Because of the retrospective nature of this study and others reported in the literature, a prospective, randomized study of femoral shaft fractures was undertaken between 1984 and 1986 in order to clarify these issues.[1,6–9] In this study, all femoral fractures were randomized to an early or delayed surgical stabilization group.[4] All femoral fractures were randomized, with the exception of those in patients over the age of 65 years who had a hip fracture. In this series, 178 patients with femoral shaft fractures were identified and randomly assigned into four groups: early isolated injury group (EI), early multiple injury group (EM), late isolated injury group (LI), and a late multiple injury group (LM). Statistically significant differences were noted in this study, as well, with a markedly increased rate of pulmonary complications and hospital cost in the LI and LM groups (Table 2). Pulmonary complications consisted of adult respiratory distress syndrome, pulmonary dysfunction, fat emboli, abnormal blood gases, pulmonary embolism, and pneumonia, all of which occurred at a higher rate in the LI and LM groups (Table 3). Recommendations, following this study, were that blood gases should be performed in the emergency room on all patients with a femoral shaft fracture and on all multiply injured patients. In the multiply injured patient, surgical stabilization of all major fractures, including fractures of the femur, pelvis, spine, and tibia, should be performed in the initial 24 hours. If fracture stabilization is not performed early, blood gases should be obtained every eight to 12 hours to monitor the patient's pulmonary function.[4]

Contraindications to early stabilization of long-bone fracture in the multiply injured patient are uncommon. In our series, no patient was adversely affected by a long (more than four hours) orthopaedic procedure within the initial 24 hours of injury, when the patients were carefully monitored by the anesthesia department before, during, and after this surgical procedure. This often required the placement of an intracranial pressure monitor, a Swan-Ganz catheter, a Foley catheter, and multiple venous access sites. Contraindications to early stabilization of long-bone fractures are a patient who is hemodynamically unstable despite treatment and who will not survive the anesthetic or the surgery, and a surgeon or an institution that is unable to perform the procedure rapidly and successfully. Patients with potentially fatal head injuries must be stabilized and monitored as well, but these injuries rarely contraindicate orthopaedic procedures.

Difficulties with early fracture stabilization are a possible increased incidence of orthopaedic infection,[5] surgeon or hospital inconvenience, and the need for a level I or II trauma center to perform the procedures adequately. In our retrospective study, an increased incidence of orthopaedic infection was noted in the early stabilization group, but this was not statistically significant. The early stabilization group had a statistically significant increase in the number of open tibial shaft fractures that was thought to predispose this group to a higher infection rate. Complications of delayed fracture stabilization in the multiply injured patient include an increased incidence of adult respiratory distress syndrome and other pulmonary complications, increased mortality, increased systemic infection rate, increased cost of care, and an increased incidence of musculoskeletal complications.

Fractures of the Femur

All fractures of the femur in multiply injured patients should be stabilized within 24 hours if possible. The exact type of fracture stabilization depends on whether the fracture is a proximal fracture involving the femoral neck, intertrochanteric area, or subtrochanteric area; a diaphyseal fracture that may be open or closed; or a distal-third fracture that may be intra-articular.

Proximal femoral fractures can be difficult to handle because they often occur in combination with a femoral shaft fracture or involve the hip joint. Isolated femoral neck fractures are best treated by closed reduction and multiple screw or pin fixation. Isolated intertrochanteric fractures are best treated with a compression hip screw. Although retrograde flexible intramedullary nails can be used to treat intertrochanteric fractures, these have not been perfected to the point that this can be recommended as a routine treatment for the isolated intertrochanteric fracture in a patient with multiple injuries. Subtrochanteric fractures are best treated by an intramedullary nail.[10]

Subtrochanteric fractures have been the subject of several presentations over the last several years. Three separate studies by Shifflett and Bray,[11] Brien and associates,[12] and Garbarino and associates[13] demonstrated that the best possible treatment for a subtrochanteric fracture is closed intramedullary nailing. Of a total of 132 patients in their combined series, there were no cases of hardware failure and only three nonunions. These nonunions were successfully treated either by bone grafting or by replacing the nail with a larger reamed nail. A recent study by Wiss and associates[14] comparing a closed intramedullary nailing technique with an angle blade plate or a Zickel nail, showed better long-term results with less surgical time and less blood loss with the closed intramedullary nailing technique in subtrochanteric fractures.

Subtrochanteric fractures can be classified according to their trochanteric extension (Fig. 1).[11] Three zones can be identified: (1) fractures below the lesser trochanter, (2) fractures at or including the lesser trochanter, and (3) fractures that extend into the greater

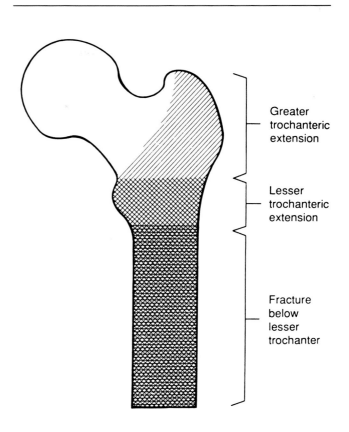

Fig. 1 Subtrochanteric fracture classification by trochanter extension.

trochanter. All fractures below the lesser trochanter should be stabilized with closed intramedullary nailing. Even fractures at the level of the lesser trochanter may be treated by locked intramedullary nailing (Fig. 2). Nailing of these fractures may result in a slight varus caused by the muscle pull that dictates a slightly lateral starting position. This generally leads to solid union without significant patient complaints or abnormalities. Unfortunately, when the subtrochanteric fracture includes extension into the greater trochanter, locked intramedullary nailing cannot be recommended (Fig. 3). These fractures may be treated by means of a fixed-angle side-plate device such as an angle-blade plate or a compression hip screw or by a new generation of locked intramedullary nail, with cross-screw fixation that is inserted into the femoral head.[15] Compression hip screws need to be keyed. The side plate should be long enough to allow fixation of the shaft with at least four solid bicortical screws. Place cancellous bone graft on the medial aspect of femur opposite the plate to enhance early union. The new reconstruction-type nails with screws into the femoral head are technically difficult to use and require extensive previous experience with the use of closed intramedullary nailing techniques

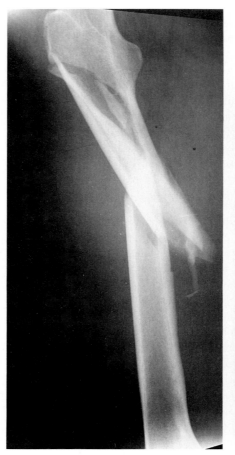
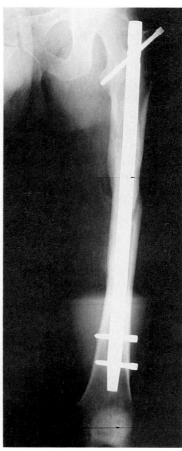

Fig. 2   Left, Subtrochanteric fracture at the level of the lesser trochanter with intramedullary nail. **Right**, Treated by intramedullary nail with proximal and distal interlocking screws.

(Fig. 4).[11,16] Any intramedullary nail placed in a subtrochanteric fracture should have static locking to ensure stability, both in control of length and of rotation. This is absolutely necessary because of the overreaming required to place these large nails. Distal locking may be performed at a later time if there is a great hurry to remove the patient from the operating table.

Diaphyseal femoral shaft fractures are best treated by closed intramedullary nailing technique.[10] Treat stable, transverse midshaft or short oblique fractures with an unlocked intramedullary nail. All others should have a statically locked nail placed.[17,18] If the patient is on a regular operating table, modified open nailing may be necessary to facilitate fixation. Open the fracture just enough to assist reduction and passage of the guide pin. Monitor the procedure with a C-arm. The wound at the fracture can be closed after placing the guide pin.

Distal Femoral Fractures

I will discuss extra-articular fractures, intra-articular fractures, open fractures, and fractures associated with a vascular injury. If possible, extra-articular fractures of the distal femur are best treated by closed intramedullary nailing. Most frequently, I use a locked intramedullary nail, but occasionally a Zickel supracondylar device is required.[19] A Zickel nail is quick and easy to apply and gives good stability in stable noncomminuted fractures. Comminuted intra-articular fractures usually require open reduction and internal fixation using some type of side-plate device. My personal preference is the AO-condylar buttress plate (Fig. 5), which has a fixed angle at the junction of the side plate and the cloverleaf section that allows for the normal valgus alignment of the distal femur. This device allows multiple screws to be placed across the most comminuted intra-articular distal femoral fractures without removing further bone from the distal femur for placement of a large blade or screw. It does have the drawback of being slightly weaker than the angle blade plate or dynamic condylar screw. Therefore, if the patient stands and applies full weight to this device, it may bend and deform into a varus alignment. Generally speaking, most patients can protect themselves from full weight-bearing until early fracture union has occurred and

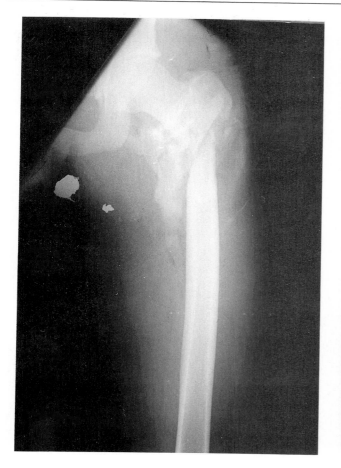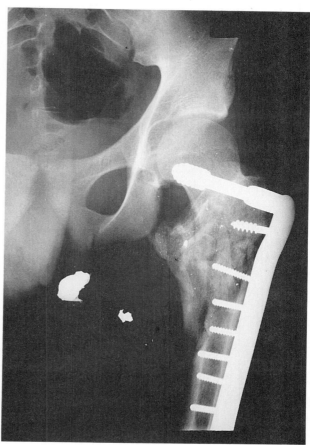

Fig. 3   **Left**, Subtrochanteric fracture with greater trochanter extension. **Right**, Treated with compression screw and side plate.

then progress from partial to full weightbearing as fracture healing allows.

Open fractures of the distal femur require meticulous irrigation and debridement. Anatomic reconstruction of the articular portion of the femur is usually possible using internal fixation. An external fixator is recommended only for highly contaminated wounds, because of the potential for pin-tract infection, as well as interference with knee motion caused by the pins.

Repair of a fracture of the distal third of the femur with a concomitant vascular injury can be a most difficult undertaking in the multiply injured patient. Restoration of peripheral vascular flow takes first priority. This requires an extensive medial approach to the artery. Fracture stabilization must be done in the presence of a long medial incision extending from mid-thigh to mid-calf with the patient supine on a regular operating table. Rather than perform an extensive surgical dissection on the lateral side or apply a medial plate, a simpler solution has been to insert Zickel supracondylar nails (Fig. 6). Do a closed reduction of the fracture through the medial incision. The medial tine

can be inserted from the medial condyle without any further dissection. Make a 1-inch incision over the lateral femoral condyle, and drill a hole in the lateral femoral condyle for insertion of the lateral tine. Then advance the medial and lateral tines up the femoral shaft, holding the fracture reduced. Finally, insert the two cross-bolts through the nails. This will resolve this difficult problem if the fracture is not excessively comminuted. Repair of a severely comminuted fracture in the face of a vascular injury is a most trying undertaking and requires consultation between the orthopaedic surgeon and vascular surgeon before undertaking the surgical repair of both injuries.

Ipsilateral Femoral Shaft and Concomitant Hip Fracture

The ipsilateral femoral shaft and concomitant hip fracture has been described extensively by Casey and Chapman[20] in 1979, as well as Swiontkowski and associates[21] in 1984. Both studies noted a high incidence of this injury in multiply injured patients, and advised early surgical stabilization of both fractures. A 25% incidence of pulmonary complications occurred

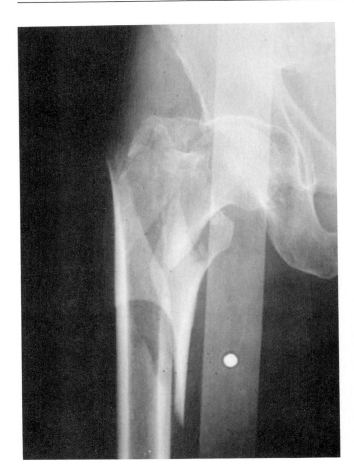 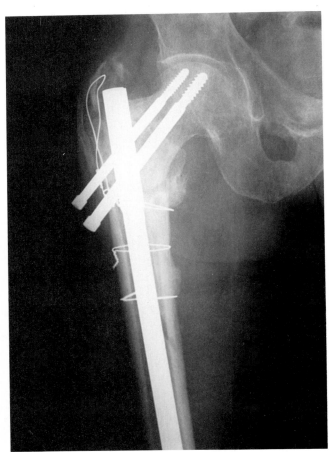

Fig. 4 **Left**, Subtrochanteric fracture with greater trochanter extension. **Right**, Treated with reconstruction nail.

when the patient was treated in traction. Probably the most significant factor noted in these series was the fact that making the correct diagnosis is crucial. In 30% of patients, the initial diagnosis was missed for numerous reasons. Any multiply injured patient with a femoral shaft fracture must have anteroposterior radiographs of the hip with the hip internally rotated. Every trauma patient must have an anteroposterior radiograph of the pelvis performed in the emergency room.

Currently there is no single best method of treatment for the ipsilateral femoral shaft and hip fracture. Treatment protocols depend to a large extent on the status of the patient, the fracture patterns, and the surgeon's experience. Treatment of the hip always takes precedence over the femoral shaft fracture. This is because complications related to the femoral neck fracture can lead to loss of hip function.

Fracture of the femoral shaft and femoral neck is the most common combination. Current protocol at my institution is closed reduction of both the femoral neck and shaft fractures, closed intramedullary nailing of the femoral shaft fracture, and multiple-screw fixation of

the femoral neck. Screws are placed anterior to the intramedullary nail (Fig. 7). Steinmann pins can be placed in an oblique manner from anterior on the femoral shaft directed posterior into the head to hold the head and neck fracture in place during closed intramedullary nailing of the shaft. Following intramedullary nailing of the femoral shaft fracture, replace the pins used for reduction and temporary fixation of the femoral head with cannulated 6.5- or 7-mm screws.

Other surgical techniques include closed reduction and internal fixation of the femoral neck fracture using multiple pins or screws with plating or retrograde intramedullary nailing of the femoral shaft. The newer locked nails with large screws or nails that run obliquely up into the femoral head are difficult to use. Current experience with these devices is so limited that no recommendation for their use can be made.

A femoral shaft and intertrochanteric fracture is the second most common concomitant ipsilateral femoral shaft and hip fracture. This fracture pattern is handled by one of three methods. If the intertrochanteric fracture is nondisplaced, an attempt may be made to fix

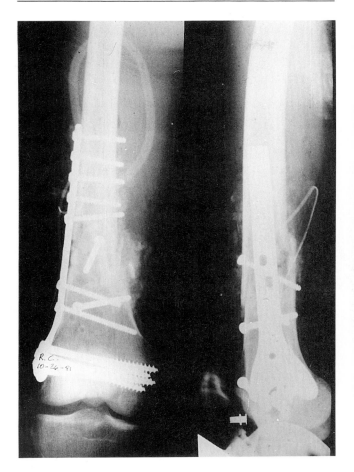

Fig. 5 Comminuted distal femoral fracture treated with condylar buttress plate.

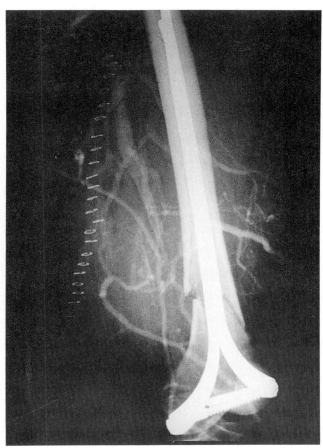

Fig. 6 Zickel devices used with concomitant cross-bolts in vascular injury.

the femoral shaft with an intramedullary nail and the intertrochanteric fracture by compression screws inserted anterior to the intramedullary nail up the femoral neck in the manner previously described for the ipsilateral femoral shaft and femoral neck fracture. Displaced intertrochanteric fractures in the presence of a femoral shaft fracture can be stabilized with an angle blade plate, compression hip screw, or a second-generation locked intramedullary nail. Cancellous bone grafting on the medial side of the femur to hasten union is advisable when plates are used. The second-generation locked intramedullary nail with fixation up into the femoral head and neck has demonstrated good results with this particular fracture pattern (Fig. 8). Use of this type of locked intramedullary nail is technically difficult and may require an open reduction and pin or clamp fixation of the proximal fracture during placement of the intramedullary nail. Open reduction of the proximal fracture is recommended if displacement of the fracture occurs during placement of the intramedullary nail.

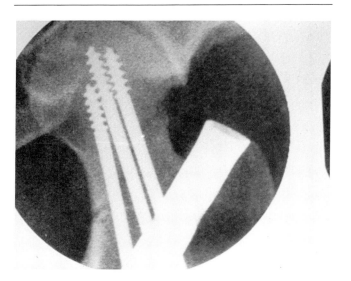

Fig. 7 Screws anterior to nail with ipsilateral neck and shaft.

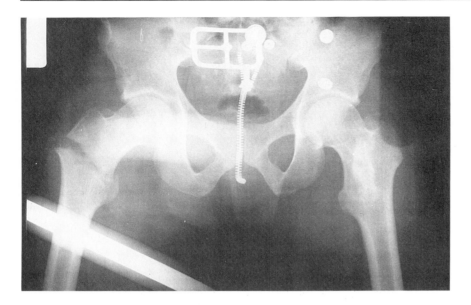

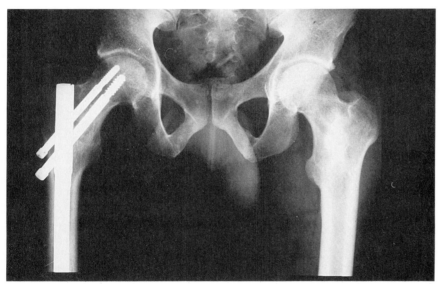

Fig. 8 Top, Ipsilateral shaft and inter-trochanteric fracture with second generation nail. **Bottom,** Fracture treated by closed reduction and fixation by second generation nail.

Ipsilateral Concomitant Fracture of the Femur and Tibia (the Floating-Knee Lesion)

This combination was first described by Blake and McBryde in 1965.[22,23] The incidence of the lesion in the multiply injured patient with fractures approximates 50%. In one retrospective series, 132 patients had 67 ipsilateral tibial and femoral shaft fractures and 32 patients had three or more fractures in one extremity.[5] Veith and associates[24] in 1984 described 57 consecutive cases. Their complications included one death and two fat emboli. All of these occurred before stabilization of the femoral fracture. Three pulmonary emboli occurred in patients who averaged ten days to femoral fracture stabilization. Decreased function occurred when only one of the fractures, generally that in the femur, was surgically stabilized. Floating-knee lesions do best with surgical fracture stabilization within 24 hours of injury. In the case of ipsilateral diaphyseal fractures of the femur and tibia, the best treatment is closed intramedullary nailing of both femur and tibia. Unfortunately, these fractures are often comminuted. Various combinations of nails, plates, and external fixation may be necessary. In grade III open fractures about the knee, immediate plate fixation may be necessary, but this is a risky procedure because the infection rate averages 15%.

The Open Femoral Shaft Fracture

Open fractures of the femur occur approximately 80% of the time in multiply injured patients.[25] Treatment methods, such as traction, that limit patient mobility and wound access should be avoided if possible. Currently there is controversy as to whether open femoral shaft fractures should be stabilized immediately or delayed, or whether stabilization should be by internal or external fixation. Dabezies and associates,[26] using external fixation, noted a 30% incidence of soft-tissue infection (generally secondary to pin-tract problems), 50% loss of knee motion, and a 15% rate of malunion (Fig. 9). Because of these problems and the difficulty of converting from external fixation to internal fixation because of contaminated pin sites, I have avoided external fixation in the femur except in extreme cases of contamination. Intramedullary nailing has proven to be the most consistent and dependable method for handling femoral shaft fractures and is my treatment of choice in the open fracture.

Recent studies[25,27–29] have given us better information as to the timing of intramedullary nailing of open femoral fractures (Table 4). From these articles and presentations several factors can be noted. External fixation in the femoral shaft has been problematic and is in-

Table 4
Infection rate with intramedullary nailing of open femoral shaft fracture

Study	Type I	Type II	Types IIIA and IIIB	Overall
Lhowe and Hansen[28]*				
No.	25	19	8	42
Rate	0	10%	0	5%
Brumback and associates[12,18]†				
No.	27	16	46	89
Rate	0	0	6%	3%
Templeman and associates[25]†				
No.	31	16	21	68
Rate	0	0	4.8%	1.5%
Overall				
No.	73	51	75	199
Rate	0	4%	5%	3%

*All immediate.
†Delayed and immediate.

creasingly avoided. The infection rate (1% to 4%) following reamed intramedullary nailing of open femoral fractures has been acceptable. In type I and II fractures, there is little difference in the infection rate between delayed intramedullary nailing at approximately ten days and immediate intramedullary nailing. The advantages of immediate reamed intramedullary nailing in all multiply injured patients with open femoral fractures offsets the slightly increased risk of infection.

I recommend that grade I and II open fractures have immediate irrigation and debridement and placement of a locked intramedullary nail. Static locking of the nail is recommended to prevent motion at the fracture site and allow uncomplicated wound healing. In the multiply injured patient, I recommend that grade III open femoral shaft fractures be treated similarly. In patients with an isolated type III open femoral fracture, consider delayed nailing. In instances of extreme contamination, such as in a farm injury or an open fracture with a vascular injury, consideration should be given to external fixation as opposed to intramedullary nailing. A stacked half-pin frame is recommended (Fig. 10).

Tibial Fracture Stabilization

Early fracture stabilization of the tibia is not as crucial as in the femoral shaft fracture. Increasingly, however, we stabilize tibial shaft fractures nearly as frequently as those of the femoral shaft. This is because many of these are open fractures that require immediate irrigation and debridement with fracture stabilization, or are part of the floating-knee lesion that occurs frequently in the multiply injured patient.

Tibial fractures can be categorized as proximal metaphyseal fractures, diaphyseal fractures, distal metaphyseal fractures, and open fractures. The proximal tibial fracture can occur as a simple depressed tibial plateau fracture that may require simple elevation and

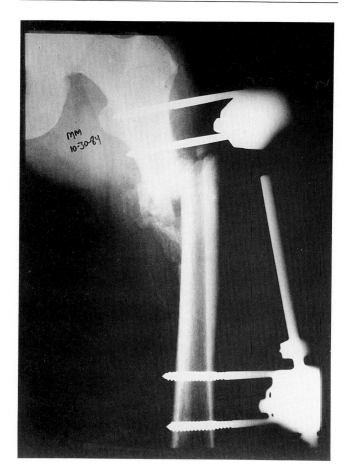

Fig. 9   Malunion of an open femoral fracture treated by external fixation.

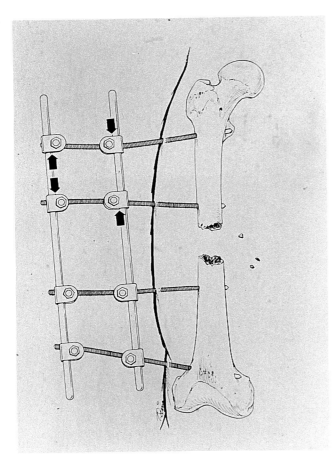

Fig. 10 Stacked half-pin frame on open femoral fracture.

stabilization by means of a single medial or lateral buttress plate with screws. Those proximal fractures that are of major concern are the tibial plateau fracture with marked depression and displacement, or those with significant diaphyseal extension. Surgical procedures on these fracture patterns can lead to major soft-tissue complications if care is not taken. Avoid the use of medial and lateral incisions; instead, perform a long midline incision. If simultaneous access to both the medial and lateral aspects of the proximal tibia is necessary, an osteotomy can be performed on the tibial tubercle or the patellar tendon can be incised by means of a Z-plasty. Avoid the simultaneous use of medial and lateral plates on proximal tibial fractures. Place the most logical plate, either medial or lateral, and then use an external fixator on the contralateral side if necessary. Remove the external fixator approximately three to four weeks after injury, following early fracture consolidation. This will prevent the extensive soft-tissue and infection problems associated with the application of dual plates.

In the multiply injured patient, give strong consid-

eration to intramedullary nailing of diaphyseal fractures of the tibia. I usually use a reamed nail in closed fractures and an unreamed nail in open fractures.[30] If compartment syndrome is a concern with acute tibial fractures, an unreamed locked nail may be used in closed fractures as well. Grades II and III open fractures of the tibia can be treated with Ender nails, a Lottes nail, or, more recently, an unreamed locked intramedullary nail. Infection rates with all of these appear to be similar to those with external fixation. The use of nails avoids some of the problems of external fixation, such as nonunion (7% to 20%), malunion (9% to 37%), contaminated pin sites (50%), and infection (2% to 10%).[31] Wound access and patient mobility can also be a problem with external fixation.

External fixation of open tibial fractures is still the standard nationally, particularly for grades II and III open fractures, fractures that require fasciotomies for release of compartment syndrome, vascular injuries, and the multiply injured pediatric patient with multiple fractures. Use a half-pin unilateral frame. Unilateral frames with half pins can be combined to form a triangulated frame that has strength of fixation equivalent to a normal tibia.

Distal tibial metaphyseal fractures present a situation similar to the proximal tibial metaphyseal fractures. Two fracture patterns occur, simple ankle fracture patterns that follow rotation or inversion forces and explosion (pilon) fractures caused by axial loading. Simple ankle fractures are treated in the usual fashion. If internal fixation is indicated, it should be done immediately. Repair of a pilon fracture can be a difficult undertaking in the multiply injured patient.[32] The major problem is marked immediate soft-tissue swelling, which can result in extensive fracture blisters within eight to ten hours of the fracture. These fractures should all undergo immediate closed reduction with application of a compression dressing and evaluation as soon as possible. If surgical stabilization of the fracture cannot be performed within eight hours of injury, severe fracture blisters may limit access to the fracture for a period of two to three weeks.

Current recommendations are for immediate open reduction and internal fixation of the pilon fracture using two incisions, one placed posteriorly along the distal fibula and the other placed anteromedially along the distal tibia with a minimum 7.5-cm skin bridge between the two incisions. The technique of fixation of the pilon fracture has been described by Rüedi and Allgöwer.[33] Step 1 is open reduction and internal fixation of the fibula, step 2 is reconstruction of the distal tibial articular surface, step 3 is bone grafting of large metaphyseal defects with cancellous bone graft, and step 4 is stabilization of the tibial fracture with plates and screws. Soft-tissue swelling may make it impossible to close the wound primarily. If this is the case, an attempt should be made to close the most significant wound and leave the other wound open with the intention of performing delayed primary closure. Under no circumstances should wounds in this area be closed under tension.

Upper-Extremity Fractures

Most upper-extremity fractures are of significantly lower priority than those in the lower extremity. Once again, open fractures in the upper extremity are relatively common in the multiply injured patient. As opposed to the lower extremity, fine motor function is crucial and the anatomic restoration of long bones, particularly in the forearm, should be achieved if possible.

The floating elbow, an ipsilateral fracture of the humerus and forearm (Fig. 11), occurs with relative frequency in the multiply injured patient. Surgical stabilization of both the humeral shaft fracture and the forearm fracture is almost always indicated. It is virtually impossible to obtain near-normal elbow function without surgical stabilization of both fractures.

It seems that fractures of the humeral shaft are seen with increasing frequency in the multiply injured patient. Often this fracture is complicated by injury of the radial and ulnar nerves. Humeral shaft fractures require surgical stabilization more frequently in the multiply injured patient than in patients with isolated fractures. I recommend compression-plate fixation. Commonly I apply the plate posteriorly through a triceps-splitting incision, which allows exploration of the radial nerve as well as the ulnar nerve if indicated. I routinely plate distal-third fractures of the humerus in the multiply injured patient. Other options for fixation of humeral shaft fractures include unreamed intramedullary nails, which can make stabilization of the humerus a less time-consuming procedure in the multiply injured patient. Some newer nails allow cross-locking.

In the patient under consideration, the simple transverse humeral shaft fracture is a high-energy injury with avulsion of the triceps tendon from the olecranon and major injury to the brachialis muscle in conjunction with radial and ulnar nerve deficits. The radiograph does not reflect the severity of injury.

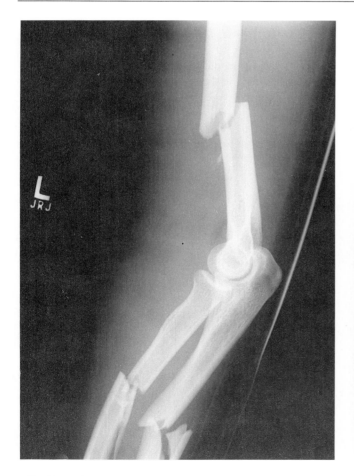
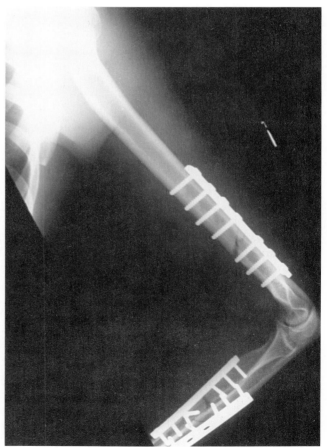

Fig. 11 **Left,** Floating elbow. **Right,** Fractures of humerus and forearm treated by plate fixation.

Surgical treatment of intra-articular fractures of the distal humerus is a difficult undertaking in the multiply injured patient. Because of the required prone positioning of the patient and the difficult, extensive nature of the procedure, this treatment should be reserved for a more controlled, quiet setting.

Treat both-bone forearm fractures with compression plating and bone grafting of large defects. Proximal ulnar fractures are treated by means of a tension-band wire or a small fragment plate as indicated. I generally treat unstable comminuted intra-articular fractures of the distal radius by closed reduction and external fixation. This usually permits excellent function and good access to open fractures.

References

1. Seibel R, LaDuca J, Hassett JM, et al: Blunt multiple trauma (ISS 36), femur traction, and the pulmonary failure-septic state. *Ann Surg* 1985;202:283–295.
2. American College of Surgeons Committee on Trauma: Field categorization of trauma patients and hospital trauma index. *Bull Am Coll Surg* 1980;65:32–33.
3. Baker SP, O'Neill B, Haddon W Jr. et al: The injury severity score: A method of describing patients with multiple injuries and evaluating emergency care. *J Trauma* 1974;14:187–196.
4. Bone LB, Johnson KD, Weigelt J, et al: Early versus delayed stabilization of femoral fractures: A prospective randomized study. *J Bone Joint Surg* 1989;71A:336–340.
5. Johnson KD, Cadambi A, Seibert GB: Incidence of adult respiratory distress syndrome in patients with multiple musculoskeletal injuries: Effect of early operative stabilization of fractures. *J Trauma* 1985;25:375–384.
6. Goris RJA, Draaisma J: Causes of death after blunt trauma. *J Trauma* 1982;22:141–146.
7. Goris RJ, Gimbrère JS, Van Niekerk JL, et al: Early osteosynthesis and prophylactic mechanical ventilation in the multitrauma patient. *J Trauma* 1982;22:895–903.
8. Riska EB, Myllynen P: Fat embolism in patients with multiple injuries. *J Trauma* 1982;22:891–894.
9. Wolff G, Oittman M, Ruedi T, et al: Koordination von chirurgie und intensivmedizin zur vermeidun per posttraumatischen respiratorische insuffizienz. *Monats Unfallheilkd* 1978;81:425–442.
10. Winquist RA, Hansen ST Jr, Clawson DK: Closed intramedullary nailing of femoral fractures: A report of five hundred and twenty cases. *J Bone Joint Surg* 1984;66A:529–539.
11. Shifflett MW, Bray TJ: Subtrochanteric femur fractures treated by Zickel and Grosse-Kempf nailing. Presented at the 54th Annual Meeting of the American Academy of Orthopaedic Surgeons, San Francisco, Jan 25, 1987.
12. Brien W, Wiss DA, Peter K, et al: Subtrochanteric fractures of the femur: Treatment with locked medullary nails. Presented at the 54th Annual Meeting of the American Academy of Orthopaedic Surgeons, San Francisco, Jan 25, 1987.
13. Garbarino JL, Brumback RJ, Poka A, et al: Closed interlocking intramedullary nailing of subtrochanteric fractures. Presented at

the 54th Annual Meeting of the American Academy of Orthopaedic Surgeons, San Francisco, Jan 25, 1987.
14. Wiss DA, Brien W, Becker V, et al: Subtrochanteric femur fractures: A comparison between the Zickel nail, 95° blade plate, and interlocking nail. Presented at the 56th Annual Meeting of the American Academy of Orthopaedic Surgeons, Las Vegas, Feb 11, 1989.
15. Johnson KD: Current techniques in the treatment of subtrochanteric fractures. *Techn Orthop* 1988;3:14–24.
16. Henry SL, Williams M, Seligson D: The Williams interlocking Y nail for fixation of proximal femoral fractures. *Techn Orthop* 1988;3:25–32.
17. Brumback RJ, Reilly JP, Poka A, et al: Intramedullary nailing of femoral shaft fractures: Part I. Decision-making errors with interlocking fixation. *J Bone Joint Surg* 1988;70A:1441–1452.
18. Brumback RJ, Uwagie-Ero S, Lakatos PR, et al: Intramedullary nailing of femoral shaft fractures: Part II. Fracture healing with static interlocking fixation. *J Bone Joint Surg* 1988;70A:1453–1462.
19. Zickel RE, Fietti VG Jr, Lansing JF III, et al: A new intramedullary fixation device for the distal third of the femur. *Clin Orthop* 1977;125:185–191.
20. Casey MJ, Chapman MW: Ipsilateral concomitant fractures of the hip and femoral shaft. *J Bone Joint Surg* 1979;61A:503–509.
21. Swiontkowski MF, Hansen ST Jr, Kellam J: Ipsilateral fractures of the femoral neck and shaft: A treatment protocol. *J Bone Joint Surg* 1984;66A:260–268.
22. Blake R, McBryde A Jr: The floating knee: Ipsilateral fractures of the tibia and femur. *South Med J* 1975;68:13–16.
23. McBryde AM Jr, Blake R: The floating knee: Ipsilateral fractures of the femur and tibia, abstract. *J Bone Joint Surg* 1974;56A:1309.
24. Veith RG, Winquist RA, Hansen ST Jr: Ipsilateral fractures of the femur and tibia: A report of fifty-seven consecutive cases. *J Bone Joint Surg* 1984;66A:991–1002.
25. Templeman DC, Sweeny C, Chapman MW, et al: Critical analysis of the management of open femur fractures at two regional trauma centers. Presented at the 56th Annual Meeting of the American Academy of Orthopaedic Surgeons, Las Vegas, Feb 13, 1989.
26. Dabezies EJ, D'Ambrosia R, Shoji H, et al: Fractures of the femoral shaft treated by external fixation with the Wagner device. *J Bone Joint Surg* 1984;66A:360–364.
27. Chapman MW: The role of intramedullary fixation in open fractures. *Clin Orthop* 1986;212:26–34.
28. Lhowe DW, Hansen ST: Immediate nailing of open fractures of the femoral shaft. *J Bone Joint Surg* 1988;70A:812–820.
29. Brumback RJ, Ellison PS, Jr, Poka A, et al: Intramedullary nailing of open fractures of the femoral shaft. *J Bone Joint Surg* 1989;71A:1324–1330.
30. Bone LB, Johnson KD: Treatment of tibial fractures by reaming and intramedullary nailing. *J Bone Joint Surg* 1986;68A:877–887.
31. Karlström G, Olerud S: Percutaneous pin fixation of open tibial fractures: Double-frame anchorage using the Vidal-Adrey method. *J Bone Joint Surg* 1975;57A:915–924.
32. Kellam JF, Waddell JP: Fractures of the distal tibial metaphysis with intra-articular extension: The distal tibial explosion fracture. *J Trauma* 1979;19:593–601.
33. Rüedi TB, Allgöwer M: The operative treatment of intra-articular fractures of the lower end of the tibia. *Clin Orthop* 1979;138:105–110.

Evaluation and Treatment of Trauma to the Vertebral Column

Daniel R. Benson, MD

Timothy L. Keenen, MD

Introduction: Incidence, Etiology, and Demographics

When vertebral column injury occurs, some degree of neurologic deficit is present in a significant percentage of cases. Neurologic damage occurs in 40% of patients with fracture at the cervical level[1-3] and in 15% to 20% of patients with fracture at thoracolumbar levels.[1,4] Each year about 11,000 new spinal cord injuries require treatment.[5,6] This chapter segment will outline methods for initial evaluation and treatment of vertebral column injuries with emphasis on minimizing risk of further damage and maximizing the likelihood of neurologic recovery.

In patients who have had trauma or multiple injuries, there is a risk of overlooking fracture of the spine. For this reason, it is important that an accurate history, a thorough physical examination, and proper roentgenograms be done on these patients. Frequently, diagnosis of vertebral injury is delayed because the patient is unconscious, has life-threatening polytrauma, or has used alcohol and/or intravenous drugs and is intoxicated. Of vertebral column injuries, 45% are caused by motor-vehicle accidents, 20% by falls, 15% as a result of sports injuries, and 15% from acts of violence.[1-4,6,7] Among patients aged 75 years and older, falls account for 60% of spinal fractures.[6] The incidence of such injuries is four times greater among males than females.

Relevant Anatomy and Pathophysiology

Drawing the correct conclusions from the initial physical examination of the spine-injured patient requires a basic knowledge of the spinal column osseous and neurologic structures. Knowledge of the fracture patterns in each anatomic area of the spine (cervical, thoracic, lumbar) allows the examining physician to determine the relative stability of the injury, the risk of an associated neurologic deficit, and the specific type of treatment needed.

Spinal Cord Anatomy

The spinal cord fills about 35% of the canal at the level of the atlas,[8] and approximately 50% of the canal in the lower cervical spine—vertebrae C2 through C7—and in the thoracolumbar segments (Fig. 1). The remainder of the canal is filled with cerebrospinal fluid, epidural fat, and dura mater. The spinal cord has a variable diameter, with swelling in the cervical and lum-

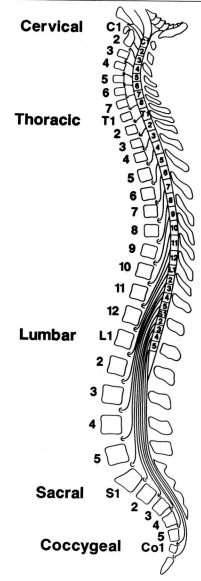

Fig. 1 The myelomere, or segment of cord from which a nerve root arises, lies one level above the same numbered vertebral body. The lumbar and sacral myelomeres are concentrated between the T11 and L1 vertebral bodies. The end of the spinal cord (conus medullaris) is usually found at the levels of the L1-L2 intervertebral disk.

bar regions for the exiting nerve roots of the cervical and lumbosacral plexi. The myelomere, or segment of cord from which a nerve root arises, lies one level above the same numbered vertebral body. For example, the

T5 myelomere lies at the level of the T4 vertebral body. The lumbar and sacral myelomeres are concentrated between the Tll and Ll vertebral bodies. The end of the spinal cord, or conus medullaris, is usually found at the level of the L1-L2 intervertebral disk. The conus medullaris contains the myelomeres of the five sacral nerve roots.

The relative positions of gray and white matter structures are consistent throughout the length of the cord, but the proportions of the two vary at different levels. The white matter carries the long-tract fibers from the cervical, thoracic, lumbar, and sacral levels, and occupies more cross-sectional area cervically than it does sacrally. The gray matter, with its concentration of lower motor neurons, is prominent in the cervical and lumbar swellings where the axons exit to innervate the upper and lower extremities.

The upper motor neurons originate in the cerebral cortex, cross to the opposite side in the mid-brain, and then descend in the lateral corticospinal tract to connect synaptically with the respective lower motor neurons in the anterior horn of the gray matter. The sacral fibers of the corticospinal tract are most peripheral and the cervical most central (Fig. 2).

The ascending sensory input originates in an axon from the cell body located in the dorsal root ganglion within the vertebral foramen. Sensory input enters the posterior horn of the gray matter and travels cephalad by routes that depend on the type of sensation. Pain and temperature sensation immediately cross to the opposite side of the cord and ascend in the lateral spinothalamic tract. Touch, which also crosses immedi-

ately, ascends in a diffuse manner, primarily in the ventral or anterior spinothalamic tract. Proprioceptive position and vibratory sensation ascend in the fibers of the posterior column and cross higher in the brain stem. In the posterior column, the sacral elements are once again more peripheral than the lumbar, thoracic, or cervical ones (Fig. 2).

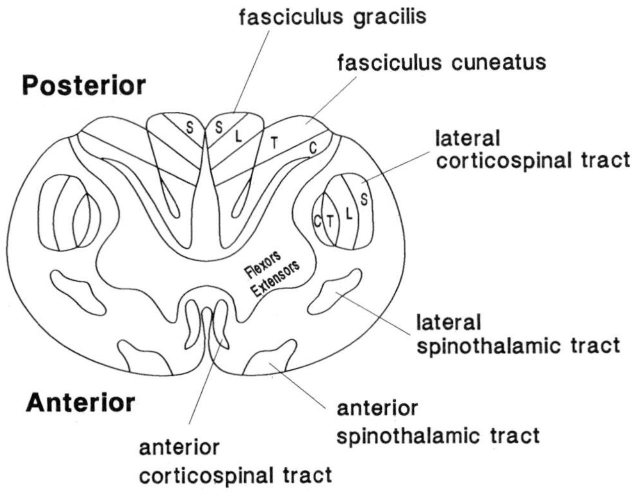

Reflex Arc

The reflex arc, such as the bulbocavernosus, is a simple sensory motor pathway that can function without using either ascending or descending white matter long-tract axons. If the level of the reflex arc is both physiologically and anatomically intact, then the reflex will function despite disruption of the spinal cord at a higher level (Fig. 3).

Cauda Equina

Below the level of the conus medullaris at the interspace between L1 and L2, the spinal canal is filled with the cauda equina (the motor and sensory roots). These roots, which exit caudally through their respective foramen, are less likely to be injured because they have more room in the canal and are tethered to a lesser degree than the spinal cord. Furthermore, because the motor nerve root is distal to the lower motor neuron axon and is therefore a peripheral nerve, it is more

Fig. 2 Transverse view of the spinal cord in the cervical region. Note that the sacral structures are most peripheral in both the posterior columns and in the lateral corticospinal tracts. The extensors are also more lateral than the flexors in the gray matter. These anatomic features are important in understanding injury to the spinal cord.

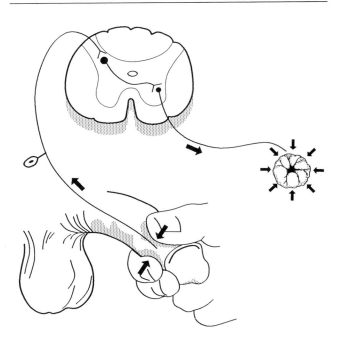

Fig. 3 The bulbocavernosus, a reflex arc that is a simple sensorimotor pathway, can function without using ascending or descending white matter long-tract axons. After spinal shock is over, if the level of the reflex arc is both physiologically and anatomically intact, the reflex will function despite complete spinal cord disruption at a higher level.

resilient to trauma than is central nervous tissue (Fig. 1).

Pathophysiology of Spinal Cord Injury

Spinal cord deficit is more frequently caused by contusion and compression than by complete transection. The initial blunt injury sets off a sequence of molecular-level events that result in ischemia, tissue hypoxia, and secondary tissue degeneration.[9] The secondary post-traumatic tissue degeneration has in the past been attributed, at least in part, to edema. It appears from animal research that 10% of the axons in the ventral funiculus are enough for near-normal ambulation.[10] If the initial insult spares these fibers, and secondary damage to them can be prevented, a better recovery from spinal cord injury can be expected.

The term "spinal shock" is defined as a spinal cord nervous tissue dysfunction based on physiologic rather than structural disruption. Spinal shock has resolved when the reflex arcs below the level of the injury begin to function again. The term neurogenic shock is defined as vascular hypotension with bradycardia as a result of spinal injury. The first few minutes after spinal cord injury are associated with hypertension and tachycardia, followed by a drop in pressure and pulse rate. Neurogenic shock is attributed to traumatic disruption of sympathetic outflow at vertebrae T1 through L2 and unopposed vagal tone.

Patterns of Neurologic Injury

One of the most important initial responsibilities of the examining physician in evaluating spinal cord injury is to distinguish between complete and incomplete neurologic deficit. With complete neurologic deficit, functional motor recovery is seen in only 3% of such injuries in the first 24 hours and drops to virtually none after 24 to 48 hours.[2,11] An incomplete neurologic deficit has a good prognosis for at least some functional motor recovery. The incomplete deficit is evidenced by one of several patterns of partial neurologic function. A well-established method of recording the functional degree of neurologic deficit is the Frankel classification (Outline 1). First described in 1969 by Frankel and associates,[12] this classification is probably the most widely used method to record the patient's level of neurologic deficit.

Complete Deficit

A complete neurologic deficit is evidenced by absence of motor and sensory function caudal to the spinal column injury, and presence of the bulbocavernosus reflex. The presence of the bulbocavernosus reflex indicates that the S3, S4 region of the conus

Outline 1
Frankel classification

A. Absent motor and sensory function
B. Sensation present, motor absent
C. Sensation present, motor active but not useful
D. Sensation present, motor active and useful
E. Normal motor + sensory function

medullaris of the spinal cord is physiologically and anatomically functional, and that there is no spinal shock. So long as bulbocavernosus reflex is absent, and motor and sensory function are likewise absent below the level of the spine injury, the lesion cannot be classified until return of the bulbocavernosus reflex signals the end of spinal shock. In 99% of patients, the bulbocavernosus reflex will return within 24 hours.[13] A lack of neurologic function below the level of the spinal column injury after cessation of spinal shock indicates that the lesion is a complete one and that the prognosis for recovery is bleak.

Incomplete Neurologic Deficit

If some degree of neurologic function persists below the level of the injury, the lesion is incomplete. As a general rule, the greater the function distal to the lesion and the more rapid the recovery, the better is the prognosis.[14]

The concept of sacral sparing in the incomplete spinal cord injury is important, as it represents at least partial structural continuity of the white-matter long tracts (corticospinal and spinothalamic tracts). Sacral sparing is evidenced by perianal sensation, rectal and motor function, and great-toe flexor activity. A comparison of Figure 2, representing the normal anatomy, with Figure 4, representing an incomplete lesion, shows how preservation of the peripheral fibers helps to preserve the sacral white matter despite damage to the central fibers. Sacral sparing allows continued function of the lower sacral motor neurons in the conus medullaris, and spares their connections via the spinal cord to the cerebral cortex. Presence of sacral sparing therefore indicates an incomplete cord injury and leaves the potential for more function at resolution of spinal shock. During physical examination in the emergency room, sacral sparing may be the only indication that the lesion is incomplete. Documentation of its presence or absence is essential.

On the other hand, because absence of sacral neurologic function may be the only neurologic deficit at the time of examination, a failure to include specific testing of perianal sensation, rectal tone, and great-toe flexion may result in a misdiagnosis of normal. A patient whose injury is limited to the conus medullaris will be able to move both lower extremities, and the pain of injury can prevent subjective detection of perianal sensory loss. Whenever there is a possibility of

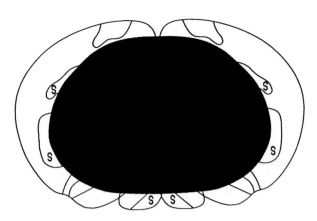

Fig. 4 This illustration of a central-cord syndrome can be compared with Figure 2 to appreciate the spinal cord abnormality. Here, an incomplete spinal injury affects the more central but not the peripheral fibers, thereby preserving the sacral white fibers. This is why sacral sparing can occur despite an otherwise seemingly complete neurologic lesion. The sparing indicates an incomplete lesion and therefore potential for more return of function after the resolution of spinal shock.

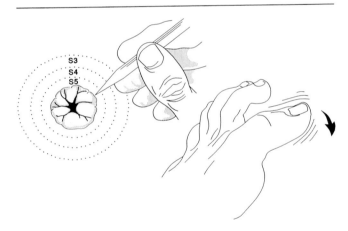

Fig. 5 Sacral sparing may include the triad of perianal sensation, rectal tone, and great toe flexion. The examiner must complete and record his findings of sacral-root function in all patients with spinal cord injuries.

spine injury, the examiner must complete testing of sacral root function and record the findings (Fig. 5).

Specific Incomplete Neurologic Syndromes

Central Cord Syndrome

The most common pattern of incomplete neurologic injury, this represents central gray-matter destruction with preservation of only the peripheral spinal cord structures—the sacral spinothalamic and corticospinal tracts (Table 1). Usual symptoms are distal motor and sensory paralysis with preserved perianal sensation and an early return of bowel and bladder control. Any return of motor function generally begins with the sacral elements of toe flexion and then extension, followed by the lumbar elements of the ankle, knee, and hip. Return of upper-extremity function is usually minimal and depends on the degree of central gray-matter destruction. The chance of some functional motor recovery is reported to be about 75%.[15]

Anterior Cord Syndrome

With anterior cord syndrome, the patient has complete motor and sensory loss except for retained trunk and lower-extremity deep pressure, pain sensation, and proprioception.[16] This syndrome carries the worst prognosis for return of function, with only a 10% chance of functional motor recovery.[17]

Posterior Cord Syndrome

Posterior cord syndrome is a rare syndrome that consists of loss of deep pressure, deep pain, and proprioception with otherwise normal cord function. The result is usually a patient who ambulates with a foot-slapping gait, similar to that described in tabes dorsalis.

Brown-Séquard Syndrome

This syndrome, caused by a unilateral cord injury, is characterized clinically by a motor deficit ipsilateral to the spinal cord injury in combination with a contralateral pain and temperature hypoesthesia. Virtually all of these patients show partial recovery and regain near-normal bowel and bladder function and the ability to ambulate.[15]

Root Injury

The spinal nerve root exiting at the level of the fracture may be injured, either alone, or in conjunction with the spinal cord at that level. The prognosis for motor return of that nerve root is good, with high cervical lesions having a 30% chance, mid-cervical lesions a 60% chance, and lower cervical injuries a 100% chance of recovery of at least one nerve root level.[15,17] Injuries to the cauda equina are root injuries and therefore have a reasonable prognosis for recovery (Table 1).

Initial Evaluation

The initial evaluation of any trauma patient begins at the scene of the accident with the time-honored ABCs of resuscitation, such as the Advanced Trauma Life Support method described by the American College of Surgeons.[18] The Airway, Breathing, and Circulation method might in fact better be called Airway and Cervical Spine, Breathing, and Circulation. All patients with potential spine injuries should be brought to the emergency room on a backboard with the cervical

Table 1
Incomplete cord syndromes

Syndrome	Frequency	Description	Functional Recovery
Central	Most common	Usually quadriplegic with sacral sparing. Upper extremities affected more than lower.	75%
Anterior	Common	Complete motor deficit. Trunk and lower-extremity deep pressure and proprioception preserved.	10%
Posterior	Rare	Loss of deep pressure, deep pain and proprioception	—
Brown-Séquard	Uncommon	Ipsilateral motor deficit. Contralateral pain and temperature deficit.	>90%
Root	Common	Sensorimotor deficit in dermatonal distribution	30% to 100%*

*See text

spine immobilized. A spinal column injury should be suspected in all polytrauma patients, especially those who are unconscious, intoxicated, or have head-and-neck injuries. The only part of the initial assessment that pertains solely to the spine is the lateral cervical spine radiograph showing the areas from the occiput to the superior end plate of T1. This radiograph serves to determine the safest means of establishing and maintaining an airway.

Neurogenic shock is evidenced by hypotension associated with bradycardia or a normal heart rate. When hypotension is associated with tachycardia, some cause other than neurogenic shock must be sought. A review of 228 cervical spine-injury patients revealed that, of 58 patients whose systolic blood pressure was less than 100 mm Hg, 40, or 69%, had neurogenic shock. In the other 18 patients the hypotension was caused by other associated major injury.[19]

Neurogenic shock is treated initially by volume replacement, followed by a vasopressor if hypotension without tachycardia persists despite volume expansion.[18] Overinfusion of the patient with hypotensive spinal cord injury can cause fatal pulmonary edema.[20] The degree of hypotension, bradycardia, and incidence of cardiac arrest is directly related to the Frankel grade. For example, in a study of 45 patients with acute cervical spinal cord injury, 87% of the Frankel A patients had a daily average pulse rate of less than 55 bpm, 21% had cardiac arrest, and 39% required the use of atropine or a vasopressor. In Frankel B patients, by comparison, 62% had average pulses of less than 55 bpm and none had cardiac arrest or a need for vasopressors.[21] Endotracheal suctioning is a cause of severe bradycardia and may induce cardiac arrest, attributable to vagal stimulation. Repeated doses of atropine may be necessary to restore the heart rate.

The patient wearing a helmet at the time of injury should arrive in the emergency room with it still in place unless a face shield obstructed ventilation and could not be removed separately or the helmet was too loose-fitting to allow adequate cervical spine immobilization.[22] In preparing for intubation, a patient with a suspected spine injury should have the airway maintained using a jaw-thrust maneuver rather than a head-tilt method.

Secondary assessment includes evaluation of the spinal column and spinal cord function. It is recommended that a flow sheet be used to record the initial findings (Fig. 6). Evaluation usually begins with a physical examination. A more detailed history is elicited later.

History

A minimal history should note any symptoms such as transient paralysis or even numbness or tingling of an extremity that might suggest an injury to the spinal cord or its roots. Alternately, a patient who seems completely paralyzed, but reports a period of perianal or lower-extremity sensation or any movement of the lower extremities, may have an incomplete spinal cord injury and a chance for some neurologic recovery.

Physical Examination

With an unconscious or intoxicated patient, it is difficult to assess pain and sensorimotor function. Careful observation of spontaneous extremity motion may be the only source of information indicating spinal cord function, and a detailed examination must wait until the patient is able to cooperate. With the unconscious patient, response to noxious stimuli, reflexes, and rectal tone may provide some information on the status of the cord. Similarly, spontaneous respiration with elevation and separation of the costal margins on inspiration indicates normal thoracic innervation and intercostal function. The unconscious patient should be rolled onto his side with the cervical spine immobilized while using the full-length backboard, and the entire length of the spine inspected for deformity, abrasions, and ecchymosis. The spinous processes should be palpated, noting any step-off or interspinous widening. A well-executed, four-person log roll without the use of a full-length backboard has been associated with both anterior and lateral translation of thoracolumbar frac-

SPINE FRACTURE FLOW SHEET

MEDICAL REC NO.:

NAME:

BIRTH DATE:

ADMIT DATE:

INJURY DATE:

DISCHARGE DATE:

SEX:

DIAGNOSIS:

TREATMENT

    NON-SURGICAL:

    SURGICAL:

2 YR	1 YR	6 MO	3 MO	1 MO	1 WK	INIT.	Date LEFT	Muscles		Date RIGHT	INIT.	1 WK	1 MO	3 MO	6 MO	1 YR	2 YR
								Diaphragm	C-4	+/-							
							0-5	BICEPS	C-5	0-5							
							0-5	WRIST EXT	C-6	0-5							
							0-5	TRICEPS	C-7	0-5							
							0-5	FINGER FLEX	C-8	0-5							
							0-5	INTRINSIC	T-1	0-5							
								Intercost	2-9	+/-							
								Abdominal	10-12	+/-							
								Cremasteric	T12-L1	+/-							
							0-5	ILIOPSOAS	L-2	0-5							
							0-5	QUADRICEP	L-3	0-5							
							0-5	TIB ANTER	L-4	0-5							
							0-5	EX HALLIC	L-5	0-5							
							0-5	GASTROC	S-1	0-5							
								Blad sph	S-2	+/-							
								Anal sph	S-3	+/-							
								B-C reflex	S-3,4	+/-							

0 = No contraction
1 = Contracts without motion
2 = Contracts with motion (gravity eliminated)
3 = Motion against gravity
4 = Motion against resistance
5 = Normal motor strength

SENSORY:

DATE: _____   DATE: _____   DATE: _____

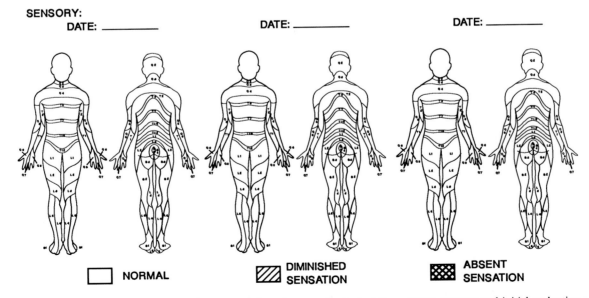

☐ NORMAL   ▨ DIMINISHED SENSATION   ▧ ABSENT SENSATION

Fig. 6 A neurologic examination time-oriented flow sheet can be devised for emergency room and initial evaluation use. This example lists the motor function of the major muscle groups and allows the examiner to illustrate the sensory loss over a period of time. A sheet like this can be invaluable when making surgical decisions or when evaluating results retrospectively.

tures.[23] For this reason, it is best to use a backboard during lateral turning. Any associated head-and-neck trauma increases the likelihood of cervical spine injury. Signs of thoracic or abdominal trauma, such as marks made by shoulder or lap seat belts, often indicate thoracolumbar spine injury.

The responsive patient who is hemodynamically stable may be examined in greater detail. The entire spine should be inspected and palpated as described above. Ask the patient to report the location of any pain, and to move upper and then lower extremities to help locate any gross neurologic deficit. As depicted in Figure 7 for the upper extremity and Figure 8 for the lower extremity, the extremities are examined for motor function by nerve root level. The motor examination includes a digital rectal examination for voluntary or reflex anal sphincter contraction. A flow sheet may be used to grade the strength of each muscle (Fig. 6).

The sensory examination tests the dermatomal pattern of the proprioception and pain and temperature pathways as previously described (Fig. 9). The sharp/dull sensation of a pin tests the pain pathway in the lateral spinothalamic tract. Proprioception, which travels the posterior columns, is tested easily by having the patient report the position of the toes as up, down, or neutral as the examiner moves them. Temperature sensation, which also passes through the lateral spinothalamic tract, is difficult to establish in emergency room settings, and is commonly deferred to a later time. Areas of sensory deficit should be accurately recorded, dated, and timed, using the medical record progress note or a spinal injury flow sheet (Fig. 6). It is recommended that the sensory level also be marked, dated, and timed in ink on the patient's skin at the affected level. This practice can avoid much uncertainty when multiple sequential examiners are involved.

Figure 10 reviews the locations of the upper- and lower-extremity stretch reflexes and their respective nerve roots of origin. Spinal shock may cause absence of all reflexes for up to 24 hours, followed by hyper-reflexia, muscle spasticity, and clonus. When a spine-injured patient with a neurologic deficit has a concomitant head injury, it is important to determine which is injured: a cranial upper motor neuron, a spinal cord lower motor neuron, or both. The presence of extremity stretch reflexes in the patient without spontaneous motion of the extremities or a response to noxious stimuli implies an upper motor neuron origin. The absence of these reflexes in the same setting implies a lower motor neuron injury.

The plantar reflex in the lower extremity is elicited by stroking the plantar aspect of the foot firmly with pointed object, and watching the direction of a motion of the toes. A normal plantar reflex is plantar flexion of the toes. An abnormal plantar reflex, in which the great toe extends and the toes splay out, is called the Babinski sign and represents an upper motor neuron

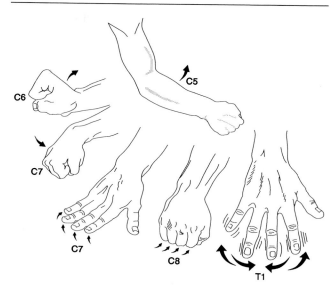

Fig. 7 An examination of the upper extremities must include, at a minimum, the muscle groups that are designated by their respective nerve root innervation. These are C5, elbow flexion; C6, wrist extension; C7, finger extension; C8, finger flexion; and T1, finger abduction. The strength (0 to 5) should be listed on the time-oriented flow sheet.

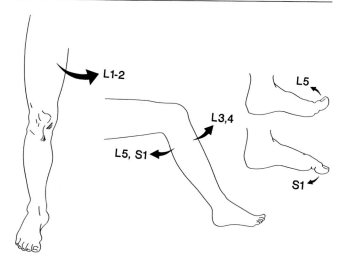

Fig. 8 An examination of the lower extremities needs to include at least these muscle groups. Designated by their respective nerve root innervation, they are L1-2, hip abductors; L3-4, knee extension; L5, S1, knee flexion; L5, great toe extension; and S1, great toe flexion.

lesion. Similar information is gained by firmly running a finger down the tibial crest.

Other important reflexes include the cremasteric, the anal wink, and the bulbocavernosus reflexes. The cremasteric reflex, which tests nerve root T12-L1, is elicited by stroking the proximal inner thigh with a pointed instrument while observing the scrotal sac. A normal

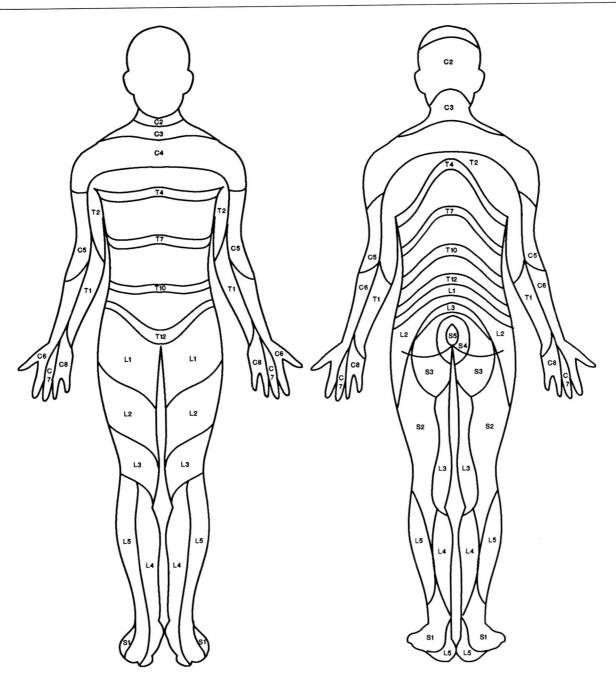

Fig. 9 Pain temperature dermatome chart. Note that C4 includes the upper chest just superior to T2. The rest of the cervical and T1 roots are represented in the upper extremities.

reflex involves contraction of the cremasteric muscle and an upward motion of the scrotal sac. An abnormal reflex involves no motion of the sac. The anal wink, which tests nerve roots S2, S3, and S4, is elicited by stroking the skin around the anal sphincter, and watching it contract. An abnormal reflex involves no contraction. Another test involving nerve roots S3 and S4 is the bulbocavernosus reflex (Fig. 3), which in the male

involves squeezing the glans penis and in the female applying pressure to the clitoris. Normal response is contraction of the anal sphincter. This can usually be elicited more easily in the male or female by gently pulling the Foley catheter balloon against the bladder wall while feeling for contraction of the anal sphincter.

Not uncommonly, a more detailed history is delayed until the patient is hemodynamically stable and the overall neurologic status is determined. In addition to the routine review of systems, the patient should be specifically questioned as to previous spine injury or neurologic deficits and the details of the mechanism of the current injury. If the patient is unable to respond, an attempt should be made to interview family members or observers of the accident personally or by telephone.

At some time during the physical examination the initial lateral cervical spine radiograph should be available for review. It should first be examined to insure that the interval from the occiput to the superior end plate of Tl can be seen clearly. If it is normal, the remainder of the cervical spine series is obtained. Spine precautions must be kept in place until after the cervical spine and any suspicious areas of the thoracolumbar spine have been cleared radiographically.

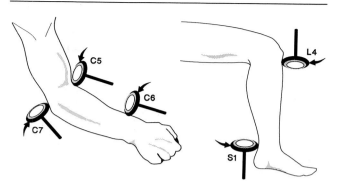

Fig. 10 The stretch reflexes shown on this illustration are represented by their respective nerve roots of origin. These are C5, biceps; C6, brachioradialis; C7, triceps; L4, patellar; and S1, Achilles tendon. In the presence of spinal shock, all reflexes may be absent for as long as 24 hours, only to be replaced by hyperreflexes, muscle spasticity, and clonus.

Management

Treatment

Underlying any treatment for the patient with spinal cord injury is the need to prevent further injury to an already compromised cord and to protect uninjured cord tissue. This is achieved primarily by immobilizing the spinal column during transport and evaluation. If indicated, immobilization should continue during surgical decompression and stabilization. Treatment begins at the scene of the accident, where trained paramedical personnel immobilize all areas of potential spinal injury. Specific extrication methods are used to remove patients from damaged vehicles.[22]

For patients with either an isolated injury or complicated polytrauma, a simple, reliable method of cervical and thoracolumbar immobilization is necessary to allow a complete, safe evaluation. The most effective method of initial cervical immobilization uses bilateral sand bags with the patient taped across the forehead to a spine board. Addition of a Philadelphia collar serves to limit extension.[24] In the cervical spine, the use of a soft collar, extrication collar, hard collar, or Philadelphia collar alone probably will not achieve sufficient immobilization.[24,25] A poster brace or cervicothoracic brace is not practical for use in emergency settings. A standard long spineboard is adequate for the immobilization and turning of the thoracolumbar spine.[2] Immobilization gear may be removed only after the radiographs have been interpreted as normal.

The unstable and/or dislocated cervical spine requires either a more stable immobilization or axial traction to achieve reduction. The concept of skull traction was introduced by Crutchfield in 1933,[26] but Crutchfield traction tongs have been replaced by the Gardner-Wells tongs and by halo immobilization devices. Although Gardner-Wells tongs are easy to use and are an effective means of applying axial traction for reduction, they do not significantly limit voluntary rotation, flex-

ion, or extension in the uncooperative patient. Gardner-Wells tongs can be applied after a brief skin preparation and without assistance. The halo ring allows axial traction for reduction and, with application of a vest, provides stable immobilization. The fact that it requires two people and takes longer to apply can be a disadvantage in a busy polytrauma setting.

Technique of Gardner-Wells Tong Application

Crutchfield tongs,[26] now largely superseded by the Gardner-Wells tongs, are applied higher on the skull (5 cm to either side of the midline). They facilitate turning the patient, but are more likely either to pull out or to penetrate the inner table of the skull.[20]

The Gardner-Wells tongs can be applied quickly and easily without assistance. A point 2 cm above the external auditory canal is selected, above the temporalis muscle. No shave or preparation is necessary, and the skin is infiltrated with local anesthetic after application of an antiseptic solution. In tightening the screws, care must be taken to do so symmetrically. The tongs are secure when the metal pressure pin protrudes 1 mm. It is recommended that the pin be tightened the next day to 1 mm, but not again thereafter.

Pharmocologic Treatment

The drugs with potential benefit to the patient with spinal cord injury include glucocorticoid steroids[9,11,27]; opiate antagonists, such as thyrotropin-releasing hormone[28,29,30]; opiate receptor antagonists, such as naloxone[28,20,31]; and osmotic diuretics, such as mannitol.[30,32] In animal studies, a significantly greater recovery from neurologic injury has been achieved with these as compared with controls. The clinical use of corticosteroids was based initially on the observation that their use significantly reduced cerebral edema around brain tumors.[33] Although benefits of steroids in neurooncology with spinal cord compression have been reported, no clinical study to date has documented the efficacy of steroids in spinal cord trauma.[9,11,33,34] Clinical studies are underway that attempt to correlate the efficacy of naloxone and thyrotropin-releasing hormone in spinal cord trauma.[29]

A higher incidence of gastrointestinal hemorrhage is associated with head and spinal cord injuries than with other types of trauma. The incidence is higher in cervical cord injuries than in lower-level injuries, and is higher in complete deficits than in incomplete ones.[35] A causative relationship between the short-term use of steroids and gastrointestinal hemorrhage has not been clearly established and remains controversial.[2,36,37,38] Given the absence of data documenting the efficacy of steroids in spinal cord injury, and the possibility of associated gastrointestinal hemorrhage, the routine use of steroids is not recommended.

Special Considerations in Polytrauma

Pediatrics

The spine is considered to become biomechanically mature at about 8 to 10 years of age.[39,40-42] Until that time injuries usually involve the soft tissues, and spinal column fracture is uncommon. Soft-tissue injuries cannot be seen on plain radiographs. Before the age of 10 years, the most common injury is in the occiput to C3 region.[40,41] The spectrum of neurologic involvement is associated with these injuries, including cranial-nerve lesions and vertebral-basilar signs such as vomiting and vertigo. Spinal cord injury without radiographic abnormality (SCIWORA) is most common in children under 10 years of age. Flexion, extension, and distracting cervical spine views may be useful in identifying the level, but extreme care must be taken to avoid further injury.[40] After the age of 10 years, the pattern of injury is similar to that seen in adults.

Recent attention has been paid to the techniques of initial immobilization in the pediatric patient, and a phenomenon called supine kyphosis anterior translation (SKAT) has been described.[42] In the normal development of the child, the head diameter grows at a logarithmic rate, achieving 50% of adult size by age 18 months; and the chest diameter grows at an arithmetical rate, achieving 50% of adult size at 8 years. Because of this, a young child supine on a standard backboard may have his head forced into kyphosis as a result of the normal disproportionate size of the large head and smaller trunk. Cases have been reported in which this forced kyphosis caused an anterior translation of the unstable pediatric spine.[42] The problem can be avoided by using a folded sheet to elevate the thorax of a child on a spineboard until the shoulders are level with the external auditory meatus. In the future it may be possible to use a specially designed pediatric backboard that has a cutout for the prominent occiput in the young child.

Missed Spine Fracture:

Delay in diagnosis of spinal trauma is not unusual. Between 22% and 33% of cervical spine injuries[2,43] and about 5% of thoracolumbar spine injuries are not diagnosed until later. In one series, as many as 22% of such injuries were not diagnosed until after arrival at a tertiary referral center. The main causes for delay are first, failure to take radiographs; second, not seeing a fracture on the radiograph; and third, which is less common, failure of the patient to seek medical attention. A secondary neurologic deficit developed in 10% of patients who had delayed diagnosis, compared with 1.5% of those diagnosed on initial evaluation.[43] Other factors associated with delayed diagnosis include intoxication, polytrauma, decreased level of consciousness, and noncontiguous spine fractures. Patients with spinal cord injuries who have hemiparesis have been admitted and discharged with the erroneous diagnosis of stroke.[2] Noncontiguous spine fractures account for about 4% to 5% of all spine fractures.[1,44]

Approximately 50% to 60% of spine-injured patients have an associated nonspinal injury ranging from a simple closed extremity fracture to a life-threatening thoracic and abdominal injury.[1,44] For the patient, a severe life-threatening injury has, in addition to the immediate danger, a significant risk of subsequent disability. Another source of disability lies in the small-bone fracture of an extremity, which may remain undiagnosed because of attention focused on the polytrauma. The potential for malunion or nonunion can prohibit or delay a patient's return to ambulation or employment. The reverse is also true, as for example when severe bilateral calcaneal fractures divert attention from an associated lumbar spine fracture. Craniofacial trauma is usually associated with cervical spine injuries and abdominal seat-belt ecchymosis associated with thoracolumbar injuries, but the opposite can also be true. It is important to remember that a patient may have severe facial injury and lumbar spine injury, or abdominal trauma and cervical spine injury.

Imaging

Transportation to Special Studies The patient with cervical spine injury who is in skull traction can be safely moved using a hospital bed, gurney, or Stryker frame, as long as a traction-pulley unit is used. Use of a Stryker frame alone has been associated with loss of reduction after turning and with worsening of neurologic deficit.[45] Traction may be compromised while the patient lies on the radiographic table with the rope temporarily disconnected from the pulley. Disturbance of magnetic resonance imaging by the ferrous elements of traction equipment can also present a problem, but solutions are being proposed. A patient with a high cervical spine injury, who is ventilator-dependent, will have to be hand ventilated or use a nonferrous ventilator during imaging.[46] The patient with thoracolumbar spine injury is easier to manage because plastic backboards are available that can remain in place while radiographs are made or magnetic resonance imaging is done.

Radiographic Examination Radiographs are the basic diagnostic tool for examining most patients. Cervical spine radiographs should include lateral, anteroposterior, and open-mouth views. If the lower cervical vertebrae are not observable through the standard views, then tomograms or a swimmer's view may be used for the lower cervical and upper thoracic area. For the thoracic lumbar spine, anteroposterior and lateral radiographs must to be done. In order to rule out trauma to the entire cervical spine, all seven cervical vertebrae must be visualized. The open-mouth view is necessary in order to demonstrate dens fractures and fractures of the ring of C1.

Tomography Computed tomographic scanning gives better visualization of the vertebral arches, facet joints, and the neural canal. It can be used for reconstruction in the coronal, sagittal, or oblique planes. Tomography is particularly helpful in evaluating fractures and can be used for clarification in the case of odontoid fractures, unilateral facet dislocations, and thoracic fractures. It is also helpful in determining the integrity of the canal when computed tomography is not available.

Myelography Although myelography is seldom used in acute trauma, in some situations it can be helpful. The main indication in an acute injury is an incomplete cord lesion caused by nonosseous material, such as a disk herniation or a hematoma. It is particularly helpful in examining a bilateral facet dislocation of the cervical spine in a patient with incomplete paraplegia. If the disk space is completely lost, there is a possibility of extrusion of the disk. Magnetic resonance imaging or a myelogram can help demonstrate the disk herniation and suggests that reduction of the dislocation may completely occlude the spinal cord, which would make the paralysis complete.

Magnetic Resonance Imaging Magnetic resonance imaging scans permit visualization of the spinal cord in the acutely injured patient. Because intramedullary lesions such as cysts, hematomas, or edema can be visualized, prognosis for recovery can be made more accurately. In most hospital settings, it can be difficult to perform magnetic resonance imaging on the acutely injured patient. Also, the need to keep traction apparatus or tubes in place may preclude placing the patient in the scanner.

Soft-Tissue Injury to the Neck

There can be severe soft-tissue injury to the neck even though the radiographs are absolutely negative.

Patients who sustain neck injuries in auto accidents may have pain immediately, or the pain can be delayed for 24 to 48 hours. The pain generally remains in the neck but can also affect the shoulders, arms, or the suboccipital area. Symptoms may include dysphagia, retro-ocular pain, or otologic symptoms. There can also be a significant amount of soft-tissue swelling with normal radiographic findings. Soft-tissue radiology is used to determine any reversal of the cervical or thoracic curves suggesting spinal spasm and pain. Also, the spine can be checked for any prevertebral swelling; the normal measurement anterior to C2 in the retropharyngeal area is 1 mm to 7 mm, and anterior to C6 the retrotracheal area is 9 mm to 22 mm. In children, retrotracheal area measurements are slightly smaller, 5 mm to 14 mm.

Soft-tissue injury to the cervical spine can have serious long-term consequences. In patients so injured, symptoms will never resolve completely in 12% and cervical disk disease will develop in 39%. In the general population, the incidence of cervical disk disease is only 6%.

In evaluating the cervical or thoracic lumbar spine, it is important to look for injuries at more than one level. The discovery of a lesion at one level should not end the diagnostic and clinical examination, as association with a fracture at another level is common. A significant soft-tissue injury can lead to later vertebral deformity. Therefore, if a patient's symptoms exceed those that are expected, a repeat radiographic examination should be performed.

Philosophy of Treatment of the Spine in the Patient With Polytrauma

Although it is important to identify and stabilize the fractured or dislocated spine in the patient with multiple injuries, spinal injuries do not necessarily take priority over fractures in scheduling surgery. There are only two absolute indications for emergency spinal surgery: an open fracture (extremely rare) or an incomplete neurologic lesion that has shown documented deterioration over a period of time. The need to document any deterioration makes the physical examination and its recording especially important (Fig. 6). Confusion over this issue usually stems from questionable examination or incomplete documentation. In fact, it is unusual for deterioration to take place after hospital admission.

With this in mind, the cervical spine can be stabilized or reduced and held using Gardner-Wells tongs or a halo ring. The halo ring can later be attached to a plastic vest as treatment or as a preliminary to spinal surgery. Thoracic and lumbar injuries can be treated in a regular hospital bed, provided good nursing care is available to logroll the patient carefully from side to back to side every two hours to avoid pressure injury. This can be done either as the final treatment, a common practice in Europe, or while organizing the definitive surgical procedure for stabilization.

If other bones, such as the pelvis or extremities, need open reduction and internal fixation, decisions must be made. At the University of California, Davis, we have found it practical to attend to the pelvis and lower extremities first. Then, after they have been fixed, the patient can more easily be rolled into position to expose the vertebral column. Also, fractures of the extremities and pelvis are more likely to contribute to blood loss in the polytraumatized patient. Once vascular stability is attained, the spine surgery can be done deliberately, taking time to avoid any further risk to the spinal cord. On occasion we have performed surgery on the spine while maintaining an extremity in traction. Use of an external pelvic fixator can make it possible for the patient to be placed in a prone position for surgery.

The major point to be made regarding treatment of the patient with multiple injuries is that all the specialists must communicate with each other. Through mutual understanding, a total plan can be developed, optimizing the patient's care. This is most effectively done in a manner that respects each of the surgical disciplines and offers appropriate priorities as the team identifies them.

Most spine operations can be delayed for at least a few hours if not for a day or two. The operation must be performed by a knowledgeable and experienced team, using instruments that they are familiar with and can handle well. Any deviation from this can do more to harm than to help the patient.

Advice on the treatment of individual fracture types exceeds the intent of this chapter. Suffice it to say that spinal surgery for trauma is a rapidly developing area in orthopaedic surgery. The surgeon who performs this type of surgery must be able to stabilize and decompress the vertebral column and cord both anteriorly and posteriorly. Techniques, instrumentation, and types of graft materials and implants are wide-ranging and change constantly. A clear understanding of the biomechanics of the vertebral column and the dynamics of the injury are essential before selection of the surgical procedure or instrumentation type. It is far better to proceed conservatively than to try to use the latest technique or vertebral implant to see how it works. Success depends more on the surgeon's knowledge than on any specific type of instrumentation.

References

1. Benson DR, Keenen TL, Anthony J: Unsuspected associated lesions in the fractured spine. Presented at the meeting of the Orthopaedic Trauma Association, October 1988.
2. Bohlman HH: Acute fractures and dislocations of the cervical spine: An analysis of three hundred hospitalized patients and review of the literature. *J Bone Joint Surg* 1979;61A:1119–1142.
3. Riggins RS, Kraus JF: The risk of neurologic damage with fractures of the vertebrae. *J Trauma* 1977;17:126–133.
4. Denis F: The three column spine and its significance in the classification of acute thoracolumbar spinal injuries. *Spine* 1983;8: 817–831.
5. Ergas Z: Spinal cord injury in the United States: A statistical update. *Cent Nerv Syst Trauma* 1985;2:19–32.
6. Stover SL, Fine PR: *Spinal Cord Injury: The Facts and Figures*. Birmingham, University of Alabama, 1986.
7. Bosch A, Stauffer ES, Nickel VL: Incomplete traumatic quadriplegia: A ten-year review. *JAMA* 1971;216:473–478.
8. Steel HH: Anatomical and mechanical considerations of the atlanto-axial articulations, abstract. *J Bone Joint Surg* 1968;50A: 1481–1482.
9. Hall ED, Braughler JM: Non-surgical management of spinal cord injuries: A review of studies with the glucocorticoid steroid methylprednisolone. *Acta Anaesthesiol Belg* 1987;38:405–409.
10. Sabel BA, Stein DG: Pharmacological treatment of central nervous system injury. *Nature* 1986;323:493.
11. Bracken MB, Shepard MJ, Hellenbrand KG, et al: Methylprednisolone and neurological function 1 year after spinal cord injury: Results of the National Acute Spinal Cord Injury Study. *J Neurosurg* 1985;63:704–713.
12. Frankel HL, Hancock DO, Hyslop G, et al: The value of postural reduction in the initial management of closed injuries of the spine with paraplegia and tetraplegia. *Paraplegia* 1969;7:179–192.
13. Stauffer ES: Diagnosis and prognosis of acute cervical spinal cord injury. *Clin Orthop* 1975;112:9–15.
14. Lucas JT, Ducker TB: Motor classification of spinal cord injuries with mobility, morbidity and recovery indices. *Am Surg* 1979;45: 151–158.
15. Stauffer ES: A quantitative evaluation of neurologic recovery following spinal cord injuries. Presented at the Third Annual Meeting of the Federation of Spine Associations, Atlanta, 1988.
16. Schneider RC: The syndrome of acute anterior spinal cord injury. *J Neurosurg* 1955;12:95–122.
17. Stauffer ES: Neurologic recovery following injuries to the cervical spinal cord and nerve roots. *Spine* 1984;9:532–534.
18. *Advanced Trauma Life Support Manual*. Chicago, American College of Surgeons, 1984.
19. Soderstrom CA, McArdle DQ, Ducker TB, et al: The diagnosis of intra-abdominal injury in patients with cervical cord trauma. *J Trauma* 1983;23:1061–1065.
20. Grundy D, Swain A, Russell J: ABC of spinal cord injury: Early management and complications. Part I. *Br Med J* 1986;292:44–47.
21. Piepmeier JM, Lehmann KB, Lane JG: Cardiovascular instability following acute cervical spinal cord trauma. *Cent Nerv Syst Trauma* 1985;2:153–160.
22. American Academy of Orthopaedic Surgeons: *Emergency Care and Transportation of the Sick and Injured*, ed 4. Park Ridge, Illinois, American Academy of Orthopaedic Surgeons, 1987.
23. McGuire RA, Neville S, Green BA, et al: Spinal instability and the log-rolling maneuver. *J Trauma* 1987;27:525–531.
24. Podolsky S, Baraff LJ, Simon RR, et al: Efficacy of cervical spine immobilization methods. *J Trauma* 1983;23:461–465.
25. Johnson RM, Hart DL, Simmons EF, et al: Cervical orthoses: A study comparing their effectiveness in restricting cervical motion in normal subjects. *J Bone Joint Surg* 1977;59A:332–339.
26. Crutchfield WG: Skeletal traction for dislocation of the cervical spine: Report of a case. *South Surgeon* 1933;2:156–159.
27. Bracken MB, Collins WF, Freeman DF, et al: Efficacy of methylprednisolone in acute spinal cord injury. *JAMA* 1984;251:45–52.
28. Faden AI: Opiate antagonists and thyrotropin-releasing hor-

mone: II. Potential role in the treatment of central nervous system injury. *JAMA* 1984;252:1452–1454.

29. McIntosh TK, Faden AI: Opiate antagonist in traumatic shock. *Ann Emerg Med* 1986;15:1462–1465.

30. Hill RG: Neuropharmacology of the injured spinal cord. *Paraplegia* 1987;25:209–211.

31. Hamilton AJ, McBlack PM, Carr DB: Contrasting actions of naloxone in experimental spinal cord trauma and cerebral ischemia: A review. *Neurosurgery* 1985;17:845–849.

32. Reed JE, Allen WE III, Dohrmann GJ: Effect of mannitol on the traumatized spinal cord: Microangiography, blood flow patterns, and electrophysiology. *Spine* 1979;4:391–397.

33. Kobrine AI: The question of steroids in neurotrauma: To give or not to give, editorial. *JAMA* 1984;251:68.

34. Braakman R, Schouten HJA, Blaauw-van Dishoeck M, et al: Megadose steroids in severe head injury: Results of a prospective double-blind clinical trial. *J Neurosurg* 1983;58:326–330.

35. Soderstrom CA, Ducker TB: Increased susceptibility of patients with cervical cord lesions to peptic gastrointestinal complications. *J Trauma* 1985;25:1030–1038.

36. Dunn EJ, LeClair WE: How to reduce complications in treatment of cervical spine trauma, in Stauffer ES (ed): American Academy of Orthopaedic Surgeons *Instructional Course Lectures, XXXIV*. St. Louis, CV Mosby, 1985, pp 155–162.

37. Epstein N, Hood DC, Ransohoff J: Gastrointestinal bleeding in patients with spinal cord trauma: Effects of steroids, cimetidine, and mini-dose heparin. *J Neurosurg* 1981;54:16–20.

38. Fadul CE, Lemann W, Thaler HT, et al: Perforation of the gastrointestinal tract in patients receiving steroids for neurologic disease. *Neurology* 1988;38:348–352.

39. Apple JS, Kirks DR, Merten DF, et al: Cervical spine fractures and dislocations in children. *Pediatr Radiol* 1987;17:45–49.

40. Hensinger RN: The pediatric cervical spine I. Presented at the 55th Annual Meeting of the American Academy of Orthopaedic Surgeons, Atlanta, Feb 5, 1988.

41. Hill SA, Miller CA, Kosnik EJ, et al: Pediatric neck injuries: A clinical study. *J Neurosurg* 1984;60:700–706.

42. Herzenberg JE, Hensinger RN, Dedrick DK, et al: Potential hazards of backboards in transport of children with neck injuries. Presented at the 55th Annual Meeting of the American Academy of Orthopaedic Surgeons, Atlanta, Feb 6, 1988.

43. Reid DC, Henderson R, Saboe L, et al: Etiology and clinical course of missed spine fractures. *J Trauma* 1987;27:980–986.

44. Kewalramani LS, Taylor RG: Multiple non-contiguous injuries to the spine. *Acta Orthop Scand* 1976;47:52–58.

45. Slabaugh PB, Nickel VL: Complications with use of the Stryker frame. *J Bone Joint Surg* 1978;60A:1111–1112.

46. Mirvis SE, Borg U, Belzberg H: MR imaging of ventilator-dependent patients: Preliminary experience. *Am J Radiol* 1987;149:845.

Fractures of the Pelvic Ring and Acetabulum in Patients With Severe Polytrauma

Michael W. Chapman, MD

Introduction

This brief chapter is not designed to teach you how to manage fractures and dislocations of the pelvic ring and acetabulum. I assume that you understand the basic principles and techniques for treatment of these injuries. Rather, it is my purpose to put into perspective the treatment of these important and difficult injuries in the patient with severe multiple injuries. In the patient with an Injury Severity Score of 18 or more, it is critically important to treat unstable injuries of the pelvis in a way that will allow immediate mobilization of the patient. If neither internal nor external fixation is feasible, and traction or other nonsurgical treatment becomes necessary, it is essential to use methods that will allow the nursing staff to move the patient in bed as freely as possible and, ideally, also be able to get the patient into a bedside chair while maintaining traction.

Hemorrhage in patients with unstable injuries of the pelvic ring is often a major contributor to death within the first 24 hours after injury. Immediate stabilization of the pelvis can be a critical factor in reducing hemorrhage and controlling shock, often taking precedence over the treatment of open fractures and peripheral vascular injuries.

Initial Assessment

In the emergency room, rapid but efficient physical examination of the pelvis and an immediate anteroposterior radiograph of the pelvis, one that includes both hips, is essential. Palpate the bony landmarks of the pelvis looking for a proximally migrated hemipelvis or other distortion, and for evidence of free-floating segments of the pelvis. Palpation along the iliac crest and posteriorly over sacroiliac joints can reveal evidence of a displacement or defect suggestive of a fracture or dislocation. Palpation of the pubic symphysis commonly reveals evidence of separation. Grasp the anterosuperior iliac spines and "book" the pelvis, open and closed, to detect "open-book" instability. With your hands on the iliac crest, have an assistant do a push-pull stress test of the extremities to look for evidence of vertical instability. Before doing this test, of course, carefully examine the hips and lower extremities to rule out other fractures or dislocations.

As pointed out in the chapter on initial management, careful evaluation of the abdomen and genitourinary structures is essential, because these areas are commonly injured with pelvic fractures.

It is absolutely essential to rule out the presence of an open fracture by inspecting the genitalia, vagina in women, and perineum and rectal area in all persons for evidence of lacerations. Examine the vaginal vault with a speculum. Careful rectal examination is essential. If the stool guaiac is positive, anoscopy is indicated. Any suspicion of an open pelvic fracture, particularly involving the orifices or perineum, requires general surgical consultation. Colostomy is indicated if any evidence of rectal rupture is found or if there is a laceration of the perineum that communicates with the pelvis. Urethral injuries and bladder ruptures may require suprapubic cystostomy. A urethral catheter is placed in nearly all cases, if for no other reason than fluid management.

Radiographs

Although an anteroposterior radiograph of the pelvis will reveal most major fractures or dislocations, unstable injuries, if undisplaced, may be difficult to detect. Indicators of potentially unstable vertical shear fractures of the pelvic ring include avulsion fractures of the fifth lumbar transverse process and the medial corner of the ilium, secondary to rupture of the ligament that connects these structures, and avulsions of the ischial spine. Sacral fractures can be very difficult to diagnose, particularly if considerable fecal material or rectal gas is present. Internal and external oblique views (Judet views) are very helpful, but may not be possible in the initial assessment of the multiply injured patient. If an abdominal computed tomographic scan is ordered as a part of the initial assessment of the patient, a few cuts through the pelvis may be quite revealing, particularly for hidden fractures of the sacrum. If there is suspicion of injury to the pelvic ring, a full pelvic radiographic survey should be completed some time after the initial stage of resuscitation. Instability of the pelvis should be detected early, because stabilization at the time of emergency laparotomy is often indicated. It is frustrating to find an unstable separation of the pubic symphysis, suitable for plate fixation, after the wound from an emergency laparotomy has been closed. Often it is possible to fix the symphysis through the abdominal wound. This possibility must always be kept in mind by general surgeons, and preparation of the patient's abdomen should always include shaving the upper portions of the pubic hair and preparation of the abdomen to well below the pubic symphysis.

Uncontrolled Hemorrhage

Management of uncontrolled hemorrhage from the pelvis requires a dual general surgical and orthopaedic approach. Patients with hemodynamic instability and evidence of intra-abdominal bleeding usually require immediate laparotomy. If the source of bleeding is an unstable pelvic fracture or dislocation, then a nonpulsatile retroperitoneal hematoma is commonly found. At this point it is vital to achieve immediate stabilization of the pelvis by either external or internal fixation. Most authorities advise external fixation because this technique is more familiar to the average orthopaedic surgeon and can be accomplished with minimal risk. More recently, internal fixation techniques have been employed. Entering a retroperitoneal hematoma rarely results in additional major hemorrhage as long as the pelvic fracture is stabilized immediately. If, after stabilization of the pelvis, the patient shows continued evidence of hemorrhage, then a coagulopathy or disseminated intravascular coagulation must be searched for and treated. Evidence of continuing hemorrhage in the absence of a coagulopathy usually indicates the presence of hemorrhage from a major vessel, which might be amenable to embolization. Therefore, angiography of the pelvis is the next step. In our institution, we have not had to embolize a single vessel in the past five years, probably because all pelvic fractures are stabilized immediately. This would indicate that the incidence of hemorrhage from major vessels is rare.

The "Open-Book" Pelvis

Separation of the pubic symphysis with rupture of the anterior sacroiliac ligaments, but with intact posterior ligaments, can be treated nonsurgically if the separation is less than 2.5 cm. No stabilization is necessary and the patient can be mobilized as tolerated. The only indication for stabilization is unremitting severe pain caused by instability. Symphysis diastasis of more than 2.5 cm usually requires stabilization. I prefer internal fixation to external fixation. In my experience, internal fixation is much better accepted by the patient, eliminates the problem of pin-tract infection and skin erosion commonly associated with external fixation frames, is easier to apply, often requires less surgery time, and carries a lower complication rate. If the abdomen is explored, fixation can be done through the lower end of the abdominal incision. If the abdomen is not explored, fixation is best performed through Pfannen-

stiel's incision. I prefer a four- or five-hole AO 4.5-cm reconstruction plate, prebent to a smooth curve of approximately 35 degrees. This is fixed to the top of the pubic symphysis after subperiosteal exposure. Place two 6.5-mm cancellous screws into the dense bone at the junction of the inferior and superior pubic rami on each side of the symphysis. The outer screws are 4.5-mm cortical screws of appropriate length inserted without tapping. This fixation is stable enough to allow most patients to be mobilized immediately with crutches and weightbearing as tolerated.

If significant residual opening of the sacroiliac joint is evident, fixation is possible anteriorly through a retroperitoneal approach. An incision placed just above the iliac crest and the iliacus is reflected subperiosteally anteriorly to reveal the sacroiliac joint. I prefer fixation with two three-hole 4.5-cm AO reconstruction plates with appropriately sized cortical screws. Take care to avoid injury to the fifth lumbar nerve root.

Malgaigne Injuries

The Malgaigne disruption of the pelvic ring with vertical instability is often accompanied by life-threatening hemorrhage and poses a major challenge in the patient with multiple injuries. If initial radiographs show an undisplaced fracture, perform a careful examination to rule out instability. If the lesion is stable, nonsurgical treatment with frequent postoperative follow-up for detection of any displacement is necessary. Unstable fractures are difficult. Immediate external or internal fixation is nearly always indicated to control hemorrhage and permit mobilization of the patient. Unfortunately, external fixation frames, although capable of closing the "open-book" portion of such injuries and providing life-salvaging stabilization, do not adequately control vertical instability. Even if an anatomic reduction is achieved acutely, loss of reduction later is common. As no external fixation frame of any type adequately controls vertical instability, a simple basic quadrilateral or triangular frame with two pins in each iliac wing is adequate. Use supplemental skeletal traction to try to maintain length. I use single-line traction and allow the nurses to remove the traction temporarily as needed for respiratory care. The patient can even be mobilized to a chair at bedside and the traction placed while sitting.

When the patient's general condition has stabilized, internal fixation of the posterior break in the pelvic ring is indicated. The external fixator usually controls the anterior disruption. Using fluoroscopic control, stabilize iliac wing fractures and sacroiliac joint disruptions with plates and screws or with interfragmentary screws. Unstable sacral fractures are more difficult to manage and usually require fixation between the two iliac wings, either using a large plate or double Harrington sacral rods. On occasion, immediate internal fixation of Malgaigne disruptions is possible. I prefer to do these through two anterior approaches as described above for the "open-book" pelvis. A combination of a plate on the pubic symphysis and posterior fixation can be done as well.

Acetabular Fractures

Stable fractures may require no treatment other than careful observation or perhaps protection in single-line traction as described above. Unstable fractures, particularly if comminuted, are difficult to manage in the acute situation, because the extensive surgical procedure necessary is often not feasible on the day of injury. Posterior wall fractures, usually caused by a posterior dislocation, and simple transverse fractures often can be internally fixed immediately through a Kocher-Lan-

genbeck approach. Simple-pattern, anterior-column fractures that are unstable can usually be fixed immediately through an ilioinguinal approach. Treatment of more complex fractures usually must be delayed until the patient is more stable. Perform internal fixation as soon as possible, however. In severely injured patients, if the fracture is not fixed within the first 24 hours, a delay of two to three weeks is often necessary, because the patient becomes septic and has other complications. One can temporize with longitudinal skeletal traction, but if mobilization of the patient becomes imperative, external fixation from the iliac wing to the shaft of the femur may save a life in a difficult situation. We try to avoid external fixation, however, because infection in the pin tracts may contraindicate subsequent open reduction. Fortunately, as our skills and equipment for the management of acetabular fractures have improved, we have been able to fix many of these quite early.

Index